Respiratory Medicine

Series Editor

Sharon I. S. Rounds

For further volumes:
http://www.springer.com/series/7665

Jeffrey P. Kanne
Editor

Clinically Oriented Pulmonary Imaging

Springer

Jeffrey P. Kanne
Department of Radiology
University of Wisconsin
School of Medicine and Public Health
600 Highland Ave.
Madison, WI 53792
USA
e-mail: jkanne@uwhealth.org

ISBN 978-1-4939-5959-4 ISBN 978-1-61779-542-8 (eBook)
DOI 10.1007/978-1-61779-542-8
Springer New York Dordrecht Heidelberg London

Printed on acid-free paper

Humana Press is a part of Springer Science+Business Media (www.springer.com)

To Drs. J. David Godwin, Eric J. Stern, Julie E. Takasugi, John R. Mayo, and Nestor L. Müller, all of whom mentored me and taught me to recognize the beauty hiding beneath all of the "white stuff" in the lungs.

Preface

Imaging is central to the diagnosis and management of patients with known or suspected pulmonary disease. Advances in imaging technology, particularly computerized tomography (CT), have broadened our understanding of pulmonary disease and have changed how we care for our patients.

Chest radiography remains the most commonly performed medical imaging examination because it is widely available, relatively inexpensive, uses very low doses of ionizing radiation, and often can answer the clinical question at hand. Radiography has been enhanced by the transition from film-screen to digital imaging and the subsequent electronic distribution of images and radiologic reports. Newer technologies such as dual-energy radiography and computer-aided detection (CAD) can further enhance the utility of radiography.

The impact that CT has had on our understanding of pulmonary disease cannot be summarized in this brief introduction. CT has become a standard component of assessing respiratory tract disease. With current scanner technology, volumetric high-resolution CT (HRCT) images can readily be generated from routine chest CT scans at the time of imaging with little or no change in acquisition parameters. In fact, some institutions, such as mine, routinely generate thin-section images with all chest CT scans performed. CT pulmonary angiography has changed the paradigm for evaluating patients with suspected pulmonary thromboembolic disease, providing more definitive diagnosis and frequently identifying other causes of patients' presenting signs and symptoms. CT is also used to guide transthoracic needle biopsies.

The utility of magnetic resonance (MR) imaging for pulmonary disease has been relatively limited not only because of technical limitations but also because of overshadowing by the rapid growth in CT technology and applications. However, MR imaging techniques currently under development show promise for evaluation of the lungs. Furthermore, the ability to integrate cardiac and pulmonary imaging with a single MR imaging examination has the potential to revolutionize how we think about the intimate relationship between the heart and lungs.

While we can expect many exciting developments in pulmonary imaging in the future, one still needs to understand how imaging available today fits into the evaluation of our patients. This text aims to provide a clinically oriented approach to imaging the lungs and is by no means a comprehensive thoracic imaging text. Rather, the authors focus on specific clinical problems such as pulmonary thromboembolic disease, hemoptysis, or lung cancer, and they discuss the utility of imaging in addition to illustrating the imaging findings commonly encountered. It is my hope that the novice reader will find this text a useful introduction to how imaging fits into the evaluation of patients with known or suspected pulmonary disease. Additionally, more experienced readers may benefit from the focused approach to specific clinical problems or patient care settings and better understand the imaging tools available to improve care for their patients.

October 2011 Jeffrey P. Kanne

Acknowledgments

I would first like to acknowledge Linda Jacobs, my developmental editor at Springer, who kept this project organized and on schedule. Linda ensured that every piece of the puzzle was in place throughout the entire process. Second, this book would not exist without the hard work and dedication from the contributing authors. Finally, I would like to thank my thoracic imaging colleagues at the University of Wisconsin School of Medicine and Public Health for their never waning support of me during my work on this project.

Contents

Contributors

Gopal Allada Department of Medicine, Division of Pulmonary and Critical Care, Oregon Health and Science University, Portland, OR, USA

Kayvan Amjadi Department of Medicine, The Ottawa Hospital, Ottawa, ON, Canada

Daniel Barnes Directorate of Clinical Radiology, Central Manchester University Hospitals NHS Foundation Trust, Manchester, UK

Helen Katrina Busby Department of Pulmonary/Critical Care, University of New Mexico School of Medicine, Albuquerque, NM, USA

George Chandy Department of Medicine, Division of Respirology, Heart Institute Pulmonary Hypertension Clinic, The Ottawa Hospital, Ottawa, ON, Canada

Jonathan Hero Chung Institute of Advanced Biomedical Imaging, National Jewish Health, Denver, CO, USA

Carole Dennie Department of Medical Imaging, University of Ottawa, The Ottawa Hospital, Ottawa, ON, Canada

Stuart M. Garay Department of Medicine, NYU Langone Medical Center, New York, NY, USA

Barry H. Gross University of Michigan Hospitals, Ann Arbor, MI, USA

Kristie Guite Department of Radiology, University of Wisconsin Hospital and Clinics, Madison, WI, USA

Shailaja J. Hayden Division of Pulmonary and Critical Care Medicine, University of Washington, Seattle, WA, USA

Todd R. Hazelton Department of Radiology, University of South Florida College of Medicine, Tampa, FL, USA

Trina J. Hollatz Division of Pulmonary and Critical Care, University of Wisconsin School of Medicine and Public Health, Madison, WI, USA

Leif Jensen Diagnostic Radiology, University of Wisconsin–Madison, Madison, WI, USA

Jeffrey P. Kanne Department of Radiology, University of Wisconsin School of Medicine and Public Health, Madison, WI, USA

Loren Ketai Department of Radiology, University of New Mexico Health Science Center, Albuquerque, NM, USA

Jean Kuriakose Department of Radiology, University of Michigan Medical Center, Ann Arbor, MI, USA

James Lockey Department of Environmental Health, University of Cincinnati College of Medicine, Cincinnati, OH, USA

Cris A. Meyer Department of Radiology, University of Wisconsin Hospital and Clinics, Madison, WI, USA

Jie C. Nguyen Department of Radiology, University of Wisconsin Hospital and Clinics, Madison, WI, USA

Elena Peña, Department of Medical Imaging, University of Ottawa, The Ottawa Hospital, Ottawa, ON, Canada

Sudhakar N. J. Pipavath Department of Radiology, University of Washington, Seattle, WA, USA

Elie Portnoy Department of Radiology, NYU Langone Medical Center, New York, NY, USA

Steven L. Primack Department of Radiology, Oregon Health and Science University, Portland, OR, USA

Stephen A. Quinet Department of Radiology, University of Wisconsin School of Medicine and Public Health, Madison, WI, USA

A. Keith Rastogi Department of Radiology, University of Wisconsin Hospital and Clinics, Madison, WI, USA

James R. Runo Department of Pulmonary and Critical Care Medicine, University of Wisconsin School of Medicine and Public Health, Madison, WI, USA

Megan Saettele Department of Radiology, University of Missouri-Kansas City, Saint Luke's Hospital, Kansas City, MO, USA

Tim Saettele Department of Pulmonary/Critical Care, Truman Medical Center/Saint Luke's Hospital, Kansas City, MO, USA

Mark L. Schiebler Department of Radiology, University of Wisconsin School of Medicine and Public Health, Madison, WI, USA

Jean M. Seely Department of Medical Imaging, University of Ottawa, The Ottawa Hospital, Ottawa, ON, Canada

Maria C. Shiau Department of Radiology, NYU Langone Medical Center, New York, NY, USA

Arlene Sirajuddin Department of Radiology, Northwestern University, Chicago, IL, USA

Amie J. Tucker Department of Medicine, Division of Pulmonary and Critical Care, Oregon Health and Science University, Portland, OR, USA

Frank W. Walsh Pulmonary Department, Moffitt Cancer Center, Tampa, FL, USA

Normal Thoracic Anatomy and Common Variants

1

Arlene Sirajuddin

Abstract

The normal anatomy of the thorax includes anatomy of the airways, lung parenchyma, pleura and fissures, mediastinum, great vessels, and diaphragm. This chapter will describe normal anatomy of the thorax as well as anatomic relationships of these structures to each other. Common congenital anatomic variants of the thorax will also be discussed.

Keywords

Normal thoracic anatomy • Variant anatomy • Trachea • Airways • Lung parenchyma • Mediastinum • Great vessels • Pleura • Hila • Diaphragm

Airways and Lung Parenchyma

Trachea and Central Airways

The trachea is an air-conducting tube that begins at the inferior margin of the cricoid cartilage, just below the level of the true vocal cords, and extends to the level of the carina, a ridge where the trachea bifurcates into right and left main bronchi. The trachea is lined by pseudostratified ciliated columnar epithelium. This epithelial layer also contains secretory goblet cells as well as specialized neuroendocrine cells. Fibroelastic lamina propria and the submucosa, made of both cartilage and muscle, compose the subepithelial tissue. There are approximately 16–22 C–shaped tracheal cartilages that are linked together by annular ligaments of fibrous and connective tissue. These cartilage rings can calcify with age (Fig. 1.1) [1, 2].

Sympathetic innervation of the trachea by the recurrent laryngeal nerve contracts the smooth muscle of the trachea, while parasympathetic innervation by the vagus nerve relaxes the smooth muscle of the trachea. The trachea vascular supply consists of tracheal branches of the inferior thyroid and bronchial arteries, and venous drainage is via the inferior thyroid veins. The lymphatics of the trachea drain into the pretracheal and right paratracheal nodes [1].

The shape of the trachea is always round in children. In adults, the extrathoracic portion of the trachea can be circular, elliptical, or horseshoe shaped. The intrathoracic adult trachea is usually round or oval. Tracheal length is approximately 5.7 cm long from birth to 3 years

A. Sirajuddin (✉)
Department of Radiology, Northwestern University, Suite 800, 676 North St. Clair Street, Chicago, IL 60611, USA
e-mail: asirajud@nmff.org

J. P. Kanne (ed.), *Clinically Oriented Pulmonary Imaging*, Respiratory Medicine, DOI: 10.1007/978-1-61779-542-8_1,

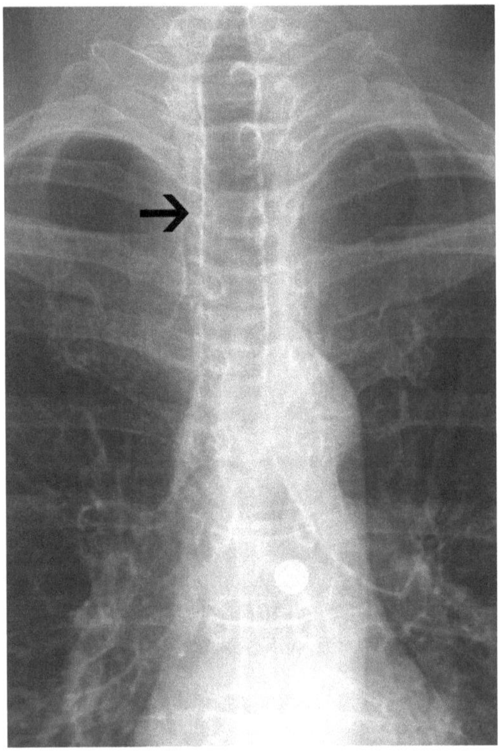

Fig. 1.1 Coned-down frontal radiograph shows a normal trachea bifurcating into right and left main bronchi. Note calcification in the wall of the trachea in this older individual. The arrow points to a normal right paratracheal stripe

and continues to lengthen until the age of 14 years. In boys, the trachea can continue to widen after the age of 14 years. In the adult, the tracheal length ranges from 8.5 to 15 cm, with an average length of 10 cm in women and 11 cm in men. Tracheal length is dynamic, and can change up to 3 cm with respiration [1]. Breatnach et al. describe normal tracheal measurements on PA and lateral radiographs as averaging 25 to 27 mm in men, and 21 to 23 mm in women, respectively. They report a lower limit of normal of 10 mm in women and 13 mm in men in both dimensions [3].

The trachea is essentially a midline structure. However, a study by Bhalla et al. describes normal deviation of the trachea to the right by up to 1.6 cm or to the left up to 0.7 cm [4]. The aortic arch also makes a mild impression on the intrathoracic trachea.

At the carina, the trachea bifurcates into the left and right main bronchi. The main bronchi subsequently give rise to the lobar bronchi. The right main bronchus gives rise to the right upper lobe bronchus, right middle lobe bronchus, and the right lower lobe bronchus. The left main bronchus gives rise to the left upper lobe bronchus, the lingular bronchus, and the left lower lobe bronchus. The lobar bronchi then give rise to segmental bronchi, listed below [5].

- right upper lobe: apical, anterior, posterior
- right middle lobe: medial, lateral
- right lower lobe: superior, anterior basal, medial basal, lateral basal, posterior basal
- left upper lobe: apicoposterior and anterior
- lingula: superior and inferior
- left lower lobe: superior, anteromedial basal, lateral basal, posterior basal

The anatomic relationships of the trachea, main bronchi, and the branching pattern of these airways are depicted in Fig. 1.2.

Several important landmarks have been described in relation to the lobar bronchi. At the level of the right upper lobe bronchus, the right superior pulmonary vein is reliably present just lateral to this bronchus (Fig. 1.3). Distal to the origin of the right upper lobe bronchus is a short segment of bronchus known as the bronchus intermedius, which lies directly posterior to the right pulmonary artery (Fig. 1.4). The bronchus intermedius gives rise to the right middle lobe and right lower lobe bronchi [5].

The left upper lobe bronchus arises at a lower level than the right upper lobe bronchus and forms a sling over which the left pulmonary artery crosses. The posterior wall of the left upper lobe bronchus is concave secondary to the presence of the left pulmonary artery (Fig. 1.4). The lingular bronchus has an oblique course and, thus, is not as clearly depicted on cross-sectional imaging. The descending left pulmonary artery always lies directly posterior to the lingular bronchus [5, 6]. The left lower lobe bronchus is similar to the right lower lobe bronchus, though its origin is higher [5].

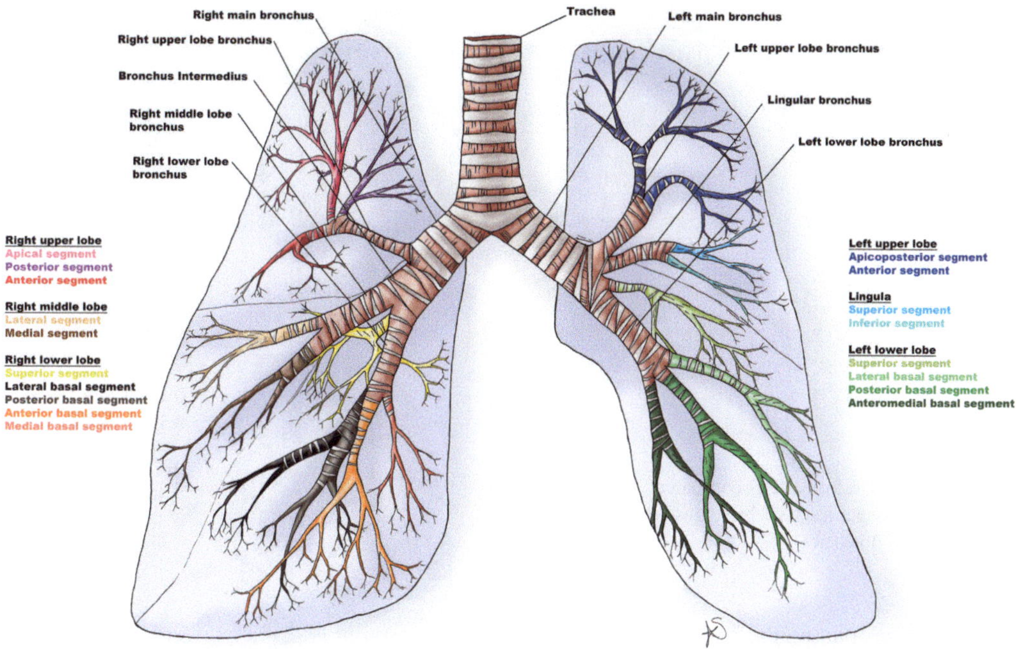

Fig. 1.2 Illustration depicting the relationship of the trachea, main bronchi, lobar bronchi, and segmental bronchi

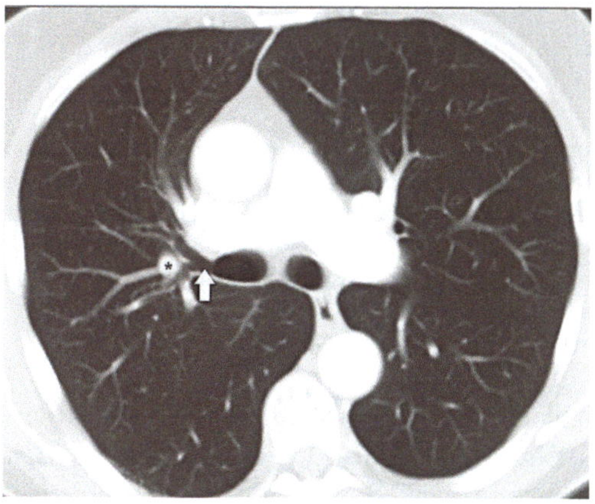

Fig. 1.3 Transverse computed tomography image shows the superior right pulmonary vein (*asterisk*) just lateral to the right upper lobe bronchus (*arrow*)

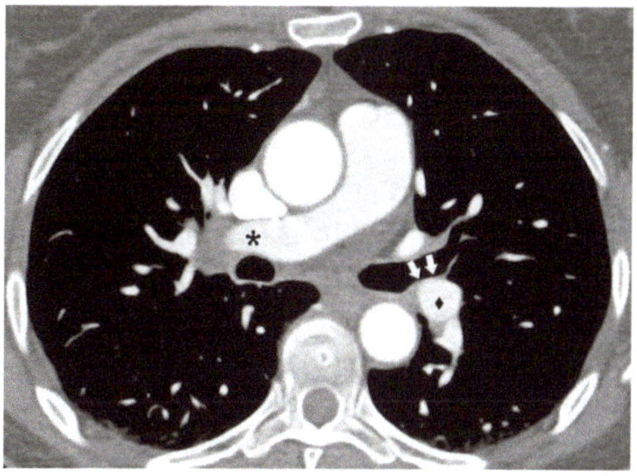

Fig. 1.4 Transverse computed tomography image shows the right pulmonary artery (*asterisk*) anterior to the bronchus intermedius. Also note the concave wall of the left upper lobe bronchus (*white arrows*) secondary to the left pulmonary artery (*diamond*)

Central Airway Anomalies

Anomalies of the airways include both major abnormalities of the lobar bronchi and minor abnormalities of the segmental bronchi. Bronchial anomalies are more common on the right [7]. These anomalies include displaced airways arising from nonstandard locations, supernumerary airways, absent or atretic airways, and airway abnormalities associated with abnormalities of situs.

The tracheal bronchus is a bronchus arising from the trachea, almost always on the right (Fig. 1.5), and is usually a displaced right upper lobe bronchus or displaced apical segmental

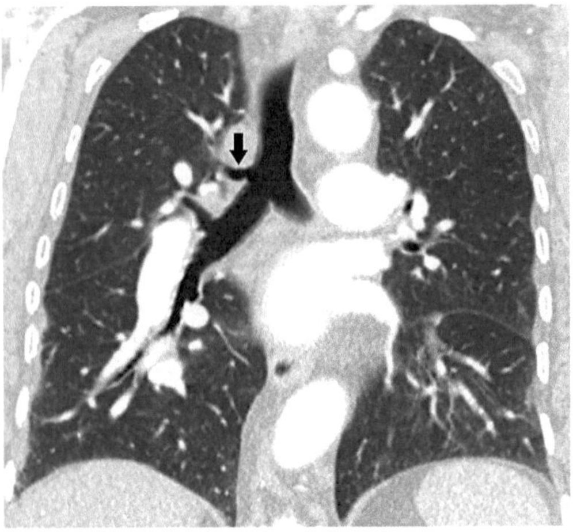

Fig. 1.5 Coronal reformatted computed tomography image demonstrates a tracheal bronchus (*arrow*) arising directly from the trachea

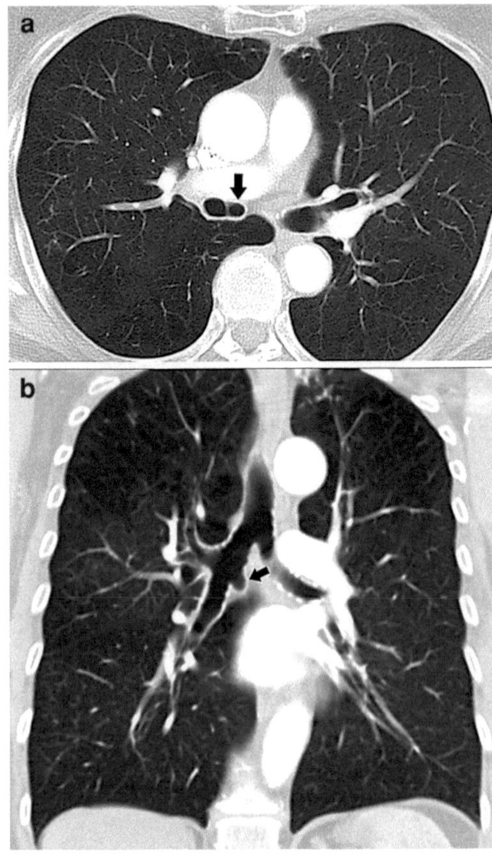

Fig. 1.6 **a** Transverse computed tomography image shows a cardiac bronchus (*arrow*) arising medially from the bronchus intermedius. **b** Coronal reformatted computed tomography image shows a blind-ending cardiac bronchus (*arrow*) arising from the medial aspect of the bronchus intermedius

bronchus. Occasionally, the tracheal bronchus is a supernumerary bronchus with a normal right upper lobe bronchus also present [8–12]. The lung tissue aerated by a supernumerary tracheal bronchus has been described as the tracheal lobe. A tracheal bronchus usually produces no signs or symptoms. However, it can be associated with infection, cough, dyspnea, and hemoptysis [9–12]. In children, it is a recognized cause of recurrent right upper lobe pneumonia [13].

A cardiac bronchus is a true supernumerary bronchus. It occurs in 0.09–0.5% of patients and is more common in men. It is a short segment bronchus arising from the medial wall of the bronchus intermedius. This bronchus usually is blind ending but occasionally supplies a rudimentary lobe of lung tissue (Fig. 1.6). As with the tracheal bronchus, the cardiac bronchus usually produces no signs or symptoms but can be associated with cough, recurrent infection, empyema, and hemoptysis [9–11, 14, 15]. A combination of a tracheal bronchus and a cardiac bronchus has been described in the same patient [16].

A bridging bronchus is rare. The bridging bronchus is a bronchus intermedius that arises from the left main bronchus, crosses the midline, and supplies the lower right lung [9, 10].

Bronchial anomalies also occur with abnormalities of situs. In the case of situs inversus, the right and left lungs are switched in positions. In situs ambiguous, left isomerism or right isomerism can be present. In left isomerism, there are bilateral morphologic left lungs and polysplenia. In right isomerism, there are bilateral morphological right lungs, asplenia, and frequently congenital heart disease [9, 17].

Bronchial atresia is most common in the left upper lobe. The cause of bronchial atresia is unknown but may be secondary to ischemic insult or developmental dysfunction. The bronchi distal to the atretic segment are often impacted with mucus. Distal alveoli are aerated via collateral pathways and usually are hyperlucent secondary to air-trapping (Fig. 1.7) [10].

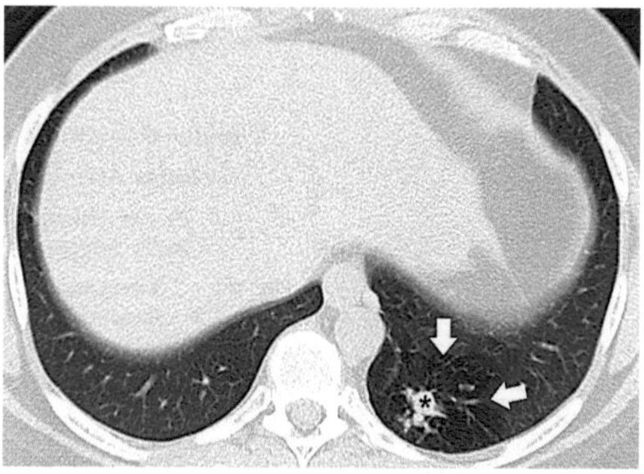

Fig. 1.7 Transverse computed tomography image of bronchial atresia shows a mucus distended bronchus (*asterisk*) with surrounding hypoattenuating lung (*arrows*)

Distal Airways and Lung Parenchyma

The segmental airways continue to divide into several generations of subsegmental bronchi and bronchioles. Eventually, bronchiole size reaches approximately 1 mm at the secondary pulmonary lobule of the lung [18].

The secondary pulmonary lobule is a polyhedral shaped structure and is considered to be the fundamental unit of lung structure. It is the smallest lung unit that is surrounded by thin septa of connective tissue. Each secondary pulmonary lobule is supplied by a bronchiole approximately 1 mm in size and a pulmonary artery branch, both of which are located in the center of the secondary pulmonary lobule. Lymphatics and veins travel within the peripheral connective tissue septa surrounding the secondary pulmonary lobule (Fig. 1.8) [18].

Within the secondary pulmonary lobule, preterminal and terminal bronchioles travel within intralobular septa. The terminal bronchiole is the final purely air-conducting bronchiole. The terminal bronchiole bifurcates into two respiratory bronchioles that supply a pulmonary acinus (Fig. 1.8). A respiratory bronchiole contains alveoli within its walls, and thus, the acinus is the largest unit within the lung in which all the airways are involved in gas exchange. Approximately 10–12 acini are present within each secondary pulmonary lobule [18, 19].

Pleura and Fissures

The pleura is formed by two thin layers, parietal pleura and visceral pleura, and is a potential space [20, 21]. Each pleural layer is a monolayer of flattened ovoid to columnar cells that lie over a substructure of pleural basement membrane containing capillaries arising from bronchial vessels and lymphatic vessels [21]. The parietal pleura covers the diaphragm, chest wall, and mediastinum [22]. The visceral pleura covers the lung [22]. The lymphatic drainage of the parietal pleura is to the internal thoracic (mammary), subpleural, costophrenic, and cardiophrenic angle nodes. The lymphatic drainage of the visceral pleura is to bronchopulmonary, hilar, mediastinal, scalene, and supraclavicular nodes. There are normally approximately 8 mL of fluid within the pleural space [20].

Pleural fissures are double layers of invaginations of visceral pleura that separate the lung into five lobes: right upper lobe, right middle lobe, right lower lobe, left upper lobe (including the lingula), and left lower lobe [23–27]. There are three normal fissures. The right major fissure separates the right lower lobe from the right middle lobe and right upper lobe [23–26]. The anterior surface of the right major fissure is divided into upper and lower parts at the interfissural crest, which separates the areas that contact the right upper and right middle lobes [28]. The left major fissure separates the left lower lobe from the left upper lobe. The right minor fissure separates the right middle lobe from the right upper lobe (Fig. 1.9) [23–26]. Fissures are often incomplete, more often on the right, and the lobes are fused at the site of the incomplete fissure, allowing for spread of disease and collateral air drift [23–28].

Fissures are undulating structures that appear as linear bands of avascular lucency on conventional CT and as thin white lines on high resolution CT [23, 24, 29]. The major and minor fissures are not well seen in their entirety on radiography, but sometimes portions of them are apparent. The superolateral major fissure is a curving edge or line sometimes present in the upper lateral aspect

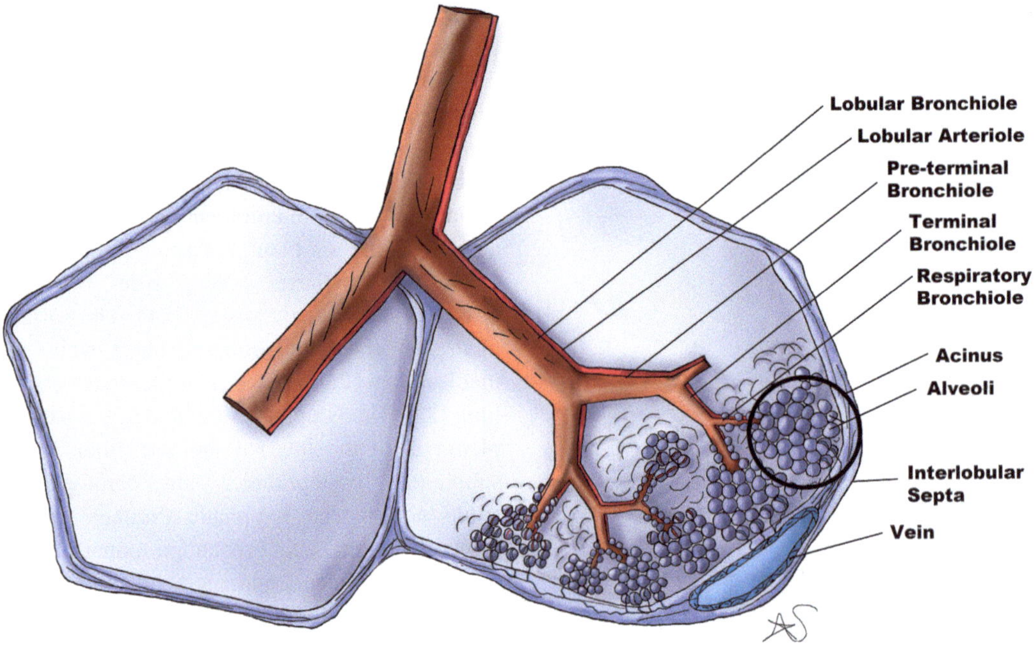

Fig. 1.8 Illustration depicting the anatomy of the secondary pulmonary lobule

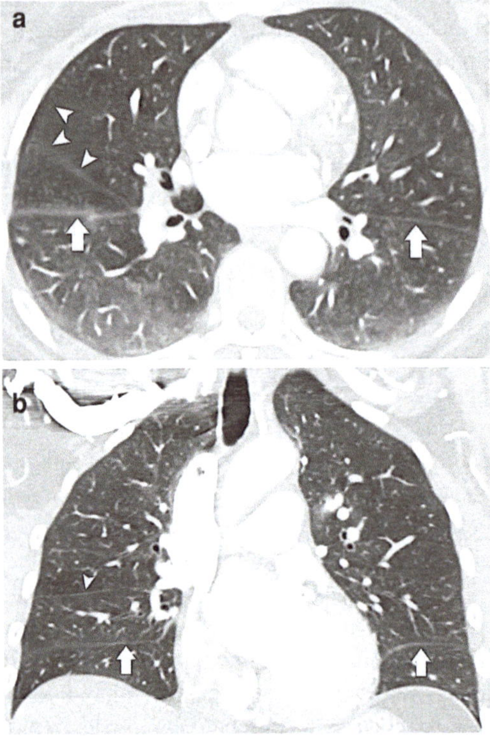

Fig. 1.9 Transverse computed tomography image (**a**) and coronal reformatted computed tomography image (**b**) show normal major (*arrows*) and minor (*arrowheads*) fissures

of the hemithorax on a PA radiograph. It represents the major fissure as it courses laterally along the superior segment of the lower lobe [23, 29]. Proto et al. reported the superolateral major fissure present on 14% of radiographs in their study [30]. The vertical fissure line on a PA radiograph is a thin linear opacity coursing from the costophrenic angle superiorly and medially toward the hilum and represents a segment of the major fissure. When extrapleural, intrafissural fat is present along the lateral aspects of the major fissure, the fissure has the appearance of an edge rather than a thin line [23, 29].

Multiple accessory fissures have been described: inferior accessory fissure, superior accessory fissure, left minor fissure, and azygos fissure [23, 26, 31]. The inferior accessory fissure separates the medial basal segment of the lower lobe from the remainder of the lower lobe (Fig. 1.10). This segment has been called the inferior accessory lobe, cardiac lobe, infracardiac lobe, and retrocardiac lobe. The superior accessory fissure separates the superior segment of the lower lobe from the basal segments of the lower lobe (Fig. 1.11). On a PA radiograph, the superior

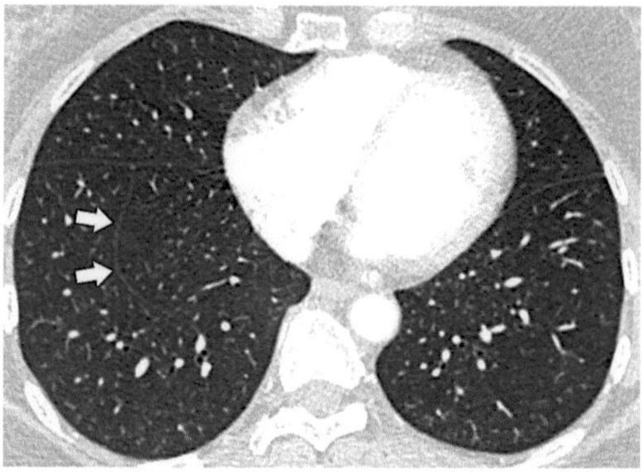

Fig. 1.10 Transverse computed tomography image shows a right inferior accessory fissure (*arrows*)

accessory fissure has an appearance similar to the minor fissure, but on the lateral radiograph, it extends posteriorly from the major fissure. The left minor fissure separates the lingula from the rest of the left upper lobe (Fig. 1.12) [25, 26, 31]. The azygos fissure is almost always on the right and extends from the posterior aspect of the first vertebral body to the superior vena cava (Fig. 1.13) [25, 26]. Other accessory fissures are less common, but often involve separating segments of a lobe [25, 26, 31]. For example, Godwin et al. described an accessory fissure separating the posterior and lateral segments of the lower lobe [31].

The inferior pulmonary ligament is a double layer of pleura formed by reflection of both the parietal and visceral pleural layers at the hilum that become continuous with intervening connective tissue and extend caudally, attaching the medial aspect of the lower lobe to the mediastinum (Fig. 1.14) [22, 32]. This leaves a linear bare area with no pleural cover along the mediastinum and lower lobe below the level of the hilum. On the right, the inferior pulmonary ligament arises between the IVC and the azygos vein, while it arises along the esophagus on the left [32].

Intrapulmonary lymph nodes are often subpleural in location and appear as pulmonary nodules less than 2 cm in size. They are associated with smoking and dust exposure and likely represent hyperplastic lymphoid nodules secondary to irritant dust. These are difficult to reliably distinguish from lung carcinoma on the basis of imaging alone and require pathology [33–35].

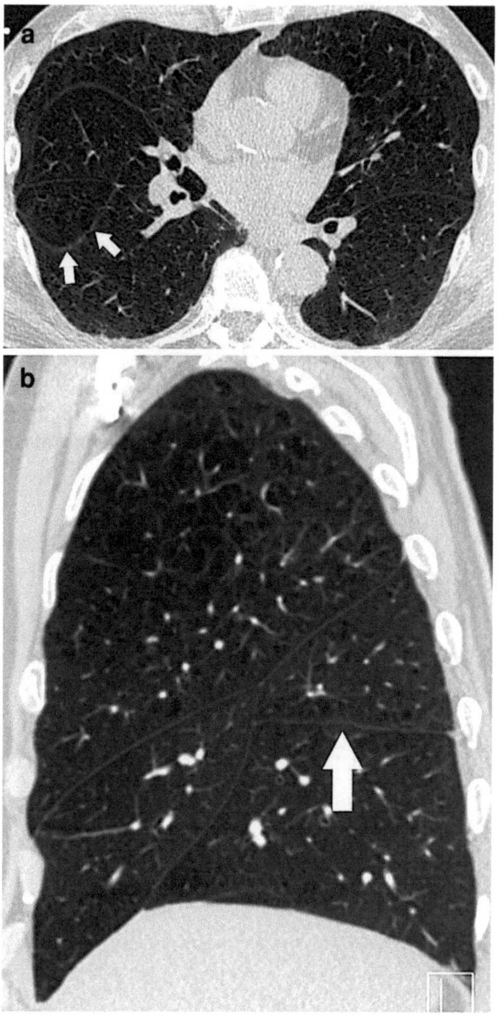

Fig. 1.11 Transverse (**a**) and sagittal reformatted (**b**) computed tomography images show a right superior accessory fissure (*arrows*)

Mediastinum and Great Vessels

Mediastinum

There are many normal contours, lines, and stripes of the mediastinum that are present on the chest radiograph. The trachea makes four of these contours: the right paratracheal stripe, anterior

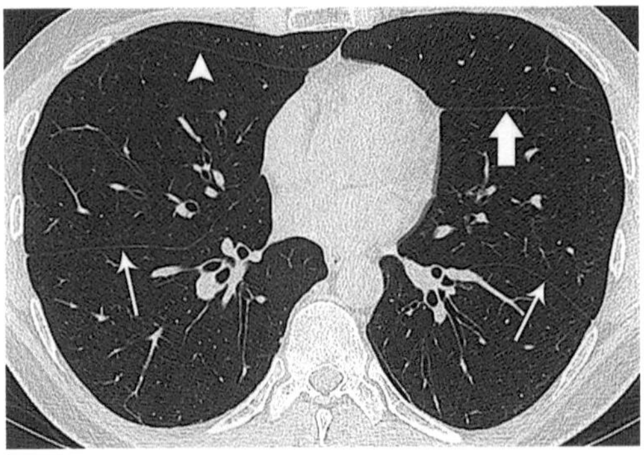

Fig. 1.12 Transverse computed tomography image shows an accessory left minor fissure (*wide arrow*). Note normal right minor fissure (*arrowhead*) and normal major fissures (*thin arrows*)

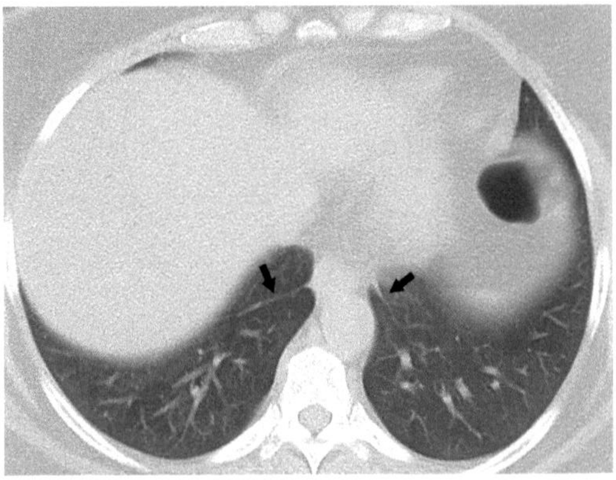

Fig. 1.14 Transverse computed tomography image shows the inferior pulmonary ligaments (*arrows*)

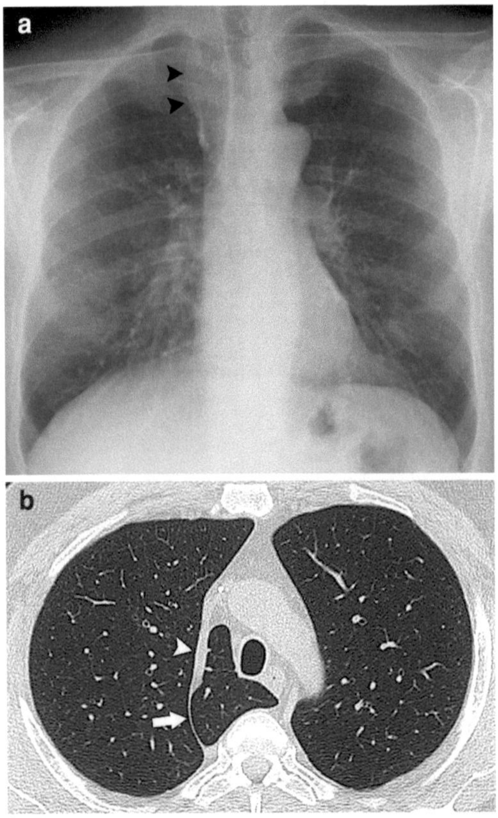

Fig. 1.13 **a** Frontal radiograph shows an azygos fissure (*arrowheads*). **b** Transverse computed tomography image shows an azygos fissure (*arrow*) with azygos vein (*arrowhead*) traveling within it

tracheal stripe, retrotracheal stripe, and the retrotracheal triangle. The right paratracheal stripe is a thin soft tissue band located just to the right of the tracheal wall and apparent on the frontal radiograph. This stripe consists of tracheal wall, mediastinal connective tissue, and parietal and visceral pleura. Its normal size is 1–4 mm (Fig. 1.1) [1, 36]. The anterior tracheal stripe is appreciated on the lateral radiograph and is created by the interface of anterior tracheal wall and lung. The posterior tracheal stripe, also known as the retrotracheal stripe, consists of posterior tracheal wall, mediastinal tissue, and parietal and visceral pleura. This stripe is abnormal if it is greater than 2.5 mm in width. A variation of this is the tracheoesophageal stripe, which also includes the anterior wall of the esophagus in the case of an air-distended esophagus [1, 36]. Finally, the retrotracheal triangle (Raider's triangle) is a lucent triangle behind the trachea. The borders of this triangle are the posterior tracheal wall anteriorly, the vertebral bodies posteriorly, the thoracic inlet superiorly, and the aortic arch inferiorly (Fig. 1.15). Both lungs contribute to the lucency within this triangle [1, 37]. Abnormal opacity within this space should prompt further investigation.

Other important mediastinal lines include the anterior junction line, which is formed by the apposition of the two lungs behind the upper two-thirds of the body of the sternum. It appears as an oblique line crossing the superior two-thirds of the sternum from the upper right to the left. It is often deviated up to 2 cm to the left secondary to levoposition of the heart, but

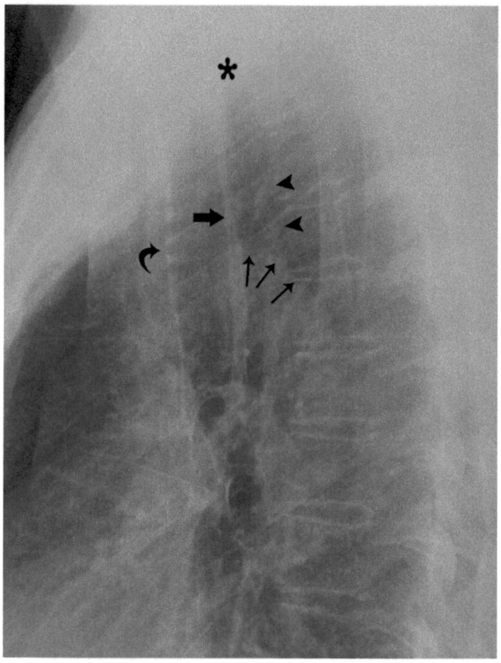

Fig. 1.15 Coned down lateral radiograph of Raider's triangle, formed by the posterior tracheal stripe (*arrow*), top of the aortic arch (*small arrows*), anterior aspect of the vertebral bodies (*arrowheads*) and the thoracic inlet (*asterisk*). Also note the anterior tracheal stripe (*curved arrow*)

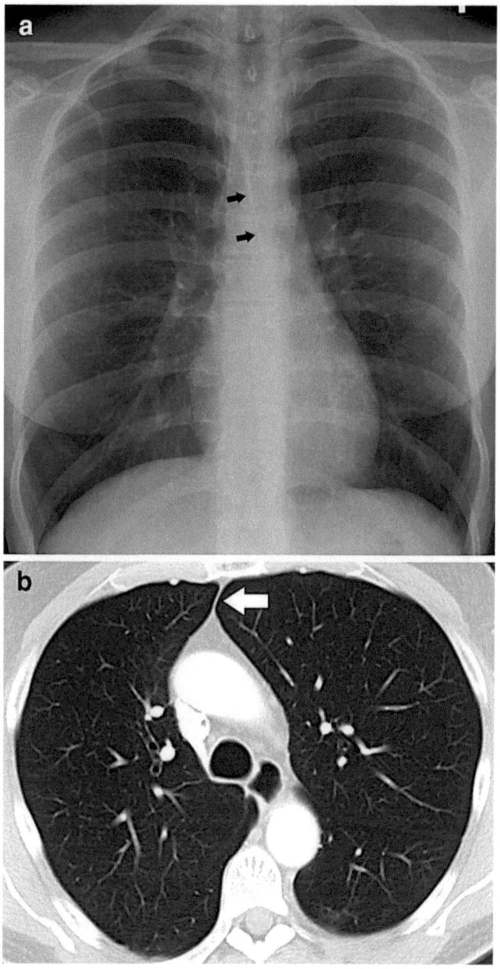

Fig. 1.16 Frontal radiograph (**a**) and transverse computed tomography image (**b**) show the anterior junction line (*arrows*)

remains straight (Fig. 1.16). Convexity of the anterior junction line is abnormal and needs further evaluation [4, 36]. The posterior junction line is a result of the apposition of the posterior aspects of the lungs and appears as a straight line projecting through the tracheal air column, above the level of the clavicles (Fig. 1.17). As with the anterior junction line, abnormal bulging of the posterior junction line should be viewed with suspicion for an underlying posterior mediastinal mass [36]. The right and left paraspinal lines represent the location where the lung and pleura contact the right and left posterior mediastinal fat and paraspinal muscles, respectively. The azygoesophageal recess is an area extending from the azygos arch caudally to the aortic hiatus. The medial aspect of the right lower lobe abuts this area, creating the azygoesophageal recess (Fig. 1.18). The contour of the azygoesophageal recess is convex to the left in adults, but in children it is often convex to the right [36, 38]. Finally, there is the aortopulmonary window. This window is bordered superiorly by the inferior wall of the aortic arch and inferiorly by the superior wall of the left pulmonary artery. It appears as a small concave contour with lung projecting within it (Fig. 1.19) [36].

There are four compartments of the mediastinum. The three compartments based on the lateral radiograph include the anterior, middle, and posterior mediastinum compartments. The anterior mediastinum includes everything anterior to a vertical line drawn anterior to the trachea and posterior to the heart. The middle mediastinum includes everything posterior to

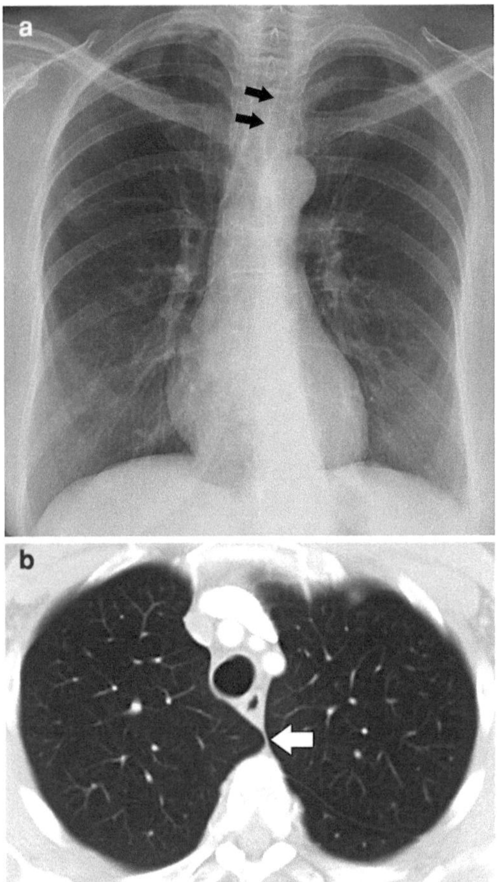

Fig. 1.17 **a** Frontal radiograph shows a thin vertical line of the posterior junction line seen through the tracheal air column (*arrows*). **b** Transverse computed tomography image shows the posterior junction line (*arrow*)

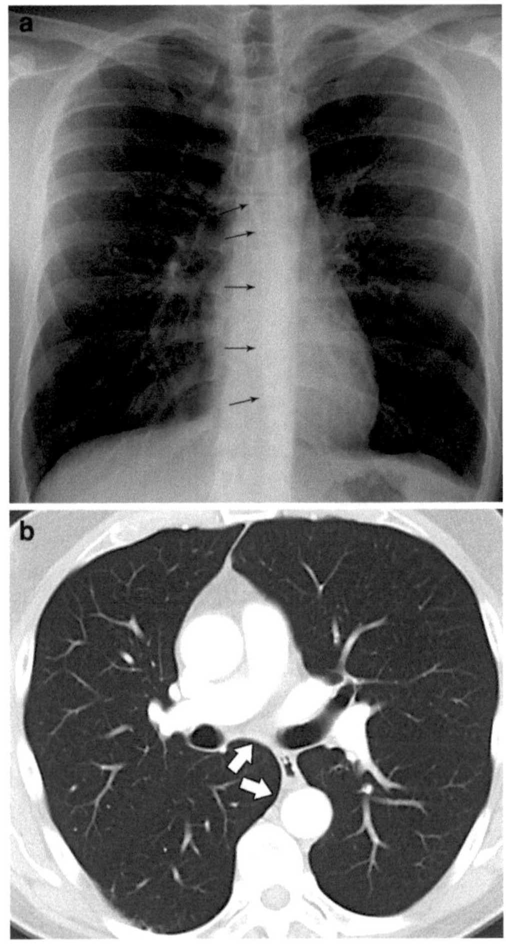

Fig. 1.18 Frontal radiograph (**a**) and transverse computed tomography image (**b**) show the azygoesophageal recess (*arrows*)

the anterior mediastinum and anterior to a vertical line drawn 1 cm posterior to the vertebral bodies. The posterior mediastinum includes everything posterior to the middle mediastinum. Some authors prefer to separate the superior mediastinum into all things in the mediastinum above the level of the T4–5 disk space [39].

Spaces within the mediastinum include the pretracheal space, prevascular space, aortopulmonary window, subcarinal space, azygoesophageal recess, and the retrocrural space. The pretracheal space is the space anterior to the trachea. The prevascular space is a triangular shaped space anterior to the great vessels. The aortopulmonary window is a small space that is bordered by the inferior aorta superiorly and the left pulmonary artery inferiorly. The subcarinal space is located just below the carina and is bordered by the main bronchi laterally and the left atrium inferiorly. The azygoesophageal recess has been described above. The retrocrural space is a small space that is located medial to the diaphragmatic crura (Fig. 1.20) [39]. All of these spaces contain lymph nodes. Normal lymph node size has been studied by several groups. Maximal short axis mediastinal lymph node diameters reported range from 10 to 11 mm [40]. There are 14 lymph node stations numbered by Mountain et al. for lung cancer staging purposes [41].

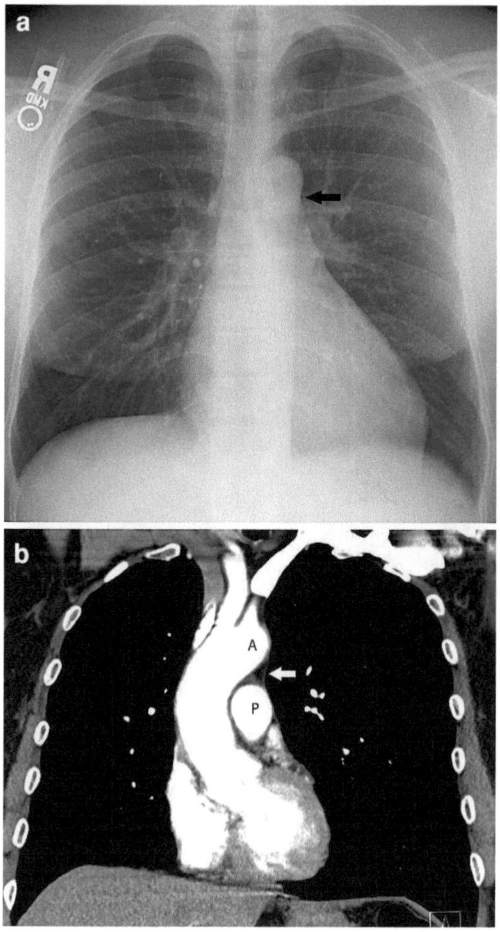

Fig. 1.19 **a** Frontal radiograph shows a small concave contour along the left mediastinal silhouette (*arrow*), consistent with the normal radiographic contour of the aortopulmonary window. **b** Coronal reformatted computed tomography image shows a small triangle of fat (*arrow*) between the aorta (A) and pulmonary artery (P), which is the aortopulmonary window

The thymus is a bilobed organ in the superoanterior mediastinum and can extend from the level of the left brachiocephalic vein to the aortic root [42]. The thymus becomes increasingly fatty with age. Under the age of 20 years, there is no significant fatty replacement; however, over the age of 40 years, approximately 75% of the thymus has been fatty replaced [42]. The shape of the thymus is often biconvex in children less than 5 years old. Between the ages of 5–15 years old, it can have a convex, straight, or concave morphology. After the age of 15 years, biconcave morphology is most common [43]. Although the thymus is usually in the superoanterior mediastinum, it can extend into retrocaval and paratracheal spaces, extend between the right brachiocephalic vein and artery, and be located ectopically within the posterior mediastinum [44–46].

Great Vessels

The venous system is more variable than the arterial system of the thorax. The subclavian vein, a continuation of the axillary vein, drains the upper extremity, shoulder, and part of the chest wall. It combines with the internal jugular vein, which drains the brain, and forms the brachiocephalic vein. Several veins drain into the brachiocephalic vein. The vertebral vein, which drains the cervical vertebral bodies, and the internal mammary vein, which drains intercostal veins, both drain into the brachiocephalic vein. The left and right brachiocephalic veins then combine at the level of the first intercostal space behind the sternum just to the right of midline into the superior vena cava (SVC), which drains into the right atrium (Fig. 1.21) [47].

The azygos venous system consists of the azygos vein, hemiazygos vein, accessory hemiazygos vein, and the left superior intercostal vein. The azygos vein is a continuation of the right ascending lumbar vein and enters the thorax via the aortic hiatus and courses anteriorly along the spine. The azygos vein drains the right intercostal veins and empties into the SVC (Fig. 1.22). The hemiazygos vein continues from the ascending left lumbar vein and also enters the thorax via the aortic hiatus. The hemiazygos vein drains the lower left intercostal veins, crosses the midline at the level of T8, and empties into the azygos vein. The accessory hemiazygos vein drains intercostal veins from the middle left hemithorax and crosses the midline at the level of T7 to empty into the azygos vein [47, 48]. The left superior intercostal vein, which drains the third and fourth

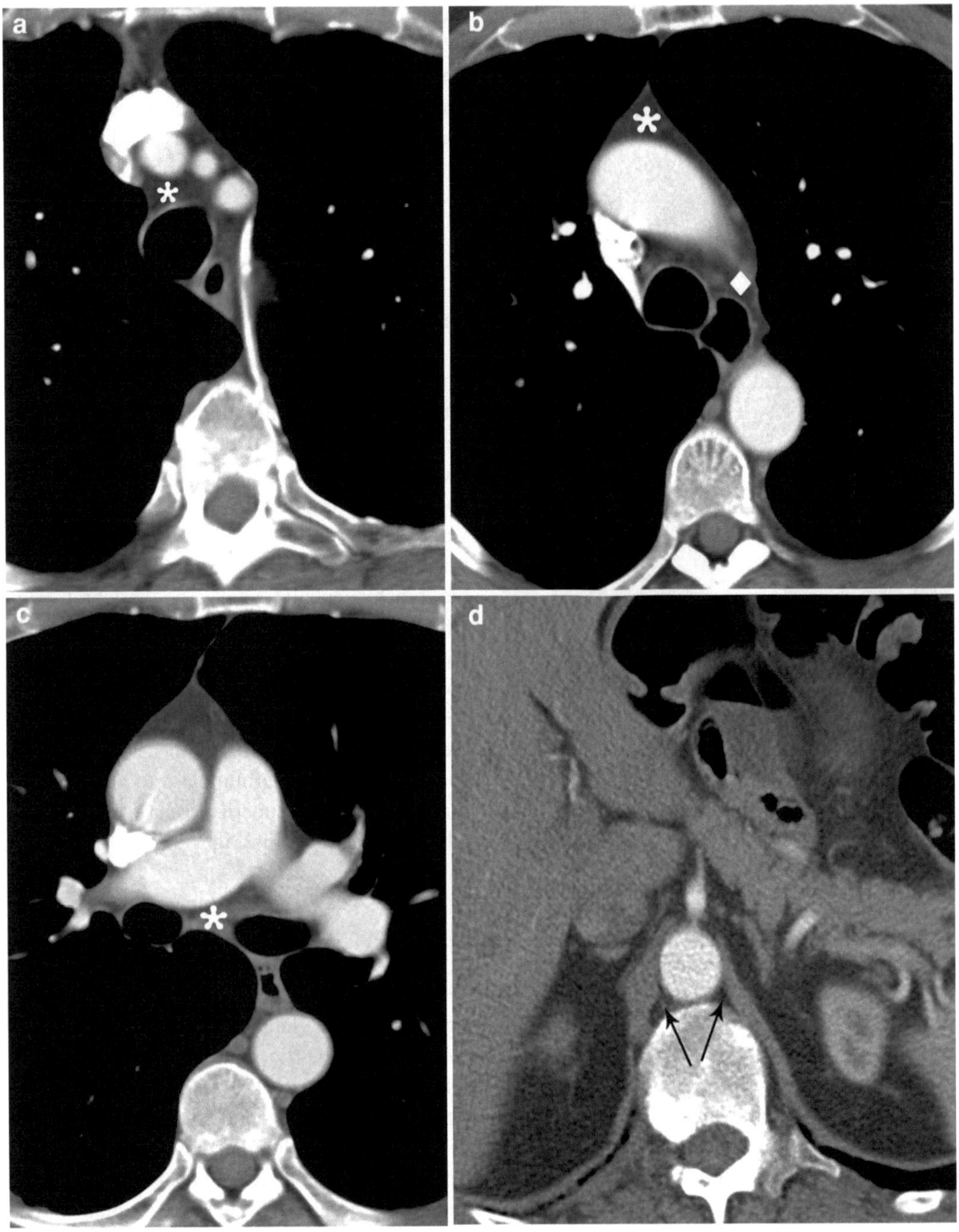

Fig. 1.20 Multiple transverse computed tomography images demonstrate the mediastinal spaces. **a** Pretracheal space (*asterisk*). **b** Prevascular space (*asterisk*) and aortopulmonary space (*diamond*). **c** Subcarinal space (*asterisk*). **d** Retrocrural space (*arrows*)

posterior intercostal veins, makes a small arch along the left lateral margin of the mediastinum. It may be visible on the PA radiograph adjacent to the aorta as a tiny bulge and is referred to as an "aortic nipple." (Fig. 1.23) [47, 49]. The left superior intercostal vein drains into the left

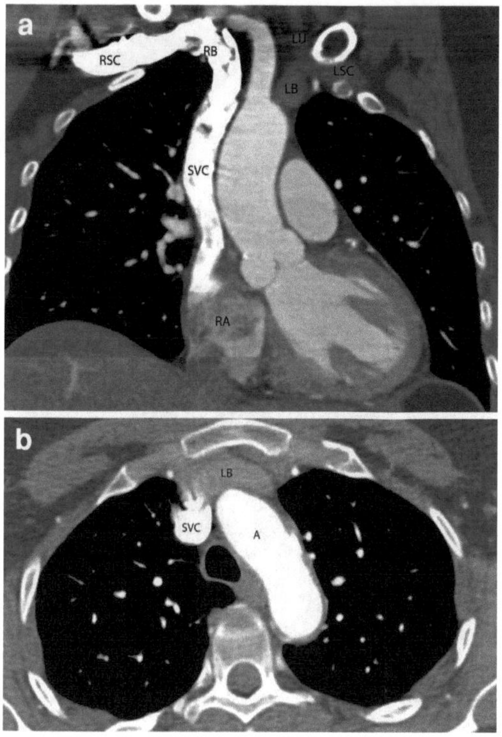

Fig. 1.21 **a** Coronal reformatted contrast enhanced computed tomography image shows the right subclavian vein (RSC) joining the right internal jugular vein (not imaged here) to form the right brachiocephalic vein (RB). The right brachiocephalic vein empties into the superior vena cava (SVC) and then into the right atrium (RA). On the left, the unenhanced left internal jugular vein (LIJ) and the left subclavian vein (LSC) join and empty into the left brachiocephalic vein (LB). **b** Transverse contrast enhanced computed tomography image shows the left brachiocephalic vein (LB) cross anterior to the aorta (A) and empty into the SVC

brachiocephalic vein but connects to the hemiazygos vein in up to 75% of patients [47, 48]. Sometimes the hemiazygos and the accessory hemiazygos veins are absent, and the left intercostal veins will then course behind the aorta and drain directly into the azygos vein [48].

Notable venous anomalies include the persistent left superior vena cava and partial anomalous pulmonary venous return. A persistent left superior vena cava occurs when there is failure of regression of parts of the left anterior and common cardinal veins. The left superior vena cava typically drains into the

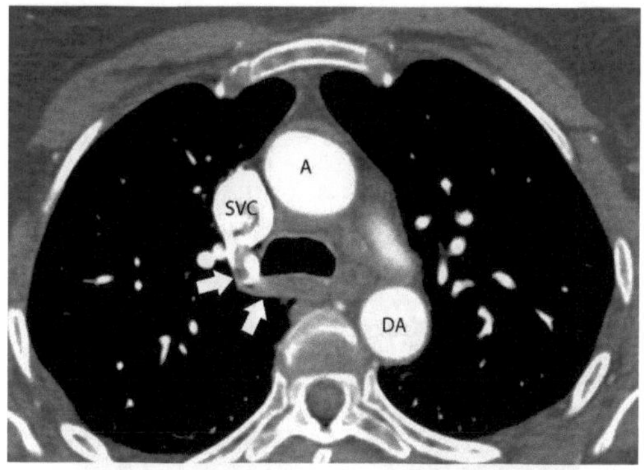

Fig. 1.22 Transverse image from a contrast enhanced CT shows the azygos vein (*arrows*) draining into the superior vena cava (SVC). A = ascending thoracic aorta, DA = descending thoracic aorta

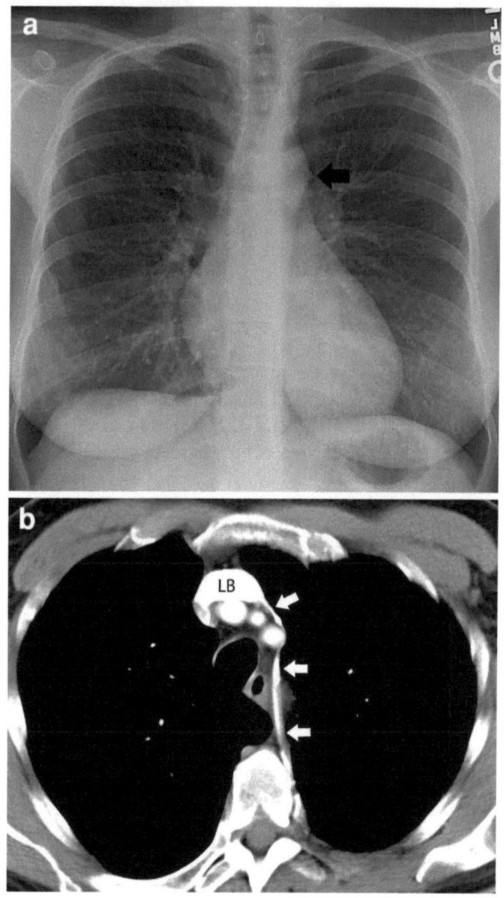

Fig. 1.23 **a** Frontal radiograph shows the left superior intercostal vein as a small nodular opacity adjacent to the aortic arch (*arrow*), giving the appearance of an aortic nipple. **b** Transverse image from a contrast enhanced CT shows the left superior intercostal vein (*arrows*) draining into the left brachiocephalic vein (LB)

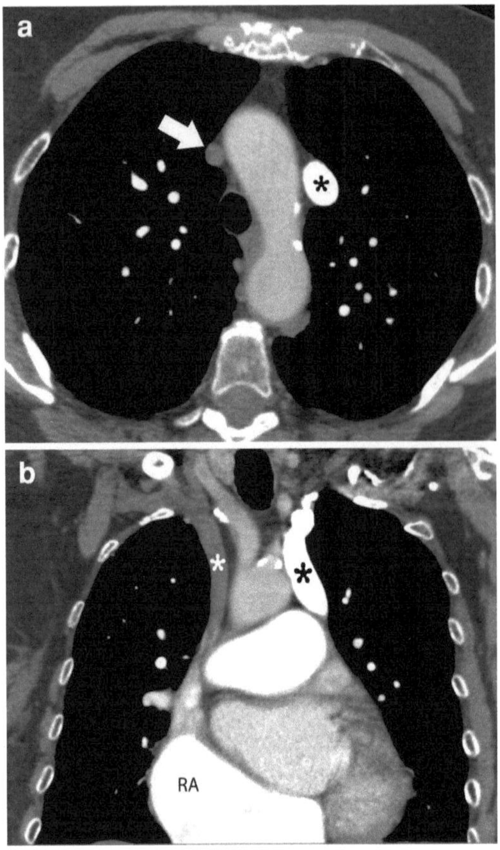

Fig. 1.24 **a** Transverse image from a contrast enhanced CT shows a persistent left superior vena cava (*asterisk*) and the right superior vena cava (*arrow*). **b** A coronal reformatted image from a contrast enhanced CT shows a right superior vena cava (*white asterisk*) and a persistent left superior vena cava (*black asterisk*). RA = right atrium

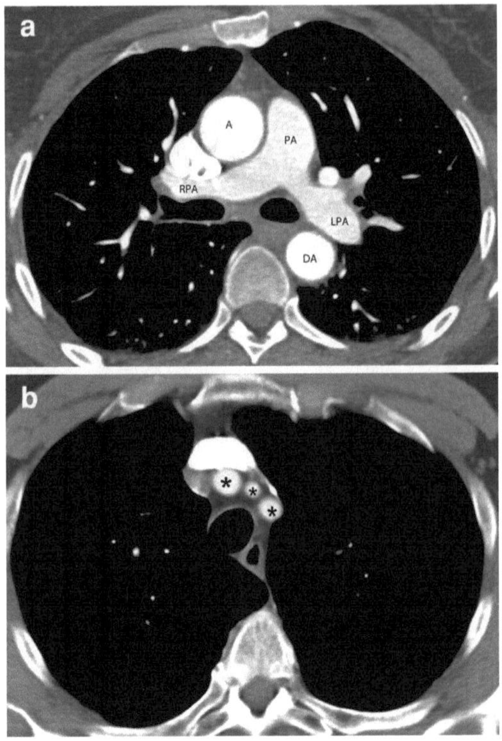

Fig. 1.25 **a** Transverse image from a contrast enhanced CT shows the ascending aorta (A), descending thoracic aorta (DA), main pulmonary artery (PA), right pulmonary artery (RPA), and the left pulmonary artery (LPA). **b** A second transverse image from a contrast enhanced CT at a slightly higher level shows the three arch vessels (*asterisks*). Going from the left side of the image to the right, these vessels are the right brachiocephalic artery, left common carotid artery, and the left subclavian artery

coronary sinus (Fig. 1.24) [47, 50]. Partial anomalous venous return occurs when the pulmonary veins fail to make a normal connection to the heart and is more common on the right than the left. The anomalous pulmonary veins may drain into the SVC, right atrium, left brachiocephalic vein, coronary sinus, and the azygos vein [47, 50].

The main arteries include the main pulmonary artery, aorta, and the arch vessels arising from the aorta. The main pulmonary artery normally measures up to 2.9 cm in transverse diameter [51] and bifurcates into the right and left pulmonary arteries. The aortic arch is normally on the left and gives rise to the right brachiocephalic artery, left common carotid artery, and the left subclavian artery. The ligamentum arteriosum courses from the left pulmonary artery to the descending aorta and may be calcified (Fig. 1.25) [52]. There are many anomalies involving the aorta and its arch vessels, including right aortic arch, the presence of both a right and left aortic arch (double arch) as well as anomalies of number, origin, and course of the arch vessels [52, 53].

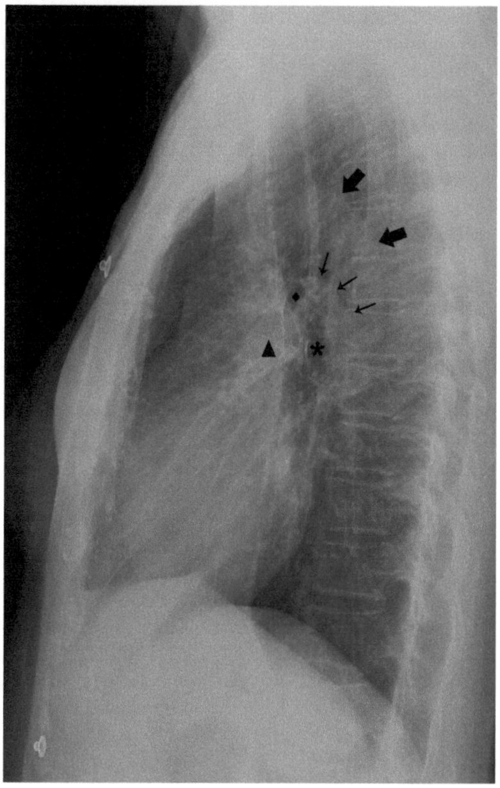

Fig. 1.26 Lateral radiograph demonstrating characteristic appearance of the hilum. Left pulmonary artery forms a smaller arch (*small arrows*) inferior to the aortic arch (*large arrows*) as it drapes over the left upper lobe bronchus (*black asterisk*). Right pulmonary artery (*arrowhead*) is anterior to the right upper lobe bronchus (*diamond*) and the left upper lobe bronchus (*black asterisk*)

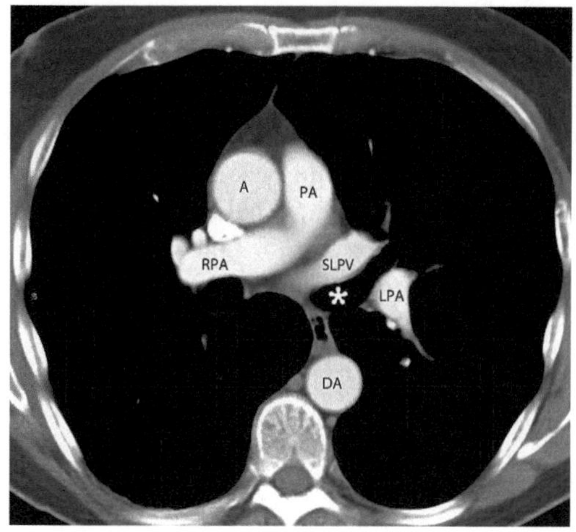

Fig. 1.27 Transverse image from a contrast enhanced CT shows the superior left pulmonary vein (SLPV) anterior to the left main bronchus (*white asterisk*). A = ascending thoracic aorta, DA = descending thoracic aorta, PA = main pulmonary artery, RPA = right pulmonary artery, LPA = left pulmonary artery

Hila

The main structures in the pulmonary hila are the pulmonary arteries, pulmonary veins, airways, and lymph nodes. The main pulmonary artery bifurcates into the right and left pulmonary arteries. The right pulmonary artery is longer and passes in front of the right main bronchus and behind the SVC (Fig. 1.3), where it bifurcates into the truncus anterior and the right interlobar artery (right descending pulmonary artery). The left pulmonary artery passes over the left main bronchus and gives off the left ascending branch artery before it continues caudally as the left descending pulmonary artery [54, 55]. The relationship between the pulmonary arteries and the main bronchi creates the characteristic hilar appearance on the lateral radiograph (Fig. 1.26).

The right upper lobe segmental veins form the right superior pulmonary vein, which drains into the posterior left atrium. The right middle vein typically joins the right superior pulmonary vein near left atrium. The left upper lobe segmental veins form the left superior pulmonary vein, which combines with the lingular vein and courses anterior to the left main bronchus before emptying into the left atrium (Fig. 1.27). The segmental veins of the lower lobes form pulmonary venous confluences medial to the lower lobe bronchi before draining into the left atrium. These can sometimes be confused with pulmonary nodules on chest radiographs [54, 55].

Diaphragm

The diaphragm consists of peripheral muscle fibers attaching to a central tendon. The central tendon fuses to the caudal portion of the pericardium. There are a number of openings including the aortic hiatus, esophageal hiatus, and the SVC hiatus. The diaphragm attaches anteriorly to the xiphoid process and anterior lower six ribs. Posteriorly, the diaphragmatic crura attach to the anterolateral aspects of the lumbar vertebral bodies. The crura extend inferiorly where the median arcuate ligament connects them anterior to the aorta just above the level of the celiac trunk. The inferior pulmonary ligament also attaches to the diaphragm [56].

References

1. Holbert JM, Strollo DC. Imaging of the normal trachea. J Thorac Imaging. 1995 Summer;10(3):171–9.
2. Gamsu G, Webb WR. Computed tomography of the trachea: normal and abnormal. Am J Roentgenol. 1982;139(2):321–6.
3. Breatnach E, Abbott GC, Fraser RG. Dimensions of the normal human trachea. Am J Roentgenol. 1984;142(5):903–6.
4. Bhalla M, Noble ER, Shepard JA, McLoud TC. Normal position of trachea and anterior junction line on CT. J Comput Assist Tomogr. 1993;17(5):714–8.
5. Naidich DP, Terry PB, Stitik FP, Siegelman SS. Computed tomography of the bronchi: 1. Normal anatomy. J Comput Assist Tomogr. 1980;4(6): 746–53.
6. Lee KS, Im JG, Bae WK, Kim YH, Jung SY, Lee BH, Han MC, Kim CW. CT anatomy of the lingular segmental bronchi. J Comput Assist Tomogr. 1991;15(1):86–91.
7. Atwell SW. Major anomalies of the tracheobronchial tree: with a list of the minor anomalies. Dis Chest. 1967;52(5):611–5.
8. Freeman SJ, Harvey JE, Goddard PR. Demonstration of supernumerary tracheal bronchus by computed tomographic scanning and magnetic resonance imaging. Thorax. 1995;50(4):426–7.
9. Wu JW, White CS, Meyer CA, Haramati LB, Mason AC. Variant bronchial anatomy: CT appearance and classification. Am J Roentgenol. 1999;172(3):741–4.
10. Desir A, Ghaye B. Congenital abnormalities of intrathoracic airways. RadiolClin North Am. 2009; 47(2):203–25.
11. Ghaye B, Szapiro D, Fanchamps JM, Dondelinger RF. Congenital bronchial abnormalities revisited. Radiographics. 2001;21(1):105–19.
12. Hosker HS, Clague HW, Morritt GN. Ectopic right upper lobe bronchus as a cause of breathlessness. Thorax. 1987;42(6):473–4.
13. Setty SP, Michaels AJ. Tracheal bronchus: case presentation, literature review, and discussion. J Trauma. 2000;49(5):943–5.
14. Endo S, Saitoh N, Murayama F, Sohara Y, Fuse K. Symptomatic accessory cardiac bronchus. Ann Thorac Surg. 2000;69(1):262–4.
15. Bentala M, Grijm K, van der Zee JH, Kloek JJ. Cardiac bronchus: a rare cause of hemoptysis. Eur J Cardiothorac Surg. 2002;22(4):643–5.
16. Jackson GD, Littleton JT. Simultaneous occurrence of anomalous cardiac and tracheal bronchi: a case study. J Thorac Imaging. 1988;3(1):59–60.
17. Landay MJ, Chaw C, Bordlee RP. Bilateral left lungs: unusual variation of hilar anatomy. AJR Am J Roentgenol. 1982;138(6):1162–4.
18. Webb WR. High resolution lung computed tomography. Normal anatomic and pathologic findings. RadiolClin North Am. 1991;29(5):1051–63.
19. Berend N, Rynell AC, Ward HE. Structure of a human pulmonary acinus. Thorax. 1991;46(2):117–21.
20. Helm EJ, Matin TN, Gleeson FV. Imaging of the pleura. J MagnReson Imaging. 2010;32(6):1275–86. doi: 10.1002/jmri.22372.
21. Jantz MA, Antony VB. Pathophysiology of the pleura. Respiration. 2008;75(2):121–33.
22. Cooper C, Moss AA, Buy JN, Stark DD. CT appearance of the normal inferior pulmonary ligament. Am J Roentgenol. 1983;141(2):237–40.
23. Hayashi K, Aziz A, Ashizawa K, Hayashi H, Nagaoki K, Otsuji H. Radiographic and CT appearances of the major fissures. Radiographics. 2001;21(4):861–74.
24. Aziz A, Ashizawa K, Nagaoki K, Hayashi K. High resolution CT anatomy of the pulmonary fissures. J Thorac Imaging. 2004;19(3):186–91.
25. Cronin P, Gross BH, Kelly AM, Patel S, Kazerooni EA, Carlos RC. Normal and accessory fissures of the lung: evaluation with contiguous volumetric thin-section multidetector CT. Eur J Radiol. 2010; 75(2):e1–e8.
26. Ozmen CA, Nazaroglu H, Bayrak AH, Senturk S, Akay HO. Evaluation of interlobar and accessory pulmonary fissures on 64-row MDCT. Clin Anat. 2010;23(5):552–8.
27. Mahmut M, Nishitani H. Evaluation of pulmonary lobe variations using multidetector row computed tomography. J Comput Assist Tomogr. 2007;31(6): 956–60.
28. Raasch BN, Carsky EW, Lane EJ, O'Callaghan JP, Heitzman ER. Radiographic anatomy of the interlobar fissures: a study of 100 specimens. Am J Roentgenol. 1982;138(6):1043–9.
29. Proto AV, Ball JB Jr. Computed tomography of the major and minor fissures. Am J Roentgenol. 1983; 140(3):439–48.
30. Proto AV, Ball JB Jr. The superolateral major fissures. Am J Roentgenol. 1983;140(3):431–7.
31. Godwin JD, Tarver RD. Accessory fissures of the lung. Am J Roentgenol. 1985;144(1):39–47.
32. Godwin JD, Vock P, Osborne DR. CT of the pulmonary ligament. Am J Roentgenol. 1983;141(2):231–6.
33. Oshiro Y, Kusumoto M, Moriyama N, Kaneko M, Suzuki K, Asamura H, Kondo H, Tsuchiya R,

Murayama S. Intrapulmonary lymph nodes: thin-section CT features of 19 nodules. J Comput Assist Tomogr. 2002;26(4):553–7.
34. Perez N, Lhoste-Trouilloud A, Boyer L, Michel JL, Escande G, Kemeny JL. Computed tomographic appearance of three intrapulmonary lymph nodes. Eur J Radiol. 1998;28(2):147–9.
35. Bankoff MS, McEniff NJ, Bhadelia RA, Garcia-Moliner M, Daly BD. Prevalence of pathologically proven intrapulmonary lymph nodes and their appearance on CT. Am J Roentgenol. 1996;167(3):629–30.
36. Gibbs JM, Chandrasekhar CA, Ferguson EC, Oldham SA. Lines and stripes: where did they go?–From conventional radiography to CT. Radiographics. 2007;27(1):33–48.
37. Franquet T, Erasmus JJ, Giménez A, Rossi S, Prats R. The retrotracheal space: normal anatomic and pathologic appearances. Radiographics. 2002;Spec No:S231–46.
38. Miller FH, Fitzgerald SW, Donaldson JS. CT of the azygoesophageal recess in infants and children. Radiographics. 1993;13(3):623–34.
39. Ferdele MP, Rosado-de-Christenson ML, Woodward PJ, Abbott GF, Shaaban AM. Diagnostic and Surgical Imaging Anatomy: Chest, Abdomen, Pelvis: Published by Amirsys®.
40. Genereux GP, Howie JL. Normal mediastinal lymph node size and number: CT and anatomic study. Am J Roentgenol. 1984;142(6):1095–100.
41. Mountain CF, Dresler CM. Regional lymph node classification for lung cancer staging. Chest. 1997;111(6):1718–23.
42. Moore AV, Korobkin M, Olanow W, Heaston DK, Ram PC, Dunnick NR, Silverman PM. Age-related changes in the thymus gland: CT-pathologic correlation. Am J Roentgenol. 1983;141(2):241–6.
43. St Amour TE, Siegel MJ, Glazer HS, Nadel SN. CT appearances of the normal and abnormal thymus in childhood.J Comput Assist Tomogr. 1987;11(4): 645–50.
44. Heiberg E, Wolverson MK, Sundaram M, Nouri S. Normal thymus: CT characteristics in subjects under age 20. Am J Roentgenol. 1982;138(3):491–4.
45. Swischuk LE, John SD. AJR Normal thymus extending between the right brachiocephalic vein and the innominate artery. Am J Roentgenol. 1996; 166(6):1462–4.
46. Rollins NK, Currarino G. MR imaging of posterior mediastinal thymus. J Comput Assist Tomogr. 1988;12(3):518–20.
47. Godwin JD, Chen JT. Thoracic venous anatomy. Am J Roentgenol. 1986;147(4):674–84.
48. Takasugi JE, Godwin JD. CT appearance of the retroaortic anastomoses of the azygos system. Am J Roentgenol. 1990;154(1):41–4.
49. Friedman AC, Chambers E, Sprayregen S. The normal and abnormal left superior intercostal vein. Am J Roentgenol. 1978;131(4):599–2.
50. Ratliff HL, Yousufuddin M, Lieving WR, Watson BE, Malas A, Rosencrance G, McCowan RJ. Persistent left superior vena cava: case reports and clinical implications. Int J Cardiol. 2006;113(2):242–6.
51. Kuriyama K, Gamsu G, Stern RG, Cann CE, Herfkens RJ, Brundage BH. CT-determined pulmonary artery diameters in predicting pulmonary hypertension. Invest Radiol. 1984;19(1):16–22.
52. Jakanani GC, Adair W. Frequency of variations in aortic arch anatomy depicted on multidetector CT. ClinRadiol. 2010;65(6):481–7.
53. Hernanz-Schulman M. Vascular rings: a practical approach to imaging diagnosis. PediatrRadiol. 2005; 35(10):961–79.
54. Genereux GP. Conventional tomographic hilar anatomy emphasizing the pulmonary veins. Am J Roentgenol. 1983;141(6):1241–57.
55. Naidich DP, Khouri NF, Scott WW Jr, Wang KP, Siegelman SS. Computed tomography of the pulmonary hila: 1. normal anatomy. J Comput Assist Tomogr. 1981;5(4):459–67.
56. Panicek DM, Benson CB, Gottlieb RH, Heitzman ER. The diaphragm: anatomic, pathologic, and radiologic considerations. Radiographics. 1988;8(3): 385–25.

2 Management of Solitary Pulmonary Nodules

Maria C. Shiau, Elie Portnoy, and Stuart M. Garay

Abstract

The workup and management of the solitary pulmonary nodule is an increasingly common and confounding clinical problem for which a uniformly accepted approach has yet to be established. Conventional radiologic literature has suggested a number of imaging characteristics of nodules such as size, cavitation, growth rate, and margin morphology to guide the physician in clinical management. More recent literature emphasizes nodule attenuation, as well as size, growth, etc., in correlation with patient risk factors for disease to guide the most appropriate course of follow-up. Risk factors include age greater than 35 years, smoking history, occupational exposures, and history of malignancy. In this chapter, based on a review of the established recommendations and the authors' clinical experiences, an approach to the management of the solitary pulmonary nodule is put forth.

Keywords

Solitary pulmonary nodule · Nodule management · Lung cancer · Ground-glass opacity · Sub-solid nodule

Management of solitary pulmonary nodules (SPN) is a vexing clinical issue augmented by rising rate of nodule detection due to more pervasive use of CT imaging in medicine. In addition, newer generation scanners allow for thin-slice imaging of the entire thorax in a few seconds resulting in improved resolution and nodule detection. The role of the radiologist is to help the clinician determine the most appropriate management strategy for these indeterminate and often incidental pulmonary nodules.

The term solitary pulmonary nodule refers to a rounded lesion 30 mm or smaller in diameter with at least two-thirds of its margins

M. C. Shiau (✉)
Department of Radiology, Thoracic Imaging, NYU Langone Medical Center, 560 1st Avenue, Room: Rusk 236, New York, NY 10016, USA
e-mail: maria.shiau@nyumc.org

E. Portnoy
Department of Radiology, NYU Langone Medical Center, 560 1st Avenue, New York, NY 10016, USA

S. M. Garay
Department of Medicine, NYU School of Medicine, NYU Langone Medical Center, 530 1st Avenue, New York, NY 10016, USA

J. P. Kanne (ed.), *Clinically Oriented Pulmonary Imaging*, Respiratory Medicine, DOI: 10.1007/978-1-61779-542-8_2,

surrounded by lung parenchyma and not associated with atelectasis or lymphadenopathy [1, 2]. On CT imaging, the term focal opacity is frequently encountered encompassing a range of nodules, which may be categorized as solid, semisolid (part solid), or nonsolid (ground-glass). The incidence of SPNs on standard chest radiographs is approximately one in every 500 chest radiographs [3] or 150,000 new cases per year in the United States. Review of eight large lung cancer screening trials revealed a variable prevalence rate of at least one nodule to be 8–51% of which 1.1–12% were malignant [4].

The first concern regarding SPNs is the exclusion of malignancy. The majority of incidental and screen-detected nodules are benign granulomas (both healed and active) (40%) and hamartomas (15%) [5]. Less common causes of benign nodules include nonspecific inflammation and fibrosis, round pneumonia, arteriovenous malformations, healed pulmonary infarcts, hemangiomas, intrapulmonary lymph nodes, tuberculoma, bronchogenic cysts, rounded atelectasis, mucoid impaction, dog "heartworm" (rare) [6], etc. Because bronchopneumonia is a very uncommon cause for SPN, a course of antibiotic therapy in a patient without symptoms is discouraged. It may cause avoidable delays in diagnosis [6]. However empiric antibiotic treatment has been recommended in cases of clustered nodules, which are more likely to represent inflammation rather than malignancy. Follow-up at 1 month after adequate treatment would facilitate distinction of inflammation from a dominant SPN with satellite nodules [1].

The majority of malignant SPNs are lung carcinomas. Imaging features of SPNs, which were subsequently characterized as bronchogenic carcinoma, include poorly defined or spiculated margins, frequently upper lobe location, and corona radiata sign. One-third to 50% may represent metastatic lesions, particularly with a known history of an extrathoracic malignancy [1, 4]. Metastases tend to occur in the subpleural regions of the lower lobes.

Various radiographic features of nodules aid in the estimation of the probability of cancer and thus affect management.

Size

Small solitary pulmonary nodules are likely benign. A screening study by Henschke et al. in 2004 found that none of the detected malignancies were less than 5 mm in diameter [7]. The prevalence of malignancy correlates with nodule size (0–1% for nodules <5 mm, 6–28% for nodules 5–10 mm, 33–60% for nodules 11–20 mm, and 64–82% for nodules greater than 20 mm) [5, 6].

Margins

Margins are classified as smooth, lobulated, spiculated, or irregular. Although most smoothly marginated nodules are benign, this feature may be present in up to 21% of malignant nodules [8]. Lobulated contour, signifying uneven growth, is often associated with malignant nodules but can be seen in 25% of benign nodules [9]. A spiculated or irregularly marginated nodule displaying a corona radiata sign indicating neoplastic infiltration and distortion on neighboring tissues is almost certainly a sign of malignancy.

Calcifications

Calcifications are found more frequently within benign SPNs. Patterns of calcification characteristic of benign nodules are laminated, dense-central, and popcorn. Stippled, punctate, and eccentric calcifications are suggestive of malignancy [10] (see Fig. 2.1).

Fatty Attenuation

The presence of fat tissue (attenuation between -40 and -120 Hounsfield units) within a SPN is suggestive of a hamartoma.(see Fig. 2.2) Caution is required to accurately measure pixel attenuation within the center of lesion since volume averaging with adjacent aerated lung

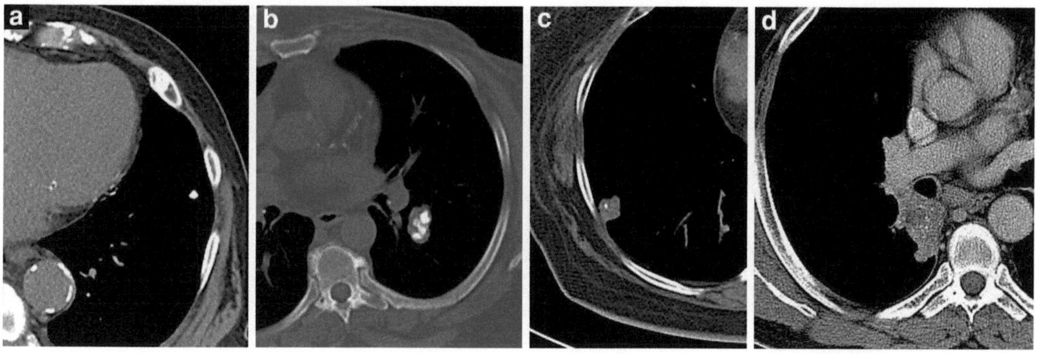

Fig. 2.1 Axial CT images demonstrate varying nodule calcification patterns: **a** dense, **b** popcorn, **c** eccentric, and **d** stippled

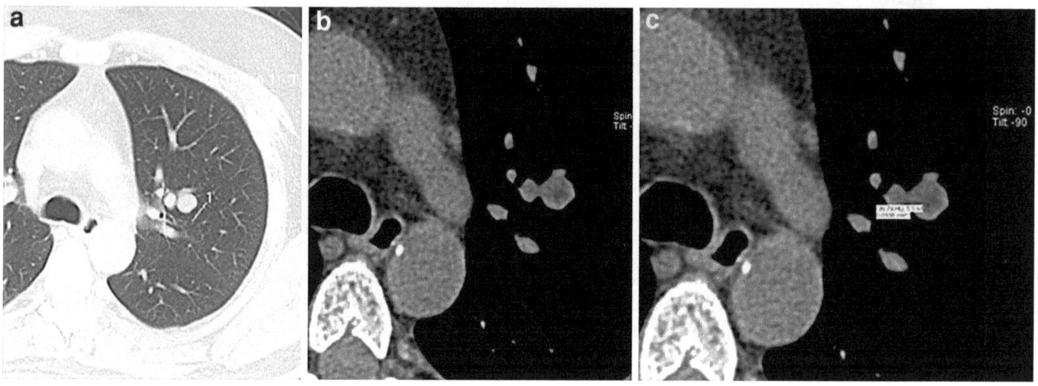

Fig. 2.2 Axial non-enhanced CT images of a left upper lobe 1.4 cm nodule in lung window setting (**a**) and soft tissue window setting on CT (**b, c**) measures fatty attenuation (−36.8 Hounsfield units (HU)), consistent with a hamartoma

may artifactually result in a low-attenuation measurement. Other diagnostic considerations when encountering a SPN containing fat attenuation are lipoid pneumonia and liposarcoma metastases. Correlation with clinical history is usually sufficient to distinguish these two from hamartoma.

Cavitation

Cavitation may be seen with both benign and malignant nodules. Unfortunately, the thickness of the wall is unreliable in distinguishing benign from malignant, although malignancy is associated with thicker and more irregular walls. Pseudocavitation is a descriptor frequently used in describing features of bronchioloalveolar carcinoma (BAC). It is the result of lepidic growth, not necrosis, as tumor cells grow along the lung scaffolding sparing the alveoli. Diagnostic considerations for cavitary nodules include pulmonary infarct, fungal infection, Wegner granulomatosis, and solitary metastasis.

Attenuation

Careful analysis of the attenuation of SPNs has revolutionized management. There is a correlation between ground-glass attenuation SPNs and histologic findings of adenocarcinoma [11] (see Fig. 2.3). The ground-glass component represents lepidic growth or mucin production. Aoki et al. showed that increasing solid components within a ground-glass nodule correlated

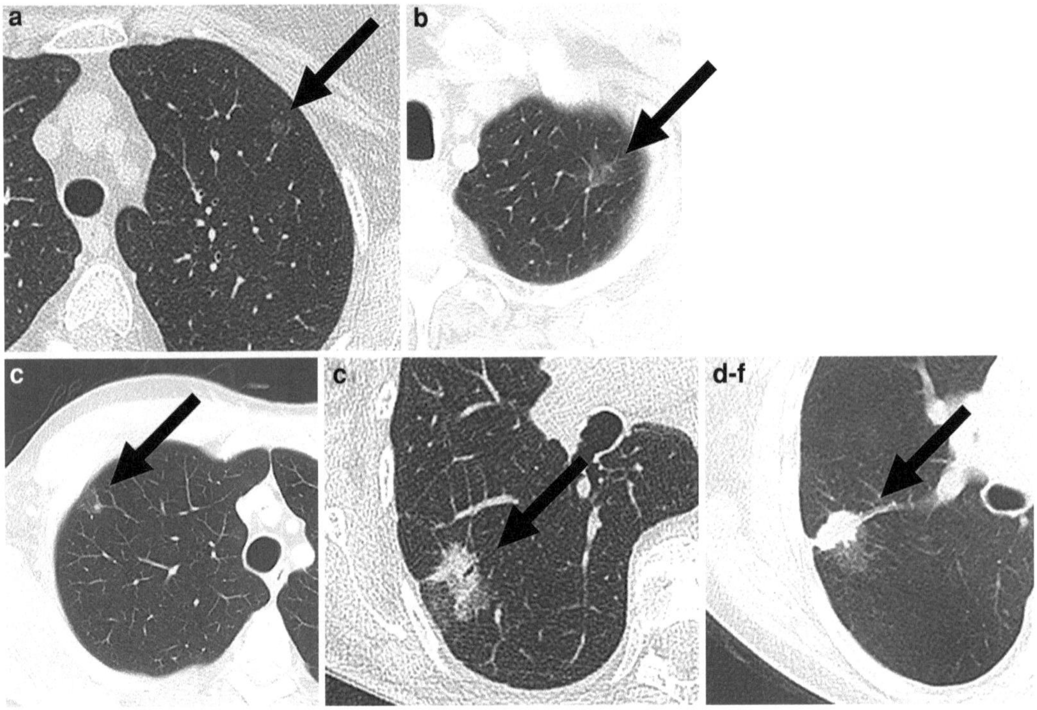

Fig. 2.3 CT appearance of the Noguchi classification of adenocarcinoma of the lung (ground-glass and part-solid nodules). **a** Localized AAH, premalignant. **b** Localized BAC. **c** Likely mixed BAC/ invasive adenocarcinoma. **d-f** Poorly differentiated tubular, papillary adenocarcinoma

with more aggressive behavior [12]. Furthermore, a screening study by Henschke et al. showed a higher rate of malignancy among mixed SPNs (63%) compared with nonsolid (18%) and solid SPNs (7%) [13]. The tumor shadow disappearance rate (TDR) ratio is a measure of the percentage of the SPN that disappears when comparing the size of the nodule on mediastinal versus lung window settings on CT. A correlate of this measurement is the pathologic non-BAC ratio, which measures the percentage of solid component of the mixed attenuation lesion on histologic specimens rather than CT. A study by Lee et al. showed that this pathologic ratio was an independent risk factor for poor prognosis in patients with SPN adenocarcinomas [14]. Differences in the predictive value of the pathologic versus radiologic analysis were likely the result of the ability to subtract out the scar component within the lesion in the ratio calculation on the histologic analysis.

Growth Rates (Volume Doubling Times)

Volume doubling time (DT) is the time required for a nodule to double in volume. For most malignant SPNs, DT is between 30 and 400 days and corresponds to a 26% increase in diameter. DT may be used to stratify nodules into different categories with differing probabilities for malignancy. For example, nodules with a DT less than 20–30 days are usually acute infectious processes. Slow growing nodules with DT greater than 450 days are likely benign. Lack of two-year growth on chest imaging was thought to confirm benignity. However, this

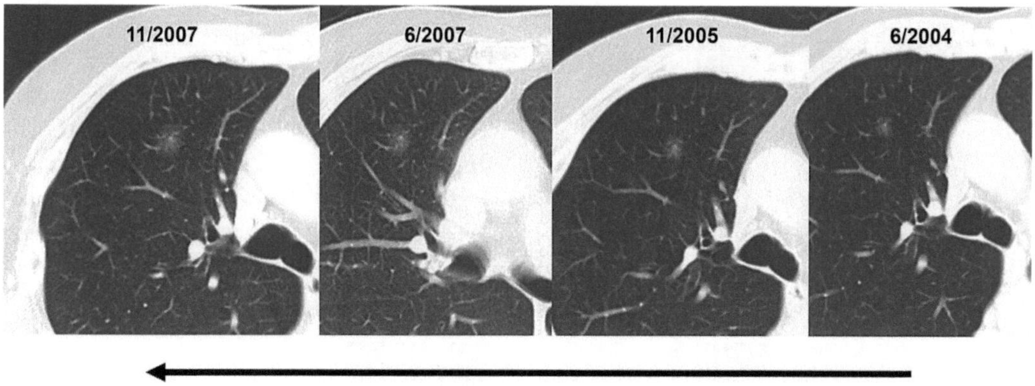

Fig. 2.4 Series of CT images of a right upper lobe ground glass nodule over a period of 3.5 years showed progression in size and density. Subsequent right upper lobe resection confirmed mixed type adenocarcinoma

longstanding dictum on categorization of nodules based on growth measurement has been challenged. Hasegawa et al. [15] reported the DT for malignant SPNs on the basis of their morphologic features: 813 ± 375 days for pure ground-glass opacities, 457 ± 260 days for mixed or partial ground-glass opacities, and 149 ± 125 days for solid nodules. From these data, the two-year stability rule signifying benignity is no longer valid, particularly for pure ground-glass or predominately ground-glass nodules. Appropriate management of these slow growing nodules is an important topic for current investigation.

Preliminary results from a retrospective review of ground-glass attenuation nodules at NYU Langone Medical Center over an 8-year period (2003–2011) showed that 23% of nodules progressed (in size, attenuation, or both) in a median of 14.8 months, with the time to progression as short as 2.8 months and as long as 61.4 months (5 years). Stable ground-glass nodules were followed for a median of 45.8 months (see Fig. 2.4)

Contrast Enhancement

Dynamic contrast-enhanced CT is a tool to assess malignant potential of a SPN. However, this tool is limited to predominately solid nodules for which contrast enhancement can be reliably measured. This technique may be under utilized given lack of screening potential nodules for this protocol and additional time and supervision required at the time of scan acquisition. Quantitative contrast enhancement consist of repeated imaging of the nodule using contiguous thin collimation sections (1–3 mm) following administration of intravenous contrast administration at a rate of 2 mL/sec. Scans are acquired every 30 s for 5 min, and maximum peak enhancement is measured. Enhancement values <15 HU strongly suggest benignity, whereas enhancement values >20 HU usually indicate malignancy (sensitivity 98%, specificity 73%, diagnostic accuracy 85%) [16]. (see Fig. 2.5). Factors that limit reliability of this technique include small nodule size (<8 mm) and necrosis within the nodule that would underestimate enhancement.

Magnetic Resonance Imaging

Similar to contrast-enhanced dynamic CT, MR has been used to measure peak contrast enhancement and assess the enhancement curve slopes for SPNs. Most benign lesions have a low peak enhancement whereas infections show higher enhancement peak, even higher than those for malignant nodules [17]. However, the

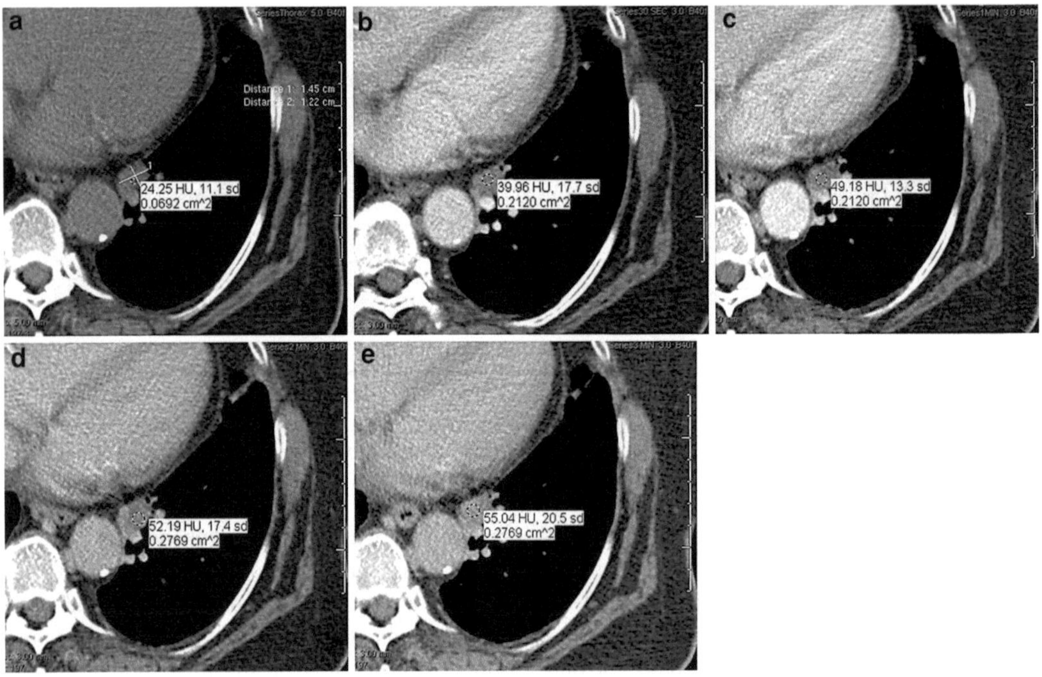

Fig. 2.5 Dynamic contrast enhanced nodule study: sequential CT images through a LLL nodule were obtained precontrast (**a**) then 30 s (**b**), 1 min (**c**), 2 min (**d**), and 3 min (**e**) following the start of intravenous contrast administration. Attenuation measurements of the nodule demonstrate enhancement greater than 15 HU, worrisome for malignancy

lower spatial resolution of MR, somewhat higher cost, lower accessibility, and similar predictive value as dynamic CT contrast-enhanced imaging have made MR less desirable as an assessment tool.

PET-CT Imaging

PET-CT has become commonplace in the assessment of pulmonary nodules that are predominately solid and measure $\geq$ 8 mm. Reported rates for both sensitivity and specificity are $\geq$ 90% [18]. However there are limitations to the use of PET. False-positive results may be encountered with infectious and inflammatory processes such as tuberculosis and fungal infections. Dual phase imaging with the first scan obtained at 1 h after injection and the second scan obtained 2–4 h later may improve specificity since infectious and inflammatory processes show reduced uptake with time whereas malignant lesions continue to accumulate FDG [19]. False-negative results can be seen with bronchioloalveolar carcinoma and carcinoid tumors (see Fig. 2.6). The accepted threshold for standard uptake value (SUV) for malignant nodules is 2.5, although any uptake in a ground-glass or subsolid nodule may suggest malignancy.

Risk Assessment

Calculating the risk of malignancy of an SPN requires not only analysis of nodule size, morphology, location, and growth rate but also defining a patient's underlying risk factors such as age, smoking history, and history of malignancy. A validated model developed by investigators at the Mayo Clinic identified six independent predictors of malignancy in patients with non-calcified nodules measuring between 4 mm and 30 mm

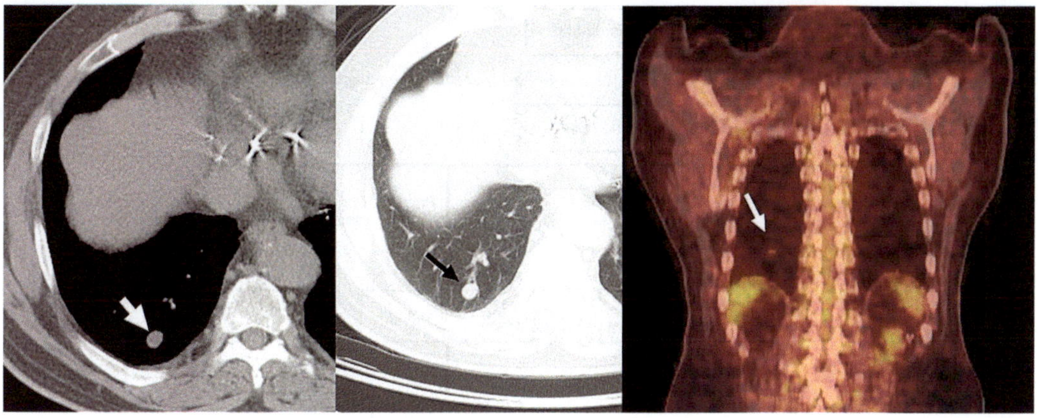

Fig. 2.6 Patient is a 71 year old man with a history of renal cancer treated with surgery and prostate cancer-treated with brachytherapy. Axial CT of the chest demonstrates a round solid 1.2 cm nodule in the right lower lobe posteriorly. There was mild metabolic activity (SUV 1.0) within the nodule, indeterminate. Subsequent right lower lobe resection revealed a carcinoid tumor

in diameter on chest radiography. Independent predictors of malignancy include age, current or past smoking, history of extrathoracic malignancy, nodule diameter, spiculation, and upper lobe location [20]. Although specific models exist for the calculation of the probability of malignancy of an SPN, they are comparable to the accuracy of expert clinicians' assessments [6].

MacMahon et al. stratified patient's risk levels as low and high as follows: for low risk: age less than 35 years, minimal or absent history of smoking, and no other risk factors [21].

Of note, follow-up CT imaging for a pulmonary nodule should be performed without contrast and utilizing low dose technique (approximately 80 mAs) and thin collimation. Although limited longitudinal coverage is advocated by the Fleischner Society, often the entire thorax is imaged due to logistical and medicolegal reasons.

Recommendations (Adopted from Reference [5])

1. Assess pretest probability (patient's age, smoking history, occupational exposures, nodule size, location, and morphology).
2. For SPN visible on a chest radiograph, compare to previous chest radiographs or other relevant imaging.
3. For SPNs that show growth within the expected time growth for malignancy, tissue diagnosis should be obtained unless contraindicated.
4. If a nodule has 2-year stability, except for patients with pure ground-glass nodules on CT, no additional evaluation recommended.
5. SPN with classic benign calcification pattern, no additional diagnostic evaluation recommended.
6. For every indeterminate SPN on chest radiograph, further characterization with chest CT recommended. Compare to prior CTs if available.
7. Small (<8 mm) solid nodule on CT in a patient without a history of malignancy and at least one risk factor for malignancy (follow Fleischner Society Recommendations [21]):
   a. ≤4 mm: 1 year low dose follow-up CT (no follow-up if stable)
   b. >4–6 mm: 6–12 month follow-up low dose CT and again at 18–24 months if stable
   c. >6–8 mm: initial follow-up at 3–6 months, then 9–12 and finally at 24 months if unchanged
8. For a solid SPN at least 8 mm in size, dynamic contrast enhancement technique recommended if patient has normal renal function.

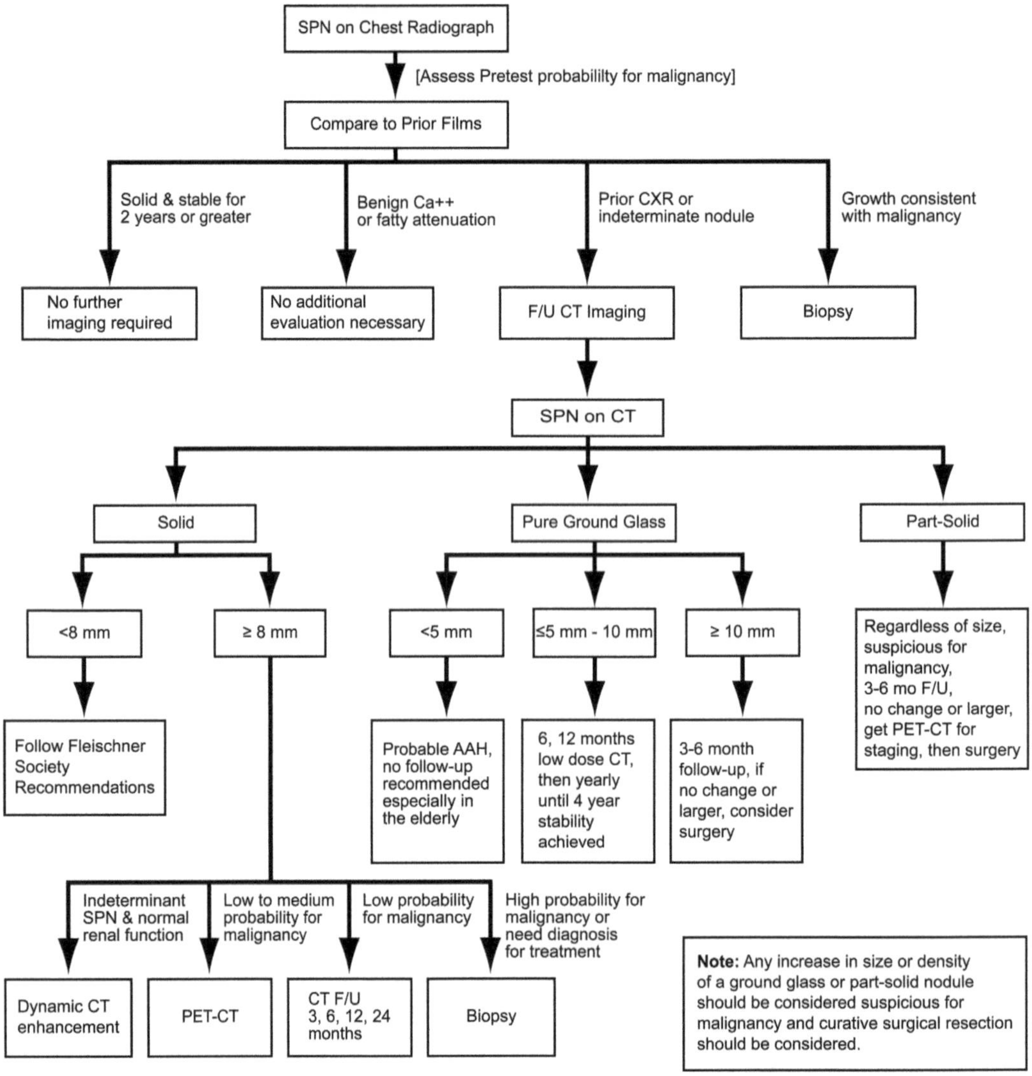

Fig. 2.7 Recommended management algorithm for SPNs

9. For SPN (at least 8 mm in size) with low to moderate pretest probability for malignancy, PET-CT may be helpful given high negative predictive value.
10. Serial (3, 6, 12, and 24 month) follow-up CT imaging may be performed for indeterminate ($\geq$8 mm) SPNs if
    a. Patient is a candidate for curative surgery
    b. Clinical probability of malignancy is low
    c. SPN is not hypermetabolic on PET
    d. SPN peak enhancement is <15 HU
    e. Patient prefers a non-aggressive approach
11. Needle biopsy should be considered when
    a. Discordant clinical pretest probability and imaging findings
    b. Suspected benign diagnosis requires treatment (i.e. tuberculosis or fungal infection)
    c. If proof of a malignant diagnosis required prior to surgery or radiation therapy
12. For ground-glass and part-solid nodules, recommended follow-up based on NYU preliminary research data on ground-glass nodule progression (described above) and published recommendations by Godoy and Naidich [22] (see Fig. 2.7).

References

1. Cardinale L, Ardissone F, Novello S, et al. The pulmonary nodule: clinical and radiological characteristics affecting a diagnosis of malignancy. Radiol Med. 2009;114:871–89.
2. Hansell DM, Bankier AA, MacMahon H, et al. Fleischner Society: Glossary of Terms for Thoracic Imaging. Radiology. 2008;246:697–722.
3. Good CA, Wilson TW. The solitary circumscribed pulmonary nodule: study of seven years. JAMA. 1958;166:210–5.
4. Wahidi MM, Govert JA, Goudar PK, et al. evidence for the treatment of patients with pulmonary nodules: when is it lung cancer? ACCP evidence-based clinical practice guidelines (2nd Edition). Chest. 2007;132:94S–107S.
5. Gould MK, Fletcher J, Iannettoni MD, et al. Evaluation of patients with pulmonary nodules: when is it lung cancer? ACCP evidence-based clinical practice guidelines (2nd Edition) Chest 2007;132:108S–130S.
6. Darrow JC, Lack EE. Solitary lung nodule due to Dirofilariaimmitis (dog 'heartworm'). J Surg Oncol. 1981;132:108S–30S.
7. Henschke CI, Yankelevitz DF, Naidich DP, et al. CT Screening for lung cancer: suspiciousness of nodules according to size on baseline scans. Radiology. 2004;231:164–8.
8. Siegleman SS, Zerhouni EA, Leo FP, et al. CT of the solitary pulmonary nodule. AJR. 1980;135:1–13.
9. Zwirewich CV, Vedal S, Miller RR, et al. Solitary pulmonary nodule: high resolution CT and radiologic-pathologic correlation. Radiology. 1991;17:469–76.
10. Fishman AP. Pulmonary disease and disorders 2nd ed. New York: McGraw-Hill; 1988. p 1947.
11. Mirtcheva RM, Vazquez M, Yankelevitz DF, Henschke CI. Bronchioloalveolar carcinoma and adenocarcinoma with bronchioloalveolar features presenting as ground glass opacities on CT. Clin Imaging. 2002;26(2):95–100.
12. Aoki T, Nakata H, Watanabe H, et al. Evolution of peripheral adenocarcinomas: CT findings correlated with histology and tumor doubling time. AJR. 2000;174:763–8.
13. Henschke CI, Yankelevitz DF, Mirtcheva R, et al. CT screening for lung cancer: frequency and significance of part-solid and nonsolid nodules. AJR. 2002;178:1053–7.
14. Lee HY, Han J, Lee KS, et al. Lung adenocarcinoma as a solitary pulmonary nodule: prognostic determinants of CT, PET and histopathologic findings. Lung Cancer. 2009;66:379–85.
15. Hasegawa M, Sone S, Takashima S, et al. Growth rates of small lung cancers detected on mass CT screening. Br J Radiol. 2000;73:1252–9.
16. Swenson SJ, Brown LR, Colby TV, et al. Lung nodule enhancement at CT: prospective findings. Radiology. 1996;194:399–405.
17. Kono R, Fujimoto K, Terasaki H, et al. Dynamic MRI of solitary pulmonary nodules: comparison of enhancement patterns of malignant and benign small peripheral lung lesions. AJR. 2007;188: 26–36.
18. Herder GJ, Golding RP, Hoekstra OS, et al. The performance of (18) F-Fluorodeoxyglucose positron emission tomography in small solitary pulmonary nodules. Eur J Nucl Med Mol Imaging. 2004;31: 1231–6.
19. Conrad GR, Sinha P. Narrow time-window dual point 18F-FDG PET for the diagnosis of Thoracic malignancy. Nucl Med Comm 2003;24 1129–37.
20. Herder GJ, van Tinteren H, Goldberg RP, et al. Clinical prediction model to characterizepulmonary nodules: validation and added value of 18-F-FDG positron emission tomography. Chest. 2005;128: 2490–6.
21. MacMahon H, Austin JH, Gamsu G. Guidelines for Management of small pulmonary nodules detected on CT scans: a statement from the Fleischner Society. Radiology. 2005;237:395–400.
22. Godoy MC, Naidich DP. Subsolid pulmonary nodules and the spectrum of peripheral adenocarcinomas of the lung: recommended interim guidelines for assessment and management. radiology. 2009;253(3): 606–22.

Lung Cancer

3

Todd R. Hazelton and Frank W. Walsh

Abstract

As the most common type of malignancy, lung cancer is regularly encountered by primary care physicians, pulmonologists, as well as radiologists during their routine practice. Many lung cancers are detected incidentally or when patients present with symptoms related to either local or systemic effects of a tumor. Imaging plays an important role in lung cancer staging through the characterization of the primary tumor, evaluation of nodal disease, and the detection of distant metastases. Imaging guidance can also provide a means for obtaining tissue diagnosis, both for the primary or metastatic lesions.

Keywords

Lung cancer · Computed tomography · CT · FDG-PET · PET/CT · Staging · Screening

Introduction

Primary care physicians, pulmonologists, and radiologists routinely encounter lung cancer in their daily practice. For the year 2010, the American Cancer Society estimated about 222,520 new cases of lung cancer with 53% occurring in males and 47% in females. Lung cancer accounts for around 28% of all cancer deaths—more than colon, breast, and prostate cancers combined. The majority of lung cancer cases occur in older people, with less than 3% of all cases found in individuals less than 45 years of age [1]. The higher risk for developing lung cancer in smokers is well established.

T. R. Hazelton (✉)
Department of Radiology, University of South Florida College of Medicine, 2 Tampa General Circle, STC 6072, Tampa, FL 33606-3571, USA
e-mail: thazelto@health.usf.edu

F. W. Walsh
Department of Internal Medicine,
Division of Pulmonary/Critical Care Medicine,
USF College of Medicine, 12902 Magnolia Drive, Tampa, FL 33612, USA

F. W. Walsh
Moffitt Cancer Center, Tampa, FL, USA

J. P. Kanne (ed.), *Clinically Oriented Pulmonary Imaging*,
Respiratory Medicine, DOI: 10.1007/978-1-61779-542-8_3,

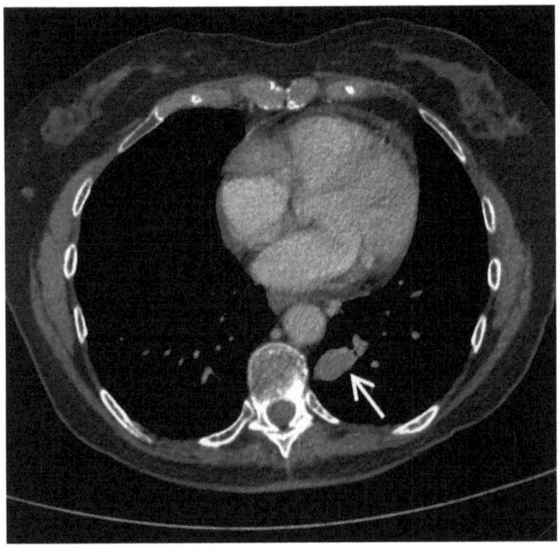

Fig. 3.1 Axial 2-minute delayed post-contrast CT image through an incidentally detected pulmonary nodule (*arrow*). The nodule showed an enhancement difference of 61 Hounsfield units compared to non-contrast imaging and was confirmed to be typical carcinoid after left lower lobectomy

Imaging Diagnosis of Lung Cancer

Since many lung cancers are detected incidentally or when patients present with symptoms related to either local or systemic effects of a tumor, chest radiography is often the initial diagnostic imaging test. Once the moderately to highly suspicious nodule (<3 cm in diameter) or mass (>3 cm in diameter) is detected on chest radiography, the potential lung cancer is most appropriately worked up using non-contrast computed tomography (CT) of the chest [2]. Because CT allows for easier identification of hilar and mediastinal lymph nodes and distinguishing vascular structures from tumors, some physicians prefer performing chest CT with intravenous contrast to work up a suspected lung cancer (Fig. 3.1). If the results of thoracic CT are not compatible with a benign lesion, the patient can then be assessed with whole body fluorine-18-2-fluoro-2-deoxy-D-glucose positron emission tomography (FDG-PET) to evaluate for increased glucose metabolism in the suspected primary lesion and to detect increased glucose metabolism in possible metastases. The semiquantitative standard uptake value (SUV) is commonly used to determine the malignant potential of a lesion on PET. An SUV threshold of 2.5 has been used to distinguish benign from malignant lesions [3]. This value is calculated as a ratio of tissue radiotracer concentration (mCi/mL) and injected dose (mCi) at the time of injection divided by the patient's body weight (in grams). Since biological factors (patient glucose level, uptake time of the tracer, and respiratory motion) as well as technical factors (scanner variability, image acquisition, and reconstruction variability) can affect the SUV measurements, care should be taken to keep these factors as similar as possible between the initial study and any follow-up study [4, 5].

Ultimately, in suspected lung cancer, histologic diagnosis is required to confirm the presence of neoplasm and guide treatment planning. Patients with a low surgical risk and high probability of cancer can proceed directly to video-assisted thoracoscopic surgery with evaluation of a frozen section from the lesion, followed by resection if the nodule is found to be malignant [6]. For intermediate probability lung lesions that show contrast enhancement on CT or are positive on FDG-PET imaging, transthoracic needle biopsy can be performed to establish a diagnosis of malignancy [2]. Central lung lesions may be more appropriately biopsied at bronchoscopy, although CT-guided biopsy of central lesions can be safely performed if the biopsy results from bronchoscopy are inconclusive. For staging purposes, a suspected metastatic lesion should be biopsied whenever possible to establish its lung origin through histopathologic analysis and immunohistochemical stains. Biopsy from a suspected metastasis provides both diagnostic and staging information important in the choice of appropriate therapy for the patient with lung cancer [7]. In these patients, estimation of the probability of malignancy ultimately guides the clinician with regard to the performance of specific imaging tests to better characterize the lesion and evaluate for possible metastases. This information, in conjunction with various treatment risks and alternatives, as well as patient preferences, will guide the patient's diagnostic and therapeutic management [6].

Lung Cancer Screening

Despite causing more deaths each year than colon, breast, and prostate cancers combined, there are presently no professional or governmental organization guidelines that recommend routine screening for lung cancer [8]. The lack of a recommendation is based on insufficient evidence that screening high-risk populations alters mortality outcomes. Although patients who are diagnosed with localized, early stage lung cancer can undergo potentially curative surgical resection, randomized, controlled trials done during the 1970s and 1980s using chest radiography did not validate this principle [9–18]. In these studies, screening did detect more early stage cancers that were surgically resected; however, the intervention and control arms of these studies ultimately showed no statistically significant difference between the number of advanced cancer diagnoses and the number of deaths from lung cancer [19]. Given its ability to detect small lung cancers at a potentially curable stage, in the late 1990s and 2000s there was great interest in utilizing low-dose helical CT as a screening tool in high-risk populations (Fig. 3.2). Despite its promise for detecting early stage cancers as demonstrated by several single arm cohort trials, this technique remained largely unproven, with insufficient evidence to support its use to screen those at high risk for lung cancer [20–22]. In November 2010, the National Cancer Institute (NCI) released the initial results of the National Lung Screening Trial (NLST), a randomized national trial involving more than 53,000 current and former heavy smokers ages 55–74. This study compared the effects of two screening procedures for lung cancer—low-dose helical CT screening and chest radiographic screening. The initial results demonstrated a lung cancer mortality reduction of 20.3% in trial participants who were screened with low-dose helical CT [23, 24]. While the ultimate role of helical CT for lung cancer screening remains to be defined, the results of the NLST represent a significant breakthrough for early cancer detection and potential survival benefit in current and former smokers [25].

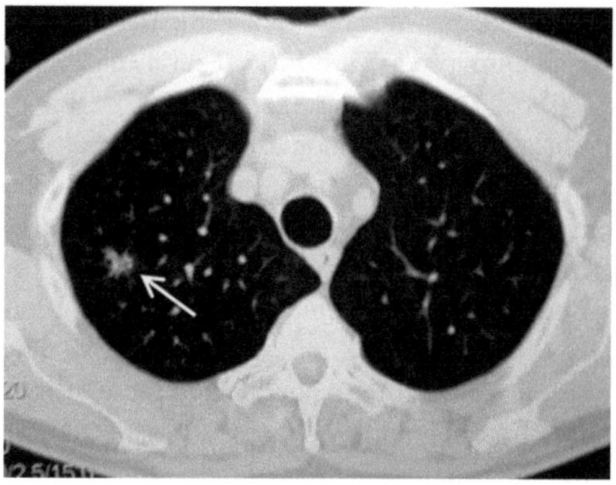

Fig. 3.2 Axial CT image of a stage Ia screening detected right upper lobe NSCLC (*arrow*) in an asymptomatic former smoker

Pathologic Classification of Lung Cancers

Lung carcinomas represent 99% of all lung neoplasms. For treatment purposes, lung carcinomas are divided into non-small-cell lung carcinomas (NSCLC) and small-cell lung carcinomas (SCLC). Histopathologically, a NSCLC is any epithelial tumor that lacks a small cell component. NSCLCs are subdivided histologically into adenocarcinomas, squamous cell carcinomas, and large cell carcinomas [26]. Adenocarcinoma is the most common histologic type of lung cancer. These tumors most commonly occur as a peripheral nodule. Cavitation is rarely observed. Occasionally, adenocarcinomas present centrally as an endobronchial tumor [26, 27]. The term bronchioloalveolar cell carcinoma (BAC) is no longer used pathologically to describe a subtype of adenocarcinoma with the introduction of the concepts of adenocarcinoma in situ (AIS) for lesions with pure lepidic growth and minimally invasive adenocarcinoma (MIA) for lesions that exhibit lepidic growth with ≤5 mm invasion [28]. Rarely, adenocarcinoma produces diffuse pleural thickening which can mimic mesothelioma [29]. Radiographically, adenocarcinomas range in appearance from ground-glass to solid opacities, with the solid component of these lesions portending a greater likelihood of invasive growth [30–32].

Squamous cell carcinoma of the lung typically occurs centrally, although up to 25% may be seen peripherally. Around 5% of these lesions demonstrate cavitation. Neuroendocrine tumors of the lung include the low-grade typical carcinoid lesions, intermediate-grade atypical carcinoids, high-grade large cell neuroendocrine carcinomas, and highly malignant SCLC. Both typical and atypical carcinoid tumors occur predominantly as endobronchial tumors that can be located centrally or peripherally [26, 33, 34].

Imaging and Lung Cancer Staging

Pre-treatment tumor staging in patients with lung carcinoma is important to distinguish patients who would benefit from potentially curative surgical resection or definitive radiation therapy from those with more advanced disease more appropriately treated with palliative therapies. The widely used TNM staging system originally proposed by Dr. Clifton Mountain and adopted by the Union Internationale Contre le Cancer (UICC) in 1973 and American Joint Committee on Cancer (AJCC) in 1974 has had multiple revisions over the ensuing decades. The most recent changes to the TNM staging system (Table 3.1) published in 2009 were made to better distinguish among tumors of different prognoses [35, 36]. In addition to classifying NSCLC, the new staging system is also used to classify both SCLC and bronchopulmonary carcinoid tumors. The TNM staging system is based on the anatomic extent of disease. In this system, the T descriptor defines the extent of the primary tumor, the N descriptor the extent of involvement of regional nodal disease based on location, and the M descriptor indicates the presence or absence of distant site metastatic disease [37–39].

Imaging Evaluation of the Primary Tumor

Factors important in the T designation for the TNM staging evaluation of the primary tumor include the anatomic location and size of the tumor as well as whether or not there is chest wall, mediastinal, or vertebral invasion. Also important is the presence or absence of satellite nodules. For the staging evaluation of lung cancer, anatomic imaging with CT is the most common examination used. The role of magnetic resonance imaging (MRI) is predominantly one of problem solving for specific cases. The role of FDG-PET in the imaging evaluation of the primary tumor is limited. Standardized measurement techniques for tumor size include the one-dimensional response evaluation criteria in solid tumors (RECIST) and the bi-dimensional World Health Organization (WHO) criteria. With the RECIST technique, tumor size is reported as a single measurement of the longest diameter of the lesion in the axial plane. To report tumor size using the WHO technique, both the longest diameter of the lesion and the greatest perpendicular diameter are obtained [40].

CT has shown disparate results in assessing chest wall invasion by tumor, with reported sensitivities ranging from 38 to 87% and specificities ranging from 40 to 90%. The most reliable indicator of primary tumor involvement of the chest wall is definite bone destruction with or without mass extending into the chest wall (Fig. 3.3) [41–47]. With regard to chest wall invasion, MRI demonstrates disruption of normal extrapleural fat by intermediate signal mass on T1-weighted images and high signal mass on T2-weighted images, although inflammatory changes can cause a false-positive appearance [48, 49]. Intravenously administered gadolinium chelates can be used to define the extent of a mass on T1-weighted MR images, usually with fat-suppression techniques applied. While thin-section multiplanar helical CT reconstructions now afford better evaluation of the vertical extent of apical tumors, MRI can be

Table 3.1 Lung cancer TNM definitions (adapted from [36])

T0	• No primary tumor
T1	• < 3 cm, surrounded by lung or visceral pleura, not more proximal than lobar bronchus
T2	• T2a if > 3–5 cm, T2b if 5–7 cm or • Invades visceral pleura, main bronchus ≥ 2 cm distal to carina or • Invades main bronchus ≥ 2 cm distal to carina, atelectasis/obstructive pneumonia extending to hilum but not entire lung
T3	• > 7 cm or • Invading chest wall, diaphragm, phrenic nerve, mediastinal pleura, parietal pericardium or • In main bronchus < 2 cm distal to carina or • Atelectasis/obstructive pneumonia of entire lung or • Separate tumor nodules in same lung lobe
T4	• Any size tumor with invasion of heart, great vessels, trachea, recurrent laryngeal nerve, esophagus, vertebral body, or carina or • Separate tumor nodules in ipsilateral different lung lobe
N0	• No regional lymph node metastases
N1	• Ipsilateral peribronchial and/or perihilar, intrapulmonary nodes
N2	• Ipsilateral mediastinal and/or subcarinal nodes
N3	• Contralateral mediastinal, contralateral hilar, ipsilateral or contralateral scalene or supraclavicular nodes
M0	• No distant metastases
M1a	• Pleural or pericardial metastases or • Separate tumor nodules in contralateral lung lobe
M1b	• Distant metastases

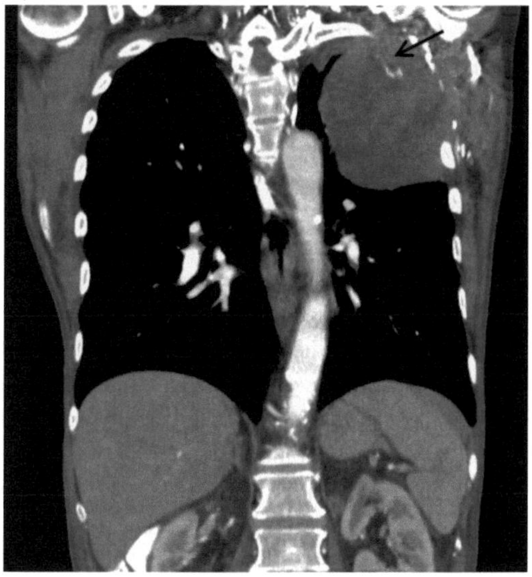

Fig. 3.3 Coronal CT image shows large left upper lobe NSCLC with rib destruction (*arrow*) indicative of definite chest wall invasion (T3)

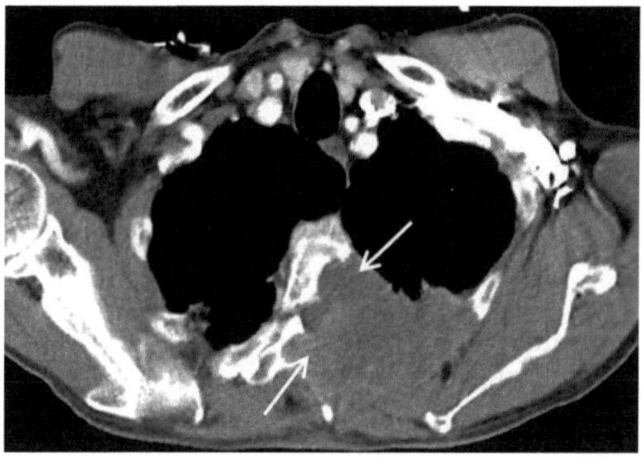

Fig. 3.4 Left upper lobe NSCLC with direct vertebral invasion (*arrows*) consistent with a T4 lesion

useful in defining chest wall invasion, encasement of the subclavian artery, and involvement of brachial plexus for superior sulcus tumors [50–54]. While tumors with minimal involvement of mediastinal fat may be considered resectable, tumor invasion of mediastinal vessels, trachea, esophagus, or vertebral body precludes surgical resection (Fig. 3.4) (T4 disease). Both CT and MRI have comparable sensitivities for detecting mediastinal involvement of the primary tumor (55% and 66%, respectively) [55]. CT criteria for resectability of a lesion that abuts the mediastinum include fewer than 3 cm of contact with the mediastinum,

Table 3.2 IASLC lymph node zones (adapted from [57])

Stations	Zones
	Supraclavicular zone
1	Low cervical, supraclavicular, and sternal notch nodes
	Upper zone (superior mediastinal nodes)
2R	Upper paratracheal (right)
2L	Lower paratracheal (left)
3a	Prevascular
3p	Retrotracheal
4R	Upper paratracheal (right)
4L	Lower paratracheal (left)
	AP zone (aortic nodes)
5	Subaortic
6	Para-aortic (ascending aorta or phrenic)
	Subcarinal zone (inferior mediastinal nodes)
7	Subcarinal
	Lower zone (inferior mediastinal nodes)
8	Paraesophageal (below carina)
9	Pulmonary ligament
	Hilar/interlobar zone (N1 nodes)
10	Hilar
11	Interlobar
	Peripheral zone (N1 nodes)
12	Lobar
13	Segmental
14	Subsegmental

fewer than 90 degrees of contact with the aorta, and a visible fat plane between the mass and adjacent mediastinal structures [56].

FDG-PET can be used to distinguish the primary mass from adjacent lung, aiding in radiation therapy planning. The use of CT and PET together has shown to be superior for T staging than either modality alone [57].

Imaging Evaluation of Nodal Disease

The nodal (N) designation in the TNM staging system is determined by the presence or absence of thoracic metastatic lymph nodes. The N classifier for nodal disease is assigned based on lymph node location in different stations defined by the relationship to adjacent anatomic structures. The IASLC International Staging Committee has adopted a new map of nodal zones and contains several traditional nodal stations (Table 3.2) [58]. For staging purposes, lymph node involvement by metastatic disease is classified as N1, N2, or N3 based on the location of the lymph nodes relative to the primary tumor (Fig. 3.5). The absence of nodal disease is designated as N0. Tumor in the ipsilateral intrapulmonary lymph nodes, peribronchial lymph nodes, or hilar lymph nodes is designated as N1. The N2

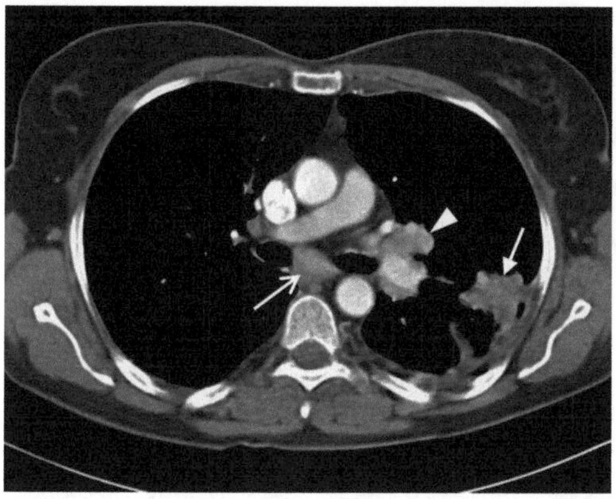

Fig. 3.5 Axial post-contrast CT image of a patient with left lung NSCLC (*closed arrow*) shows enlarged N1 interlobar zone hilar (*arrowhead*) and N2 AP zone and subcarinal zone (*open arrow*) lymph nodes

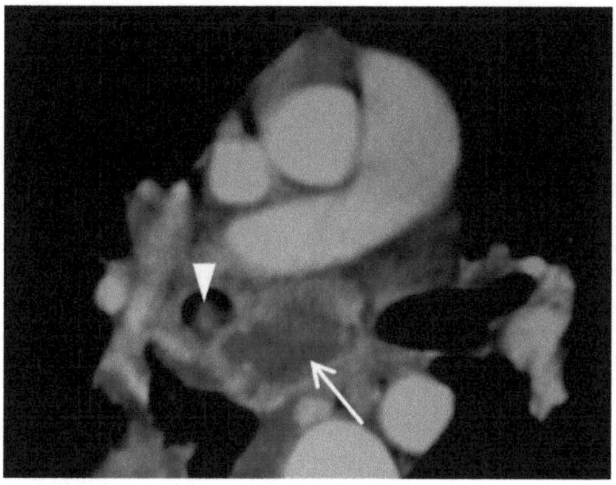

Fig. 3.6 Axial post-contrast CT image of the mediastinum shows necrotic subcarinal zone N2 nodal disease (*arrow*) in a patient with endobronchial squamous cell carcinoma (*arrowhead*)

designation refers to lymph node metastases in the ipsilateral mediastinum and subcarinal lymph node zones. N3 nodal disease refers to more distant nodal disease in the scalene and supraclavicular lymph node zones as well as lymph node metastases in the contralateral hilum or mediastinum [38, 39].

CT Criteria for Detection of Nodal Metastases

While the presence of central low attenuation in a lymph node can suggest necrosis in a malignant lymph node (Fig. 3.6) and the presence of a fatty hilum confers benignity (Fig. 3.7), the most reliable method for anatomic assessment for pathologic lymph node enlargement is based on size thresholds. The greatest short axis diameter of a lymph node is the most accurate predictor of nodal size in axial CT images [59, 60]. The consensus size threshold for pathologic lymph node enlargement is 1 cm in greatest short axis diameter [59–72]. Potential pitfalls encountered when using size threshold alone to distinguish benign from malignant lymph nodes include enlarged benign lymph nodes caused by reactive hyperplasia, anthracosis, inflammation, or infection. In addition, microscopic metastatic disease may be present in normal-sized lymph nodes. CT for hilar nodal metastases has a low sensitivity (45–63%), low positive predictive value (38–68%), and a relatively high negative predictive value (79–85%) [73]. Regarding CT for mediastinal lymph node detection, a meta-analysis of pooled data for NSCLC from 1980–1988 demonstrated approximately 80% sensitivity, specificity, and accuracy [74].

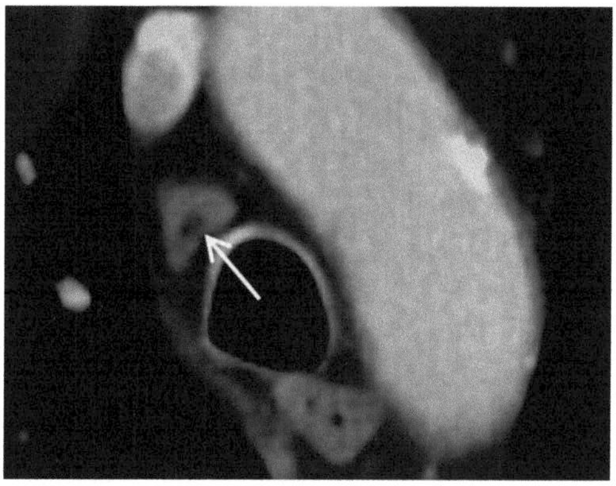

Fig. 3.7 Axial CT image of the mediastinum demonstrates a benign superior zone right lower paratracheal lymph node with a fatty hilum (*arrow*)

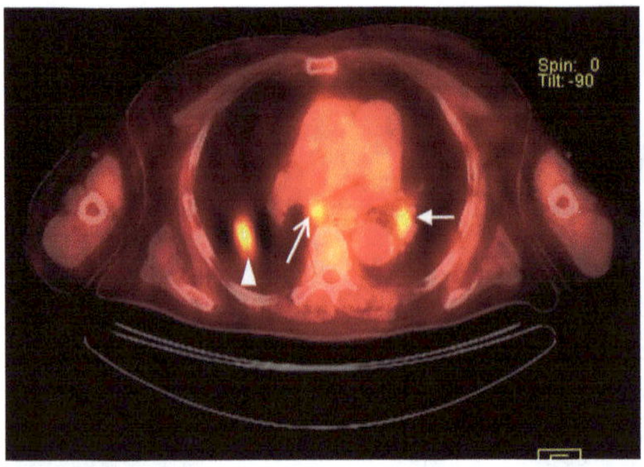

Fig. 3.8 Axial PET/CT fusion image shows FDG-avid right lower lobe NSCLC (*arrowhead*), N2 subcarinal zone lymph node (*open arrow*), and contralateral N3 interlobar zone left hilar lymph node (*closed arrow*)

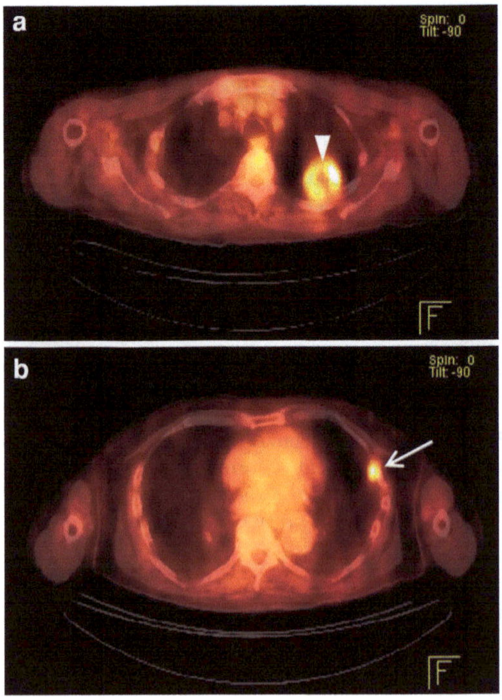

Fig. 3.9 **a**, **b** Axial PET/CT fusion images show FDG-avid left upper lobe NSCLC (*arrowhead*) and M1a pleural metastatic disease (*arrow*)

Role of FDG-PET for Detection of Nodal Metastases

Compared to the CT size threshold for lymph node enlargement of greater than 1 cm in short axis diameter, FDG-PET is superior to CT for nodal staging with reported sensitivity of 79% compared to 62% and specificity of 91% compared to 73% [75]. FDG-PET is more specific than CT for identifying tumor in normal sized lymph nodes and in distinguishing enlarged benign lymph nodes from nodal metastases (Fig. 3.8) [76]. False positives encountered with FDG-PET include follicular hyperplasia, inflammation, epithelioid granulomas, pneumoconiosis, anthracosis, and reactive lymph nodes with obstructive pneumonitis. Given the potential for false-positive results, the American Society of Clinical Oncology (ASCO) recommends mediastinal lymph node biopsy for a lymph node greater than 1 cm in short axis diameter on CT or a lymph node that is positive on FDG-PET [77]. The high negative predictive value of FDG-PET can obviate the need for more invasive tissue sampling for lymph nodes less than 15 mm in size on CT [78, 79]. The use of integrated PET and CT has been shown to improve staging accuracy compared to CT and PET interpreted separately [80].

Imaging Evaluation of Metastatic Disease

Since most lung cancers are advanced at the time of diagnosis, distant metastases have been reported to occur in up to 21% of patients with NSCLC. Common sites of metastatic disease are the adrenal glands, liver, brain, skeleton, and abdominal lymph nodes [81]. In the new staging system, metastases are classified as M1a if pleural or pericardial in location or if a separate tumor is present in a contralateral lobe (Fig. 3.9). The classification of M1b is used for distant disease. On CT, pleural disease is suggested by soft tissue nodularity and fissural thickening, although these classic findings are not always present [82]. FDG-PET is superior to CT in confirming a malignant effusion, with reported sensitivities in the 89–95% range. With regard to distant metastatic disease, whole body PET has the ability to stage both intrathoracic and extrathoracic disease in a single study. FDG-PET detects metastases in the liver, adrenal glands, and extrathoracic lymph nodes with greater sensitivity and specificity than CT [83]. Occult metastatic disease can be detected in up to 24% of patients selected for curative surgery and alters management in up to 40% of patients [75, 84, 85]. Since false positives can occur, histopathologic diagnosis should be obtained for suspected metastatic lesions that would alter patient management.

References

1. American Cancer Society. What are the key statistics about lung cancer? 2000. http://www.cancer.org/Cancer/LungCancer-Non-SmallCell/DetailedGuide/non-small-cell-lung-cancer-key-statistics. Accessed 6 June 2011.
2. American College of Radiology Appropriateness Criteria. Clinical condition: solitary pulmonary nodule. 2011. http://acsearch.acr.org/TopicList.aspx?topic_all=&topic_any='%22lung+cancer*%22'&connector=+And+&cid=0. Accessed 6 June 2011.
3. Lowe VJ, Hoffman JM, DeLong DM, et al. Semiquantitative and visual analysis of FDG-PET images in pulmonary abnormalities. J Nucl Med. 1994;35:1771–6.
4. Turkington TG, Adams MC, Wilson JM, Wong TZ. A systematic review of factors affecting accuracy of SUV measurements. Am J Roentgenol. 2010;195: 310–20.
5. Troung MT, Viswanathan C, Erasmus JJ. Positron emission tomography/computed tomography in lung cancer staging, prognosis, and assessment of therapeutic response. J Thorac Imaging. 2011;26: 132–46.
6. Gould MK, Fletcher J, Iannettoni MD, et al. Evaluation of patients with pulmonary nodules: when is it lung cancer? ACCP evidence-based clinical practice guidelines (2nd ed.). Chest. 2007; 132:108S–130S. http://chestjournal.chestpubs.org/content/132/3_suppl/108S.full. Accessed 6 June 2011.
7. Rivera MP, Mehta AC. Initial diagnosis of lung cancer: ACCP evidence-based clinical practice guidelines (2nd ed.). Chest. 2007;132:131S–148S. http://chestjournal.chestpubs.org/content/132/3_suppl/131S.full. Accessed June 6 2011.
8. American Cancer Society Guidelines for the early detection of cancer. http://www.cancer.org/Healthy/FindCancerEarly/CancerScreeningGuidelines/american-cancer-society-guidelines-for-the-early-detection-of-cancer. Accessed 6 June 2011.
9. Fontana R, Sanderson DR, Woolner LB, et al. Lung cancer screening: the Mayo program. J Occup Med. 1986;28:746–50.
10. Fontana RS, Sanderson DR, Taylor WF, et al. Early lung cancer detection: results of the initial (prevalence) radiologic and cytologic screening in the Mayo Clinic study. Am Rev Respir Dis. 1984;130:561–5.
11. Fontana RS, Sanderson DR, Woolner LB, et al. Screening for lung cancer: a critique of the Mayo Lung Project. Cancer. 1991;67:1155S–64S.
12. Marcus PM, Bergstralh EJ, Fagerstrom RM, et al. Lung cancer mortality in the Mayo lung project: impact of extended follow-up. J Natl Cancer Inst. 2000;92:1308–16.
13. Berlin N. Overview of the NCI cooperative early lung cancer detection program. Cancer. 2000;89: 2349S–51S.
14. Kubik A, Polak J. Lung cancer detection: results of a randomized prospective study in Czechoslovakia. Cancer. 1986;57:2427–37.
15. Kubik AK, Parkin DM, Zatloukal P. Czech Study on Lung cancer screening: post-trial follow-up of lung cancer deaths up to year 15 since enrollment. Cancer. 2000;89:2363S–8S.
16. Frost J, Ball WC, Levin M, et al. Early lung cancer detection: results of the initial (prevalence) radiologic and cytologic screening in the Johns Hopkins study. Am Rev Respir Dis. 1984;130:549–54.
17. Tockman MS. Survival and mortality from lung cancer in a screened population: the Johns Hopkins study. Chest. 1986;89:324S–5S.
18. Melamed MR. Lung cancer screening results in the National Cancer Institute New York study. Cancer. 2000;89:2356S–62S.
19. Bach PB, Silvestri GA, Hanger M, Jett JR. Screening for lung cancer: AACP evidence-based clinical practice guidelines (2nd ed.). Chest 2007;132:69S–77S. http://chestjournal.chestpubs.org/content/132/3_suppl/69S.long. Accessed 6 June 2011.
20. Henschke CI, Yankelevitz DF, Libby DM, et al. International early lung cancer action program investigators. survival of patients with stage I lung cancer detected on CT screening. N Engl J Med. 2006;355:1763–71.
21. Bach PB, Jett JR, Pastorino U, et al. Computed tomography screening and lung cancer outcomes. JAMA. 2007;297:953–61.
22. Swenson S, Aberle D, Kazerooni EA, et al. Consensus statement: CT screening for lung cancer. J Thorac Imaging. 2005;20:321.
23. National Cancer Institute. Lung cancer trial results show mortality benefit with low-dose CT: twenty percent fewer lung cancer deaths seen among those who were screened with low-dose spiral CT than with chest X-ray. http://www.cancer.gov/newscenter/pressreleases/2010/NLSTresultsRelease. Accessed 6 June 2011.
24. The National Lung Screening Trial Research Team. Reduced lung-cancer mortality with low-dose

computed tomographic screening. N Engl J Med. 2011;365:395–409.
25. White CS. National lung cancer screening trial: a breakthrough in lung cancer screening? J Thorac Imaging. 2011;26:86–7.
26. Beasley MB, Brambilla E, Travis WD. The 2004 World Health Organization classification of lung tumors. SeminRoentgenol. 2005;40:90–7.
27. Kodama T, Shimosato Y, Koide T, et al. Endobronchial polypoid adenocarcinoma of the lung: histopathological and ultrastructural studies of five cases. Am J Surg Pathol. 1984;8:845–54.
28. Travis WD, Brambilla E, Noguchi M, et al. International association for the study of lung cancer/ american thoracic society/european respiratory society international multidisciplinary classification of lung adenocarcinoma. J Thoracic Oncol. 2011;6:244–85.
29. Koss M, Travis W, Muran C, et al. Pseudo-mesotheliomatous adenocarcinoma: a reappraisal. Semin Diagn Pathol. 1992;9:117–23.
30. Kondo T, Yamada K, Noda K, et al. Radiologic-prognostic correlation in patients with small pulmonary adenocarcinomas. Lung Cancer. 2002;36: 49–57.
31. Takashima S, Maruyama Y, Hasegawa M, et al. CT findings in small peripheral adenocarcinoma of the lung: a retrospective study on 64 patients. Lung Cancer. 2002;36:289–95.
32. Nagao M, Murase K, Yasuhara Y, et al. Measurement of localized ground glass attenuation on thin-section computed tomography: correlation with progression of bronchioloalveolar cell carcinoma of the lung. Invest Radiol. 2002;37:692–7.
33. Colby T, Koss M, Travis WD. Tumors of the lower respiratory tract. 3rd ed. Washington: Armed Forces Institute of Pathology; 1995.
34. Soga J, Yakuwa Y. Bronchopulmonary carcinoids: an analysis of 1, 875 reported cases with special reference to a comparison between typical carcinoids and atypical varieties. Ann Thorac Cardiovasc Surg. 1999;5:211–9.
35. Union Internationale Contre le Cancer. TNM classification of malignant tumors. 7th ed. New York: Wiley-Blackwell; 2009.
36. Rami-Porta R, Crowley JJ, Goldstraw P. The revised TNM staging system for lung cancer. Ann Thorac Cardiovasc Surg. 2009;15:4–9.
37. Detterbeck FC, Boffa DJ, Tanoue LT. The new lung cancer staging system. Chest. 2009;136:260–71.
38. Kligerman S, Abbott G. A radiologic review of the new TNM classification for lung cancer. Am J Roentgenol. 2010;194:562–73.
39. Greaves SM, Brown K, Garon EB, Garon BL. The new staging system for lung cancer imaging and clinical implications. J Thorac Imaging. 2011;26:119–31.
40. Suzuki C, Jacobsson H, Hatschek T, et al. Radiologic measurements of tumor response to treatment: practical approaches and limitations. Radiographics. 2008;329–344.
41. Gdeedo A, VanSchil P, Corthouts B, VanMieghem F, VanMeerbeeck J, VanMarck E. Comparison of imaging TNM [(i)TNM] and pathological TNM [pTNM] in staging of bronchogenic carcinoma. Eur J Cardiothorac Surg. 1997;12:224–7.
42. Glazer H, Duncan-Meyer J, Aronberg D. Pleural and chest wall invasion in bronchogenic carcinoma: CT evaluation. Radiology. 1985;157:191–4.
43. Pennes D, Glazer G, Wimbish K, Gross B, Long R, Orringer M. Chest wall invasion by lung cancer: limitations of CT evaluation. Am J Roentgenol. 1985;144:507–11.
44. Ratto G, Piacenza G, Frola C. Chest wall involvement by lung cancer: computed tomographic detection and results of operation. Ann Thorac Surg. 1991;51:182–8.
45. Venuta F, Rendina E, Ciriaco P. Computed tomography for preoperative assessment of T3 and T4 bronchogenic carcinoma. Eur J Cardiothorac Surg. 1992;6:238–41.
46. Rendina E, Bognolo D, Mineo T. Computed tomography for the evaluation of intrathoracic invasion by lung cancer. J Thorac Cardiovasc Surg. 1987;94:57–63.
47. Pearlberg JL, Sandler MA, Beute GH, Lewis JW Jr, Madrazo BL. Limitations of CT in evaluation of neoplasms involving chest wall. J Comput Assist Tomogr. 1987;11:290–3.
48. Gefter W. Magnetic resonance imaging in the evaluation of lung cancer. Semin RoentgenoI. 1990; 25:73–84.
49. Webb W, Sostman H. MR imaging of thoracic disease: clinical uses. Radiology. 1992;182:621–30.
50. Castagno A, Shuman W. MR imaging in clinically suspected brachial plexus tumor. Am J Roentgenol. 1987;149:1219–22.
51. Takasugi J, Rapoport S, Shaw C. Superior sulcus tumors: the role of imaging. J Thorac Imaging. 1989;4:41–8.
52. Rapoport S, Blair D, McCarthy S, et al. Brachial plexus: correlation of MR imaging with CT and pathologic findings. Radiology. 1988;167:161–5.
53. Blair D, Rapoport S, Sostman H. Normal brachial plexus: MR imaging. Radiology. 1987;165:763–7.
54. Freundlich I, Chasen M, Dalla G. Magnetic resonance imaging of pulmonary apical tumors. J Thorac Imaging. 1996;11:210–22.
55. Martini N, Heelan R, Westcott J. Comparative merits of conventional, computed tomographic, and magnetic resonance imaging in assessing mediastinal involvement in surgically confirmed lung carcinoma. J Thorac Cardiovasc Surg. 1985;90:639–48.
56. Glazer H, Duncan-Meyer J, Aronberg D. Pleural and chest wall invasion in bronchogenic carcinoma: CT evaluation. Radiology. 1985;157:191–4.
57. De Wever W, Stroobants S, Coolen J, et al. Integrated PET/CT in the staging of nonsmall cell lung cancer: technical aspects and clinical integration. Eur Respir J. 2009;33:201–12.

58. Rusch VW, Asamura H, Watanabe H, et al. The IASLC lung cancer staging project: a proposal for a new international lymph node map in the forthcoming seventh edition of the TNM classification for lung cancer. J Thorac Oncol. 2009;4:568–577.
59. Glazer G, Gross B, Quint L, et al. Normal mediastinal lymph nodes: number and size according to American thoracic society mapping. Am J Roentgenol. 1985;144:261–5.
60. Quint L, Glazer G, Orringer M, et al. Mediastinal lymph node detection and sizing at CT and autopsy. Am J Roentgenol. 1986;147:469–72.
61. Genereux G, Howie J. Normal mediastinal lymph node size and number: CT and anatomic study. Am J Roentgenol. 1984;142:1095–100.
62. Schnyder P, Gamsu G. CT of the pretracheal retrocaval space. Am J Roentgenol. 1981;136:303–8.
63. Kiyono K, Sone S, Sakai F. The number and size of normal mediastinal lymph nodes: a postmortem study. Am J Roentgenol. 1988;150:771–6.
64. Glazer G, Orringer M, Gross B, Quint L. The mediastinum in non-small cell lung cancer: CT-surgical correlation. Am J Roentgenol. 1984;142: 1101–5.
65. Platt J, Glazer G, Gross B, Quint L, Francis I, Orringer M. CT evaluation of mediastinal lymph nodes in lung cancer: influence of the lobar site of the primary neoplasm. Am J Roentgenol. 1987;149: 683–6.
66. Faling L, Pugatch R, Jung-Legg Y. Computed tomographic scanning of the mediastinum in the staging of bronchogenic carcinoma. Am Rev Respir Dis. 1981;124:690–5.
67. Baron R, Levitt R, Sagel S, et al. Computed tomography in the preoperative evaluation of bronchogenic carcinoma. Radiology. 1982;145: 727–32.
68. Mouk G, Cockerill E, Farber M, et al. Computed tomography vs standard radiology in the evaluation of mediastinal adenopathy. Chest. 1982;82:69–75.
69. Osborne D, Korobkin M, Ravin C. Comparison of plain radiography conventional tomography, and computed tomography in detecting intrathoracic lymph node metastases from lung carcinoma. Radiology. 1982;142:157–61.
70. Rea H, Shevland J, House A. Accuracy of computed tomographic scanning in assessment of the mediastinum in bronchial carcinoma. Thorac Cardiovasc Surg. 1981;81:825–9.
71. Buy J, Ghossain M, Poirson F. Computed tomography of mediastinal lymph nodes in nonsmall cell lung cancer. J Comput Assist Tomogr. 1988;12:545–52.
72. Ikezoe J, Kadowaki K, Morimoto S. Mediastinal lymph node metastases from nonsmall cell bronchogenic carcinoma: reevaluation with CT. J Comput Assist Tomogr. 1990;14:340–4.
73. Izbicki J, Thetter O, Karg O. Accuracy of computed tomographic scan and surgical assessment for staging of bronchial carcinoma. J Thorac Cardiovasc Surg. 1992;104:413–20.
74. Dales R, Stark R, Raman S. Computed tomography to stage lung cancer. Am Rev Respir Dis. 1990;144: 1096–101.
75. Dwamena BA, Sonnad SS, Angobaldo JO, Wahl RL. Metastases from Non-small cell lung cancer: mediastinal staging in the 1990s—meta-analytic comparison of PET and CT. Radiology. 1999;213: 530–6.
76. Erasmus JJ, McAdams HP, Patz EF. Non-small cell lung cancer: FDG-PET imaging. J Thorac Imaging. 1999;14:247–56.
77. Pfister DG, Johnson DH, Azzoli CG. American society of clinical oncology treatment of unresectable non-small-cell Lung cancer guideline: update 2003. J ClinOncol. 2004; 22:330–353.
78. Lee BE, von Haag D, Lown T, et al. Advances in positron emission tomography technology have increased the need for surgical staging in non–small cell lung cancer. J Thorac Cardiovasc Surg. 2007; 133:746–52.
79. de Langen AJ, Raijmakers P, Riphagen I, et al. The size of mediastinal lymph nodes and its relation with metastatic involvement: a meta-analysis. Eur J Cardiothorac Surg. 2006;29:26–9.
80. Antoch G, Stattaus J, Nemat AT, et al. Non-small cell lung cancer: dual-modality PET/CT in preoperative staging. Radiology. 2003;229:526–33.
81. Quint LE, Tummala S, Brisson LJ, et al. Distribution of distant metastases from newly diagnosed non-small cell lung cancer. Ann Thorac Surg. 1996;62: 246–50.
82. Murayama S, Murakami J, Yoshimitsu K, et al. CT diagnosis of pleural dissemination without pleural effusion in primary lung cancer. Radiat Med. 1996;14:117–9.
83. Truong MT, Viswanathan C, Erasmus JJ. Positron emission tomography/computed tomography in lung cancer staging, prognosis, and assessment of therapeutic response. J Thorac Imaging. 2011;26: 132–46.
84. Dietlein M, Weber K, Gandjour A, et al. Cost-effectiveness of FDG-PET for the management of solitary pulmonary nodules: a decision analysis based on cost reimbursement in Germany. Eur J Nucl Med. 2000;27:1441–56.
85. Valk PE, Pounds TR, Hopkins DM, et al. Staging non-small cell lung cancer by whole-body positron emission tomographic imaging. Ann Thorac Surg. 1995;60:1573–82.

4

Pulmonary Infections in the Normal Host

Loren Ketai and Helen Katrina Busby

Abstract

Chest radiography remains the cornerstone for imaging pulmonary infections in normal hosts. It does a good, though imperfect, job of detecting pneumonia but is less effective in monitoring the response of the infection to therapy. In clinical settings where both pneumonia and noninfectious thoracic diseases are diagnostic possibilities, the addition of CT scanning to radiography can help identify imaging patterns that favor either an infectious or an non-infectious etiology. Occasionally these CT imaging patterns can narrow the differential diagnosis of possible infectious pathogens, but rarely can imaging point toward a specific organism. In most cases CT is better relied upon to identify complications of pneumonia than to identify a pathogen. Cost and radiation dose, however, argue against its indiscriminant use in patients with community acquired pneumonia. Ultrasound provides a safe low cost alternative to CT, but its utility is limited to pleural complications of pneumonia.

Keywords

Community-acquired pneumonia · Bronchiolitis · Mycoplasma · Mycobacterial infection · Lung abscess · Empyema · Chest CT

Physicians use radiology reflexively to aid the diagnosis and treatment of pneumonia but are not always aware of its strengths and weaknesses. Chest radiography does a good but surprisingly imperfect job of detecting pneumonia and is still less effective in monitoring the response of the infection to therapy. In clinical settings where both pneumonia and non-infectious thoracic diseases are diagnostic possibilities, the addition of CT scanning to radiography can help identify imaging patterns that favor one etiology over the other. Several imaging patterns can narrow the differential diagnosis of possible infectious

L. Ketai (✉)
Department of Radiology, University of New Mexico Health Science Center, MSC10 5530 1 University of New Mexico, Albuquerque, NM 87111-0001, USA
e-mail: lketai@unm.edu

H. K. Busby
Department of Pulmonary and Critical Care, University of New Mexico School of Medicine, MSC 10-5550 1 University of New Mexico, Albuquerque, NM 87131-0001, USA

J. P. Kanne (ed.), *Clinically Oriented Pulmonary Imaging*, Respiratory Medicine, DOI: 10.1007/978-1-61779-542-8_4,

pathogens, but rarely can imaging point toward a specific organism. In most cases, imaging is better relied upon to identify complications of pneumonia rather than to identify a pathogen. Both ultrasound and CT can identify these complications, but CT detects a greater range of pathology. Cost and radiation dose, however, argue against its indiscriminant use in patients with community acquired pneumonia.

Routine chest radiography is sufficiently accurate to diagnosis community acquired pneumonia (CAP) in most immunocompetent patients. Interobserver agreement in this population has been measured in the 80–90% range but is diminished by false positive interpretations in patients with chronic obstructive pulmonary disease (COPD), atelectasis, or congestive heart failure [1–3]. The presence of these co-morbidities may account for the observation that among patients admitted with the clinical diagnosis of pneumonia, the rates of septicemia and mortality did not differ between patients whose radiograph confirmed the diagnosis and those in whom it did not [2].

Among patients whose chest radiograph shows definite evidence of pneumonia, the number of lobes involved and the presence of pleural disease are predictors of disease severity and need for ICU admission [4]. The concordance for these findings between readers is high [5]. The benefit of follow-up radiographs, those taken after initial severity of disease is assessed and therapy initiated, has been more difficult to prove. Speed of radiographic improvement is related to patient age and initial extent of involvement and is often outpaced by clinical improvement (Fig. 4.1). After a week of treatment, more than 50% of hospitalized patients may experience resolution of symptoms while only 25% show radiologic resolution [6]. Conversely, progression of radiographic findings is uncommon unless accompanied by lack of clinical response to treatment [7].

Identification of specific patterns of pneumonia on chest radiographs can be as error prone as the use of radiographs to assess treatment response. Even when radiograph reader concordance for the presence of pneumonia is high, reader concordance for the presence of bronchial wall thickening, air bronchograms, or bronchopneumonia is often low [1, 4]. Because of these inconsistencies in radiograph interpretation, radiologic differentiation of pneumonia from non-infectious causes of parenchymal disease is much more difficult without the use of chest CT.

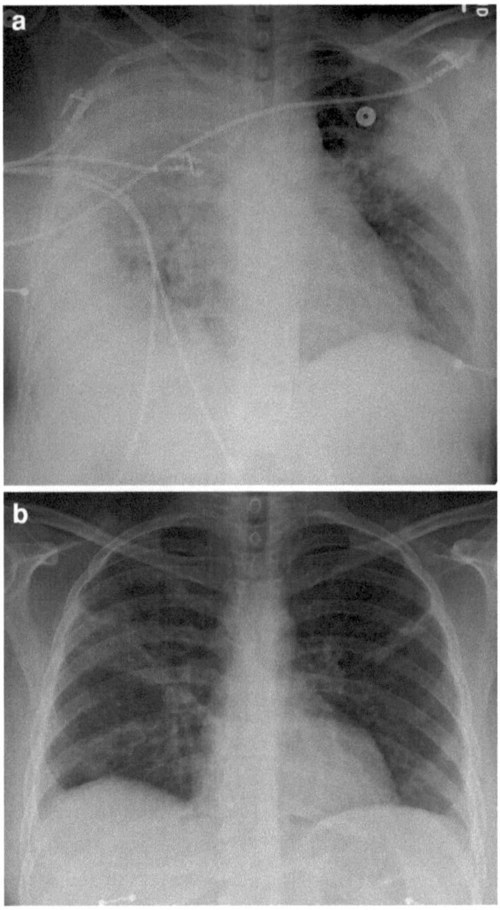

Fig. 4.1 Pneumococcal pneumonia in a young adult. **a** Admission chest radiograph shows multilobar lung consolidation. **b** Follow up radiograph two weeks later shows marked improvement. Speed of radiographic improvement is dependent both on pathogen and host factors

Differentiation of Pneumonia from Non-Infectious Diseases

Among normal hosts with suspected pneumonia, the radiologic pattern helps to determine which non-infectious diseases might also be considered

Table 4.1 Radiologic patterns shared by infectious and non-infectious disease

CT pattern	Infection	Non-infectious disease
Linear interstitial	Rare	CHF, drug reaction, acute eosinophilic pneumonia
Nodules		
Centrilobular	Common	HP, respiratory bronchiolitis, hemorrhage
Tree-in-bud	Common	Gastric aspiration
Random	Uncommon	Metastases
Lobular GGO or consolidation	Common	CHF, pulmonary hemorrhage, drug reaction
Consolidation		
Non-segmental	Common	Atelectasis, adenocarcinoma[a]
Segmental	Common	Pulmonary infarction

[a] With lepidic spreading component

in a differential diagnosis (Table 4.1). Linear interstitial pattern, micronodules, lobular ground-glass opacities (GGO) and consolidation, and segmental or non-segmental consolidation are associated with specific non-infectious diseases. On the whole, interstitial patterns are the least common radiographic manifestation of pneumonia, present on chest radiographs of 0–10% of patients with pneumonia [1, 5]. A linear interstitial pattern is readily recognized on radiography by the presence Kerley A and B lines, often accompanied by subpleural edema (thickening of the fissures), and pleural effusions. The CT equivalent of this pattern is smooth thickening of the interlobular septa. These septa are 1–2 cm in length and represent the divisions between secondary lobules, the smallest unit of lung surrounded by connective tissue. Infectious agents, including viruses, rarely cause this pattern, with the notable exception of the North American Hantaviruses and occasionally rickettsial diseases [8, 9] (Fig. 4.2). Although in most cases linear interstitial patterns are caused by hydrostatic edema, acute eosinophilic pneumonia and occasionally a drug reaction will have a similar pattern [10, 11].

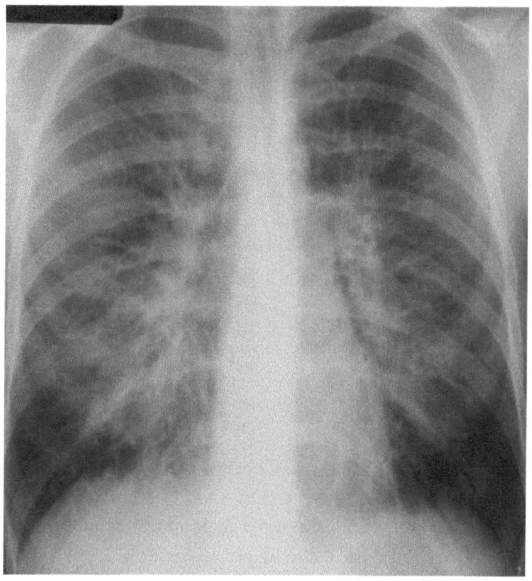

Fig. 4.2 Hantavirus cardiopulmonary syndrome. PA chest radiograph shows extensive interstitial edema manifest by Kerley A and B lines. No vascular redistribution, pleural effusions, or widening of vascular pedicle to suggest volume overload

Reticulonodular or nodular patterns are the most common "interstitial" appearance of pneumonia on chest radiographs. In the setting of pneumonia, this pattern is often the radiographic manifestation of bronchial wall thickening and bronchiolitis. Bronchiolitis results in small nodules that are individually too small to be seen on chest radiograph but become visible when multiple overlying nodules summate. On CT images, the individual 1–3 mm micronodules are readily seen. The nodules are caused by inflammation around the bronchioles, which are located in the center of the secondary lobule. Since bronchioles do not extend all the way to the pleura, the nodules that form around bronchioles (centrilobular nodules) characteristically

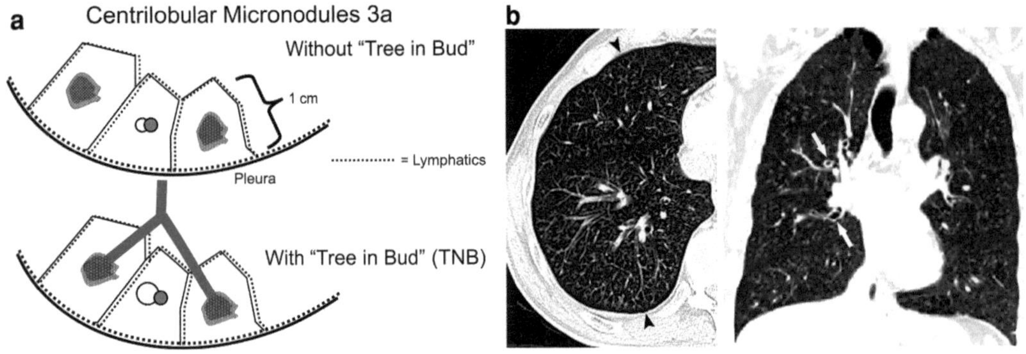

Fig. 4.3 Centrilobular nodules. **a** Diagram of appearance of centrilobular nodules, both with and without tree-in-bud. **b** Transverse and coronal reformatted CT images of *Hemophilus influenzae* bronchiolitis show bronchial wall thickening (*arrows*) and extensive tree-in-bud type centrilobular nodules that spare the pleural surfaces (*arrowheads*)

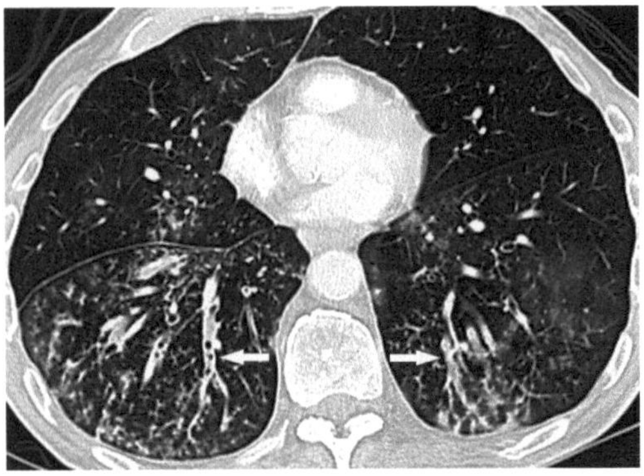

Fig. 4.4 Acute aspiration. Contrast-enhanced CT image of patient with acute aspiration shows extensive centrilobular nodules within the most dependent aspects of the lower lobes. Several bronchi are also filled with secretions (*arrows*)

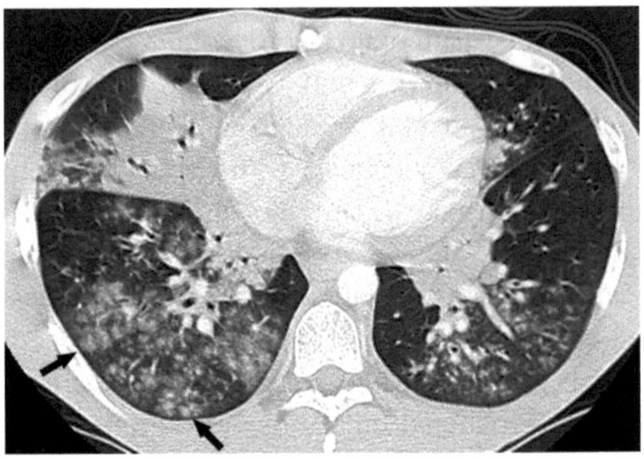

Fig. 4.5 Adenovirus pneumonia. CT image shows multiple different radiologic patterns of pneumonia. Lobar consolidation is present in the middle lobe and centrilobular micronodules with tree-in-bud pattern in the left lower lobe. Acinar nodules (*arrows*) are present in the right lower lobe

spare the pleural surfaces (Fig. 4.3). If the bronchioles connecting centrilobular nodules are thickened or filled with secretions, they may also become visible on CT. The resulting pattern of centrilobular micronodules connected by branching structures is termed a "tree- in-bud" pattern. This subset of centrilobular nodules has strong association with infection or, in acutely ill patients, gastric aspiration [12] (Fig. 4.4). The CT finding of simple centrilobular micronodules without features of tree-in-bud is less specific. It may not only be caused by infection but also occurs commonly in other diseases, particularly those caused by inhaled materials, such as hypersensitivity pneumonitis and respiratory bronchiolitis-interstitial lung disease [13]. When occurring in the setting of infection, centrilobular micronodules (without tree-in-bud pattern) are often accompanied by additional abnormalities such as consolidation and the presence of larger, acinar nodules (5–7 mm) that occupy more of the alveoli within the secondary lobule (Fig. 4.5).

CT is particularly useful in the evaluation of patients presenting with small nodular opacities on chest radiography, in part because it can distinguish nodules with a simple centrilobular pattern from centrilobular nodules with a tree-in-

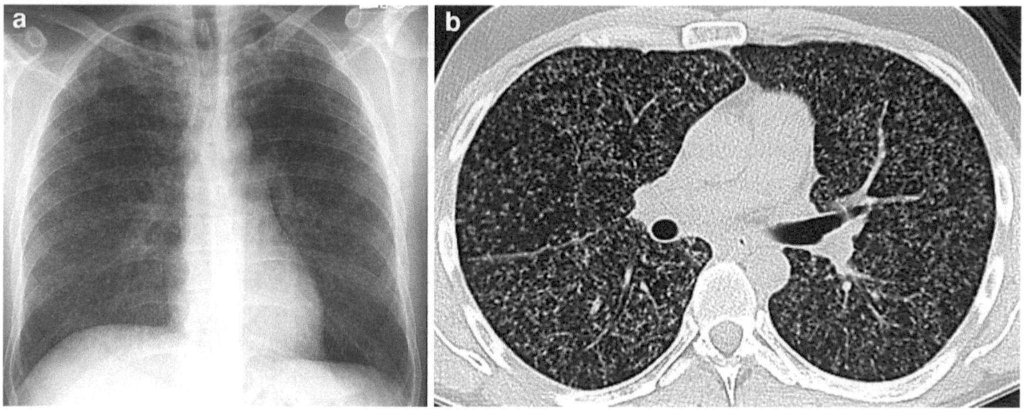

Fig. 4.6 Miliary tuberculosis. **a** PA chest radiograph of a patient with miliary tuberculosis showing diffuse micronodular opacities. The distribution pattern of the micronodules cannot be discerned on the radiograph. **b** HRCT image shows nodules to be randomly distributed, some touching the pleural surfaces, including the fissures

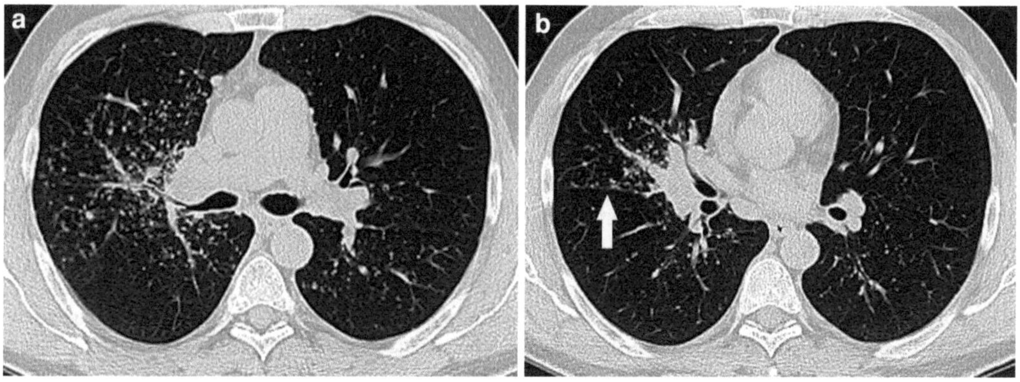

Fig. 4.7 Sarcoidosis. **a**, **b** HRCT images show micronodules in a perilymphatic distribution. Nodules are preferentially aggregated along the bronchovascular bundles and along the fissures (*arrow*)

bud pattern. Equally important, CT can distinguish both types of centrilobular nodules from nodules with either a random or a perilymphatic distribution. Randomly distributed nodules are often caused by blood borne dissemination of disease, pathogenic material reaching small capillaries in the periphery of the secondary lobules. Unlike centrilobular nodules, random nodules can touch the pleural surfaces, including the fissures [14]. Miliary tuberculosis is the classic cause of randomly distributed micronodules (Fig. 4.6). Disseminated fungal infections and metastatic neoplasms such as renal cell carcinoma, thyroid carcinoma, and melanoma may have identical appearances. While centrilobular and random micronodules can be associated with either infectious or non-infectious diseases, a third micronodule pattern, perilymphatic, is almost always noninfectious. This pattern, in which nodules show predilection for interlobular septa and pleural surfaces is common in sarcoidosis and lymphangitic spread of tumors (Fig. 4.7).

Rather than causing linear, reticulonodular, or nodular opacities, most pneumonias fill airspaces creating a bronchopneumonia or lobar pneumonia pattern. On chest radiographs, bronchopneumonia appears as patchy opacities that may be accompanied by bronchial wall thickening. Because of the bronchocentric distribution of inflammation, bronchi may be obstructed by secretions, accounting for the volume loss and absence of air bronchograms seen in some cases of bronchopneumonia.

The CT appearance of bronchopneumonia may illustrate progression from an initial bronchiolitis, with infection spreading outward from the center of the secondary lobule. As entire lobules fill with inflammatory debris, the opacities created conform to lobular architecture and are sharply marginated by borders of the secondary lobules. Opacities that are sufficiently transparent to allow visualization of underlying vasculature are termed "ground-glass opacities" (GGO), and those dense enough to obscure vessels, "consolidation" (Fig. 4.8). In addition to bronchopneumonia, a lobular pattern of GGO or consolidation may be caused by drug toxicity, chronic infiltrative lung diseases, pulmonary hemorrhage, or pulmonary edema [15]. The coexistence of tree-in-bud type centrilobular nodules or peribronchial (bronchocentric) consolidation with lobular opacities on CT favors pneumonia over these other diagnoses.

Lobar pneumonias often begin in the lung periphery and then spread centrally. Consolidation is confluent rather than patchy and often sufficient to form air bronchograms. Although early in the course of infection consolidation may be confined to a single segment, over time it can spread through a lobe of the lung without regard for segmental boundaries (the resulting opacities sometimes referred to as "non-segmental"). Most of the organisms that cause lobar pneumonia, particularly *Streptococcus pneumoniae*, can also cause bronchopneumonia, and examples of both patterns may be present in the same patient (Fig. 4.9). Distinguishing bronchopneumonia from lobar pneumonia is, therefore, usually not helpful in identifying a specific pathogen. Confluent consolidation, however, needs to be distinguished from a different spectrum of noninfectious diseases than does bronchopneumonia.

Consolidation of an entire lobe (the lobe characteristically maintaining a normal volume) almost always represents pneumonia, but less extensive disease requires a broader differential diagnosis that includes pulmonary infarction, atelectasis, and adenocarcinoma with a lepdic growth component. If atelectasis involves less than an entire lobe, definitive signs of volume loss may not be evident on chest radiographs. In these cases, CT more clearly shows displacement and crowding of fissures and bronchi. Contrast enhancement pattern may also help to distinguish atelectasis from pneumonia. On contrast-enhanced CT, the lung parenchyma in areas of passive atelectasis enhances markedly, often enough to partially obscure underlying vessels. Some pneumonias enhance to a similar degree, but a third or more of pneumonias and cases of obstructive atelectasis enhance less

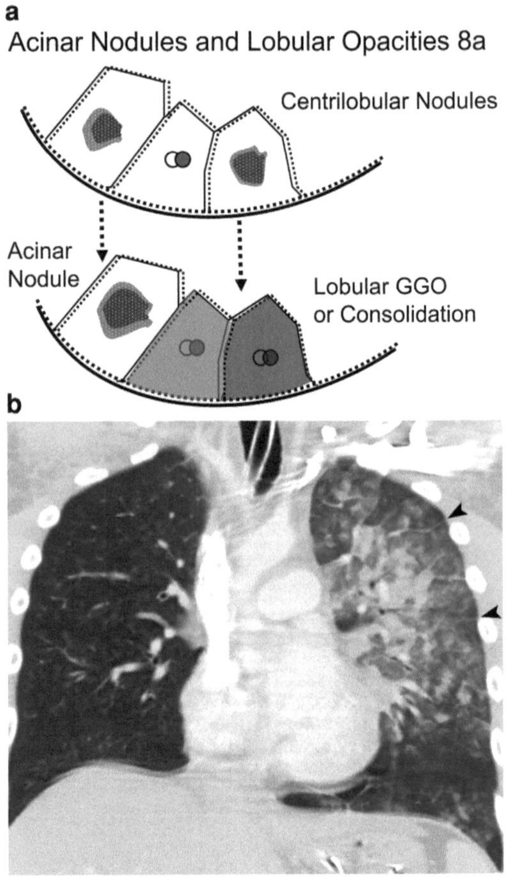

Fig. 4.8 **a** Diagram of appearance of acinar nodules and lobular opacities. **b** Coronal reformatted contrast-enhanced CT image shows lobular ground-glass opacities (GGO) and consolidation, manifesting as different attenuation lung parenchyma with geographic borders defined by septal thickening (*arrowheads*). Findings are often caused by infection but are not specific

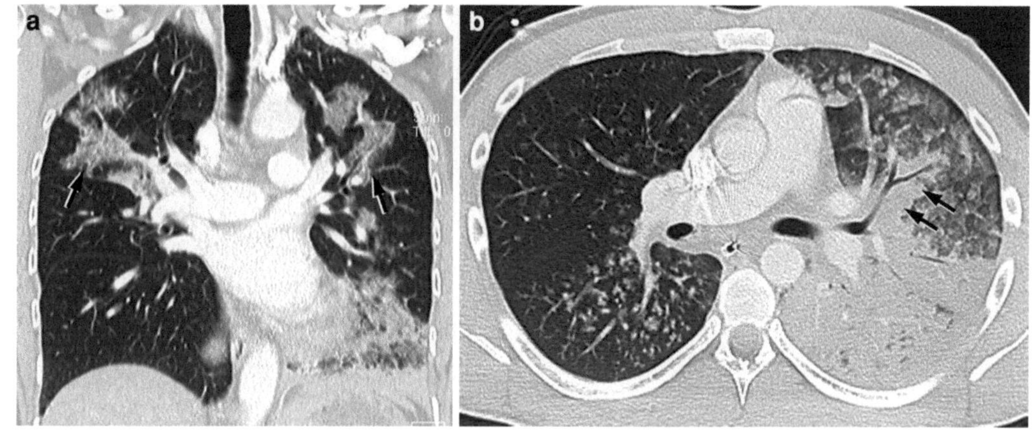

Fig. 4.9 Bronchopneumonia and lobar pneumonia. **a** Bronchopneumonia displaying predominantly peribronchovascular consolidation. **b** Contrast-enhanced CT image of a patient with community-acquired pneumonia shows a mixed radiologic pattern (a common finding). Lobar consolidation is present in the left lower lobe. Peribronchovascular consolidation (*arrows*) in the lingula is typical of bronchopneumonia. Centrilobular micronodules with a tree-in-bud pattern are present in the right lower lobe, indicative of bronchiolitis

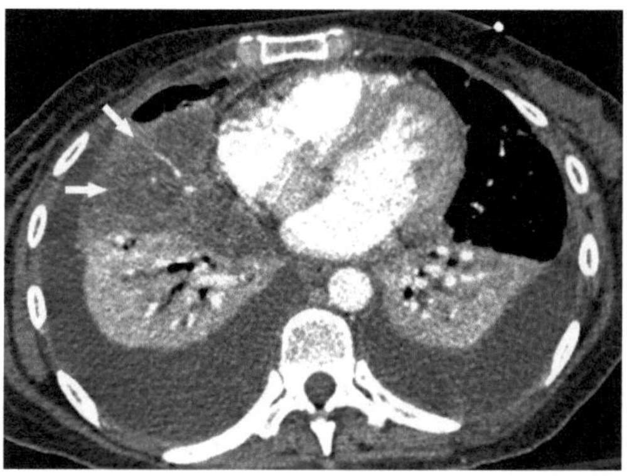

Fig. 4.10 Contrast-enhanced CT shows large bilateral pleural effusions. Passive atelectasis is present in both lower lobes, which are relatively high in attenuation. Middle lobe (*arrows*) is lower in attenuation and only slightly decreased in volume. No air bronchograms are present, favoring obstructive atelectasis over pneumonia. More superior CT sections (not shown) showed obstruction of central bronchi with secretions

intensely, allowing clear delineation of pulmonary vasculature from surrounding lung parenchyma [16]. This relatively low attenuation of lung parenchyma likely represents retained fluid within alveoli. Its presence in conjunction with air filled bronchi favors pneumonia. Relatively low attenuation lung in conjunction with airless, fluid-filled bronchi suggests obstructive atelectasis (Fig. 4.10).

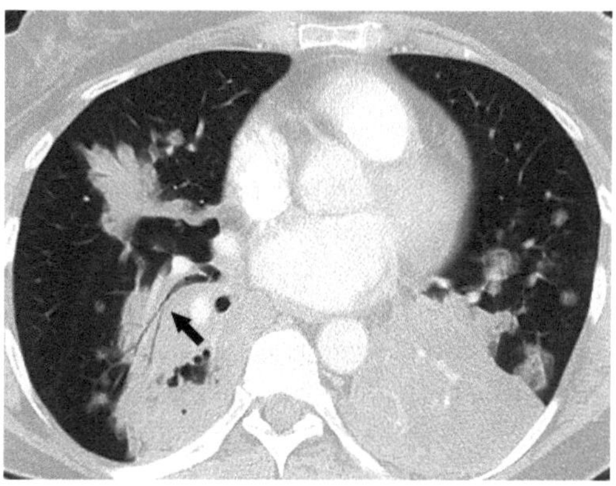

Fig. 4.11 Multifocal adenocarcinoma with pneumonic pattern. Contrast-enhanced CT image shows multifocal consolidation and scattered nodules. Bronchi in the right lower lobe (*arrow*) are distorted and stretched

Like obstructive atelectasis, adenocarcinomas with a lepidic growth component can also cause low attenuation consolidation on CT and can be difficult to distinguish from pneumonia. The presence or absence of air bronchograms on CT is not helpful in differentiating infection from neoplasm in this setting. Bronchi are more likely to be distorted, however, as they course through an area of consolidation caused by adenocarcinoma and are more likely to have thickened walls proximal to an area of consolidation caused by pneumonia [17, 18] (Fig. 4.11). Most

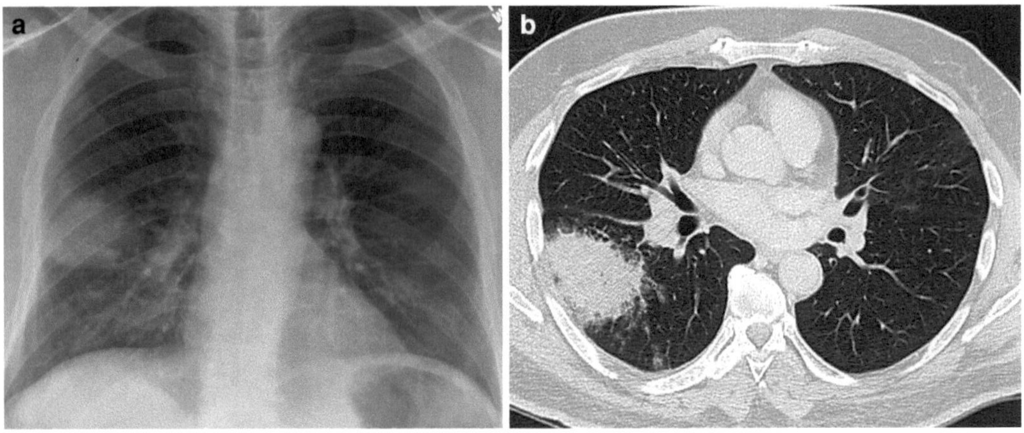

Fig. 4.12 Round pneumonia in an adult. Chest radiograph (**a**) and CT image (**b**) show round right lower lobe mass with an appearance indistinguishable from a primary lung neoplasm. The mass resolved with empiric antibiotic treatment

commonly, the patient's symptoms and the chronicity of radiologic abnormalities, rather than specific radiologic findings, are relied upon to distinguish this subtype of adenocarcinoma from infection.

Serial imaging and symptoms are also key to distinguishing round pneumonias from neoplasm. While adenocarcinoma with lepidic growth is easily mistaken for a common form of pneumonia, round pneumonias may be mistaken for a primary lung neoplasm on both chest radiography and CT (Fig. 4.12). Round pneumonias are much more common in children than adults. When they occur in adults, the diagnoses of Q fever and endemic fungal infection should be considered, depending on the exposure history [19]. As a variant of lobar pneumonia, however, round pneumonias also occur sporadically, caused by bacterial pathogens that respond to standard antibiotic treatment. Their existence also argues for a trial of antibiotics prior to biopsy of many lung masses.

Both pulmonary infarcts and early lobar pneumonia arise in the periphery of the lung and may have similar appearances on chest radiography. CT images of infarcts demonstrate a characteristic triangular opacity, with its broad base against the pleura and its apex truncated and pointing centrally. Central lucency within opacity and the absence of air bronchograms both strongly favor infarct over other causes of parenchymal lung disease [20]. The presence of opacities with this configuration on a non-contrast CT may prompt further evaluation with a CT pulmonary angiogram (Fig. 4.13).

Specific Diagnoses: Mycoplasma, Viruses, and Mycobacteria

Mycoplasma

Attention to the same patterns that aid in distinguishing infection from non-infectious disease can sometimes aid in narrowing the list of potential infectious pathogens. The presence of a reticulonodular radiographic pattern or its CT correlate, centrilobular micronodules and bronchial wall thickening, is reason to consider the diagnosis of *Mycoplasma* in adults [21–23] (Fig. 4.14). CT images of *Mycoplasma* infections also frequently reveal peribronchovascular ground-glass opacities and lobular opacities indicative of bronchopneumonia. The bronchitis/bronchiolitis and bronchopneumonia patterns may be more common in adults than in children, who frequently manifest infection as segmental and lobar pneumonias [24]. Although the bronchiolitis-bronchopneumonia

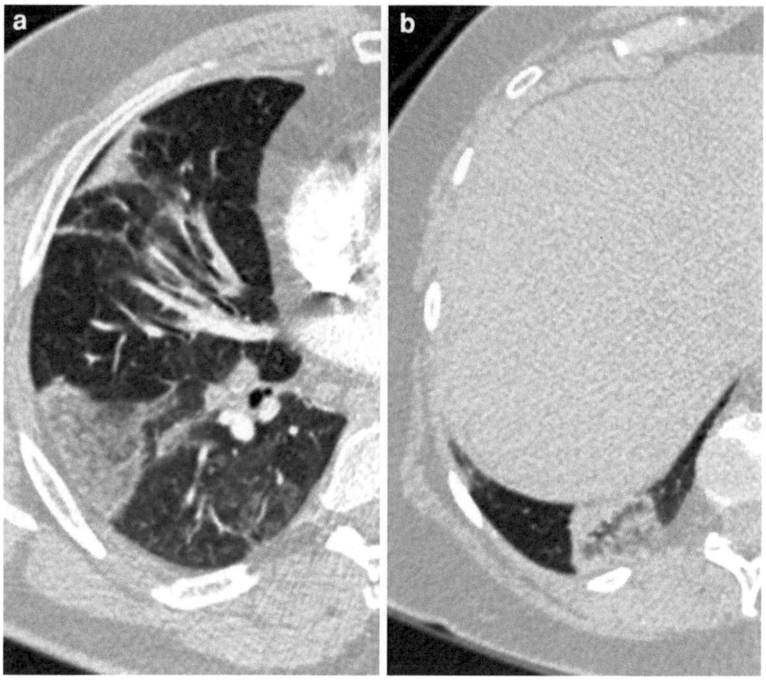

Fig. 4.13 Pulmonary infarctions. **a**, **b** Contrast-enhanced CT image of pulmonary infarctions in two different patients show peripheral opacities abutting the pleura. Attenuation is lower centrally than peripherally. No air bronchograms are present

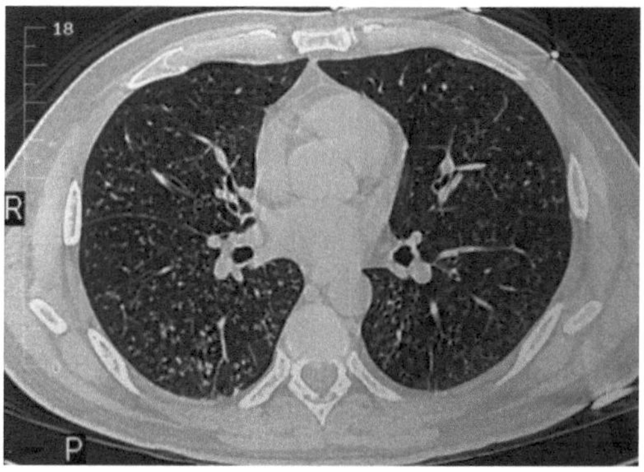

Fig. 4.14 Mycoplasma infection. HRCT image shows widespread centrilobular micronodules with a tree-in-bud pattern, indicative of a bronchiolitis. Micronodules largely spare the pleural surfaces

pattern is characteristic of *Mycoplasma* infection in adults, the pattern is not specific. Similar findings may be caused by *Chlamydia* and bacterial infections, particularly those with *Hemophilus influenzae* [25, 26]. Viral pathogens are now being more widely detected in normal hosts and may be the causative agent of bronchiolitis and bronchopneumonia in cases where no pathogen could previously have been identified.

Viral Infections

Implementation of more advanced diagnostic measures, particularly polymerase chain reactions, has driven the more frequent identification of viral pathogens. Several studies have shown that viral pathogens may cause 15–25% of lower respiratory tract infections among immunocompetent adults [27, 28]. These viral pathogens, such as influenza virus, metapneumovirus, and respiratory syncytial virus may cause a bronchitis/bronchiolitis pattern similar to *Mycoplasma*. The use of newer diagnostic techniques, however, has also shown that the radiologic manifestations of viral lower tract infections are not limited to bronchiolitis. CT imaging of patients with lower respiratory tract infection and polymerase chain reaction (PCR) positive for viral pathogens has shown that a widespread consolidation pattern occurs as frequently as the bronchitis/bronchiolitis pattern [29]. The consolidative pattern appears to be particularly common in adenovirus infections, a phenomenon that may be accentuated during outbreaks of new immunologic strains of that virus (Fig. 4.15) [30].

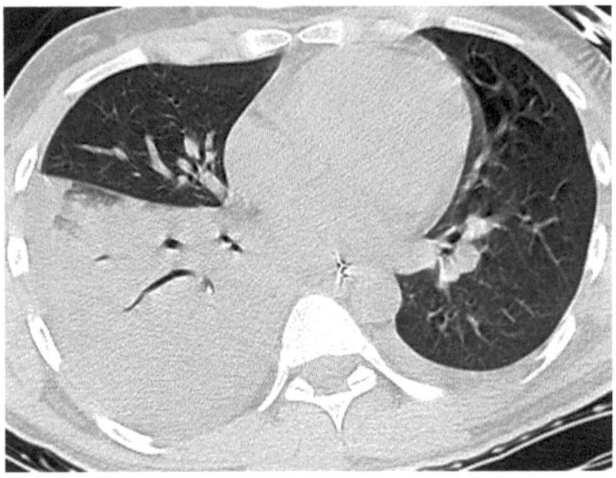

Fig. 4.15 Adenovirus pneumonia. CT image shows extensive right lower lobe consolidation without features of bronchitis/bronchiolitis or a bronchopneumonia pattern

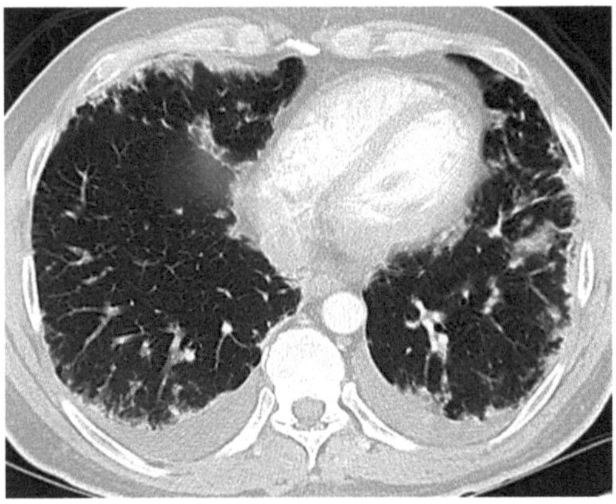

Fig. 4.16 H1N1 Influenza. Contrast-enhanced CT image shows peripheral consolidation similar to that seen in cryptogenic organizing pneumonia (COP). Small pleural effusions are present

The pleomorphic imaging appearance of viral lower tract infections is not only influenced by the infecting organism but also is influenced by the host's immune system. During the 2009 H1N1 influenza pandemic, the virus showed the ability to cause a variety of CT patterns ranging from minimal ground-glass opacity to a diffuse alveolar damage pattern. Of these presentations, bronchopneumonia was the most common, but a pattern of peribronchial and peripheral opacities similar to cryptogenic organizing pneumonia was also seen in multiple centers [31] (Fig. 4.16). Most series dominated by normal hosts reported little evidence of bronchiolitis. This pattern was subsequently reported in immunocompromised patients [32]. It is unknown whether detection of bronchiolitis in these patients represents a more limited inflammatory response or simply reflects more aggressive use of imaging earlier in the course of disease. Other work has linked the inflammatory response caused by non-protective H1N1 antibodies to severe disease among normal hosts, arguing that host inflammation plays in important role in determining the radiologic appearance in this viral disease [33].

Mycobacterial Infections

The pattern of CT abnormalities may be more useful in the diagnosis of mycobacterial disease than in distinguishing *Mycoplasma*, viral, and pyogenic disease from one another. Upper lobe predominance of centrilobular nodules is a common early manifestation of tuberculosis, representing bronchogenic spread of disease [34, 35]. This pattern is typical of what has previously been termed "reactivation" tuberculosis, but is now recognized to also be a manifestation of re-infection in immunocompetent hosts [36, 37]. Early in the course of tuberculosis, centrilobular nodules may be accompanied by macronodules (5–10 mm in diameter), lobular consolidation, and small areas of cavitation, the latter an uncommon finding in *Mycoplasma* infection and in most other causes of infectious bronchiolitis (Fig. 4.17). CT is capable of detecting early cavitation that is occult on chest radiographs and, in the setting of suspected tuberculosis, may be a useful diagnostic adjunct to interferon gamma release assays [38]. In more advanced disease, cavitation is often evident on radiographs. In these cases, CT may provide little added value unless the activity of the infection is uncertain based on clinical grounds. In these cases CT images showing cavities, consolidation, and large numbers of centrilobular nodules increase the likelihood that the infection is active and that sputum smears will be positive [39].

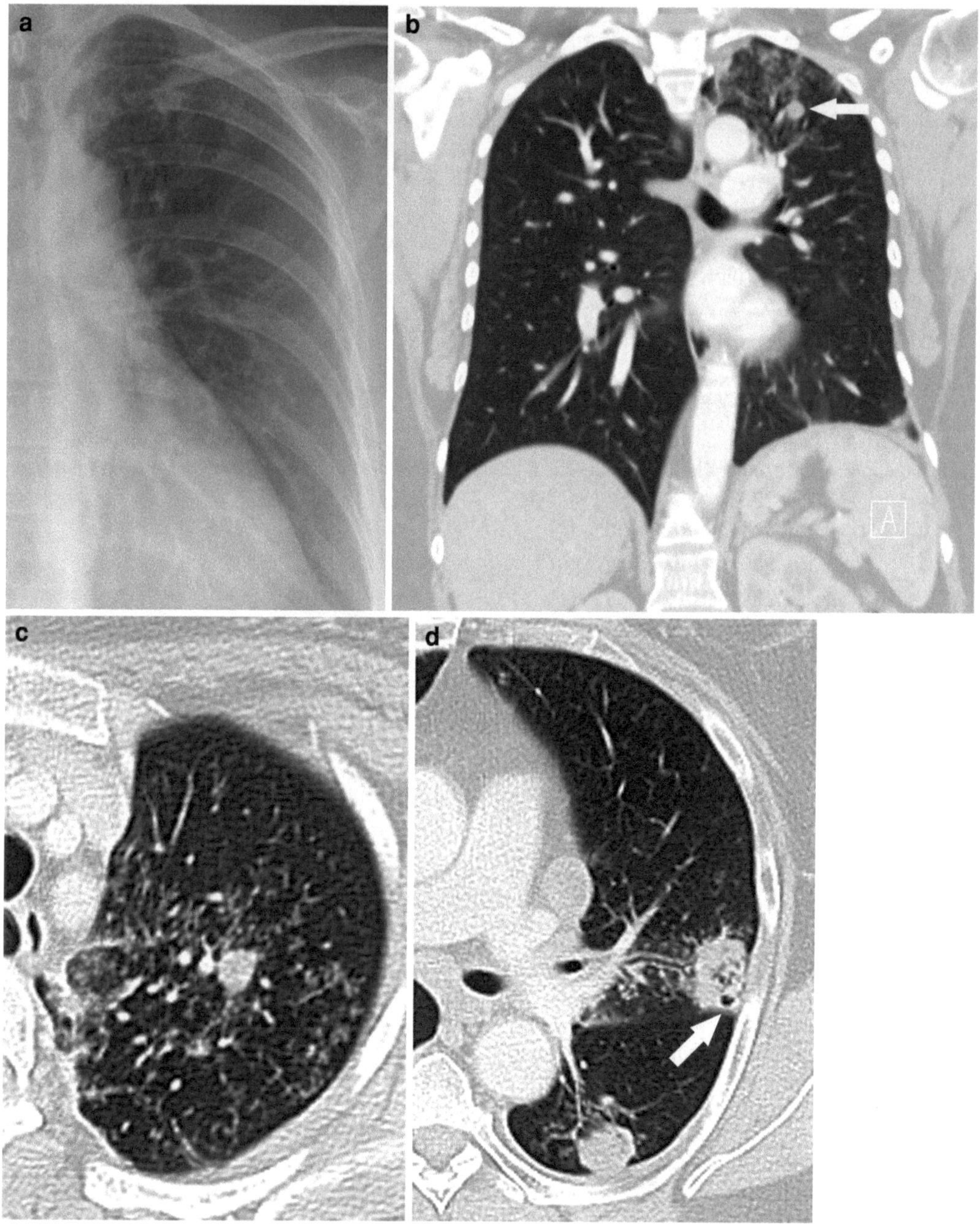

Fig. 4.17 Tuberculosis. **a** Coned down view of a PA chest radiograph shows subtle upper lobe opacities. **b** Contrast-enhanced CT coronal reformat image shows centrilobular nodules as well as a macronodule (*arrow*) in the left upper lobe. **c** Micronodules and macronodules on transverse CT image through the left upper lobe. **d** Contrast-enhanced CT image from another patient shows early cavitation (*arrow*) within upper lobe macronodules, findings that suggest the diagnosis of tuberculosis

In later stages of mycobacterial disease, lung necrosis and associated cicatricial atelectasis can cause marked volume loss and architectural distortion. Endemic fungal infections (e.g. coccidioidomycosis and histoplasmosis) and chronic necrotizing aspergillosis (the semi-invasive form

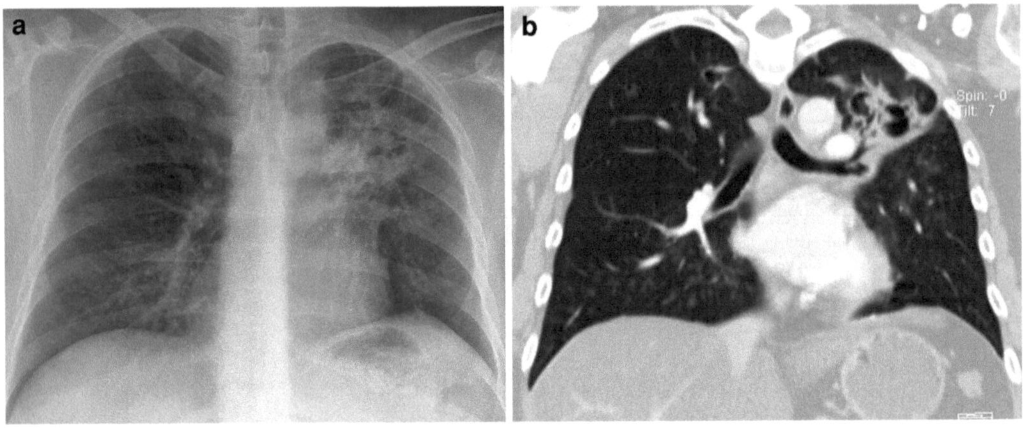

Fig. 4.18 Chronic progressive coccidioidomycosis in a patient presenting with hemoptysis. **a** PA chest radiograph and contrast-enhanced CT coronal reformat image **b** show cavitary pneumonia with volume loss in the left upper lobe and upward retraction of the left hilum

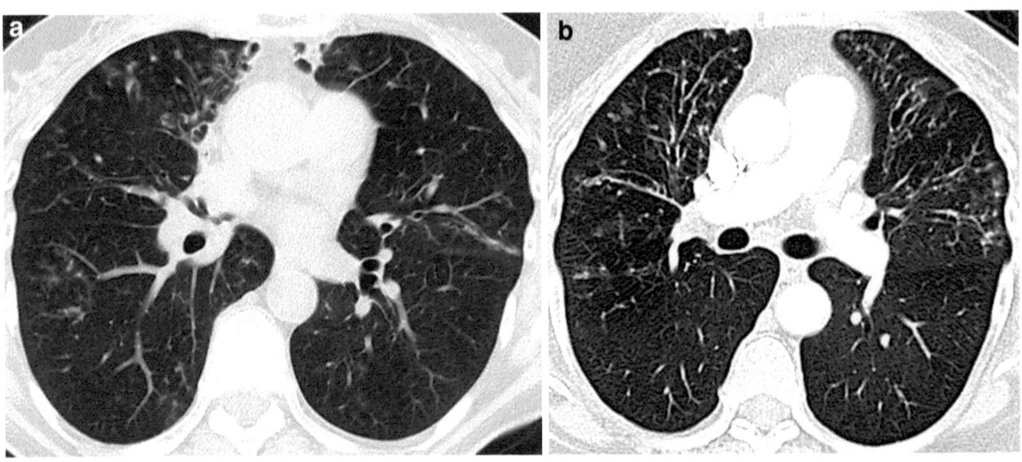

Fig. 4.19 Non-classic *Mycobacterium avium-intracellulare* infection. **a** CT image shows multiple small foci of bronchiectasis. **b** CT from a second patient from whom only a single sputum sample had been obtained. Culture was negative for mycobacteria but typical imaging appearance suggests that culture results were falsely negative

of aspergillosis seen in patients with underlying COPD) can have a similar appearance (Fig. 4.18). Lung volume loss and architectural distortion can occasionally accompany severe necrotizing pneumonias caused by pyogenic bacteria. In these cases, however, symptoms are usually more severe and more acute than in the setting of mycobacterial or endemic fungal infections.

Centrilobular nodules are also associated with non-tuberculous mycobacterial (NTMB) infections. In normal hosts, non-tuberculous mycobacterial infections can present as a classic form that mimics tuberculosis, as a bronchiectatic form, or as hypersensitivity pneumonitis [40]. All three forms of disease may have centrilobular nodules but the bronchiectatic form, seen in middle-aged women, has the most distinctive radiologic pattern. This form of disease manifests as centrilobular micronodules (both with and without tree–in-bud configuration) accompanied by cylindrical bronchiectasis (Fig. 4.19). Bronchiectasis characteristically occurs in the middle and lingular lobes, but

Table 4.2 Radiographic indications for cross-sectional imaging of pneumonia

Radiographic findings	Advantage of CT	Advantage of US
Diffuse nodular pattern	Distinguish miliary disease from airway spread	NA
	Identify perilymphatic pattern	
Rapidly increasing opacity without air bronchograms	Identify effusions and determine full extent	Identify effusions and assess their complexity
	Identify central airway obstruction	No radiation
Possible cavitation	Confirm presence in suspected tuberculosis and assess for signs of active disease	NA
	Evaluate for complications of necrotic bacterial pneumonia	
Possible lymphadenopathy	Evaluate for underlying neoplasm or sarcoidosis	NA

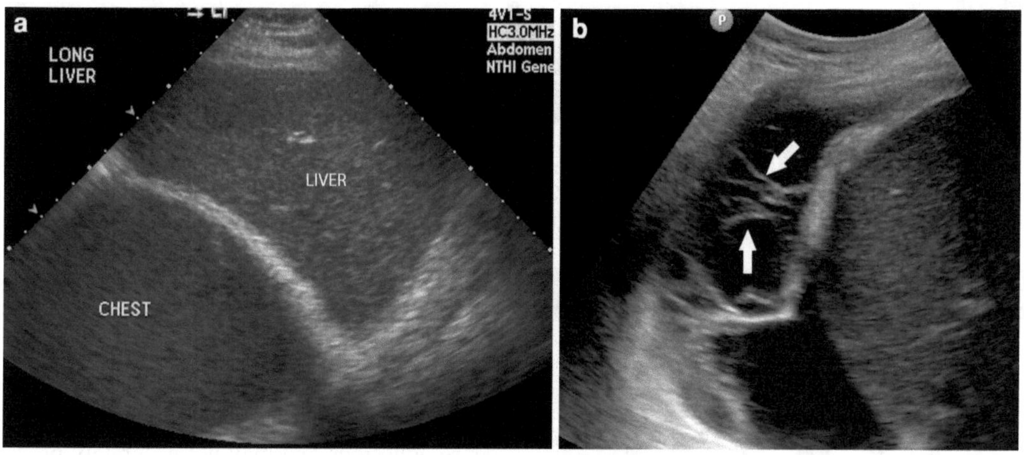

Fig. 4.20 Ultrasound of parapneumonic effusions. **a** Ultrasound image shows pleural fluid that is nearly as echogenic as the liver, suggesting fluid that is either hemorrhagic or purulent. **b** Ultrasound showing multiple adhesions (*arrows*) within a pleural effusion. Findings suggest that thoracentesis should be performed but does not predict whether or not catheter drainage will be successful

positive cultures are most commonly obtained in patients with involvement of all lobes [41].

Complications of Pneumonia

For most immunocompetent individuals, the combination of clinical and chest radiographic findings provides adequate information for diagnosis and treatment of pneumonia, without need to employ either CT or ultrasound. Although a retrospective series suggested that CT scanning of patients with suspected pneumonia frequently led to modification in treatment or an alternative diagnosis, the conclusion is likely distorted by selection bias [42]. In general, CT is most likely to be useful in patients with pneumonia that is severe or unresponsive to treatment, particularly for those patients with suspected cavitation, large pleural effusions, mediastinal or hilar lymphadenopathy, or endobronchial obstruction (Table 4.2). For instance, prompt cross-sectional imaging is warranted in patients with pleuritic chest pain and rapidly worsening radiographic or physical examination findings. These findings can indicate rapidly progressive pleural disease,

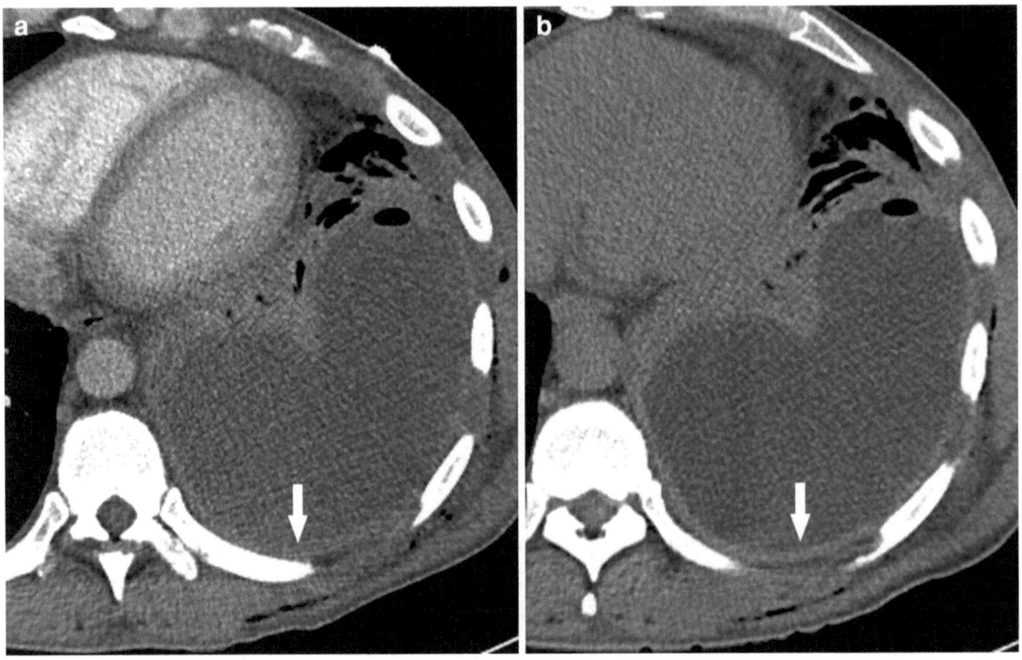

Fig. 4.21 CT images of a patient with subsequently proven empyema. **a** CT images performed with 25-second delay show modest degree of enhancement of the thickened pleura (*arrow*). **b** On delayed (70 s) imaging, the presence of pleural enhancement (*arrow*) is more conspicuous

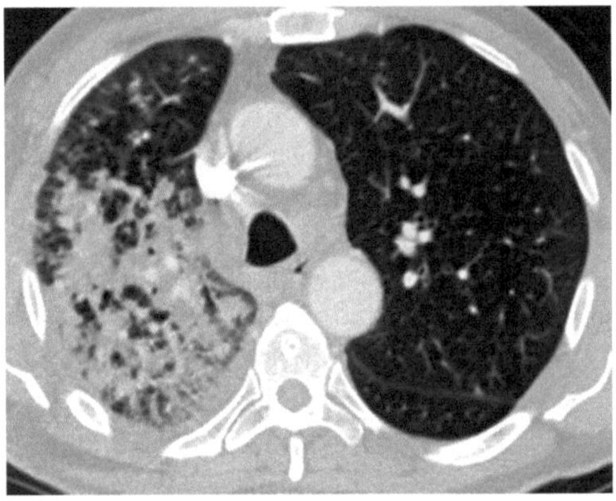

Fig. 4.22 Lobar pneumonia superimposed on emphysema. CT shows right upper lobe pneumonia that contains multiple lucencies that could be mistaken for cavitation. Inspection of the uninfected left lung shows similar small low attenuation foci indicative of centrilobular emphysema

sometimes termed "explosive pleuritis", that is most typical of beta hemolytic *Streptococcus* infections [43].

Both CT and ultrasound have advantages in evaluating suspected parapneumonic effusions. Ultrasound's principal advantages are its low cost, portability, and lack of ionizing radiation. Ultrasound images can also show septations within pleural fluid collections that are not visible on contrast-enhanced CT scanning [44]. These septations are often fibrinous strands rather than dense adhesions and may not accurately predict the failure of closed catheter drainage. They can, however, support the decision to perform a thoracentesis [45]. Anechoic effusions or effusions that contain scattered echoes but are free of septations are at relatively low risk of representing an empyema. In these cases, the decision to perform thoracentesis rests on the size of the effusions and the patient's clinical status. Complex septated or homogeneously echogenic effusions in patients hospitalized with pneumonia carry a higher risk of being infected and usually warrant prompt thoracentesis (Fig. 4.20). Sometimes, homogenous echogenic effusions may be sufficiently echogenic to be mistaken for solid tissue by inexperienced sonographers [46] (Fig. 4.20). In those cases, Doppler imaging showing the lack of blood flow can distinguish loculated echogenic fluid from solid tissue.

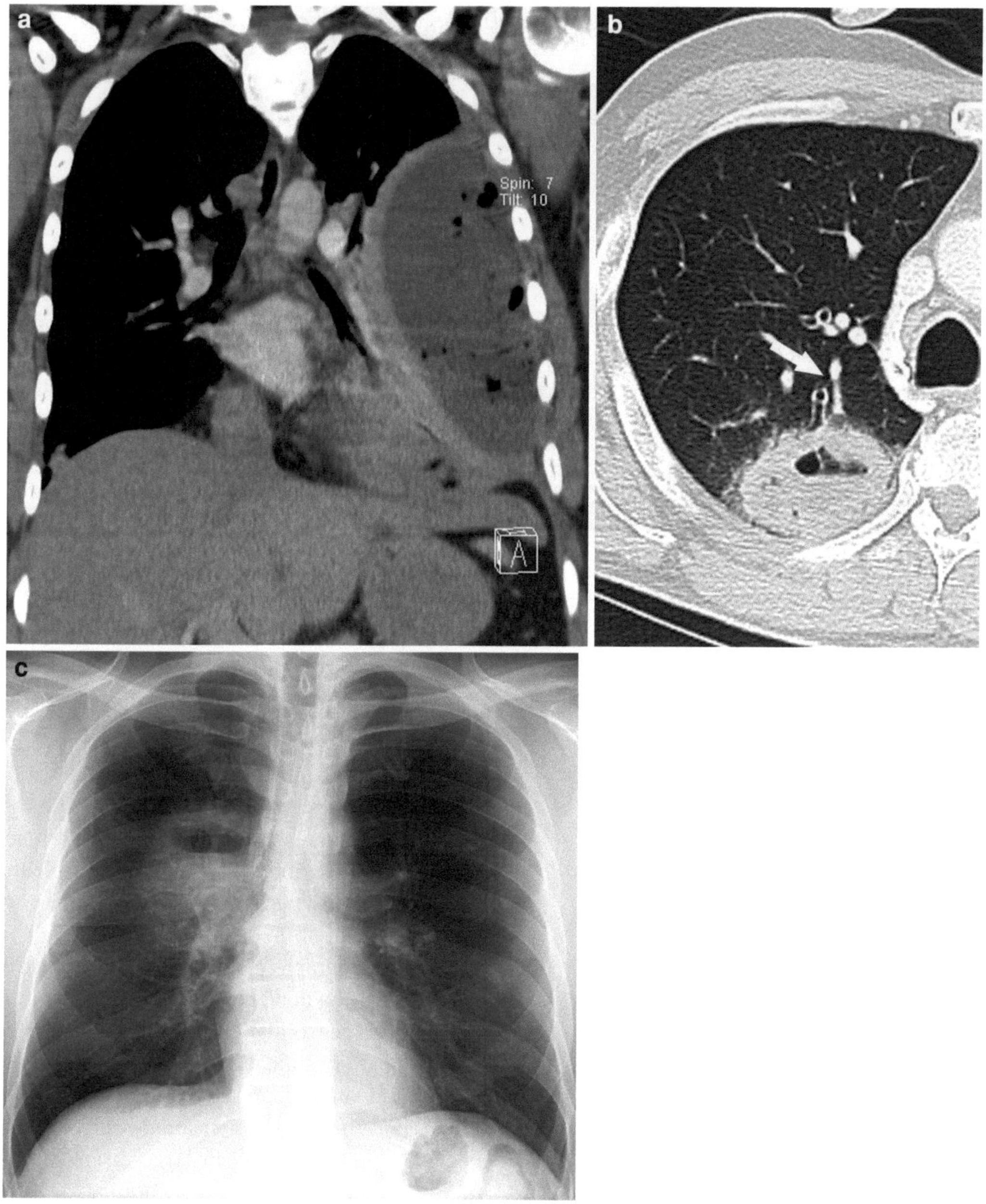

Fig. 4.23 Empyema and lung abscess. **a** Coronal contrast-enhanced CT image shows a loculated effusion containing gas bubbles, indicating empyema. Blood vessels in adjacent lung are deviated away from the lenticular shaped fluid collection. **b** CT of patient with lung abscess shows a bronchus and pulmonary artery (*arrow*) heading directly into the abscess. **c** Chest radiograph confirms that abscess is round in shape rather than lenticular

CT scanning is superior to ultrasound in providing a "global" assessment of multi loculated pleural fluid including paramediastinal collections that do not have a good ultrasonographic window. On CTs performed with intravenous contrast, the pleura enhances in the majority of uninfected parapneumonic effusions and in 85–100% of empyemas [47, 48]. Pleural enhancement is accentuated on delayed images (60–70 s) (Fig. 4.21). Absence of parietal pleural

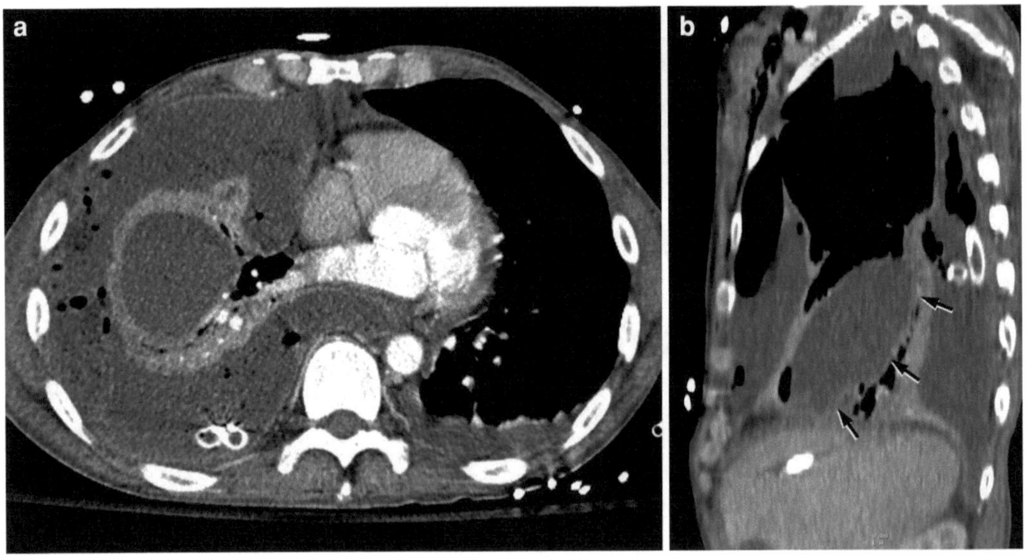

Fig. 4.24 Empyema with component loculated in the major fissure. **a** Axial section appears to show a round fluid collection in the lung that could be mistaken for abscess. **b** Sagittal reconstruction shows that fluid (*arrows*) is instead trapped between the pleural surfaces in the major fissures and has a lenticular shape

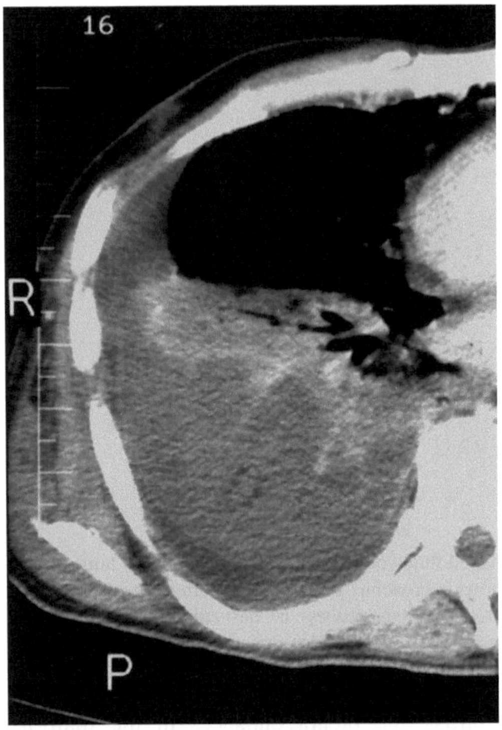

Fig. 4.25 Early lung necrosis. CT images show lung parenchyma that is only slightly greater than adjacent (pleural) fluid attenuation. Small foci of gas within the parenchyma are likely a prelude to abscess formation

enhancement in a properly performed CT argues strongly against the presence of an empyema. Thickening (>2 mm) and increased attenuation of the extrapleural fat may be a more specific sign than pleural enhancement, but only the presence of gas within previously un-instrumented pleural fluid can establish the diagnosis of empyema prior to the sampling of the pleural fluid [48].

Chest radiographs can suggest the presence of lung necrosis by depicting focal lucencies within an area of consolidation. Lucencies scattered within lobar consolidation early in the course of pneumonia often represent underlying emphysema, but their later appearance favors lung necrosis (Fig. 4.22). When large discrete areas of lung become liquefied, forming a lung abscess, distinction from an empyema can be difficult. Empyemas tend to be lenticular shaped, have smooth walls of uniform thickness, and compress adjacent lung such that adjacent bronchi and vessels are displaced around them. In contrast, lung abscesses are usually round; have irregular walls of variable thickness; and, because intervening lung has been destroyed rather than compressed, do not cause as much displacement of nearby bronchi and vessels

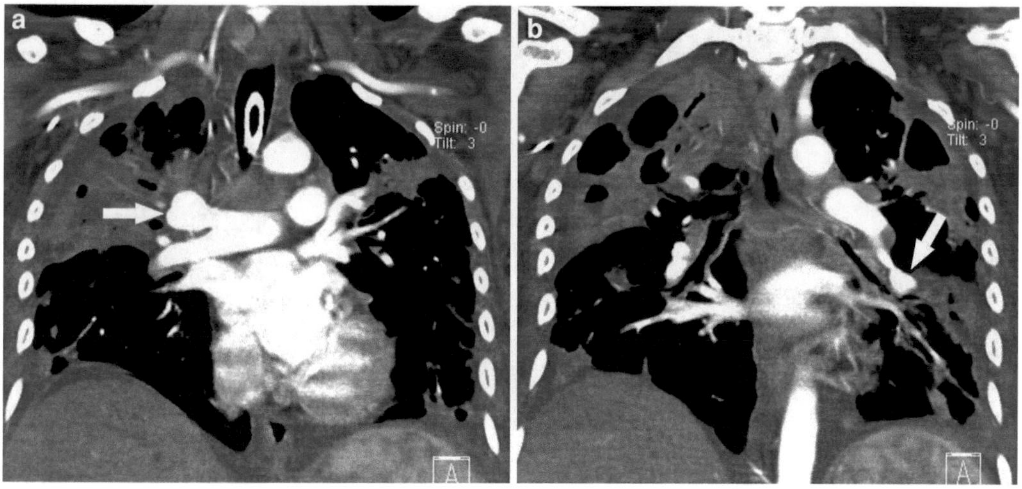

Fig. 4.26 Patient with severe staphylococcal pneumonia and pulmonary artery pseudoaneurysms. **a**, **b** Contrast-enhanced CT image shows pulmonary artery pseudoaneurysms (*arrows*), manifesting as segments of the pulmonary arteries wider than the adjacent proximal vessel

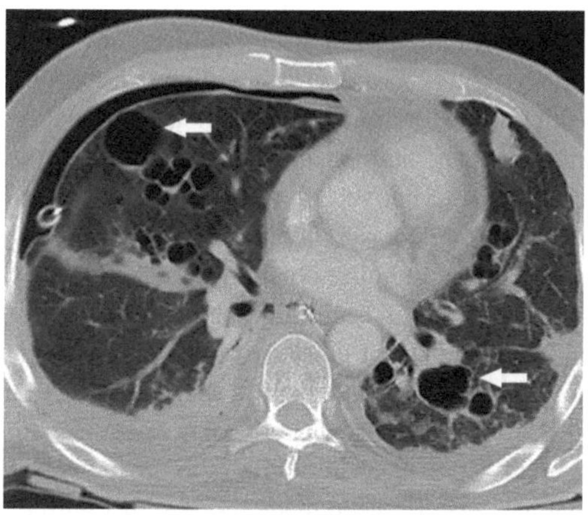

Fig. 4.27 Pneumatoceles resulting from staphylococcal pneumonia. CT image shows multiple thin walled pneumatoceles (*arrows*). One had ruptured into the pleural space causing a right pneumothorax

(Fig. 4.23). Pleural fluid loculated within a major fissure can be particularly difficult to distinguish from an abscess. Multiplanar reconstructions can help prove the intrapleural location of the fluid (Fig. 4.24).

In addition to discrete lung abscesses, contrast-enhanced CT of patients with severe infections may show large geographic areas of non-enhancing lung parenchyma that are sufficiently low in attenuation that margins between lung and adjacent pleural fluid become indistinct (Fig. 4.25). This finding presages frank abscess formation and is a predictor of prolonged hospital stay [49]. In rare cases, necrosis may extend into the pulmonary vasculature resulting in in situ thrombosis of a pulmonary artery or sufficient destruction of the arterial wall to form a pseudoaneurysm. Both complications often require surgical resection, but some cases of pulmonary artery pseudoaneurysm may be amenable to trans-catheter embolization [50] (Fig. 4.26). As necrotic pneumonias are typically caused by anaerobic or staphylococcal infections, the presence of any of the above manifestations of lung necrosis should prompt coverage for these organisms in empiric antibiotic regimens [51].

Focal areas of necrosis most commonly result in lung abscesses; however, pneumatoceles can occur when focal alveolar or bronchiolar necrosis allows air to dissect into the pulmonary parenchyma and create an air cyst. Because this cyst is formed by a ball-valve phenomenon rather than excavation of necrotic tissue, it can enlarge rapidly over several days and cause compression of adjacent structures [52]. Cysts' thin walls also predispose them to rupture into the pleural space, causing pneumothoraces. [53].

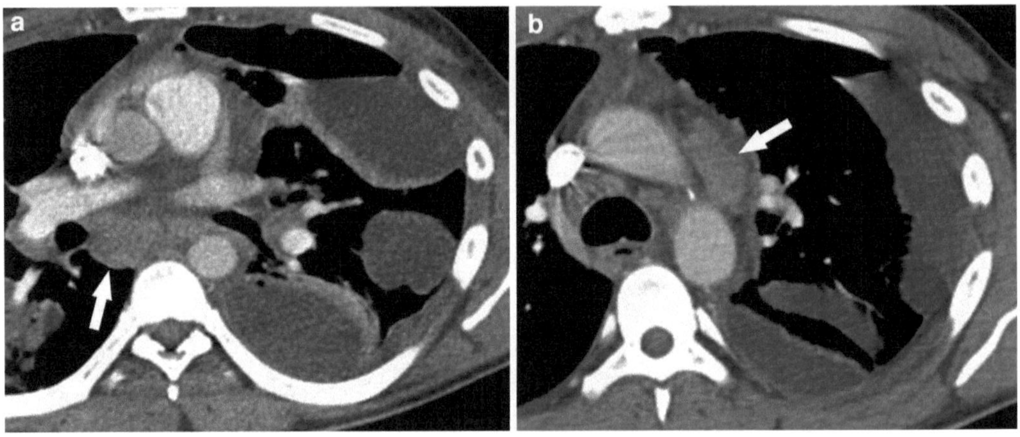

Fig. 4.28 Patient with a multiloculated empyema and lymphadenopathy. **a**, **b** Contrast-enhanced CT images show moderate subcarinal and aortopulmonary window lymph node enlargement (*arrows*)

Pneumatocele formation is more common in children than adults. Although classically associated with staphylococcal infections, it has been reported in pneumococcal and gram-negative bacterial pneumonias (Fig. 4.27).

In addition to pleural effusion and lung parenchymal necrosis, imaging of pneumonia occasionally shows accompanying hilar or mediastinal lymphadenopathy. Lymphadenopathy that is apparent on chest radiography suggests either an underlying disease such neoplasm or sarcoidosis, or a short list of infectious agents that include primary tuberculosis, endemic fungal infections, tularemia, and anthrax. Further evaluation with CT is warranted in these patients. CT detection of modest lymph node enlargement occult on radiography is a non-specific finding. Lymph nodes that exceed normal CT size criteria (1.5 cm short axis in the subcarinal area, 1 cm elsewhere) are found in about half of patients with bacteremic pneumococcal pneumonia or empyema [54] (Fig. 4.28). The enlarged nodes are usually normal in attenuation. Enlarged lymph nodes with low attenuation centers are a much less common finding and in children or HIV infected patients with pneumonia and suggest tuberculosis in a non-immune host. Enlargement of lymph nodes is rare in immunocompetent patients with the destructive fibrocavitary pattern of tuberculosis that has traditionally termed “reactivation“disease [35].

Summary

Diagnostic imaging is useful in detecting pneumonias but is less useful in following response to therapy. Combined with clinical information, imaging can answer questions about the presence of alternative, non-infectious diagnoses, including atelectasis, neoplasm, and pulmonary infarcts. The radiologic pattern of disease, better seen on CT, can sometimes narrow the differential diagnosis of causative pathogens but can only occasionally suggest a specific pathogen. In most cases, identification of a specific pathogen is better answered with laboratory analysis that has recently been made more robust with the use of polymerase chain reactions. Imaging is routinely useful in the identification of complications of pneumonia such as pleural effusions lung necrosis, and lymphadenopathy.

References

1. Boersma WG, Daniels JM, Lowenbery A, Boeve WJ, van de Jaft EJ. Reliability of radiographic findings and the relation to etiologic agents in community acquired pneumonia. Respir Med. 2006;100(5):916–32.
2. Basi SK, Marrie TJ, Huang JQ, Majumdar SR. Patients admitted to the hospital with suspected pneumonia and normal chest radiographs: epidemiologic, microbiology and outcomes. AM J Med. 2004;117(5):305–11.

3. Hopstaken RM, Witbraad T, van Engelshoven JM, Dinant GJ. Inter-observer variation in the interpretation of chest radiographs for pneumonia in community acquired lower respiratory tract infections. Clin Radiol. 2004;59(8):743–52.
4. Woodhead W, Blasi F, Ewig S, et al. Guidelines for the management of adult lower respiratory tract infections. Eur Respir J. 2005;26:1138–80.
5. Albaum MN, Hill LC, Murphy M et al. Interobserver reliability of the chest radiograph in community acquired pneumonia. Chest 1996;110(2):343–50.
6. Bruns AHW, Oosterheert JJ, Prokop M, Lammers JJ, Hak E, Hoepleman AI. Patterns of resolution of chest radiograph abnormalities in adults hospitalized with severe community-acquired pneumonia. Clin Infect Dis. 2007;45:983–91.
7. Bruns AH, Oosterheert JJ, El Moussaoui R, Opmeer HC, Hoepelman AI, Prins JM. Pneumonia recovery; discrepancies in perspectives of the radiologist, physician and patient. J Gen Intern Med. 2009;25(3):203–6.
8. Choi YH, Kim SJ, Lee JY, Pai HJ, Lee KY, Lee YS. Scrub typhus: radiological and clinical findings. Clin Radiol. 2000;55(2):140–4.
9. Boroja M, Barrie JR, Raymond GS. Radiographic findings in 20 patients with Hantavirus pulmonary syndrome correlated with clinical outcome. Am J Roentgenol. 2002;178(1):159–63.
10. Akira M, Ishikawa H, Yamamoto S. Drug-induced pneumonitis:thin-section CT findings in 60 Patients. Radiology 2002;224(3):852–60.
11. Takatani K, Miyazaki E, Nureki S, et al. High-resolution computed tomography patterns and immunopathogenetic findings in drug-induced pneumonitis. Respir Med. 2008;102(6):892–898.
12. Rossi SE, Franquet T, Volpacchio M, Giménez A, Aguilar G. Tree in bud pattern at thin-section CT of the lungs: radiologic-pathologic overview. Radiographics. 2005;25(3):789–801.
13. Okada F, Ando Y, Yoshitake S, Ono A, et al. Clinical/pathologic correlations in 553 patients with primary centrilobular findings on high resolution CT scan of the thorax. Chest. 2007;132(6):1939–48.
14. Raoof S, Amchentsev A, Vlahos I, Goud A, Naidich DP. Pictorial essay: multinodular disease. A high resolution CT scan diagnostic algorithm. Chest 2006;129(3):805–15.
15. Shah RM, Miller W. Widespread ground glass opacity of the lung in consecutive patients undergoing CT: does lobular distribution assist diagnosis? Am J Roentgenol. 2003;180(4):965–8.
16. Shah RM, Friedman AC. CT angiogram sign: incidence and significance in lobar consolidations evaluated by contrast-enhanced CT. Am J Roentgenol. 1998;170(3):719–21.
17. Jung JI, Kim H, Park SH, et al. CT differentiation of pneumonic-type bronchoalveolar cell carcinoma and infectious pneumonia. Br J Radiol. 2001;74(882): 490–4.
18. Kim TH, Kim SJ, Ryu YH, et al. Differentiation of CT features of infectious pneumonia versus bronchioloalveolar carcinoma (BAC) mimicking pneumonia Eur Radio. 2006;16(8):1763–8.
19. Anton E. A frequent error in etiology of round pneumonia. Chest. 2004;125(4):1592–3.
20. Revel M-P, Triki R, Chatellier G, et al. Is it possible to recognize pulmonary infarction on multisection CT images? Radiology. 2007;244(3):875–82.
21. Reittner P, Ward S, Heyneman L, Johkoh T, Muller NL. Pneumonia: high resolution CT findings in 114 patients. Eur Radiol. 2003;13(3):515–21.
22. Lee I, Kim TS, Yoon HK. Mycoplasma pneumoniae pneumonia: CT features in 16 patients. Eur Radiol. 2006;16(3):719–25.
23. Ito I, Ishida T, Togashi K, Niimi A, et al. Differentiation of bacterial and non-bacterial community-acquired pneumonia by thin-section computed tomography. Eur J Radiol. 2009;72(3);388–95.
24. Miyashita N, Kawai Y, Yamaguchi T, Ouchi K, Oka M. A typical pathogen study group clinical potential of diagnostic methods for the rapid diagnosis of mycoplasma pneumoniae pneumonia in adults. Eur J Clin Microbiol Infect Dis. 2011;30(3):439–46.
25. Okada F, Ando Y, Tanoue S, et al. Radiographic findings in acute Haemophilus influenza pulmonary infection. Br J Radiol. [Epub ahead of print: 11 Jan, 2011].
26. Nambu A, Saito A, Araki T, et al. Chlamydia pneumonia: comparison with findings of mycoplasma pneumonia and streptococcus pneumoniae at thin-section CT. Radiology. 2006;238(1):330–8.
27. Jennings LC, Anderson TP, Beynon KA, et al. Incidence and characteristics of viral community acquired pneumonia in adults. Thorax. 2008;63(1):42–8.
28. Johansson N, Kalin M, Annika Tiveljung-Lindell A, Giske CG, Hedlund J. Etiology of community-acquired pneumonia: increased microbiological yield with new diagnostic methods. Clin Infect Dis. 2010;50(2):202–9.
29. Shiley KT, Van Deerlin VM, Miller WT Jr., Chest CT features of community-acquired respiratory viral infections in adult inpatients with lower respiratory tract infections. J Thorac Imaging. 2010;25(1):68–75.
30. Lewis PF, Schmidt MA, Lu X, et al. A community-based outbreak of severe respiratory illness caused by human adenovirus serotype 14. J Infect Dis. 2009;199(10):1427–34.
31. Ajlan A, Quiney B, Nicolaou S, Muller N. Swine-origin influenza A (H1N1) viral infection: radiographic and CT findings. Am J Roentgenol. 2009;193(6):1494–9.
32. Elicker B, Schwartz B, Liu C, et al. Thoracic CT findings of novel influenza A (H1N1) infection in immunocompromised patients. Emerg Radiol. 2010;17(4):299–307.
33. Monsalvo AC, Batalle JP, Lopez MF, et al. Severe pandemic 2009 H1N1 influenza disease due to pathogenic immune complexes. Nat Med. 2011;17(2): 195–9.

34. Im JG, Itoh H, Shim YS, et al. Pulmonary tuberculosis: CT findings–early active disease and sequential change with anti-tuberculous therapy. Radiology. 1993;186(3):656–60.
35. Leung AN. Pulmonary tuberculosis: the essentials. Radiology. 1999;210(2):307–32.
36. Jeong YJ, Lee KS. Pulmonary tuberculosis: up to date imaging and management. AM J Roentgenol. 2008;191(3):834–44.
37. Andronikou S, Vanhoenacker FM, De Backer A. Advances in imaging chest tuberculosis: blurring of differences between children and adults. Clin Chest Med. 2009;30(4):717–44.
38. Lee SW, Jang YS, Park CM, et al. The role of chest CT scanning in TB outbreak investigation. Chest. 2010;137(5):1057–64.
39. Ors F, Deniz O, Bozlar U, et al. High resolution CT findings in patients with pulmonary tuberculosis: correlation with degree of smear positivity. J Thorac Imaging. 2007;22(2):154–9.
40. Martinez, S, McAdams HP, Batchu CS. The many faces of pulmonary non-tuberculous mycobacterial infection. AM J Roentgenol. 2007;189(1):177–86.
41. Koh WJ, Lee KS, Kwon OJ, Jeong YJ, Kwak SH, Kim TS. Bilateral bronchiectasis and bronchiolitis at thin section CT: diagnostic implications in nontuberculous mycobacterial pulmonary infection. Radiology. 2005;235(1):282–8.
42. Banker PD, Jain VR, Hamarati LB. Impact of chest CT on the clinical management of immunocompetent emergency department patients with chest radiographic findings of pneumonia. Emerg Radiol. 2007;14:383–8.
43. Johnson JL. Pleurisy, fever, and rapidly progressive pleural effusion in a healthy, 29-year-old physician. Chest. 2001;119(4):1266–9.
44. Kearney SE, Davies CW, Davies RJ, Gleeson FV. Computed tomography and ultrasound in parapneumonic effusions and empyema. Clin Radiol. 2000;55(7):542–7.
45. Heffner JE, Klein JS, Hampson C. Diagnostic utility and clinical application of imaging for pleural space infections. Chest. 2010;137(2):467–79.
46. Tu CY, Hsu WH, Hsia TC. Pleural effusions in febrile medical ICU patients: chest ultrasound study. Chest. 2004;126(4):1274–80.
47. Arenas-Jimenez J, Alonso-Charterina S, Sanchez-Paya J, Fernandez-Latorre F, Gil-Sanchez S, Lloret-Llorens M. Evaluation of CT findings for diagnosis of pleural effusions. Eur Radiol. 2000;10(4):681–90.
48. Smolikov A, Smolyakova R, Riesenberg K, et al. Prevalence and clinical significance of pleural microbubbles in computed tomography of thoracic empyema. Clin Radiol. 2006;61(6):513–9.
49. Donnelly LF, Klosterman LA. Pneumonia in children: decreased parenchymal contrast enhancement—CT sign of intense illness and impending cavitary necrosis. Radiology. 1997;205(3):817–20.
50. Mody GN, Lau CL, Bhalla S, et al. Mycotoic pulmonary artery pseudoaneurysm. J Thorac Imaging. 2005;20(4):310–2.
51. Bartlett JG. Anaerobic bacterial infections of the lung and pleural space. Clin Infect Dis. 1993;Suppl 4:S248–55.
52. Hunt JP, Buechter KJ, Fakhry SM. Acinetobacter calcoaceticus pneumonia and the formation of pneumatoceles. J Trauma. 2000;48(5):964–70.
53. McGarry T, Giosa R, Rohman M, Huang CT. Pneumatocele formation in adult pneumonia. Chest 1987;92(4):717–20.
54. Stein DL, Haramati LB, Spindola-Franco H, Friedman J, Klapper PJ. Intrathoracic lymphadenopathy in hospitalized patients with pneumococcal pneumonia. Chest. 2005;127(4):1271–5.

Pulmonary Infections in the Immunocompromised Host

5

Jean W. Kuriakose and Barry H. Gross

Abstract

Immunosuppressed patients are at high risk of developing fulminant, multiple, and recurrent infections. Some organisms are more common than others in this group of patients. Early diagnosis is essential for prompt, complete treatment. Imaging with high-resolution chest CT (HRCT) is a valuable diagnostic tool that may guide therapy. We discuss the imaging characteristics of the common organisms in the immunocompromised host as well as noninfectious causes that can have similar imaging features.

Keywords

Infection · Immunosuppressed · Atypical infections · HIV · Post transplant · Fungal infections · Kaposi's sarcoma · Post-transplant lymphoma

Immunocompromised host describes a patient who is at increased risk for life-threatening infection as a consequence of an abnormal immune system. Immunosuppression can be congenital, acquired, or iatrogenic. Congenital conditions are often the result of to T cell, B cell, or combined defects; macrophage; cytokine; complement defects, or combinations of defects. Most patients present at birth or in childhood [1]. Acquired conditions include HIV infection, chronic illness, alcoholism, drug abuse, and malnutrition. These may interfere with the immune system; trauma or burns may disrupt barrier functions.

Iatrogenic causes include therapies such as cytotoxic drugs and radiation therapy. Cytotoxic agents cause mucositis of the gastrointestinal tract, allowing gram-negative enteric bacteria to invade the intestinal wall and enter the circulation. Furthermore, these agents can cause neutropenia and monocytopenia. TNF-alpha inhibitors, monoclonal antibodies, and corticosteroids decrease the number of circulating lymphocytes and monocytes and inhibit phagocytosis and the activity of lymphocytes, especially T cells.

J. W. Kuriakose (✉)
Department of Radiology, University of Michigan Medical Center, 1500 E. Medical Center Drive, Room #TC B1 132, Ann Arbor, MI 48109-5302, USA
e-mail: jeankuri@med.umich.edu

B. H. Gross
Department of Radiology, University of Michigan Hospitals, 1500 E. Medical Center Drive, UHB1D530G, Ann Arbor, MI 48105, USA

J. P. Kanne (ed.), *Clinically Oriented Pulmonary Imaging*,
Respiratory Medicine, DOI: 10.1007/978-1-61779-542-8_5,

The population of immunocompromised hosts has expanded enormously because of immunosuppressive infections like human immunodeficiency virus (HIV), use of corticosteroids, and other immunosuppressive agents for the treatment of malignancy and collagen vascular disease, and increasing organ transplants with the resultant necessity of preventing organ rejection [2, 3]. Half of bone marrow transplant recipients and 80% of leukemic patients will develop pneumonia [4]. The role of the radiologist is to identify infection in these patients, to suggest further evaluation with HRCT when appropriate, to guide bronchoscopy or targeted biopsy, and to evaluate treatment response.

Duration and Severity of Immunocompromise

A variety of organisms cause pneumonia in transplant recipients and immunosuppressed patients. Factors that predispose the host to pneumonia include tissue ischemia during transplantation, causing damage to the mucosa and eroding its effectiveness as a barrier; impaired cough reflex; and interruption of lymphatic drainage. Lung transplant recipients are particularly susceptible to pneumonia, and infection is the most common cause of death in these patients [5, 6]. Risk factors include those related not only to the immunosuppressive therapy but also to the direct exposure of the graft to infectious agents in the atmosphere.

There are distinct periods of susceptibility to specific pathogens after chemotherapy for cancer and after bone marrow or other transplantation, so information about the duration of immunosuppression is helpful in narrowing the differential diagnosis of pneumonia [7–9]. In a patient with cancer who is neutropenic because of cytotoxic chemotherapy, major infection in the initial few days after therapy is usually caused by ordinary pathogens like gram-negative bacteria or *Staphylococcus aureus*. After 2 weeks of neutropenia, the likelihood of fungal infection, especially *Aspergillus*-related pneumonia, increases [7, 9].

In solid organ transplant recipients, 95% of infections that occur within one month after transplantation involve the same pathogenic organisms as those in noncompromised patients who have undergone thoracic or abdominal operations other than transplantation. Pulmonary infections during this period include aspiration pneumonia caused by oral flora or gram-negative bacilli and septic emboli caused by indwelling intravenous catheters.

From 1 to 6 months after transplantation, viruses such as cytomegalovirus (CMV), Epstein-Barr virus (EBV), and herpes simplex virus are potential causes of lung infection. These viruses can impair immunity and can predispose to opportunistic pneumonia caused by bacteria, *Pneumocystis*, or fungus.

Beyond 6 months after transplantation, 75% of patients who have adequate graft function develop infection only occasionally, and infections tend to be the same as those in the non-transplant population. The 10% of patients who have impaired graft function and require high levels of immunosuppressive therapy are at high risk for opportunistic infection. The 5% of patients who have chronic viral infection may develop organ failure or malignancy like post-transplant lymphoproliferative disorder, which is associated with EBV infection [10].

Nosocomial Infections

Half of nosocomial pneumonias in immunocompromised patients are caused by anaerobic gram-negative bacilli like *Pseudomonas aeruginosa* (Fig. 5.1), *Escherichia coli, Enterobacter, Klebsiella*, and *Acinetobacter* species [11]. Colonization of the oropharynx is promoted by endotracheal intubation, use of antibiotics, acute immunosuppressive therapy, and the presence of aphthous ulcers. Reduced gastric acidity allows bacteria to proliferate in the stomach. Subsequently, these bacteria colonize the oropharynx

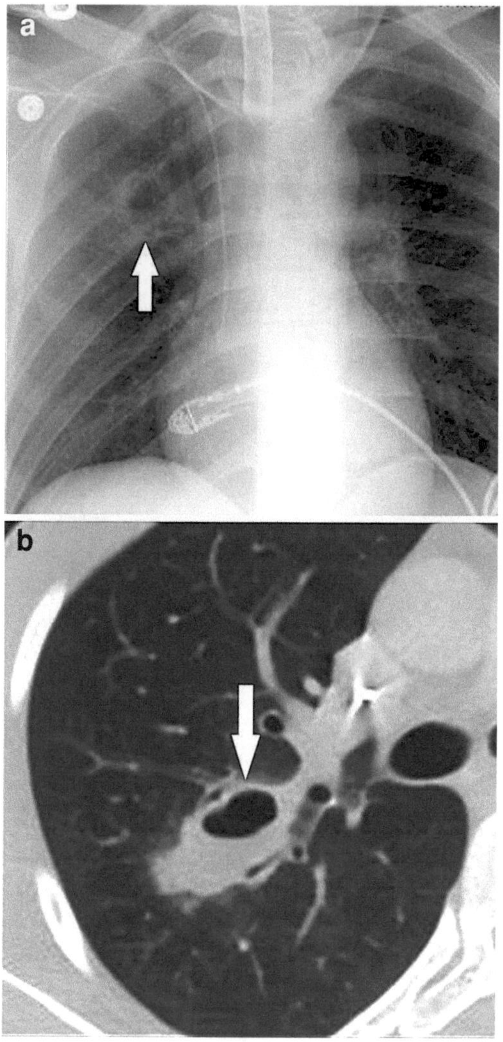

Fig. 5.1 *Pseudomonas* pneumonia resulting from aspiration. AP radiograph (**a**) and CT image (**b**) show a cavitary lesion (*arrows*) in the right upper lobe

and can be aspirated into the lungs [12]. Moisture on hospital appliances and in ventilating ducts can provide a medium for *Legionella* species and other gram-negative bacteria that cause pneumonia. Patients who are on mechanical ventilators are particularly vulnerable. Indwelling intravenous catheters increase the risk of septicemia. Catheter infection with *Staphylococcus aureus, Pseudomonas aeruginosa,* or *Candida* species can lead to septic pulmonary emboli.

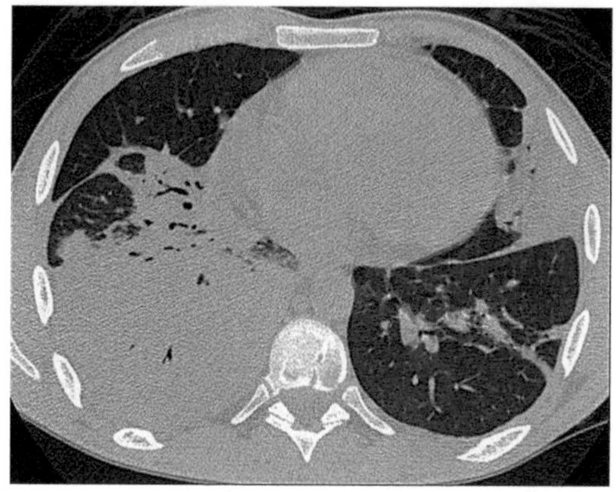

Fig. 5.2 Adrenal insufficiency secondary to corticosteroid therapy with chronic pneumonia, likely from *Burkholderia*. CT image shows dense consolidation in both lungs

Imaging Appearances of Pulmonary Infections in the Immunosuppressed

Early diagnosis and treatment of pulmonary infections is critical in immunosuppressed patients because infections in these patients can progress rapidly. Radiographic findings are often nonspecific and may not be apparent until later in the course of disease. Several studies have shown that HRCT is the most sensitive imaging method to detect early lung findings in immunocompromised patients with acute pulmonary diseases [13–20]. HRCT may detect disease not seen on radiographs, may depict features characteristic or suggestive of a specific disease, and may assist in guiding biopsy.

Lung Consolidation and Ground-Glass Opacity

Multifocal ground-glass opacity and consolidation without a lobar predilection are the primary radiographic and CT findings (Fig. 5.2). Pathologically, areas of consolidation have been shown to represent areas of bronchopneumonia, intra-alveolar hemorrhage, and alveolar edema, with diffuse alveolar septal thickening, exudates, and hyaline membranes. Superimposed multiple or recurrent infections are also possible. Cavitation may result from necrosis (Fig. 5.3),

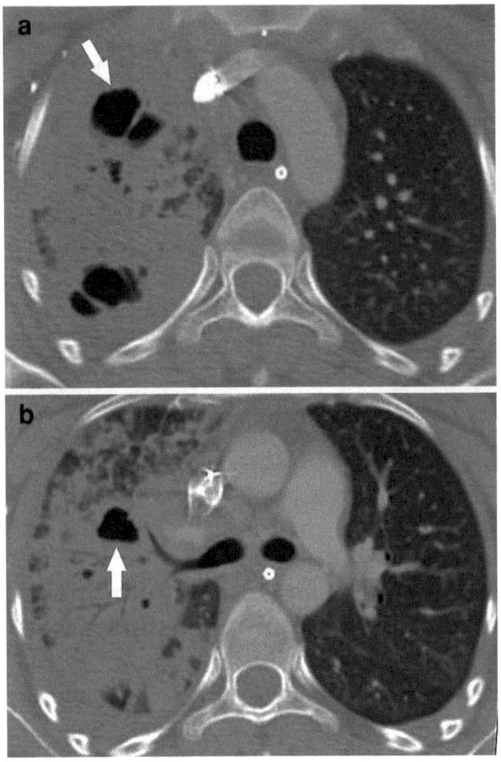

Fig. 5.3 Patient from northern Michigan with adrenal insufficiency and blastomycosis with necrotizing pneumonia. **a**-**b**. Contrast-enhanced CT images show dense right lung consolidation with foci of cavitation (*arrows*)

associated bacterial infection, or hemorrhagic lung infarcts.

Tree-in-Bud Opacities

Small-airway infection leads to inflammatory changes in the walls of bronchioles, resulting in airway wall thickening and dilatation [21, 22]. CT findings of infectious bronchiolitis consist of centrilobular nodules and tree-in-bud opacities. Tree-in-bud opacities are small Y- and V-shaped opacities typically located in the lung periphery and represent bronchioles impacted with inflammatory secretions (Fig. 5.4). Although bacteria are the most common cause of infectious bronchiolitis, in immunocompromised patients, mycobacterial, viral, and fungal organisms can also give this appearance [23–26].

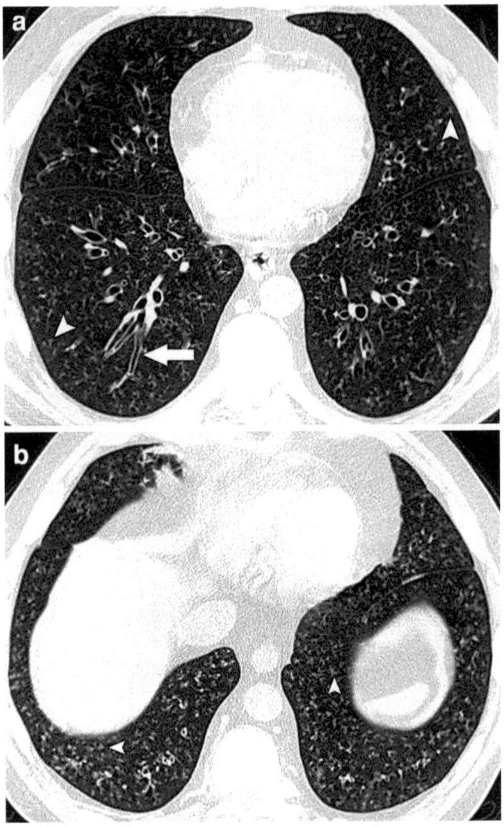

Fig. 5.4 Renal transplant recipient with pulmonary nocardiosis. **a**-**b**. HRCT images show diffuse tree-in-bud opacities (*arrowheads*) and mild bronchial dilation (*arrow*)

Nodules and the CT Halo Sign

Nodules are a common presentation of atypical infection and are often seen in fungal infections. Well-defined granulomas and pulmonary nodules correlate pathologically to localized colonies. Microscopically, the lung parenchyma may also be edematous with hyaline membrane formation and cellular fibromyxoid organizing air-space exudates, similar to those of acute respiratory distress syndrome.

The CT halo sign describes a nodule surrounded by a discrete area of ground-glass opacity. Histological correlation shows that the dense core of the nodules corresponds to a zone of coagulative necrosis from pseudohyphae (as in *Candida* growing from a thrombosed blood

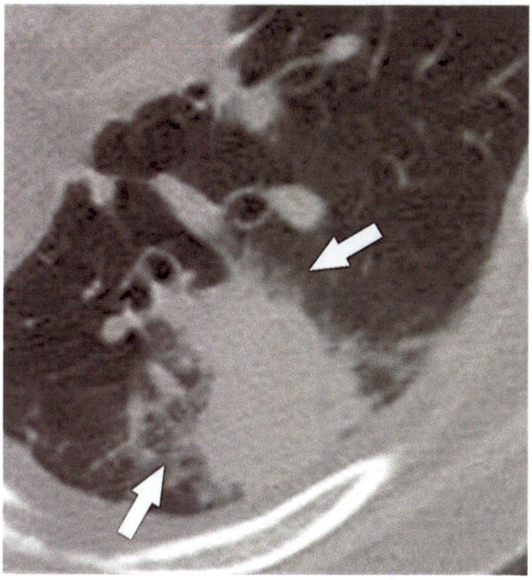

Fig. 5.5 Adenovirus infection in bone marrow transplant recipient. CT image shows an irregular nodule with surrounding ground-glass opacity (*arrows*), characteristic of the CT halo sign

vessel lumen), and the halo corresponds to a mixture of edema and hemorrhage surrounding the infarct. This sign was initially described as being characteristic of invasive aspergillosis [27], but the CT halo sign has now been shown to occur in association with hemorrhagic nodules of varying causes including candidiasis; CMV; herpes simplex virus; adenovirus; coccidioidomycosis; nocardiosis (Figs. 5.5, 5.6); non-hemorrhagic infections such as actinomycosis; and some noninfectious causes such as metastatic angiosarcoma, Kaposi sarcoma, pulmonary hemorrhage, and Wegener granulomatosis [28, 29].

Pulmonary Disease in HIV

Pulmonary infections are often the initial clinical manifestation of HIV infection. Infections in HIV, as in other causes of immunosuppression, are severe, associated with a high burden of organisms, and often disseminated; recurrent and multiple infections are common (Figs. 5.7, 5.8) [30, 31]. Many opportunistic pulmonary infections in HIV-infected patients result from endogenous reactivation of previously acquired organisms, and the prevalence of infectious agents reflects that of the local population. The most common communicable pulmonary infection is tuberculosis. Severe bacterial pneumonias are more prevalent in HIV-infected persons. In patients with AIDS, the frequency and causes of pneumonia reflect the CD4+ cell count, which is an indicator of the severity of immunocompromise. In patients with CD4+ cell counts higher than 200 cells per mm^3, bacteria like *Streptococcus pneumoniae, Hemophilus influenzae, Staphylococcus aureus,* and *Mycobacterium tuberculosis* are the typical causes of pulmonary infection. With CD4+ cell counts lower than 200 cells per mm^3, *Pneumocystis jiroveci* pneumonia and disseminated tuberculosis are common. With very low CD4+ cell counts (<100 cells per mm^3), infections with CMV, nontuberculous mycobacteria, and fungi increase (Chart 5.1) [32, 33].

Fungal, parasitic, and viral infections in HIV-infected individuals can be controlled but are often difficult to eradicate. Thus, patients may require long-term therapy. Pneumonia and respiratory failure are the most common causes of death in the late stages of HIV infection (see Chart 5.1).

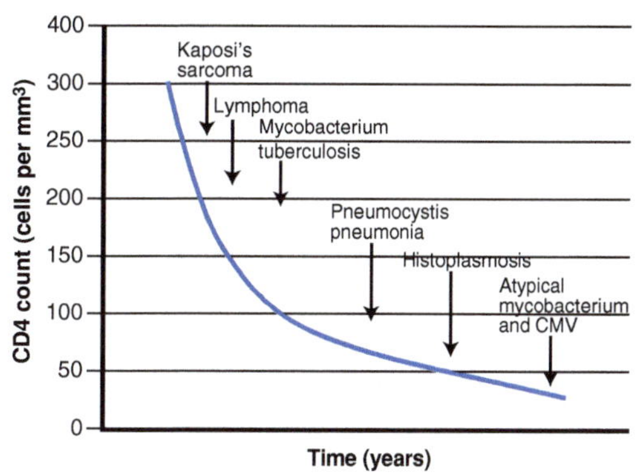

Chart 5.1 The natural history of HIV infection and CD4+ cell count decline and the occurrence of opportunistic infections and cancer

Bacterial Pneumonias in HIV

Bacterial pneumonia is the most common pulmonary complication of AIDS. Children with HIV infection and AIDS have a higher incidence

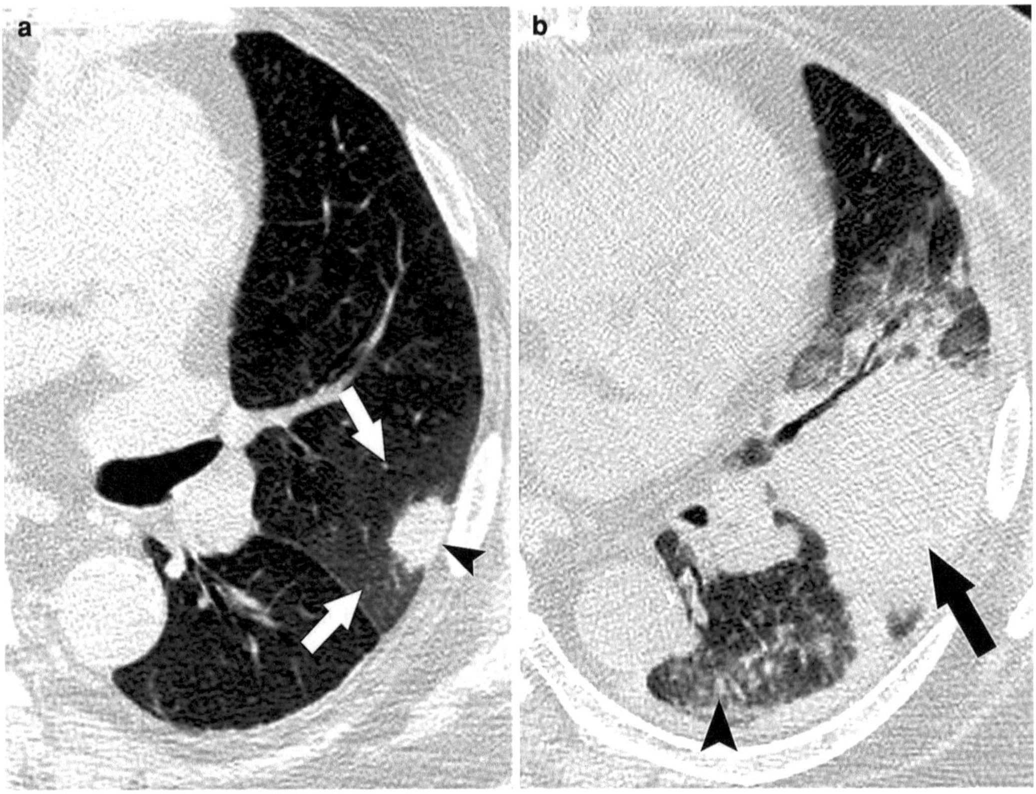

Fig. 5.6 Pulmonary nocardiosis. **a** CT image shows an irregular nodule (*arrowhead*) in the left upper lobe with a halo of ground-glass opacity (*arrows*). **b** CT image shows focal left lower lobe consolidation (*arrow*) and small nodules (*arrowhead*)

of bacterial pneumonia than HIV-infected adults. The most common causes of bacterial pneumonia in HIV-infected patients are *Streptococcus pneumoniae*, *Hemophilus influenzae*, and *Staphylococcus aureus*. Pneumococcal pneumonia is 5–6 times more common in HIV-infected individuals than in non-HIV infected individuals. Bacterial pneumonias and upper respiratory tract infections like sinusitis and bronchitis can occur at any time in the course of HIV illness but occur more frequently as HIV advances and the CD4+ cell count declines. *S. aureus* cavitary pneumonia often occurs late in the course of HIV infection. Bronchiectasis is more common in HIV-infected patients, most likely the result of recurrent and subclinical infections.

The signs and symptoms of acute bacterial pneumonia in patients with AIDS are similar to those in the non-HIV-infected patient. Failure to respond to antimicrobial therapy should raise the question of development of complications such as empyema, lung abscess, or superimposed opportunistic infection [34].

Tuberculosis

The incidence of TB has been increasing in the US since 1986, as many cases occur in patients co-infected with HIV; it is estimated that 6,000–9,000 new cases of TB in HIV occur annually in the US [35, 36]. Most cases result from reactivation of infection in the setting of waning cell-mediated immunity with progressive HIV disease. Without HIV, the lifetime risk of developing reactivation TB is 5–10%. In contrast,

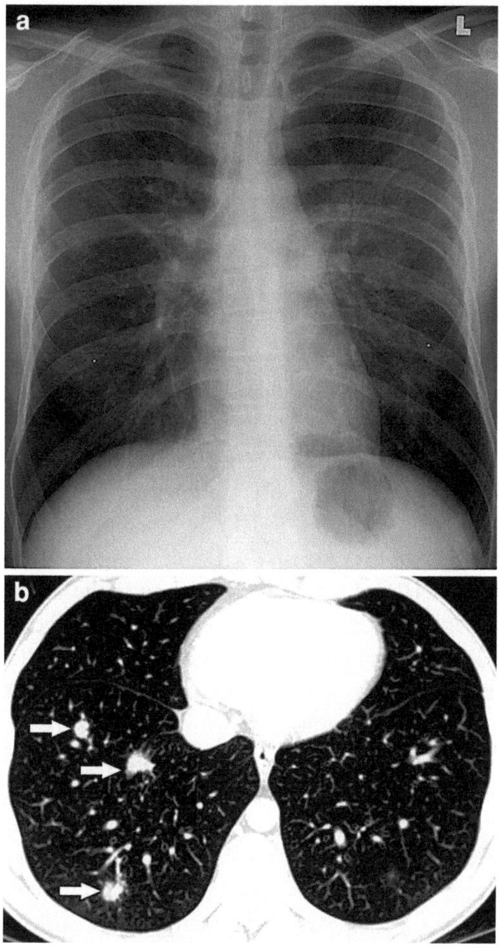

Fig. 5.7 Opportunistic infections in AIDS. **a** PA radiograph shows bilateral perihilar hazy opacities proven to reflect *Pneumocystis jiroveci* pneumonia. **b** CT scan 3 months later shows new nodules (*arrows*), which were proven to represent. *M. Kansasii* infection

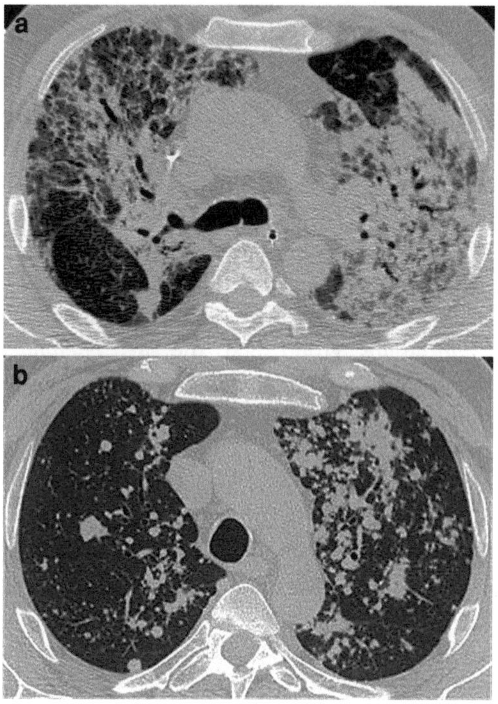

Fig. 5.8 Opportunistic infections with CLL and hypogammaglobulinemia. **a** HRCT image shows extensive consolidation and ground-glass opacity reflecting rituximab pulmonary toxicity and superimposed *P. jiroveci* pneumonia. **b** HRCT image obtained several months later shows numerous new lung nodules from histoplasmosis

patients with HIV and previous tuberculosis have an annual risk of up to 8% for developing reactivation TB. The rate is higher in endemic areas and in intravenous drug abusers.

The CD4+ cell count also affects the radiological features of tuberculosis. In the early stages of AIDS, the radiological findings are usually those of reactivation tuberculosis with apical fibrocavitary disease, whereas in patients with advanced immunocompromise, the findings are those of primary tuberculosis with focal consolidation and multiple nodules, including a miliary pattern of diffuse tiny lung nodules. Cavitation is rare at this stage. The presence of intrathoracic low attenuation lymph nodes or the appearance of a sudden large pleural effusion in a patient with AIDS is suggestive of pulmonary TB [37].

Diagnosis is made by demonstrating acid-fast bacilli (AFB) in smears of deep respiratory secretions and isolating *M. tuberculosis* in culture. It is not possible to distinguish *M. tuberculosis* from other mycobacteria on the basis of smear alone, and the diagnosis is often confirmed by gene probe analysis. Treatment is similar to patients who are not HIV infected. However, because relapse rates are higher in patients with HIV infection, a longer course of therapy may be required.

Nontuberculous Mycobacteria

Nontuberculous mycobacteria (NTM) are obligate aerobes found in the environment in soil, water, vegetables, domestic animals, and dairy products. NTM are classified based on their growth rates. Rapidly growing NTM are categorized into pigmented and non-pigmented species. Non-pigmented NTM includes the *M. fortuitum* group and the *M. chelonae/abscessus* group. The pigmented species are rarely associated with clinical infections [38].

In AIDS patients, infection is often encountered when the CD4+ cell count falls below 50 cells/mm^3 [33]. Imaging findings vary and include consolidation, lung nodules, and hilar lymph node enlargement. Cavitation is rare. The radiological appearances can be similar to *M. tuberculosis*. A normal chest radiograph is more common with NTM than in TB. Miliary disease is particularly uncommon with NTM, and lymphadenopathy is usually less florid than encountered with TB at the same stage of immunosuppression. Endobronchial disease with NTM infection is common and causes a tree-in-bud appearance on HRCT. Diagnosis is made usually by examination of bronchoalveolar lavage fluid.

Pneumocystis Jiroveci Pneumonia

Pneumocystis jiroveci was formerly considered to be protozoan but is now classified as a fungus. The environmental reservoir is unknown, but 90% of individuals have antibodies to *P. jiroveci* by age four, suggesting that infection commonly occurs in early childhood. Transmission is airborne, and the disease is almost exclusively limited to the respiratory system. The organism grows within the alveoli in great numbers, and the alveoli become filled with amorphous foamy eosinophilic exudates containing both cysts and trophozoites of the organism. This contributes to severe hypoxemia as the disease progresses [39].

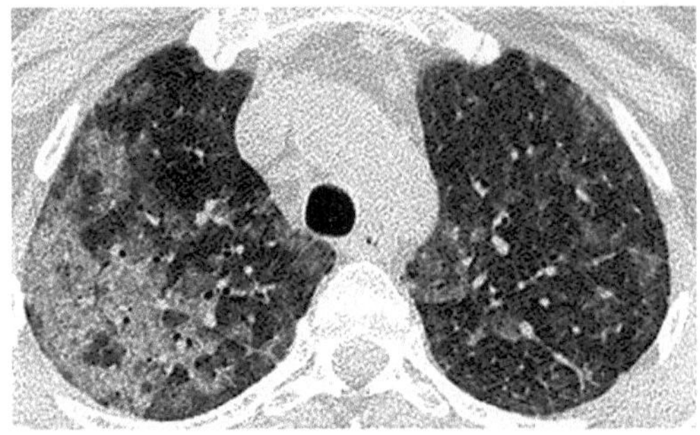

Fig. 5.9 *P. jiroveci* pneumonia in a patient on corticosteroids for seronegative inflammatory arthritis. HRCT image shows patchy lung consolidation and ground-glass opacity

P. jiroveci is the most common opportunistic pulmonary infection in HIV-infected individuals in the US and is the first AIDS-defining illness in 65% of HIV-infected persons despite the use of specific prophylaxis. *P. jiroveci* pneumonia (PJP) is an infection of later stages of HIV infection and seldom occurs with a CD4+ cell count >200 per mm^3.

In contrast to the acute respiratory illness encountered in non-AIDS immunocompromised patients, patients with AIDS and PJP typically present with a 2–6 week history of intermittent fever, non-productive cough, and progressive dyspnea on exertion. Physical examination of the thorax is often unremarkable, though a few fine crackles or wheezes may be heard. Productive cough, purulent sputum, rigors, and pleuritic chest pain are uncommon, and their presence should raise the question of an alternative diagnosis. The most important prognostic factor is the degree of hypoxemia at the time of diagnosis. The chest radiograph is normal in 10–30% of affected patients. The most common radiographic findings include diffuse perihilar haze or patchy perihilar consolidation (Fig. 5.9). Occasionally, nodules or lobar consolidation are present. Pleural effusion is rare. A necrotizing subpleural vasculitis can occur, leading to localized air cyst formation and pneumothorax [40]. Diagnosis is made by demonstrating the organism in respiratory tract secretions or lung tissue, as the organism cannot be cultured.

Fungal Pneumonia

The frequency of endemic mycotic infections in HIV depends on exposure to the organism and the prevalence of infection in the population. *Cryptococcus neoformans* is the most common deep fungal infection. It is found worldwide. Disseminated histoplasmosis is common in the Midwestern US (Ohio River Valley and Mississippi River Valley areas). *Coccidioides immitis* infections occur in the dry desert regions of the Southwestern US. Radiographic and CT findings are non-specific. However, nodules are common and may be single or multiple, sometimes occurring in a miliary pattern. Focal and lobar consolidation, pleural effusions, and lymph node enlargement are other manifestations of infection. Cavitation can occur in the nodules or foci of consolidation.

Cryptococcosis

Cryptococcosis neoformans is a dimorphic yeast found worldwide in soil, bird droppings, and decaying fruits. Infection is usually produced by inhalation of spores. The pulmonary phase of infection is typically clinically silent, and patients most often present with disseminated disease with meningitis. Chest radiographic findings include localized pulmonary consolidation with or without cavitation [41]. Diagnosis is established by examination of the CSF by India ink preparations, culture and assay of CSF, and detecting serum cryptococcal antigen. Initial treatment with amphotericin B, followed by lifelong chronic suppressive therapy with intermittent amphotericin B, fluconazole, or itraconazole is required, as the probability of relapse is extremely high.

Histoplasmosis

Histoplasmosis capsulatum grows in soil and material containing bat or bird droppings. The fungus has been found in poultry houses, caves, bird roosts, attics, basements, and construction sites. The fungus becomes airborne when contaminated soil is disturbed, and the organism can be inhaled. Outbreaks of histoplasmosis have occurred in areas where the fungus is known to live; from contact with bird, chicken, or bat droppings; or from recently disturbed contaminated soil such as at a construction site.

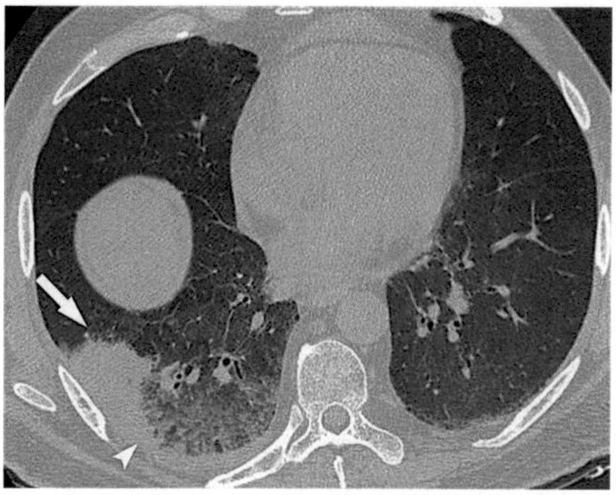

Fig. 5.10 Histoplasmosis. HRCT image shows focal dense consolidation (*arrow*) in the right lower lobe with adjacent ground-glass opacity. A small right pleural effusion (*arrowhead*) is present

Infection can occur at any age. Chronic pulmonary histoplasmosis occurs more often in older men and can mimic tuberculosis [42]. Most patients with acute histoplasmosis are asymptomatic. Symptoms, when they occur, usually develop 3–17 days after exposure and typically reflect mild respiratory or flu-like illness. Disseminated disease occurs primarily in immunosuppressed patients including those with HIV. Imaging findings are generally indistinguishable from other pneumonias (Fig. 5.10), although lung nodules and lymphadenopathy are more common than with bacterial pneumonia. Diagnosis of histoplasmosis requires bone marrow biopsy or culture, blood culture, or lung biopsy. Antigen testing of bronchoalveolar lavage or urine and antibody testing in serum are helpful adjuvants in diagnosis. Initial treatment is systemic amphotericin B, followed by chronic suppressive therapy with itraconazole.

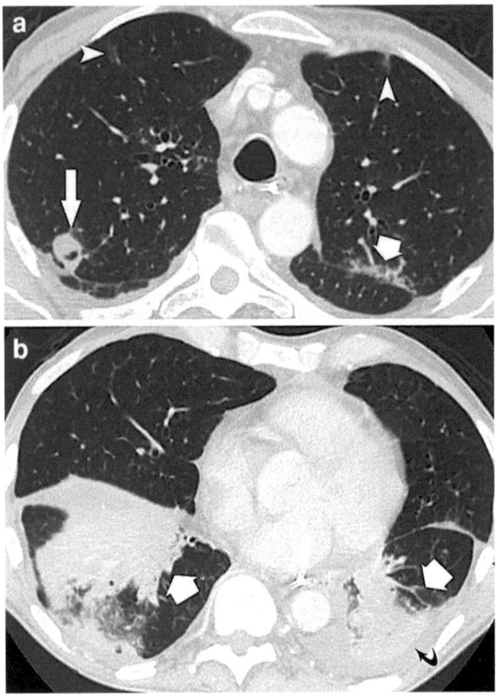

Fig. 5.11 a, b, c Chronic coccidioidomycosis pneumonia from pancytopenia resulting by leukemic bone marrow infiltration. **a-b** CT images show a cavitary nodule (*thin arrow*) in the right upper lobe, patchy foci of ground-glass opacity (*arrowheads*), and foci of lung consolidation (*wide arrows*). A small left pleural effusion (*curved arrow*) is present

Coccidioidomycosis

Coccidioidomycosis immitis is a dimorphic mold endemic in California, Arizona, New Mexico, southwestern Texas, the southern parts of Utah and Nevada, northern Mexico, Central America, and parts of South America, including Argentina, Venezuela, Colombia, and Brazil. Mycelia of *C. immitis* grow in soil during the rainy season and develop into thick-walled arthroconidia during the dry season. Wind and mechanical disruption of the soil render these arthroconidia easily airborne, and inhaling them leads to infection. Based on skin testing, one third of residents in endemic areas have been infected. The incidence of coccidioidomycosis is rising because of increased construction and drier weather in endemic areas. Military personnel and hikers are prone to the infection due to postings to endemic areas and environmental exposure.

After inhalation, *C. immitis* spores develop a thick wall, forming cyst-like spherules in the host tissue; the fungus then multiplies and forms many endospores within the spherules. The spherules eventually burst, giving rise to new spherules and spreading the infection. A granulomatous reaction similar to that in tuberculosis occurs in infected tissue. Local confinement of the infection primarily relies on T-lymphocyte response. In the immunocompetent host, the acute infection is usually confined to the lung, and resolution is rapid, even though viable fungi may survive in the tissue. In 1–2% of patients, some with no apparent immune defect, the disease can become chronic, with a waxing and waning course involving the lungs, musculoskeletal system, skin, lymph nodes, and other organs [43].

In the immunosuppressed patient, diffuse progressive involvement of the lungs and other organ systems may occur either during primary infection or as reactivation of a chronic, latent focus (Fig. 5.11). Chronic meningitis is a life-threatening complication of dissemination that occurs in a few patients following the acute primary infection. The diagnosis of coccidioidomycosis is established by detecting spherules in bronchial washings or transbronchial biopsies. Lifelong treatment is mainly with antifungals like itraconazoles; amphotericin B is required in patients with disseminated or prolonged infection.

Zygomycosis/Mucormycosis

The genera of zygomycoses most commonly causing human infection are *Rhizopus*, *Mucor*, and *Rhizomucor*, with *Mucor* causing most infections. *Cunninghamella*, *Absidia*, *Saksenaea*, and *Apophysomyces* species are less often implicated in human infection. These organisms are ubiquitous in nature and can be found in decaying vegetation and in the soil. They grow rapidly and release large numbers of spores that can become airborne. Zygomycetes are common in the environment and are relatively frequent contaminants in microbiology

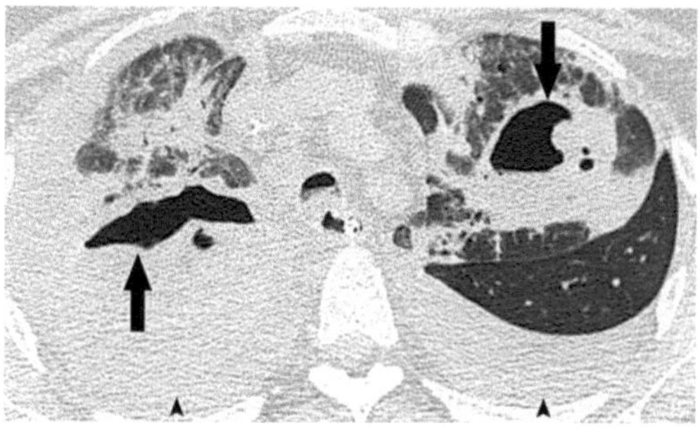

Fig. 5.12 Diabetes mellitus and pulmonary mucormycosis. HRCT image shows bilateral cavitary lesions (*arrows*) with small pleural effusions (*arrowheads*). Ground-glass opacity is also present in the upper lobes

laboratories. All humans have ample exposure to these fungi during day-to-day activities. Almost all human infections from zygomycetes occur in immunocompromised hosts (Fig. 5.12) [44].

Invasive Aspergillosis

Aspergillus is a ubiquitous fungus that is commonly found growing in decaying vegetation, stored grain, and compost piles. Infection is rare with a normal immune system. Allergic bronchopulmonary aspergillosis and intracavitary aspergilloma occur in people with a relatively normal immune system, while invasive pulmonary aspergillosis (IPA) occurs almost exclusively in people with weakened immunity. IPA often occurs at the nadir of the white blood cell count (Fig. 5.13).

Early diagnosis of angioinvasive pulmonary aspergillosis in immunosuppressed patients is critical for adequate and timely therapeutic intervention in this high-risk group. The most common CT patterns in the setting of invasive pulmonary aspergillosis are segmental areas of consolidation and ground-glass attenuation or nodules surrounded by a halo of ground-glass opacity. Although the halo sign has been considered a major sign for early diagnosis of IPA in the appropriate clinical setting, this finding is nonspecific and can occur in immunosuppressed patients with other infectious or non-infectious cause, as previously discussed [27]. Cavitation resulting in multiple fixed mural nodules is seen as the white cell count returns towards normal,

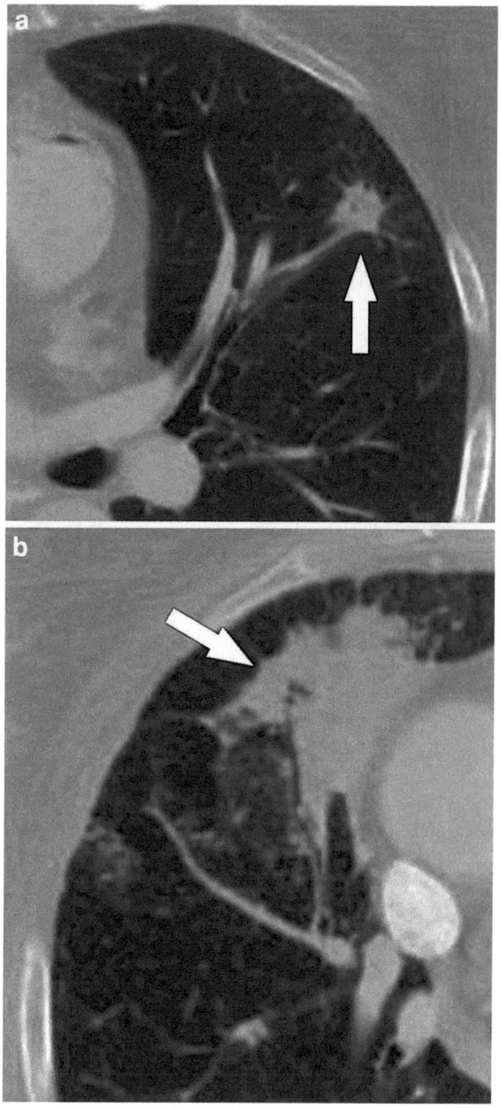

Fig. 5.13 Pulmonary aspergillosis in a bone marrow transplant recipient. **a** Contrast-enhanced CT image shows a spiculated nodule (*arrow*) in the left upper lobe. **b** Contrast-enhanced CT image more caudad shows a focus of consolidation (*arrow*) in the right upper lobe

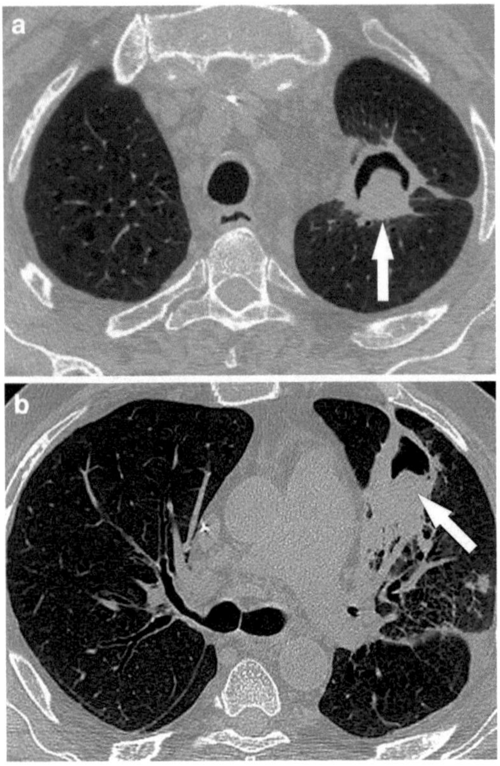

Fig. 5.14 Pulmonary aspergillosis and *Pseudomonas* pneumonia in a patient with acute myeloid leukemia. HRCT image shows cavitary lesions in the left upper lobe with mural nodules (*arrows*)

but this is a much later radiographic appearance (Fig. 5.14).

The diagnostic yield for detecting *Aspergillus* infection with bronchoalveolar lavage is only 30% [45]. Percutaneous needle biopsy may be useful for confirming the diagnosis of fungal infection but is invasive with the risk of hemorrhage, especially with IPA.

Candida

Candida species have been increasingly recognized as a source of fungal pneumonia in the immunocompromised population. A definitive diagnosis of *Candida* pneumonia is difficult to establish, as *Candida* colonization is common in immunocompromised patients.

HRCT is the most sensitive imaging method for detecting early lung changes in immunocompromised patients with acute pulmonary diseases. CT findings of candidiasis are relatively nonspecific and are similar to those described in other pulmonary infections [46]. Nodules, often multiple and ranging in size from 3–30 mm, may be associated with other parenchymal findings such as lung consolidation, tree-in-bud opacities, and ground-glass opacities. The variability of the CT findings in *Candida* pneumonia reflects the diverse patterns of pathologic reaction and the stage of disease.

Viral Pneumonia

Immunocompromised hosts are susceptible to a spectrum of viral pneumonias. The common infective organisms are CMV, herpes viruses, measles virus, adenovirus, and influenza virus types A and B. Most respiratory viral infections in lung transplant recipients are community-acquired [47].

CMV pneumonia is a frequent life-threatening infectious complication in severely immunocompromised patients, particularly in patients recovering from bone marrow or peripheral blood stem cell transplantation. CMV infection is a major cause of morbidity and mortality. The incidence of CMV pneumonia is considered to be about 20%, with a mortality rate of approximately 80% over a 10-year period after stem cell transplantation.

CMV pneumonia in allogeneic transplant recipients is caused by immune mechanisms mediated by a T cell response to virally induced antigens expressed in the lungs. Severe necrotizing pneumonitis may occur despite suppression of viral replication during ganciclovir therapy. In AIDS patients with more profound immune deficiency than transplant recipients, the direct cytopathogenic effects of CMV may cause lung damage.

CT findings of CMV pneumonia are diverse and have been described without distinction between AIDS patients and non-AIDS patients, most commonly consisting of ground-glass

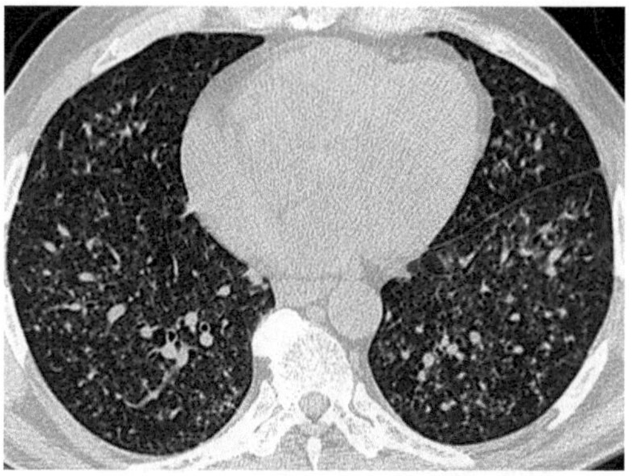

Fig. 5.15 Liver transplant recipient with CMV pneumonia. HRCT image shows diffuse tiny (miliary) nodules in both lungs

opacity, consolidation, and nodules (Fig. 5.15) [48–51].

Influenza (Seasonal and Avian)

Influenza pneumonia typically occurs during seasonal outbreaks or during pandemics. Along with very old and very young patients, the immunocompromised are at increased risk for development of fulminant influenza pneumonia with superimposed bacterial infection. The radiographic appearances of most types of viral pneumonias, including that of both seasonal and avian influenza, are quite similar and include small, poorly defined centrilobular nodules; patchy bilateral areas of peribronchial ground-glass opacity; and lung consolidation. Air trapping, septal and bronchial wall-thickening, and tree-in-bud opacities may also be present.

Diseases in the immunosuppressed that can resemble infection-specific noninfectious conditions, such as post-transplant lymphoproliferative disorder and Kaposi sarcoma (KS), have overlapping imaging features with infection. Pulmonary hemorrhage from thrombocytopenia or as a direct result of cytotoxic drugs, radiation pneumonitis, and pulmonary edema may be mistaken for infection. Graft-versus-host disease following allogeneic stem cell transplant can also mimic infection.

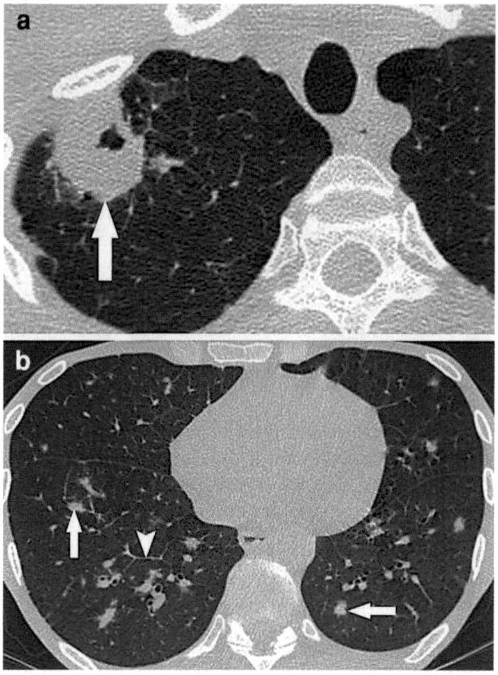

Fig. 5.16 AIDS and Kaposi sarcoma. **a** HRCT image shows a cavitary mass in the right upper lobe *(arrow)*. **b** HRCT image more inferiorly showing several nodules *(arrows)* with ill-defined margins and patchy septal thickening *(arrowhead)*

Kaposi Sarcoma

KS is a multicentric neoplasm of the lymphatics and is associated with human herpes virus 8 [52]. Lung involvement occurs in 25–75% of patients with KS and AIDS and usually occurs in the setting of extensive mucosal and cutaneous disease. The most common radiographic findings are nodular consolidation and pleural effusions. Effusions are often bloody or serosanguinous. On CT, KS lesions manifest as peribronchial or perivascular flame-shaped nodules or foci of consolidation that may coalesce to form large masses (Fig. 5.16). The nodules contain spindle-shaped cells with vascular clefts filled with red blood cells and hemosiderin that may infiltrate along the alveolar and intralobular septa. At bronchoscopy, the presence of the characteristic raised red–purple lesions similar to cutaneous KS plaques

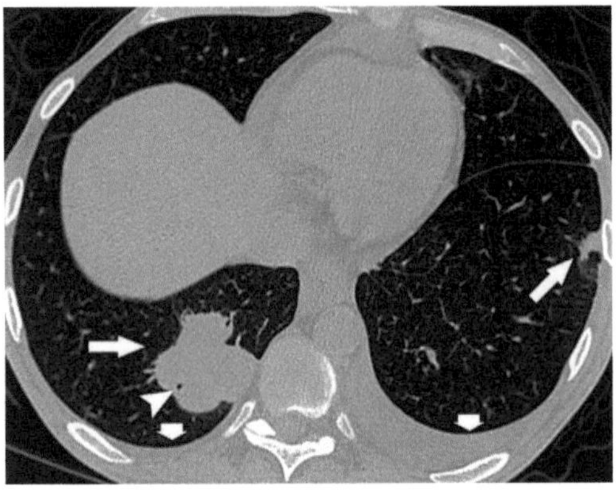

Fig. 5.17 AIDS-related lymphoma. HRCT image shows bilateral lung nodules (*thin arrows*) and small pleural effusions (*wide arrows*). Note the air bronchogram (*arrowhead*) in the right lower lobe nodule

are diagnostic. Definitive diagnosis generally requires lung biopsy. Up to 50% of patients with pulmonary KS have other potentially treatable opportunistic infections such as PJP or tuberculosis at the time of presentation with pulmonary symptoms. Prognosis for pulmonary KS is poor [53].

Pulmonary Neoplasm: Lymphoma and Lung Cancer

Transplant recipients and HIV-infected patients are at increased risk for developing lymphoma, usually high-grade B cell non-Hodgkin lymphomas [54]. These lymphomas generally present with mediastinal or hilar lymph node enlargement with or without lung involvement (Fig. 5.17). Almost all AIDS patients who develop lymphoma have serology positive for EBV. Lymphoma may also be associated with human herpes virus 8, the same virus associated with KS. Cytology of pleural effusion, if present, is diagnostic in 75–100% of effusions caused by lymphoma. The treatment of AIDS-associated lymphomas is difficult, and the prognosis is poor.

Many reports suggest that the incidence of lung cancer is increased in AIDS and often presents at a younger age (Fig. 5.18) [55].

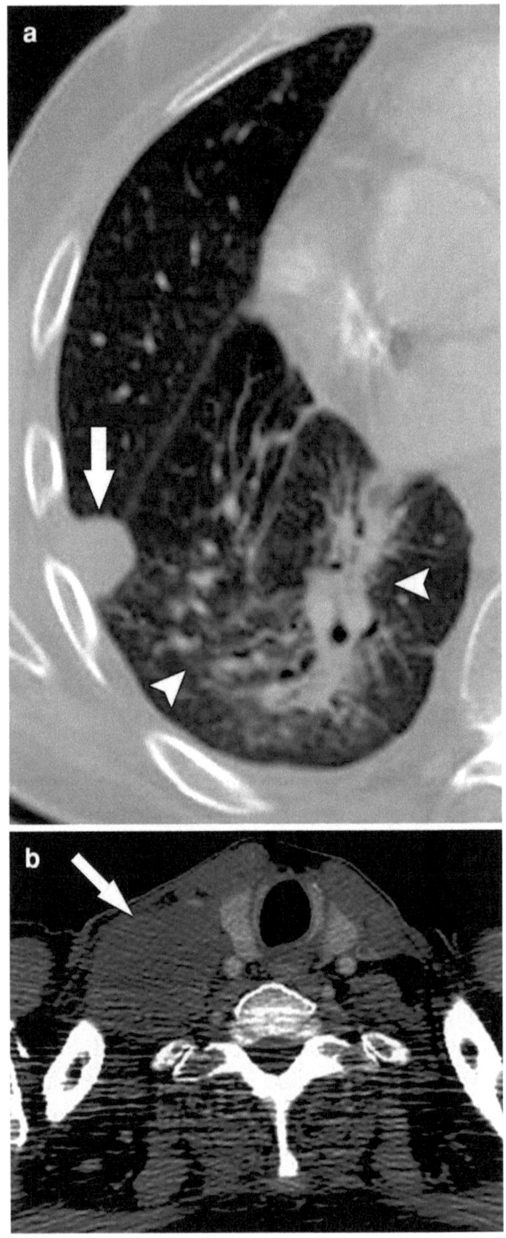

Fig. 5.18 Recurrent small-cell lung carcinoma and HIV infection. **a** Contrast-enhanced CT image shows a pleural nodule (*arrow*). Note radiation fibrosis (*arrowheads*) in the right lower lobe. **b** Contrast-enhanced CT image of the lower neck shows an enlarged right supraclavicular lymph node (*arrow*)

The diagnosis may not be suspected because of other potential causes of a lung nodule or mass such as infections, KS, and lymphoma. The prognosis is generally poor, in part from delay in diagnosis.

References

1. Hughes WT. Pneumonia in the immunocompromised child. Semin Respir Infect. 1987;2:177–83.
2. Rubin RH, Peterson PK. Overview of pneumonia in the compromised host. Semin Respir Infect. 1986;1:131–2.
3. Murray JF, Mills J. Pulmonary infectious complications of human immunodeficiency virus infection: part 1. Am Rev Respir Dis. 1990; 141:1356–72.
4. Bodey GP, Powell RD, Hersch EM, et al. Pulmonary complications of acute leukemia. Cancer. 1996; 19:781.
5. Garg K, Zamora MR, Tuder R, Armstrong JD, Lynch DA. Lung transplantation: indications, donor and recipient selection, and imaging of complications. RadioGraphics. 1996;16:355–67.
6. Maurer JR, Tullis E, Grossman RF, Vellend H, Winton TL, Patterson GA. Infectious complications following isolated lung transplantation. Chest. 1992;101:1056–9.
7. Rubin RH, Ferraro MJ. Understanding and diagnosing infectious complications in the immunocompromised host. Hematol Oncol Clin North Am. 1993;7:795–812.
8. Meyers JD. Infections in marrow transplant recipients. In: Mandell GL, Douglas RG, Bennet JE, editors. Principles and practice of infectious disease. New York: Churchill Livingstone; 1990. p. 2291–95.
9. Rubin RH, Wolfson JS, Cosimi AB, Tolkoff-Rubin NE. Infection in the renal transplant recipient. Am J Med. 1981;70:405–11.
10. Randhawa PS, Yousem SA. Epstein-Barr virus–associated lymphoproliferative disease in a heart–lung allograft. Transplantation. 1990;49:126–30.
11. Craven DE, Steger KA, Duncan RA. Prevention and control of nosocomial pneumonia. In: Wenzel RP, editor. Prevention and control of nosocomial infections. Baltimore: Williams & Wilkins; 1993. p. 580–99.
12. Rubin RH, Greene R. Etiology and management of the compromised patient with fever and pulmonary infiltrates. In: Rubin RH, Young LS, editors. Clinical approach to infection in the compromised host. New York: Plenum; 1988. p. 131–63.
13. Primack SL, Muller NL. HRCT in acute diffuse lung disease in the immunocompromised patient. Radiol Clin North Am. 1994;32:731–44.
14. Kuhlman JE, Fishman EK, Teigen C. Pulmonary septic emboli: diagnosis with CT. Radiology. 1990;174:211–3.
15. Oh YW, Kim YH, Lee NJ, et al. HRCT appearance of miliary tuberculosis. J Comput Assist Tomogr. 1994;18:862–6.
16. Graham NJ, Müller NL, Miller RR, Shepherd JD. Intrathoracic complications following allogenic bone marrow transplant: CT findings. Radiology. 1991; 181:153–6.
17. Sider L, Gabriel H, Curry DR, Pham MS. Pattern recognition of the pulmonary manifestations of AIDS on CT scans. RadioGraphics. 1993;13:771–84.
18. Worthy S, Kang EY, Muller NL. Acute lung disease in the immunocompromised host: differential diagnosis at high-resolution CT. Semin Ultrasound CT MR. 1995;16:353–60.
19. McGuinness G. Changing trends in the pulmonary manifestations of AIDS. Radiol Clin North Am. 1997;35:1029–82.
20. Heussel CP, Kauczor HU, Heussel G, Fischer B, Mildenberger P, Thelen M. Early detection of pneumonia in febrile neutropenic patients: use of thin-section CT. Am J Roentgenol. 1997;169: 1347–53.
21. Curtin JJ, Webster ADB, Farrant J, Katz D. Bronchiectasis in hypogammaglobulinemia: a computed tomography assessment. Clin Radiol. 1991;44:82–4.
22. McGuinness G, Naidich DP, Garay S, Leitman BS, McCauley DI. AIDS associated bronchiectasis: CT features. J Comput Assist Tomogr. 1993;17:260–6.
23. Im JG, Itoh H, Shim YS, et al. Pulmonary tuberculosis: CT findings—early active disease and sequential change with antituberculous therapy. Radiology. 1993;186:653–60.
24. Eisenhuber E. The tree-in-bud sign. Radiology. 2002;222:771–2.
25. Hatipoglu ON, Osma E, Manisali M, et al. High resolution computed tomographic findings in pulmonary tuberculosis. Thorax. 1996;51:397–402.
26. Collins J, Blankenbaker D, Stern EJ. CT patterns of bronchiolar disease: what is "tree-in-bud"? Am J Roentgenol. 1998;171:365–70.
27. Kuhlman JE, Fishman EK, Siegelman SS. Invasive pulmonary aspergillosis in acute leukemia: characteristic findings on CT, the CT halo sign, and the role of CT in early diagnosis. Radiology. 1985;157:611–14.
28. Gaeta M, Blandino A, Scribano E, Minutoli F, Volta S, Pandolfo I. Computed tomography halo sign in pulmonary nodules: frequency and diagnostic value. J Thorac Imaging. 1999;14:109–13.
29. Primack SL, Hartman TE, Lee KS, Muller NL. Pulmonary nodules and the CT halo sign. Radiology. 1994;190:513–5.
30. McLoud TC, Naidich DP. Thoracic disease in the immunocompromised patient. Radiol Clin North Am. 1992;30:525–54.
31. Rubin SA. Radiology of immunologic diseases of the lung. J Thorac Imaging. 1988;3:21–39.
32. Shah RM, Kaji AV, Ostrum BJ, Friedman AC. Interpretation of chest radiographs in AIDS patients: usefulness of CD4 lymphocyte counts. RadioGraphics. 1997;17:47–58.
33. Finkelstein DM, Williams PL, Molenberghs G, et al. Patterns of opportunistic infections in patients with HIV infection. J Acquir Immune Defic Syndr Hum Retrovirol. 1996;12:38–45.

HIV infection. J Acquir Immune Defic Syndr Hum Retrovirol. 1996;12:38–45.
34. Noskin GA, Glassroth J. Bacterial pneumonia associated with HIV-1 infection. Clin Chest Med. 1996;17:713–23.
35. Moore M, Onorato IM, McCray E, Castro KG. Trends in drug-resistant tuberculosis in the United States, 1993–1996. JAMA. 1997;278:833–7.
36. Raviglione MC, Dye C, Schmidt S, Kochi A. Assessment of worldwide tuberculosis control. Lancet. 1997;350:624–9.
37. Im JG, Song KS, Kang HS, et al. Mediastinal tuberculous lymphadenitis: CT manifestations. Radiology. 1987;164:115–9.
38. Silcox VA, Good RC, Floyd MM. Identification of clinically significant Mycobacterium fortuitum complex isolates. J Clin Microbiol. 1981;14(6): 686–91.
39. Walzer PD, Evans HE, Copas AJ, et al. Early predictors of mortality from Pneumocystis jirovecii pneumonia in HIV-infected patients: 1985–2006. Clin Infect Dis. 2008;46(4):625–33.
40. Amorosa JK, Nahass RG, Nosher JL, Gocke DJ. Radiologic distinction of pyogenic pulmonary infection from Pneumocystis carinii pneumonia in AIDS patients. Radiology. 1990;175:721–4.
41. Aberg JA, Mundy LM, Powderly WG. Pulmonary cryptococcosis in patients without HIV infection. Chest. 1999;115:734–40.
42. Kennedy CC, Limper AH. Redefining the clinical spectrum of chronic pulmonary histoplasmosis: a retrospective case series of 46 patients. Medicine (Baltimore). 2007;86(4):252–8.
43. McGahan JP, Graves DS, Palmer PE, Stadalnik RC, Dublin AB. Classic and contemporary imaging of coccidioidomycosis. Am J Roentgenol. 1981;136: 393–404.
44. Lee FY, Mossad SB, Adal KA. Pulmonary mucormycosis: the last 30 years. Arch Intern Med. 28 Jun 1999;159(12):1301–9
45. Orr DP, Myerowitz RL, Dubois PJ. Patho-radiologic correlation of invasive pulmonary aspergillosis in the compromised host. Cancer. 1978;41:2028–39.
46. Buff SJ, McLelland R, Gallis HA, Matthay R, Putman CE. Candida albicans pneumonia: radiographic appearance. Am J Roentgenol. 1982;138:645–8.
47. Palmer SM Jr, Henshaw NG, Howell DN, Miller SE, Davis RD, Tapson VF. Community respiratory viral infection in adult lung transplant recipients. Chest. 1998;113:944–50.
48. Kang EY, Patz EF, Müller NL. Cytomegalovirus pneumonia in transplant patients: CT findings. J Comput Assist Tomogr. 1996;20:295–9.
49. Kim HS, Lee JS. Cytomegalovirus pneumonia in immunocompromised patients: HRCT findings. J Korean Radiol Soc. 1999;41:1133–8.
50. Sakuma H, Hosoya M, Kanno H, et al. Risk of cytomegalovirus infection after peripheral blood stem cell transplantation. Bone Marrow Transplant. 1997;19:49–53.
51. Franquet T, Lee KS, Müller N. Thin-section CT findings in 32 immunocompromised patients with cytomegalovirus pneumonia who do not have AIDS. Am J Roentgenol.. 2003;181:1059–63.
52. Chang Y, Cesarman E, Pessin MS, et al. Identification of herpesvirus-like DNA sequences in AIDS-associated Kaposi's sarcoma. Science.1994; 266:1865–9.
53. Tappero JW, Conant MA, Wolfe SF, Berger TG. Kaposi's sarcoma: epidemiology, pathogenesis, histology, clinical spectrum, staging criteria and therapy. J Am Acad Dermatol. 1993;28:371–95.
54. Carignan S, Staples CA, Müller NL. Intrathoracic lymphoproliferative disorders in the immunocompromised patient: CT findings. Radiology. 1995; 197:53–8.
55. Cadranel J, Garfield D, Lavole A, Wislez M, Milleron B, Mayaud C. Lung cancer in HIV infected patients: facts, questions and challenges. Thorax. 2006;61(11):1000–8.

Pleural Disease

6

A. Keith Rastogi and Jeffrey P. Kanne

Abstract

The pleural space, which normally contains approximately 10 mL of fluid on either side, can be a host to a variety of pathologic conditions. The most common process to affect this space is increased fluid volume, known as a pleural effusion. An effusion may have a variety of causes, and both imaging and laboratory evaluation are used to distinguish among these etiologies. Other collections in the pleural space include chylothorax, hemothorax, or pneumothorax, and these are also important to consider on radiologic and clinical workup. Primary pleural malignancies, while rare, can be life threatening, and imaging can play a large part in the diagnosis and management of these entities. The most common malignancy in the pleural space is metastatic disease. The most common primary pleural malignancy is mesothelioma, a deadly neoplasm that is most often associated with asbestos exposure. Other pleural neoplasms, including solitary fibrous tumor of the pleura, are even rarer. This chapter highlights the key concepts of pleural disease, illustrates radiologic examples of these conditions, and provides a background into each disease process.

Keywords

Pleural effusion · Chylothorax · Hemothorax · Pneumothorax · Fibrothorax · Mesothelioma · Solitary fibrous tumor of the pleura (SFTP)

A. K. Rastogi (✉)
Department of Radiology, University of Wisconsin Hospital and Clinics, 600 Highland Ave, MC 3252 Madison, WI 53792-3252, USA
e-mail: arastogi@unwhealth.org

J. P. Kanne
Department of Radiology, University of Wisconsin School of Medicine and Public Health, 600 Highland Ave, MC 3252 Madison, WI 53792-3252, USA
e-mail: jkanne@uwhealth.org

Pleural Disease

Two layers of pleura surround the lung. The visceral pleura is tightly adhered to the lung surface while the parietal pleural lines the thoracic cavity. Between these two layers is the pleural cavity. This space normally contains approximately 10 mL of fluid on either side. This fluid serves as a lubricant for the lung

J. P. Kanne (ed.), *Clinically Oriented Pulmonary Imaging*, Respiratory Medicine, DOI: 10.1007/978-1-61779-542-8_6,

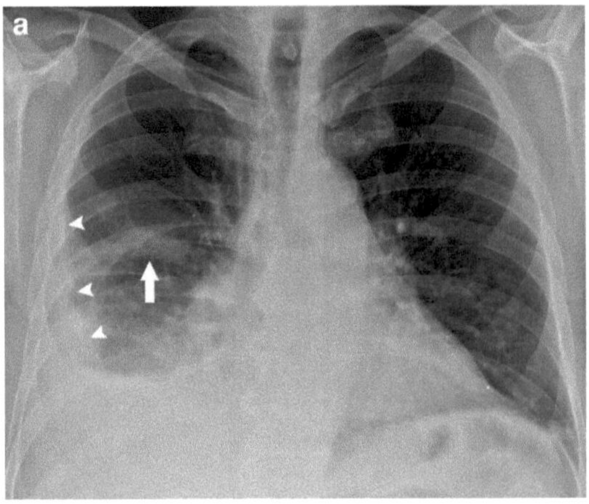

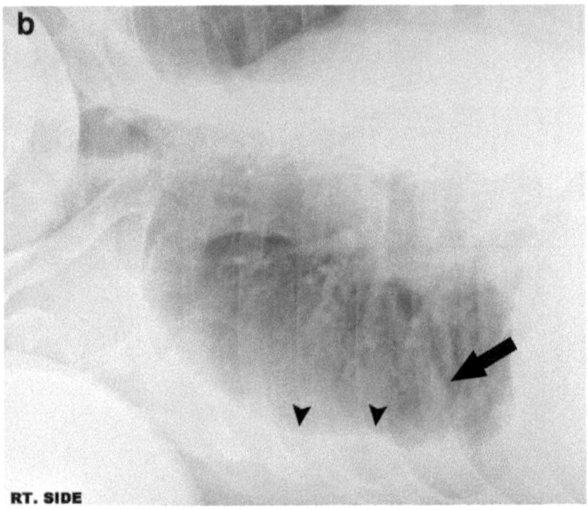

Fig. 6.1 Partially loculated pleural effusion. **a** PA radiograph shows a moderate right pleural effusion, which tracks into the major fissure (*arrow*). The lobulated contours (*arrowheads*) suggest partial loculation. **b** Right lateral decubitus radiograph shows that most of the effusion layers dependently (*arrowheads*) with a small amount of fluid loculated in the fissure (*arrow*)

during normal respiratory motion. Processes affecting either fluid production or removal may alter the state of this space and lead to an increase in pleural fluid volume. This is known as a pleural effusion.

Pleural Effusions

Pleural effusion can occur in numerous scenarios. These classically include elevated hydrostatic pressure as occurs in congestive heart failure, increased capillary permeability as occurs in the setting of infection or neoplasm, and decreased colloid osmotic pressure as occurs in cirrhosis and nephrotic syndrome. Decreased pleural fluid absorption can result from any cause of lymphatic obstruction.

Pleural effusions are classified into two broad categories, transudative or exudative, as originally described in 1972 by Light et al. [1]. Transudative effusions are generally the result of a systemic process, with common causes including cirrhosis, congestive heart failure, nephrotic syndrome, or other causes of hypoalbuminemia. Exudative effusions, in contrast, are usually associated with local disease, such as infection, malignancy, or pulmonary embolism [2].

Diagnostic Workup: Radiologic

Frontal and lateral chest radiographs are generally obtained as the screening test of choice when a pleural effusion is suspected. Pleural effusions (Fig. 6.1) obscure the costophrenic sulcus and are best seen on the lateral view. As pleural fluid volume increases, the entire ipsilateral hemidiaphragm may be obscured (Fig. 6.2). Lateral decubitus radiographs can be obtained to evaluate for the presence of very small effusions if a lateral view is not feasible or to assess whether or not a pleural effusion is loculated.

Ultrasound can be performed to further characterize and localize pleural fluid collections. Commonly, ultrasound is used to find a large pocket of fluid and suitable skin entry site in order to facilitate drainage via thoracentesis or pleural drain placement. If additional evaluation is desired, a chest CT (Fig. 6.3) can be performed for a detailed evaluation of the pleural surfaces and lung parenchyma.

An infected pleural effusion, also known as an empyema (Figs. 6.4, 6.5), can be suggested by certain CT findings, including enhancing, thick pleural surfaces, or the “split pleura sign”,

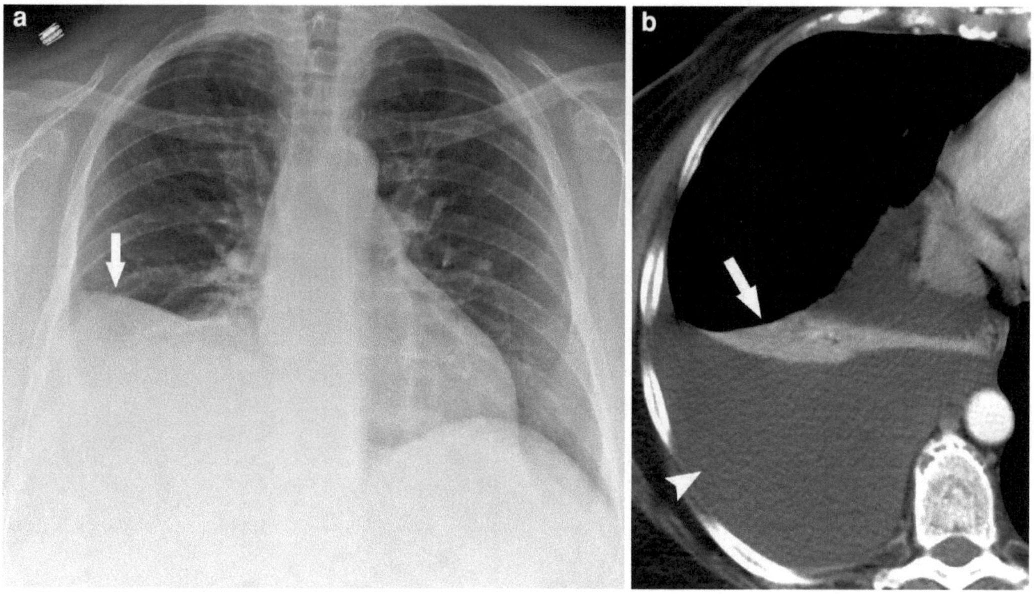

Fig. 6.2 Subpulmonic pleural effusion. **a** PA radiograph shows a dense, well-demarcated opacity (*arrow*) obscuring the hemidiaphragm and blunting the right costophrenic sulcus. **b** Contrast-enhanced CT image shows a large homogeneous pleural effusion (*arrowhead*) compressing the right lower lobe (*arrow*)

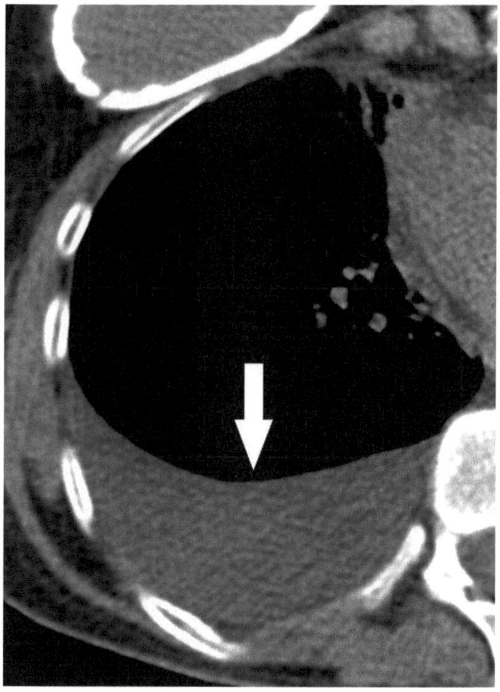

Fig. 6.3 Simple pleural effusion. Unenhanced CT image shows a moderate layering right pleural effusion (*arrow*)

which is characterized by thickened visceral and parietal pleural surfaces separated by pleural fluid [3]. In fact, parietal pleural enhancement has been shown to be highly sensitive and specific in identifying patients with complicated parapneumonic effusions or empyemas versus those with transudative effusions [4]. Increased CT attenuation of extrapleural fat is also suggestive of empyema. Direct fluid sampling, most commonly via thoracentesis, is required to confirm empyema.

Diagnostic Workup: Laboratory Analysis

If direct fluid sampling is desired for determining the etiology of the accumulation, thoracentesis can be performed. Numerous laboratory tests can be performed on a pleural fluid sample for further characterization in order to help determine its etiology. Classically, a protein level and lactate dehydrogenase (LDH) level are used to assess whether a pleural effusion is transudative or exudative.

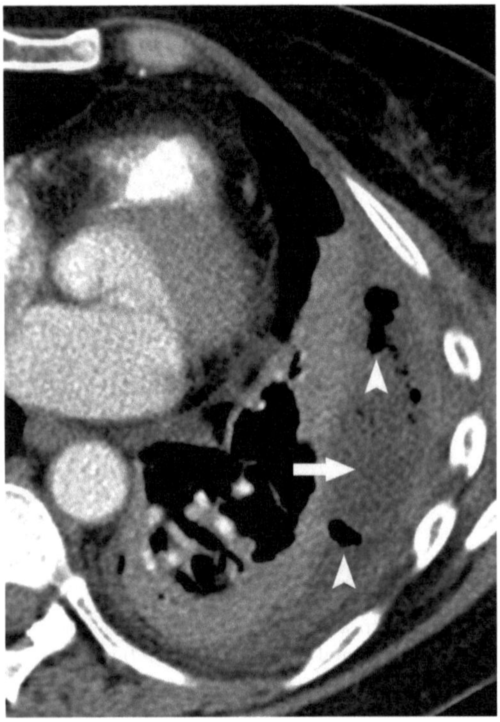

Fig. 6.4 Empyema. Contrast-enhanced CT image shows a heterogeneous left pleural collection (*arrow*) containing pockets of gas (*arrowheads*). In the absence of instrumentation, gas collections such as these are presumably from gas-forming organisms

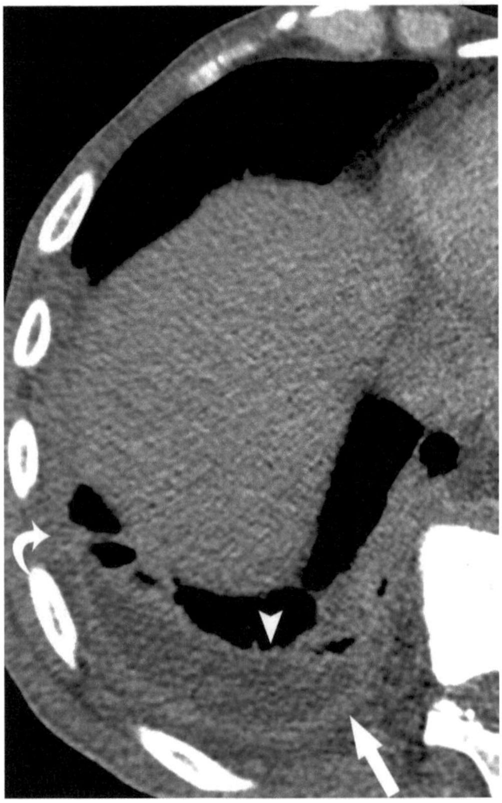

Fig. 6.5 Empyema. Contrast-enhanced CT image shows thickening and enhancement of the visceral (*arrowhead*) and parietal (*straight arrow*) pleura separated by an effusion ("split pleura") sign. Note infiltration of the extrapleural fat (*curved arrow*)

As initially described by Light et al. [1], an exudative effusion meets any of the following criteria:

- ratio of pleural fluid protein to serum protein greater than 0.5
- ratio of pleural fluid LDH to serum LDH greater than 0.6
- pleural fluid LDH greater than two-thirds the upper limit of normal for serum LDH

If none of these criteria is met, then the effusion is classified as transudative.

The serum-effusion albumin gradient (serum albumin concentration minus effusion albumin concentration) can be used as a more specific criterion in the diagnosis of an exudative effusion [5]. A value below 1.2 g/dL has been proposed to define an exudate. This information should be used with the criteria mentioned above for thorough evaluation (see Table 6.1).

Other Pleural Collections

Chylothorax

A chylothorax forms as a consequence of injury to or disruption of the thoracic duct. Potential causes include trauma, tumor, and venous thrombosis. Lymphangioleiomyomatosis, a rare disease characterized by lung cysts and renal angiomyolipomas, can also cause chylothorax. Measuring a triglyceride level in pleural fluid can assist in this diagnosis. A triglyceride level greater than 110 mg/dL confirms the diagnosis, and a level less than 40 mg/dL excludes the diagnosis [2].

Table 6.1 Differentiating transudative and exudative pleural effusions

	Transudate	Exudate
Specific gravity	<1.012	>1.020
Fluid protein: serum protein	<0.5	>0.5
Fluid LDH: serum LDH	<0.6	>0.6
Serum effusion albumin gradient (g/dL)	>1.2	<1.2
Cholesterol content (mg/dL)	<45	>45

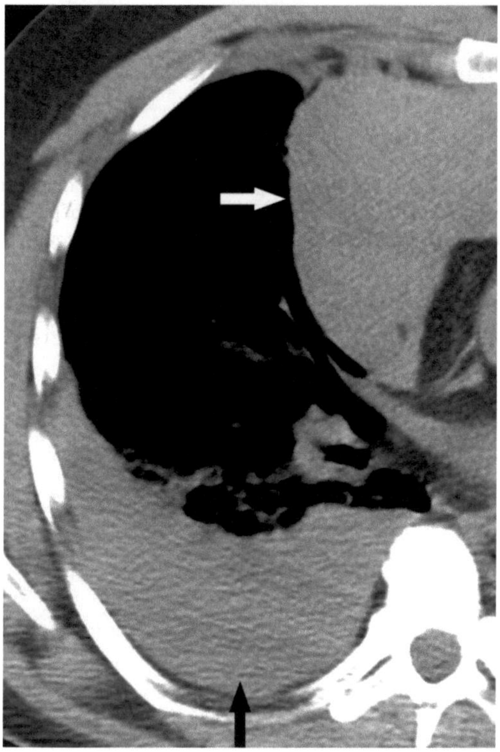

Fig. 6.6 Hemothorax. Unenhanced CT image shows a high attenuation right pleural collection (*black arrow*) similar in attenuation to skeletal muscle. A large anterior mediastinal hematoma (*white arrow*) is also present

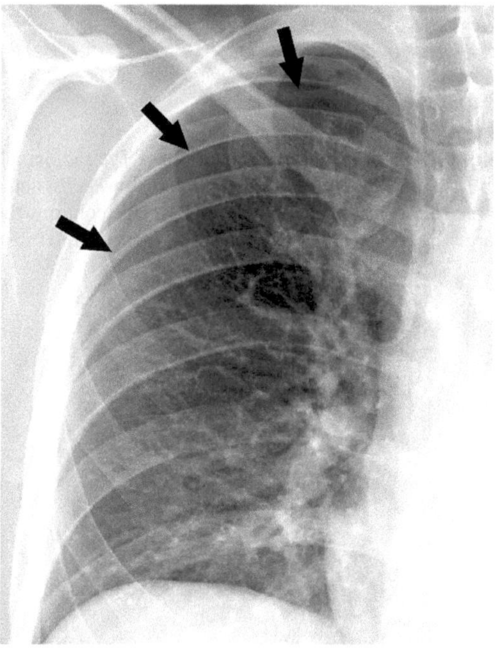

Fig. 6.7 Traumatic pneumothorax from collision in a soccer game. Coned-down view of a PA radiograph shows a sharp, thin visceral pleural line denoting the small pneumothorax

Hemothorax

Hemothorax refers to an accumulation of blood in the pleural space. This condition is most often the result of chest trauma. Non-traumatic etiologies are rare but include underlying malignancy or pulmonary embolism. On imaging, a hemothorax should be suspected if the attenuation of pleural fluid on CT imaging (Fig. 6.6) is approximately 30–70 Hounsfield units (HU). In contrast, a simple pleural effusion measures <20 HU. Furthermore, if the hematocrit level in the pleural fluid is greater than 50% of the patient's serum hematocrit level, a hemothorax is present.

Pneumothorax

Air within the pleural space is referred to as a pneumothorax. Causes include trauma, iatrogenic causes (surgery, barotrauma), chronic obstructive

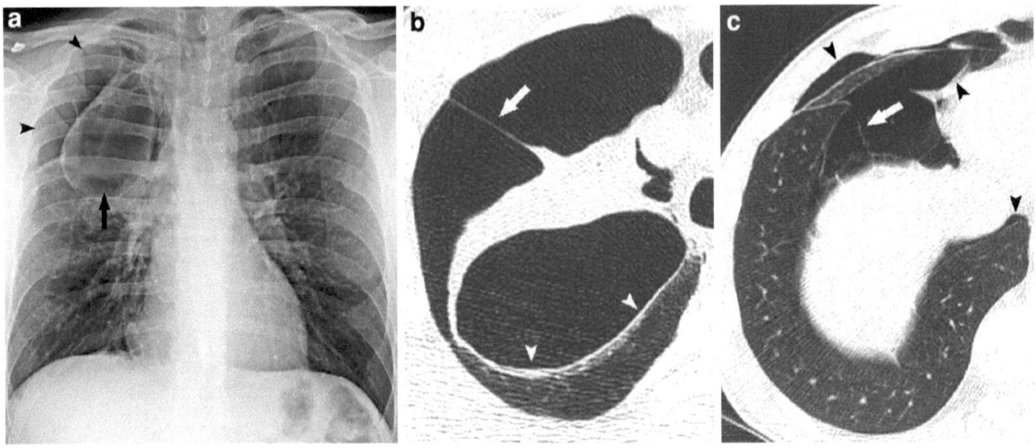

Fig. 6.8 Spontaneous pneumothorax. **a** PA radiograph shows a moderate right pneumothorax (*arrowheads*) and a large right apical bleb (*arrow*). **b** CT image confirms the large bleb, which has a thin wall (*arrowheads*). An adhesion (*arrow*) is apparent in the pneumothorax, presumably from previous pneumothorax. **c** CT image at the level of the diaphragm shows several pockets of pleural air (*arrowheads*) and small pleural adhesions (*arrow*)

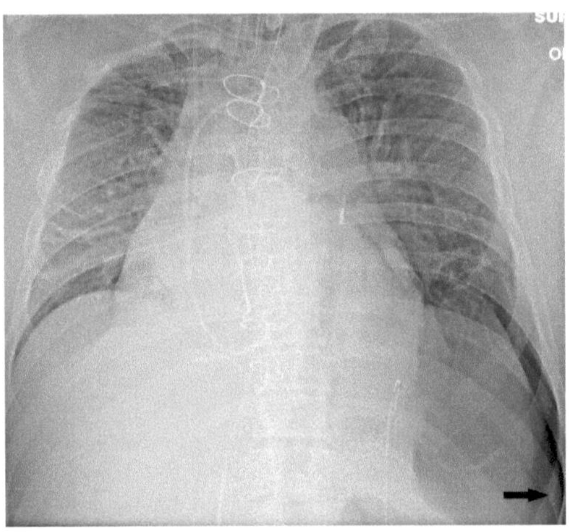

Fig. 6.9 Pneumothorax and deep sulcus sign. Supine AP radiograph shows hyperlucency in the inferolateral aspect of the left hemithorax and inferior displacement of the costophrenic sulcus (*arrow*). Note the sharpness of the left inferior mediastinal and diaphragmatic borders

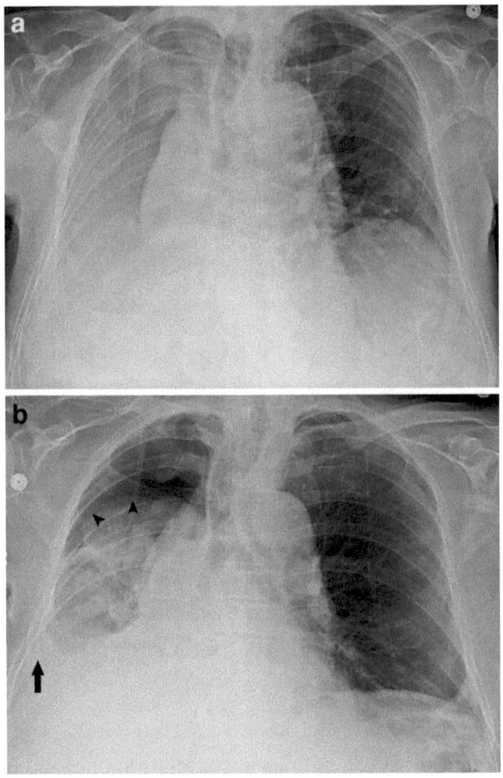

Fig. 6.10 Hydropneumothorax. **a** Supine AP radiograph shows diffuse hazy opacity in the right hemithorax. Note the sharp outline of the right heart and mediastinal borders. **b** Semiupright AP radiograph obtained shortly after A clearly shows a sharp visceral pleural line (*arrowheads*) from pneumothorax. Blunting of the right costophrenic sulcus (*arrow*) reflects the liquid component of the hydropneumothorax

pulmonary disease (often from rupture of a peripheral bleb into the pleural space), infection, and malignancy. Pneumothoraces can be small and produce no symptoms or can be life threatening.

On an upright chest radiograph, a pneumothorax is seen as a well-defined visceral pleural line usually located along the apical and lateral margins of the affected lung (Figs. 6.7, 6.8). Pulmonary vessels are usually not seen

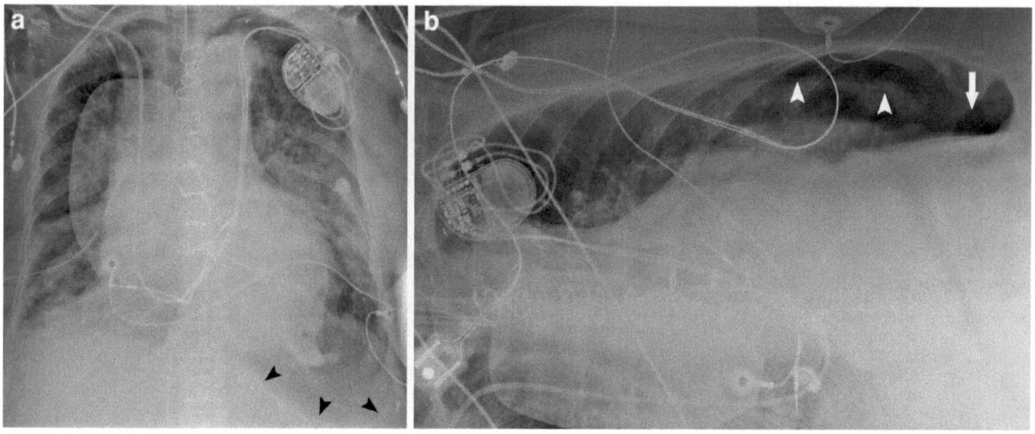

Fig. 6.11 Pneumothorax and deep sulcus sign. **a** Supine AP radiograph shows inferior displacement of the left costophrenic sulcus (*arrowheads*) with left basal hyperlucency and sharpness of the inferior left heart border. **b** Right lateral decubitus radiograph shows a sharp visceral pleural line (*arrowheads*) and the basal pneumothorax (*arrow*)

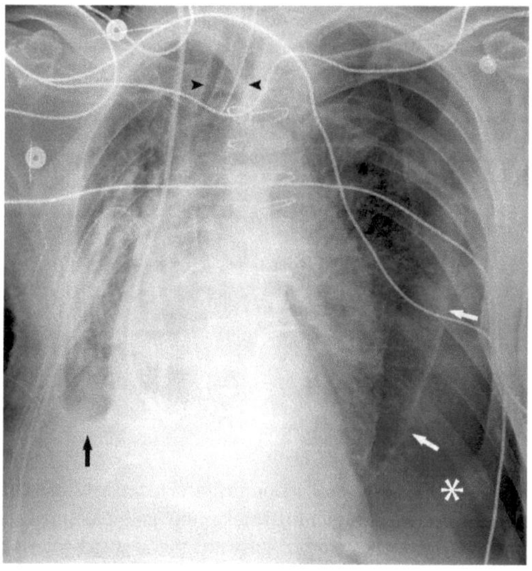

Fig. 6.12 Tension pneumothorax. Supine AP radiograph shows a sharp left visceral pleural line (*white arrows*) and large left pneumothorax (*asterisk*). The heart and trachea (*arrowheads*) are displaced to the right, indicating tension. A small right pleural effusion (*black arrow*) is also present

peripheral to the pleural line. In contrast to an upright radiograph, pneumothoraces may be extremely subtle or occult on a supine chest radiograph.

Findings suggesting pneumothorax on a supine radiograph include a very discrete and more inferiorly located costophrenic sulcus (deep sulcus sign) (Fig. 6.9), basilar hyperlucency, and sharply defined hemidiaphragm and cardiac margins on the affected side. These findings reflect that air will collect anteriorly and basally in a supine patient (Fig. 6.10). If pneumothorax is suspected in a patient who is unable to stand or sit upright, a lateral decubitus radiograph (with the suspected side up) can be useful for further evaluation (Fig. 6.11).

A tension pneumothorax (Figs. 6.12, 6.13) is a life-threatening situation in which the intrapleural pressure rises, causing contralateral mediastinal shift. Prompt identification and decompression are imperative. Tension pneumothorax can occur when there is free inflow of air into the pleural space but limited outflow such as in trauma.

Fibrothorax

Fibrothorax describes fibrosis of the pleural space secondary to a fibrous peel forming over the pleura. It can result from a number of preceding incidents that cause undrained pleural fluid collections including empyema, inflammatory pleural disease, or hemothorax [6, 7]. Specific causes include tuberculosis, empyema, asbestosis-related pleural disease, and

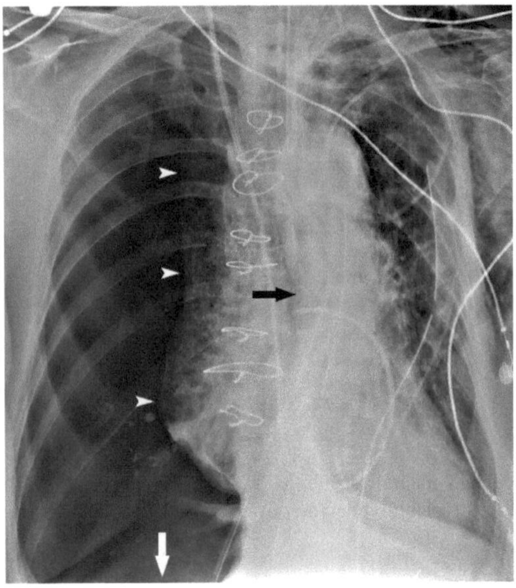

Fig. 6.13 Tension pneumothorax. Supine AP radiograph shows complete right lung collapse (*arrowheads*), right hemithorax hyperlucency and inferior displacement of the right hemidiaphragm (*white arrow*). The mediastinum (*black arrow*) is shifted to the left

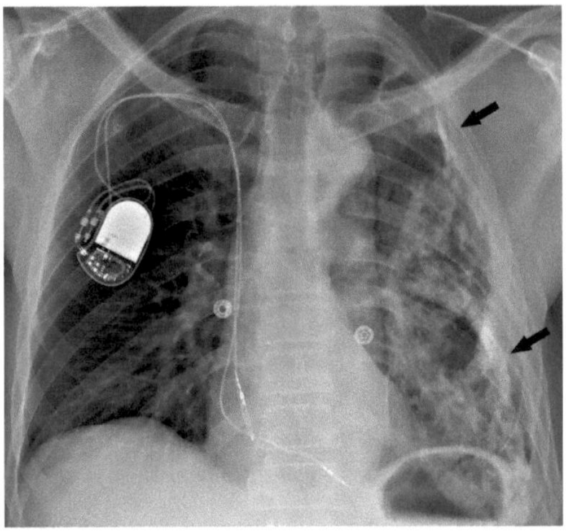

Fig. 6.14 Fibrothorax. PA radiograph shows diffuse, coarse left pleural calcification (*arrows*) resulting from remote tuberculous empyema

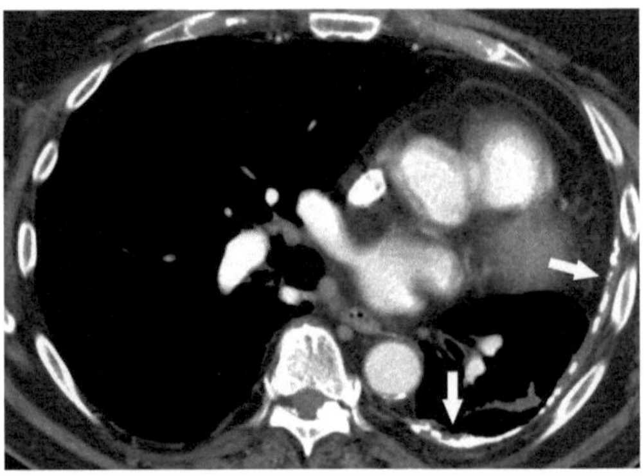

Fig. 6.15 Fibrothorax. Contrast-enhanced CT scan shows smooth left pleural thickening and calcification (*arrows*). Note the marked leftward mediastinal rotation and shift

hemothorax. Fibrothorax restricts lung motion during respiration, impairing lung function. It manifests radiographically as volume loss in the affected hemithorax with relatively smooth pleural thickening. Pleural calcification may be present (Figs. 6.14, 6.15) and can be quite extensive, especially with previous hemothorax or tuberculous empyema. Treatment often requires surgical decortication.

Pleural Malignancies

Metastases

The most common pleural malignancy is metastatic disease. Specifically, lung cancer is the most common primary malignancy to affect the pleura with direct pleural invasion being the most common route of spread. Other tumors that frequently metastasize to the pleura include breast carcinoma, ovarian carcinoma, and gastrointestinal tract malignancies. These tumors most commonly metastasize to the pleural surface via hematogenous spread. Lymphoma can arise primarily in the pleura or involve the pleura with widespread thoracic or systemic disease.

Patients with pleural metastases may present with non-specific symptoms including pleuritic chest pain and dyspnea. A pleural effusion is often present (Fig. 6.16), and there may be smooth or nodular pleural thickening (Fig. 6.17).

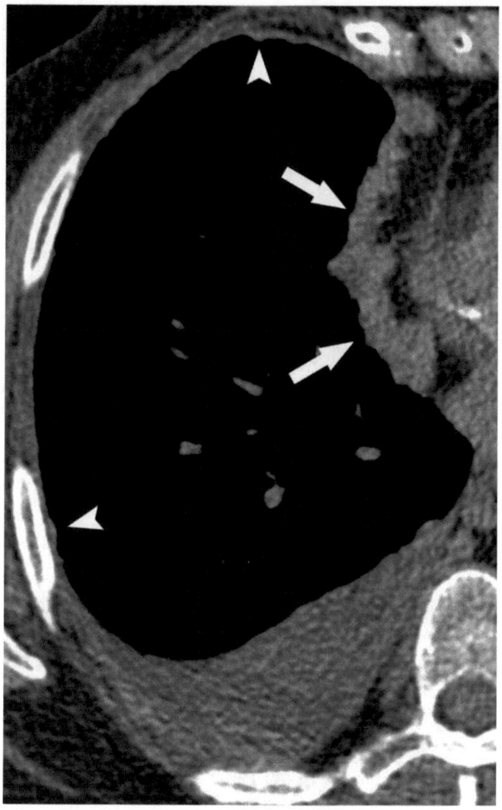

Fig. 6.16 Metastatic breast carcinoma. Unenhanced CT image shows a small right pleural effusion and nodular foci of pleural thickening (*arrowheads*). The presence of mediastinal pleural thickening (*arrows*) is highly suggestive of malignancy but can occur in tuberculous pleural disease

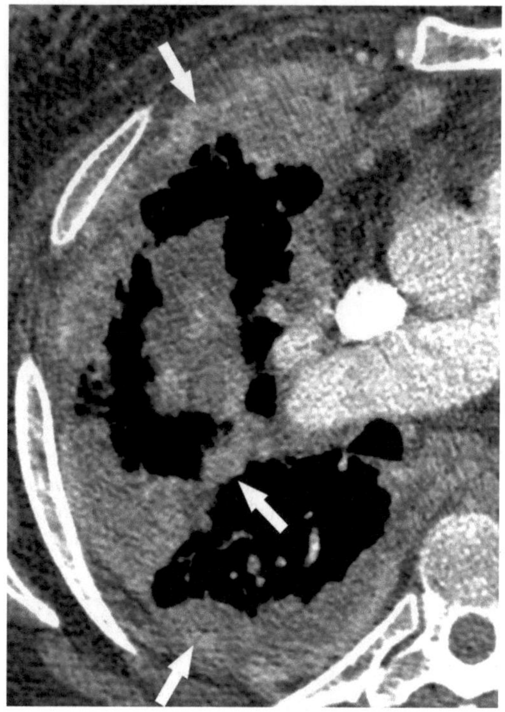

Fig. 6.17 Metastatic renal cell carcinoma. Contrast-enhanced CT image shows circumferential enhancing right pleural soft tissue thickening (*arrows*)

Mesothelioma

The most common primary pleural malignancy is mesothelioma, which has an incidence of approximately 2,500 cases per year in the US [8]. Asbestos exposure remains the number one risk factor for the development of mesothelioma, and exposure can occur in mining of asbestos fibers, as well as other occupations that involve work with asbestos containing products such as ceiling and pool tiles or automobile brake lining [9]. Most patients are middle-aged men as the latency from asbestos exposure to clinical disease is often several decades [10]. However, mesothelioma may occasionally be seen in younger patients. Patients often present with non-specific symptoms, including chest wall pain and dyspnea.

Pleural effusions are common, seen in 80–95% of patients, and may be the only radiographic finding [11]. Other findings of mesothelioma include diffuse, nodular pleural thickening and a contracted ipsilateral hemithorax (Figs. 6.18, 6.19) [12]. Although cross-sectional imaging may suggest this diagnosis, tissue sampling is required for confirmation. The most common sites of metastases include lymph nodes, bone, liver, and lung. Currently, imaging is generally used to assess disease extent, specifically evaluating for surgical resectability and any evidence of metastatic disease. Imaging can also assist in guiding biopsy and can aid in following disease course with treatment.

Unfortunately, prognosis remains poor in these patients, given the often-advanced disease at time of presentation. Median survival is approximately 4–13 months in untreated patients and 6–18 months with treatment [10].

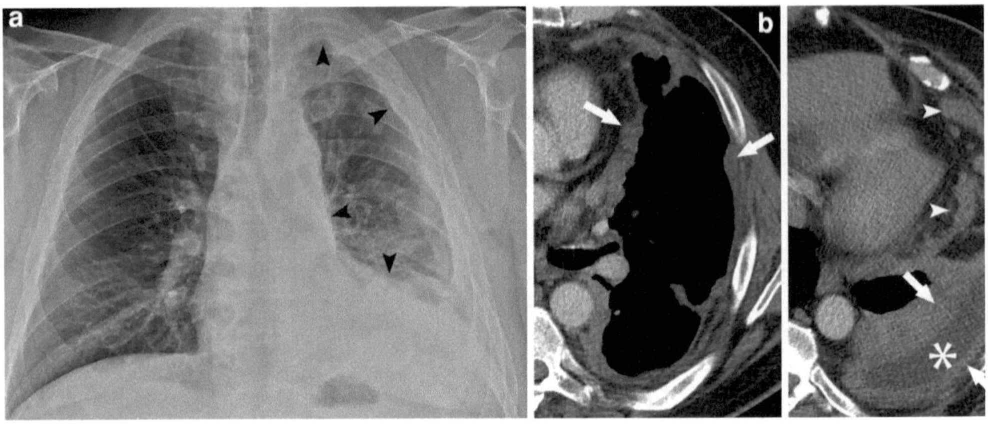

Fig. 6.18 Mesothelioma. **a** PA radiograph shows circumferential, nodular left pleural thickening (*arrowheads*) and a slightly contracted left hemithorax. **b–c** Contrast-enhanced CT images show extensive nodular and circumferential pleural soft tissue thickening (*arrows*). A small effusion (*asterisk*) is present, and tumor (*arrowheads*) has extended into the mediastinal fat

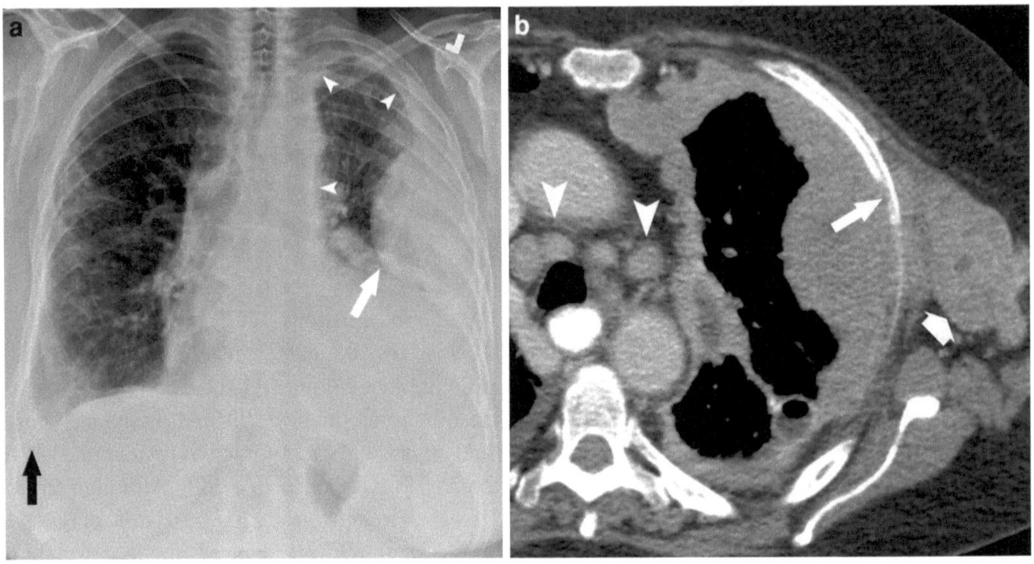

Fig. 6.19 Mesothelioma. **a** PA radiograph shows circumferential left pleural thickening (*arrowheads*) and a large left pleural mass (*white arrow*). A small right pleural effusion (*black arrow*) is also present. **b** Contrast-enhanced CT image shows extensive left pleural tumor with focal rib invasion (*thin arrow*) and mediastinal (*arrowheads*) and left axillary (*wide arrow*) lymph node metastases

Other Pleural Neoplasms

Other pleural tumors are rare. Pleural lipomas (Fig. 6.20), which rarely cause symptoms, are benign homogeneous fatty tumors that are often detected incidentally on imaging examinations obtained for other reasons. Pleural liposarcomas are extremely rare malignant soft-tissue tumors. In contrast to lipomas, liposarcomas tend to be heterogeneous with varying degrees of contrast enhancement and non-fatty soft tissue.

Solitary fibrous tumor of the pleura (SFTP) is an uncommon neoplasm that arises from the submesothelial mesenchymal layer. This tumor has previously been called by many names,

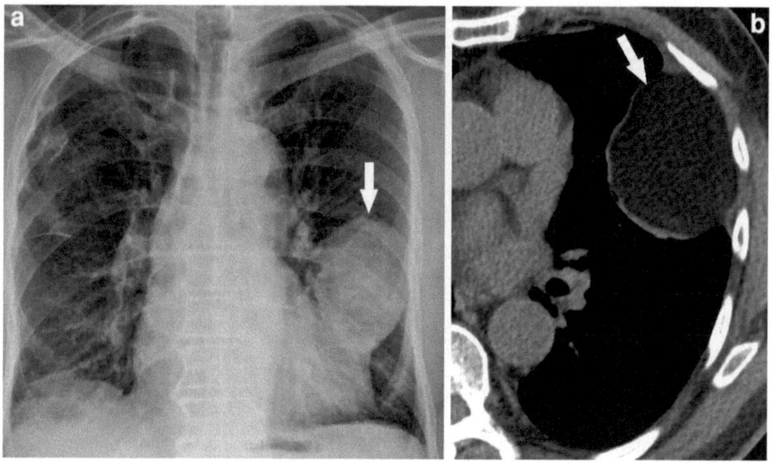

Fig. 6.20 Pleural lipoma. **a** PA radiograph shows a large, homogeneous mass (*arrow*) in the left hemithorax. **b** Unenhanced CT image shows the mass (*arrow*) to consist entirely of homogeneous fat, consistent with a pleural lipoma

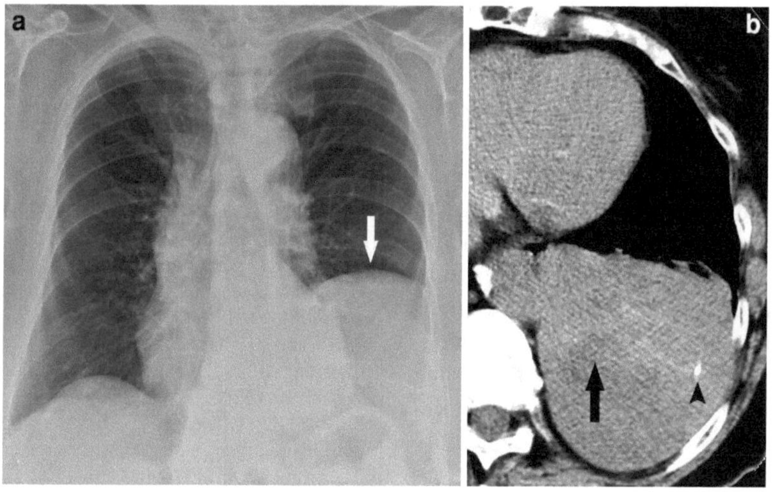

Fig. 6.21 Solitary fibrous tumor of the pleura. **a** PA radiograph shows a large mass (*arrow*). The left heart border and portions of the left hemidiaphragm remain visible, suggesting a posterior location. **b** Unenhanced CT image shows a large, somewhat heterogeneous mass containing calcification (*arrowhead*) and low attenuation foci (*arrow*)

including benign pleural fibroma, which is misleading, as it does not always have a benign course. Given its origins from pluripotent cells, SFTP can have a variety of appearances. These tumors tend to be solitary, lobulated, and heterogeneous masses ranging from 2 to 30 cm in diameter (Fig. 6.21) [3]. They often arise from a stalk and may change configuration as patient position changes (Fig. 6.22). Some patients with SFTP may present with symptomatic hypoglycemia or digital clubbing.

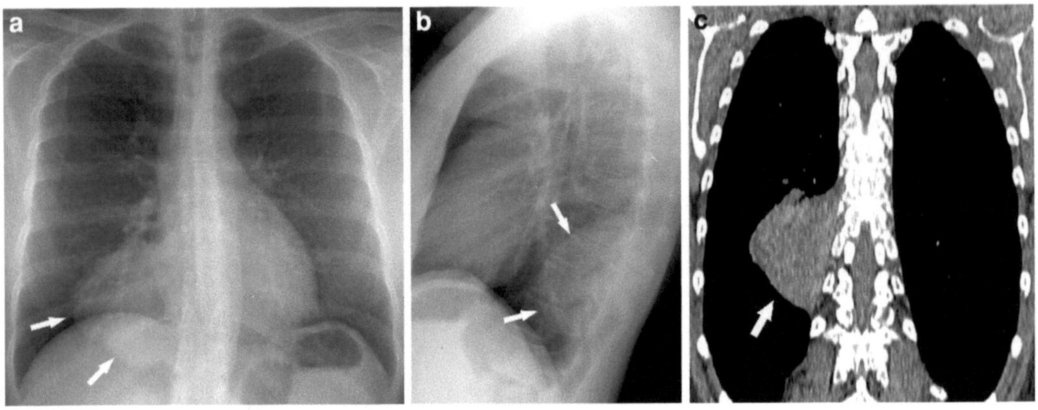

Fig. 6.22 Solitary fibrous tumor of the pleura. PA **a** and lateral **b** radiographs show a lobulated mass (*arrows*) in the lower right hemithorax. The posteromedial margins are not well defined. **c** Coronal reformatted unenhanced CT image shows a large mass (*arrow*) in the lower right hemithorax abutting the paraspinal region. The apparent slight change in shape reflects differences in patient position between radiography (*upright*) and CT (*supine*)

Radiologic Evaluation of Pleural Abnormalities

Imaging can play a significant role in detecting and determining the etiology of pleural disease, aiding in selecting optimal treatment. Upright PA and lateral chest radiographs are sensitive for pleural effusion and pneumothorax. CT can be used to evaluate for pleural thickening or nodularity. CT features most suggestive of a malignant cause include a pleural rind, circumferential pleural thickening, parietal pleural thickening of more than 1 cm, mediastinal pleural involvement, nodularity, irregularity of the pleural contours, and infiltration of the chest wall or diaphragm [8]. In contrast, pleural calcifications generally indicate a benign cause. Mediastinal pleural involvement is generally rare in benign causes. However, an important exception to this rule is tuberculous pleurisy, which is known to characteristically involve the mediastinal surface. These general rules can help to point to a more specific diagnosis in various clinical settings. In addition, imaging can help plan for biopsy or thoracic surgery, when definitive tissue diagnosis is necessary.

References

1. Light RW, MacGregor MI, Luchsinger PC, et al. Pleural effusions: the diagnostic separation of transudates and exudates. Ann Intern Med. 1972;77:507–13.
2. Dweik R. Pleural disease. Cleveland clinic center for continuing education. 2011. Web. http://www.clevelandclinicmeded.com/medicalpubs/diseasemanagement/pulmonary/pleural-disease. Accessed 23 June 2011
3. Waite RJ, Carbonneau RJ, Balikian JP, et al. Parietal pleural changes in empyema: appearances at CT. Radiology. 1990;175:145–50.
4. Rosado-de-Christenson ML, et al. From the archives of the AFIP. Localized fibrous tumors of the pleura. RadioGraphics. 2003;23:759–783
5. Roth BJ, O'Meara TF, Cragun WH. The serum-effusion albumin gradient in the evaluation of pleural effusions. Chest. 1990;98:546–9.
6. Strzalka C, Yost M. Treatment of fibrothorax using intrapleural tissue plasminogen activator. Hosp Physician. Nov. 2002;65–67.
7. Ghoshal AG. Fibrothorax: problem, profile, and prevention. J Indian Med Assoc. 1997;95(12):610–2.
8. Pistoli M, Rusthoven J. Malignant pleural mesothelioma: update, current management, and newer therapeutic strategies. Chest. 2004;126(4):1318–1329
9. Montjoy C, et al. Mesothelioma review. West Va Med J. 2009;105(3):13–6.
10. Helm EJ, et al. Imaging of the pleura. J Magn Reson Imaging. 2010;32:1275–86.
11. Ismail-Khan R, et al. Malignant pleural mesothelioma: a comprehensive review. Cancer Control. 2006;13(4):255–63.
12. Benamore RE, et al. Use of imaging in the management of malignant pleural mesothelioma. Clin Radiol. 2005;60(12):1237–47.

Pulmonary Thromboembolic Disease

7

Amie J. Tucker, Gopal Allada, and Steven L. Primack

Abstract

Diagnostic imaging for acute pulmonary embolism has evolved; CT angiography of the chest is now considered the gold standard for diagnosis. The chest radiograph has limited utility, but can occasionally detect an alternative diagnosis. Although not frequently used, ventilation/perfusion scan can be diagnostic, particularly in the setting of a normal chest radiograph. Clinical features, including risk factors and presenting signs and symptoms, should be utilized to assess pre-test probability and guide diagnostic imaging choices. Unique situations, such as renal failure and pregnancy, will potentially alter the diagnostic decisions.

Keywords

Embolism · Thromboembolism · Pulmonary · Computed tomography (CT) · Infarct

Introduction

The focus of this chapter will be on diagnostic imaging for acute pulmonary embolism. We will also address clinical features including the risk factors, clinical presentation, and diagnostic tools that assess the patient's pre-test probability of venous thromboembolism (VTE), which is critical in interpreting imaging results. Finally, we will present diagnostic algorithms for acute pulmonary embolism. Lower extremity imaging will not be a focus of this discussion.

Epidemiology

Early studies reported the incidence of deep venous thrombosis (DVT) was approximately 48–107 cases per 100,000, and the incidence of pulmonary embolism (PE) (with or without DVT) is about 23–69 in 100,000 [1–3]. A more recent population-based study indicated that the PE

A. J. Tucker · G. Allada
Division of Pulmonary and Critical Care, Department of Medicine, Oregon Health and Science University, 3181 SW Sam Jackson Park Rd, UHN 67 Portland, OR 97239, USA

S. L. Primack (✉)
Department of Radiology, Oregon Health and Science University, 3181 SW Sam Jackson Park Rd, L340 Portland, OR 97239, USA
e-mail: primacks@ohsu.edu

J. P. Kanne (ed.), *Clinically Oriented Pulmonary Imaging*, Respiratory Medicine, DOI: 10.1007/978-1-61779-542-8_7,

Table 7.1 Risk factors for VTE [7–9]

Age greater than 75
Malignancy
Previous VTE
Chronic respiratory disease
Surgery (<3 months)
Central venous instrumentation (≤3 months)
Inherited thrombophilias
Immobility
Obesity

incidence rate was 29 in 100,000, but varied greatly depending on age. Those <55 and 55–64 years old had incidence rates of 11 and 33/100,000, respectively, while ages 65–74 and ≥75 had incidence rates of 136 and 134/100,000, respectively [4]. The case fatality rate for pulmonary embolus is 4–7% [5].

Risk Factors for VTE

The randomized, double blind placebo controlled trial, MEDENOX (prophylaxis in *MED*ical patients with *ENOX*aparin) reviewed general medical hospitalized patients with VTE. The investigators found that acute infectious disease, age greater than 75, history of VTE, and cancers were significantly associated with development of VTE [6]. Other studies have noted major surgery or trauma, obesity, immobility, and inherited thrombophilias were also independent risk factors [7, 8]. A recent meta-analysis of 5,997 patients revealed only 3 risk factors for PE: active cancer, recent surgery, and current DVT [9] (see Table 7.1).

Presenting Signs and Symptoms

Extrapolated from prospective investigation of pulmonary embolism diagnosis (PIOPED) and PIOPED II data, the most common presenting signs and symptoms for patients diagnosed with PE were dyspnea, cough, leg swelling and pain, and chest pain (which occurred primarily with pulmonary infarction) [8, 10]. The absence of dyspnea and tachypnea is helpful in ruling out PE [9]. The most common clinical signs of PE were tachypnea, crackles, tachycardia, increased P2, and fever [8] (see Table 7.2).

Wells Criteria

Different clinical probability tools have been developed to assess the risk of acute PE. Wells criteria, the most cited tool, assigned a point value to a limited number of clinical features to determine the likelihood of PE. The original prediction model stratified patients into three clinical probabilities. A total score of <2 points indicated low probability, 2–6 reflected intermediate/moderate probability, and >6 suggested high probability of having a PE. Based on a prospective study of 153 patients, pulmonary embolism prevalence was 2, 15, and 43%, respectively [11, 12] (see Table 7.3).

A simplified version of the Wells criteria was developed to place patients into two clinical probabilities. A large prospective study of 3,306 patients suspected of acute PE showed that a score <4 ("PE unlikely") indicated a 12% prevalence of acute pulmonary embolism. A score ≥4 ("PE likely") indicated a 37% prevalence [13]. Several subsequent studies have validated the dichotomous version in conjunction with other testing in diagnosing acute PE [14].

Diagnostic Testing

D-Dimer

D-dimer is a degradation product of cross-linked fibrin and can be detected relatively quickly (minutes) by a variety of tests, most often using enzyme-linked immunosorbent assays (ELISA). The D-dimer test is highly sensitive, but is limited by its poor specificity in many populations. It remains a helpful tool for those with a

Table 7.2 Presenting signs and symptoms [8, 9]

Presenting sign or symptom	% Prevalence in VTE
Dyspnea	76–79
Tachypnea	59–68
Chest pain, pleuritic	47–74
Cough	42–43
Calf or thigh swelling or pain	27–42
Tachycardia	28–29
Chest pain, non-pleuritic	17
Increased P2	15–27
Hemoptysis	16
Circulatory collapse	8
Fever (>38.5°C)	2–5

Table 7.3 Wells criteria [11]

Wells criteria	Points
Signs and symptoms of DVT	3
An alternative diagnosis less likely than PE	3
Heart rate greater than 100 beats/min	1.5
Recent surgery in the past 4 weeks	1.5
Previous DVT or PE	1.5
Malignancy in the last 6 months	1
Hemoptysis	1

low pre-test probability for VTE as determined by a clinical decision tool, such as Wells criteria. A multicenter study showed that a combination of low clinical suspicion and a negative D-dimer decreases the probability of VTE to 2% [15]. The 3-month thromboembolic risk of those unlikely to have VTE was found to be as low as 0.14% [16]. If the resulting D-dimer assay is normal with a low pre-test probability, no further diagnostic imaging or continued anticoagulation is recommended. If positive, then further imaging is suggested.

D-dimer has poor specificity in many populations. D-dimer levels have been shown to significantly increase with age in those without VTE, and therefore cannot be reliably used in an aging population [17]. D-dimer is frequently nonspecific in hospitalized patients. Patients without VTE who had been hospitalized four days or more had a significantly elevated D-dimer compared with those hospitalized for 3 days or less [17]. Other populations that commonly have an elevated D-dimer without proven VTE are trauma and postoperative patients, pregnancy, heart disease, and concurrent infection.

Summary/Future Considerations

D-dimer is an excellent way to rule out PE with a negative test and potentially save the patient from unneeded cost and radiation exposure. However, many patients will have a positive test for a variety of reasons. D-dimer should not be ordered in patients with a high likelihood of a false positive result.

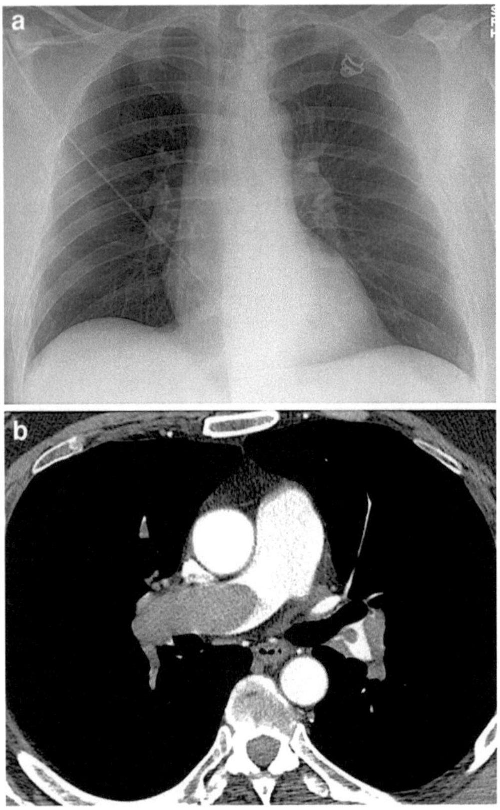

Fig. 7.1 Westermark sign. **a** AP chest radiograph shows diffuse lucency throughout the right hemithorax and decreased vascularity throughout the right lung. **b** Contrast-enhanced CT scan shows a large occlusive pulmonary embolism in the right main pulmonary artery and a small nonocclusive clot in the left lower lobe pulmonary artery

There are several different tests on the market, and familiarity with the particular test used is important in its interpretation. Different tests have different "cut-offs" for positive/negative. A level of 500 μg/L is often used, but a recent study suggested this could be increased to 1,000 μg/L [18]. Validating a higher cut-off value would result in fewer diagnostic tests needed.

Chest Radiography

A chest radiograph is usually the first imaging test obtained and is most helpful in finding an alternative diagnosis. Because PE can occur concurrently with other pulmonary diagnoses, chest radiography cannot exclude PE in a patient with a high pre-test probability.

The radiograph of a patient diagnosed with a PE is often normal or has very subtle abnormalities. In a study of 2,454 patients diagnosed with pulmonary emboli, the most common radiographic findings were cardiac enlargement (27%), normal (24%), pleural effusion (23%), elevated hemidiaphragm (20%), followed by pulmonary artery enlargement, atelectasis, consolidation, pulmonary congestion, oligemia, pulmonary infarction, and over-inflation [19].

Westermark's sign and Hampton's hump have historically been referenced with respect to pulmonary emboli; however both are very uncommon. Westermark's sign is an abrupt tapering of a blood vessel or area of oligemia due to the presence of a thrombus within that vessel with decreased vascularity distal to the obstructed pulmonary artery (Fig. 7.1). Hampton's hump is a peripheral focal area of subpleural consolidation that represents a pulmonary infarction (Fig. 7.2).

Summary/Future Considerations

The primary role for chest radiography in the diagnosis of PE is to identify alternative diagnoses. It is worth noting that VTE can occur in the presence of other pulmonary disorders and the decision to proceed to further imaging must be made on a case-by-case basis. Radiography is also valuable in determining the potential effectiveness of a ventilation/perfusion (V/Q) scan.

Ventilation/Perfusion Scan

The original PIOPED study assessed the use of V/Q scanning in diagnosing pulmonary emboli [20]. This study compared V/Q scanning to the gold standard at that time, pulmonary angiography. The study demonstrated that V/Q scanning was an effective diagnostic tool when the clinical pre-test probability of PE was low or

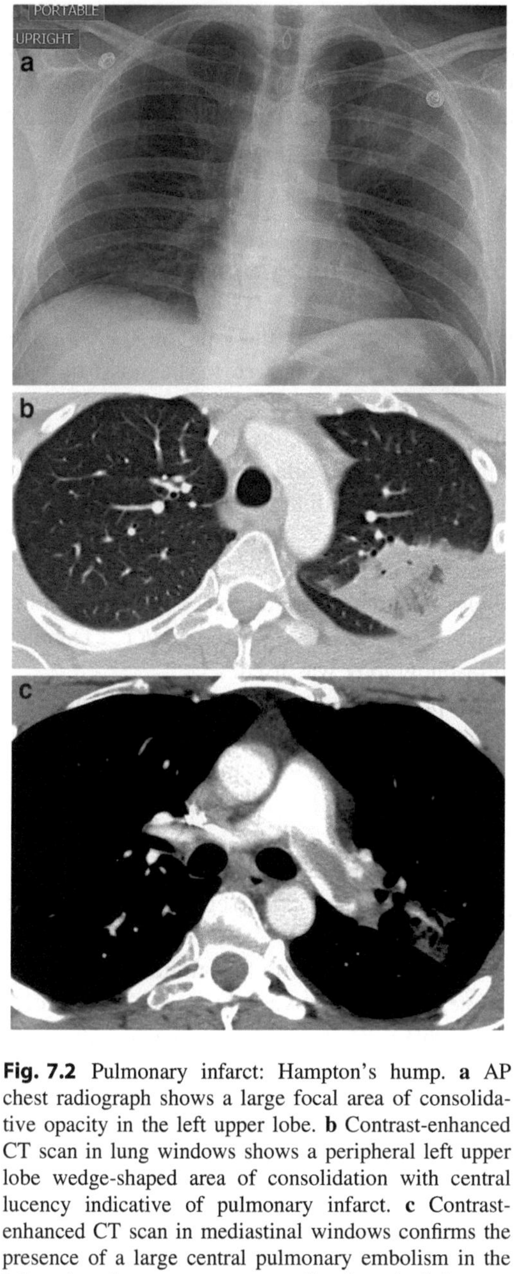

Fig. 7.2 Pulmonary infarct: Hampton's hump. **a** AP chest radiograph shows a large focal area of consolidative opacity in the left upper lobe. **b** Contrast-enhanced CT scan in lung windows shows a peripheral left upper lobe wedge-shaped area of consolidation with central lucency indicative of pulmonary infarct. **c** Contrast-enhanced CT scan in mediastinal windows confirms the presence of a large central pulmonary embolism in the left main pulmonary artery extending into the left upper lobe pulmonary artery

high, in conjunction with a low- or high-probability V/Q scan result. Unfortunately, only 14% of subjects had a normal V/Q scan and 13% had a high-probability scan (Fig. 7.3), leaving a large proportion as indeterminate (nondiagnostic).

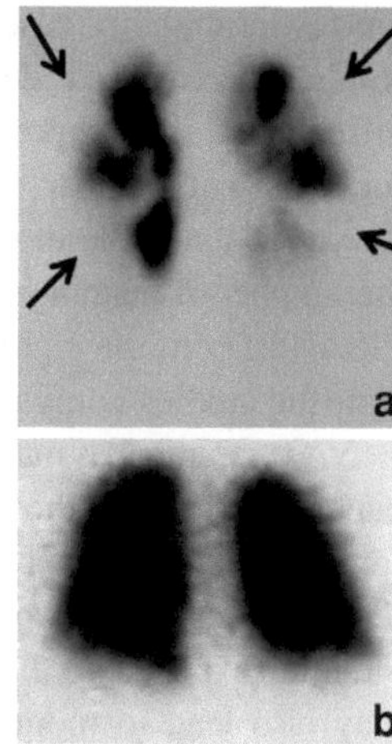

Fig. 7.3 High probability V/Q scan. **a** Perfusion scan shows multiple bilateral large perfusion defects (*arrows*). **b** Ventilation scan shows normal ventilation

Since PIOPED, modified criteria have been developed to decrease the number of nondiagnostic studies. Two such criteria, "Modified PIOPED II" and "prospective investigative study of acute pulmonary embolism diagnosis" (PISA-PED), were evaluated in subjects participating in the PIOPED II study [21]. In this study, investigators assessed chest radiography combined with perfusion scans, using pulmonary angiography or chest computed tomography angiography (CTA) results with a concordant prediction rule as the gold standard. The Modified PIOPED II criteria had more nondiagnostic readings (21%) than PISA-PED (0%), but considerably less than the original PIOPED study. In subjects with a "normal" or "near normal" chest radiograph, the modified PIOPED II criteria had only 11% nondiagnostic studies. The sensitivity/specificity using Modified PIOPED II (diagnostic tests only) and PISA-PED were 85/93% and 80/97%, respectively, which are similar to PIOPED II results for CTA (see CTA section below).

Summary/Future Considerations

The V/Q scan has been used less frequently with the increasing availability of the multidetector CT scan. Patients also have to perform a breath hold during inhalation phase of the scan. V/Q scanning limitations include intermediate pre-test probability cases and indeterminate test results, increased reader variability due to the infrequency of interpretation, and the necessity for a normal or near normal chest radiograph. However, using the modified criteria can reduce the number of nondiagnostic scans considerably. PISA-PED criteria significantly decrease nondiagnostic studies compared to PIOPED criteria.

V/Q scanning has maintained its role for certain patients, primarily those with contraindications for iodine contrast (e.g. known contrast allergy, renal dysfunction) and pregnancy. Concerns about radiation exposure to the female breast with CTA may also lead to more use in younger women. Perfusion-only studies may further reduce radiation exposure.

Infrequent use of nuclear imaging for PE may jeopardize the needed expertise for accurate interpretation. Finally, single photon emission CT (SPECT) V/Q may potentially improve on planar V/Q and may be worthwhile evaluating in future studies [22].

Pulmonary Digital Subtraction Angiography

Pulmonary digital subtraction angiography (DSA) had been considered the reference standard for diagnosis of PE since the 1960s. Since the advent of the multidetector CT scanner, pulmonary angiography is no longer considered the sole gold standard for diagnosis of acute PE. Animal models using methacrylate cast emboli (the size of human subsegmental pulmonary arteries) in porcine pulmonary vessels have confirmed equivalent sensitivity and specificity of CTA and angiography, with necropsy as the gold standard [23]. Pulmonary DSA may have improved sensitivity in detecting subsegmental clot compared with older CTA technology, but suffers from poor interobserver agreement [24].

Summary/Future Considerations

CTA has replaced pulmonary DSA as the gold standard for diagnosis of acute pulmonary embolism. While animal studies have demonstrated equivalence, several factors favor CTA, including the ability to make alternative diagnoses, less patient risk, lower cost, and greater familiarity with interpretation.

Computed Tomography Angiography

PIOPED II assessed the role of CTA in the diagnosis of PE compared to diagnosis by pulmonary angiography [25]. Investigators found that CTA was effective in assessing PE if a clinical prediction rule (Wells criteria) was used in conjunction with test results. When reviewing interpretable scans (94%), the sensitivity and specificity of CTA were 83% and 96%, respectively. A composite reference standard composed of DSA, V/Q, and/or Doppler ultrasonography was used.

In patients with a high and intermediate clinical probability, the positive predictive value (PPV) of CTA was 96% and 92%, respectively. In patients with low clinical probability, the false positive rate was 42%. The PPV was also dependent on the location of the clot [main/lobar pulmonary artery (97%), segmental (68%), and subsegmental (25%)].

Among patients with low clinical probability, the negative predictive value (NPV) was excellent (96%). However, in patients with high clinical probability, the false negative rate was 40%.

As with the original PIOPED study, PIOPED II demonstrated Bayes' theorem, which states the probability of a disease after testing relies on both the test's operating characteristics (sensitivity and specificity) and the pretest probability of the diagnosis. When clinical probability and test results are concordant, the test (in this case, CTA for PE) functions very well. Discordant results, however, warrant further clinical assessment to determine if further testing is needed. PIOPED II investigators proposed diagnostic pathways based on results of the Wells clinical prediction model [26].

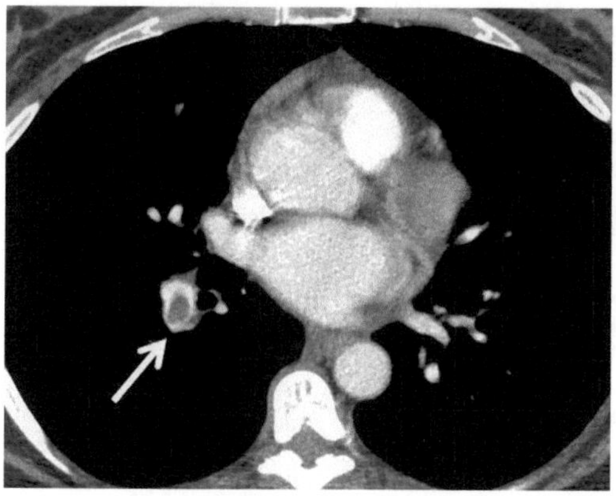

Fig. 7.4 Acute pulmonary embolism: target sign on chest CTA. Contrast enhanced CT scan shows a central filling defect in the right lower lobe pulmonary artery with a rim of contrast material (*arrow*)

Summary/Future Considerations

CTA can now be considered a gold standard for the diagnosis of acute PE. A confounding factor in assessing available data is the advancing CT technology since PIOPED II incorporated primarily four-slice CT, technology that has been largely replaced by newer 16- and 64-slice scanners in most centers. This technology has improved z-axis resolution and, therefore, improved visualization of subsegmental pulmonary arteries. Shorter scanning time has led to shorter breath hold duration for patients (previously 20–30 s; now 3–10 s) resulting in less motion artifact. Shorter scan time also allows for potential of decreased iodinated contrast volume [27].

A recent prospective study of 545 patients validated the negative predictive value using a 64-detector row scanner. Of the 367 patients with an initial negative study (received no anticoagulation), only one patient developed a symptomatic distal DVT and none developed PE in 3-month follow-up [28].

One challenge with CTA is its potential overuse. Clinical decision tools, chest radiography, and D-dimer testing can all potentially decrease unnecessary tests that have additional cost and radiation exposure. V/Q or perfusion-only scans should be considered in patients with a normal chest radiograph.

Subsegmental PE for CTA

The rapid advancement of CT technology has increased our ability to detect small, peripheral subsegmental pulmonary emboli. The clinical significance of isolated subsegmental PE is under debate. Despite these advancements, recent studies report fairly low frequencies of isolated subsegmental PE, at approximately 1–5.4% [29–32]. In a large retrospective review of 10,453 CTA studies at a single center, 93 isolated subsegmental PEs were identified. There were more adverse outcomes at 3 months in those anticoagulated compared to those that were not [33]. Further technological advancements will likely increase detection of smaller, potentially less consequential emboli.

CTA Imaging Findings of Acute PE

There are several intravascular or direct findings of acute PE on CTA. These include complete occlusion of a vessel, central filling defect, or "target sign" (Figs. 7.4, 7.5). Arterial dilatation can also be seen secondary to expansion from the intraluminal clot (Fig. 7.5).

Indirect findings of the pulmonary parenchyma include atelectasis, pulmonary infarct (Figs. 7.6, 7.7), focal hemorrhage, or focal oligemia. Small pleural effusions may be present.

In the setting of acute pulmonary embolism, the CT images should be assessed for the presence or absence of elevated right heart pressures or right heart strain. If dilation of the right ventricle and the reflux of contrast into the inferior vena cava and hepatic veins are identified on CT, there is a high likelihood of right heart strain (Fig. 7.8) [34, 35].

Enlargement of the main pulmonary artery is another finding suggestive of elevated right heart

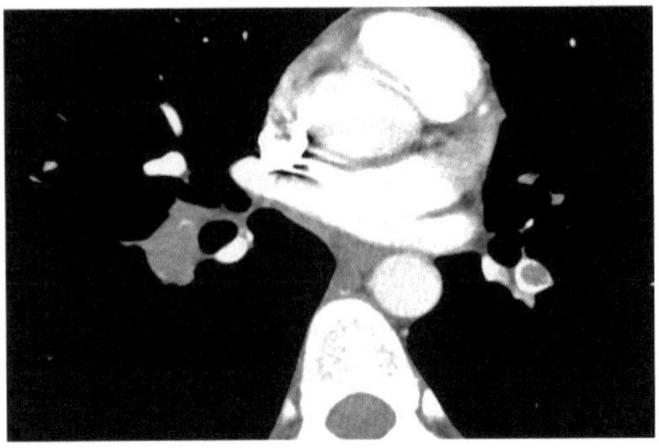

Fig. 7.5 Acute bilateral pulmonary embolism: occlusive expansile clot and target sign. Contrast-enhanced CT scan shows occlusive clot expanding the right lower lobe pulmonary artery and nonocclusive left lower lobe pulmonary embolism with central filling defect and rim of contrast material

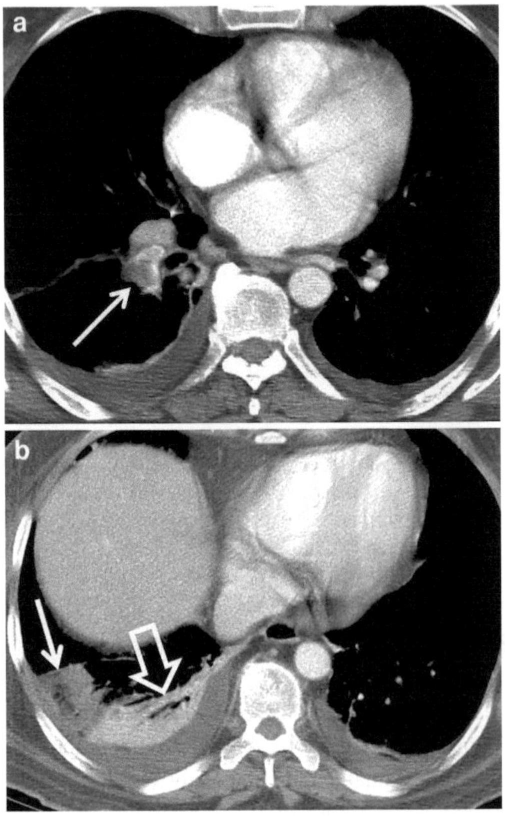

Fig. 7.6 Acute pulmonary embolism: pulmonary infarct and atelectasis. **a** Contrast-enhanced CT scan shows right lower lobe acute pulmonary embolism (*arrow*). Small pleural effusions are present. **b** Nonenhancing peripheral right lower lobe consolidation with central low attenuation represents pulmonary infarct (*thin arrow*). Enhancing posterior right lower lobe consolidation with crowded airways represents atelectasis (*open arrow*). Small bilateral pleural effusions are also present

pressures. Findings of elevated right heart pressures have clinical implications for the patient with acute PE.

Pitfalls of CTA for PE Diagnosis

While CTA is the gold standard for diagnosing PE, there are pitfalls that can lead to false positive and negative results. Contrast delivery errors include poor timing of contrast bolus, transient interruption of contrast, and streak artifact from beam hardening (dense SVC contrast, presence of intravascular catheter) (Figs. 7.9, 7.11). Respiratory and motion artifact, adjacent lymph nodes, and mucus filled bronchi can also mimic acute PE (Figs. 7.10, 7.11, 7.12).

Magnetic Resonance Angiography

In PIOPED II, 22% of patients could not undergo CT angiography due to contraindications to iodinated contrast. This spurred the PIOPED III study, which investigated the accuracy of gadolinium-enhanced magnetic resonance angiography (MRA) as an alternative to CT angiography [36]. The composite reference standard in PIOPED II was used for this study, as well. During recruitment, because of emerging evidence that gadolinium was linked to the development of nephrogenic systemic fibrosis (NSF) in patients with acute and chronic renal failure, PIOPED III investigators excluded patients with an elevated creatinine (>1.5 mg/dL for men; >1.4 mg/dL for women).

MRA was technically inadequate in 25% of patients (range 11–51% among the 7 study centers). The most common reasons for technical inadequacy were poor arterial opacification and motion artifact.

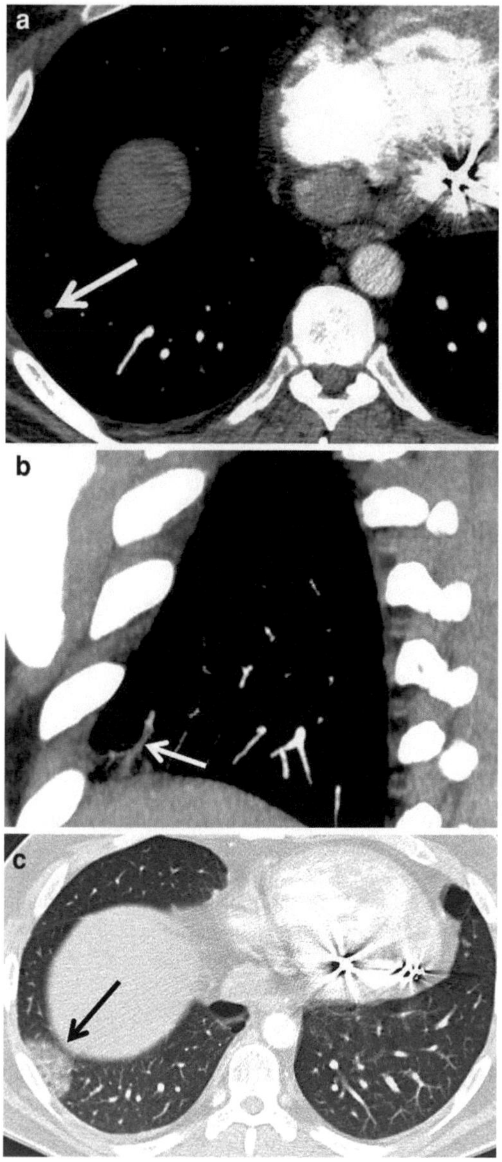

Fig. 7.7 Subsegmental pulmonary embolism with pulmonary infarct. Axial (**a**) and oblique (**b**) reconstructed contrast-enhanced CT images show an acute subsegmental pulmonary embolism (*arrows*). **c** Lung windows demonstrate a small subpleural right lower lobe pulmonary infarct (*arrow*)

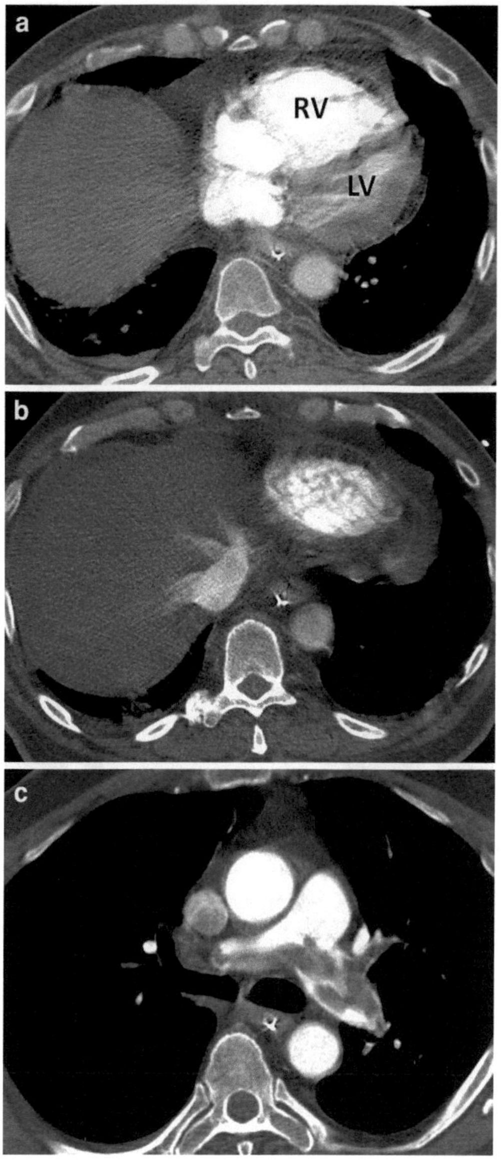

Fig. 7.8 Elevated right heart pressures due to large saddle pulmonary embolism. **a** Contrast-enhanced CT image shows a dilated right ventricle (*RV*) much larger than the left ventricle (*LV*). The interventricular septum is bowed to the left. These findings are indicators of elevated right heart pressures. **b** There is reflux of contrast material into the inferior vena cava and hepatic veins. **c** Large saddle embolism involving the left and right main pulmonary arteries

Among subjects with technically adequate studies, the sensitivity and specificity were 78% and 99%, respectively. MRA had a poor sensitivity (40%) for segmental and subsegmental emboli, which represented 8% of the emboli in this study, potentially due to poor arterial opacification in smaller vessels. Specificity remained 98% or above regardless of artery size [36].

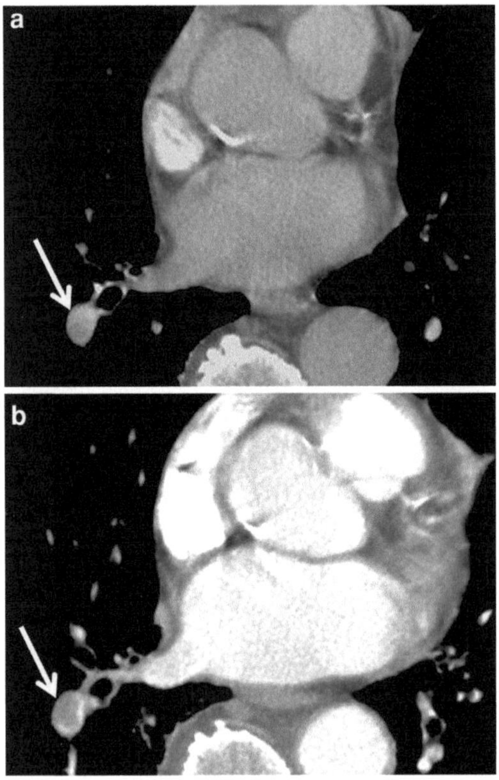

Fig. 7.9 Pitfall: inadequate pulmonary artery opacification. **a** There is inadequate contrast opacification of the right lower lobe pulmonary artery (*arrow*) on this contrast enhanced CT scan. **b** Repeat CT scan was performed 6 h later and shows a definite acute pulmonary embolism with target sign (*arrow*)

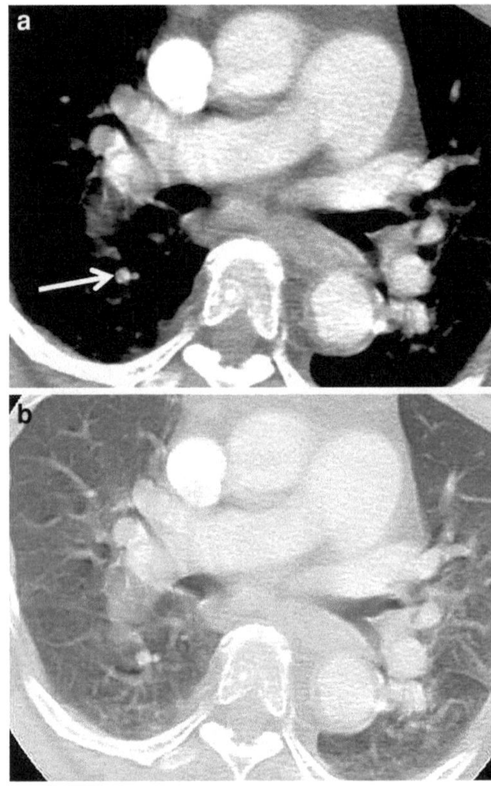

Fig. 7.10 Pitfall: respiratory motion artifact. **a** Contrast-enhanced CT scan shows a questionable filling defect in a right lower lobe segmental pulmonary artery (*arrow*). **b** Lung windows at the same level as (**a**) show substantial motion artifact indicating that the finding is likely related to blurring from motion

Summary/Future Considerations

Given the overall technical inadequacy and limitations, MRA should generally not be considered to diagnose PE. MRA is no longer considered an acceptable alternative to CTA for those with renal failure. MRA should only be considered in patients for whom standard testing is contraindicated and performed only at centers that have demonstrated both technical and diagnostic excellence. Developing a better contrast agent could potentially decrease the number of inadequate studies. Gadofosveset trisodium remains in the circulation for up to an hour and could reduce bolus-timing errors [37].

Adjuvant Diagnostic Testing

Arterial Blood Gas

PIOPED II assessed the alveolar-arterial gradient (A-a O2), PaO_2 and $PaCO_2$ in patients diagnosed with PE. While some have used a normal A-a gradient to exclude PE, PIOPED II data showed that 32% of patients with PE had a *normal* gradient (<20) [8]. The absence of hypoxia (PaO_2 >80 mm Hg) was just as prevalent in proven cases of PE (32%). $PaCO_2$ lacks sufficient diagnostic utility as it may be elevated or decreased. There is a trend toward respiratory alkalosis, likely from compensatory hyperventilation.

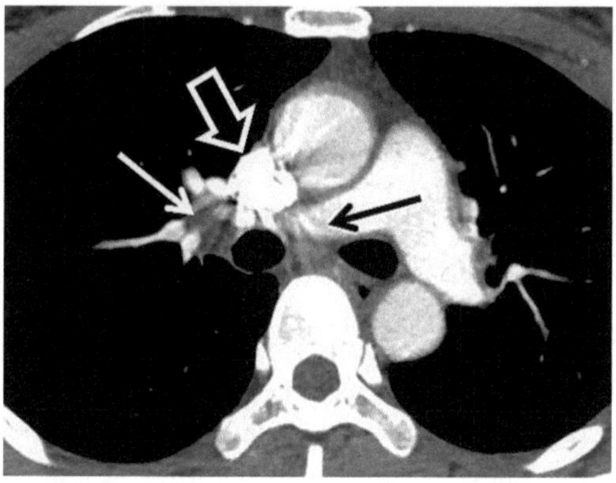

Fig. 7.11 Pitfall: Lymph node adjacent to pulmonary artery. Contrast-enhanced CT shows a normal right hilar lymph node (*thin white arrow*) adjacent to the right pulmonary artery. This should not be confused with an intraluminal filling defect. There is also dense contrast material in the superior vena cava (*open arrow*) causing streak artifact (*black arrow*) through the right main pulmonary artery

Troponin

Elevated troponin levels have been demonstrated in 30–50% of documented cases of PE [38–40]. Specificity is poor given its presence in myocardial infarctions. It therefore does not serve a purpose in PE diagnosis but may be predictive of mortality [39].

ECG

While the ECG can reveal changes secondary to PE, they are nonspecific. The well-known "S1Q3T3" pattern (prominent S in leads I and Q and inverted T in lead III) occurs in up to 50% of cases, but is not a valuable tool in establishing the diagnosis of PE given its poor specificity. The pattern reflects right heart strain, which can be present in non-PE scenarios. The ECG plays a more important role in identifying alternative diagnoses, such as myocardial infarction. Some of the more common findings associated with PE are incomplete RBBB, tachycardia, anterior T wave inversions, and nonspecific ST-T wave changes [41, 42].

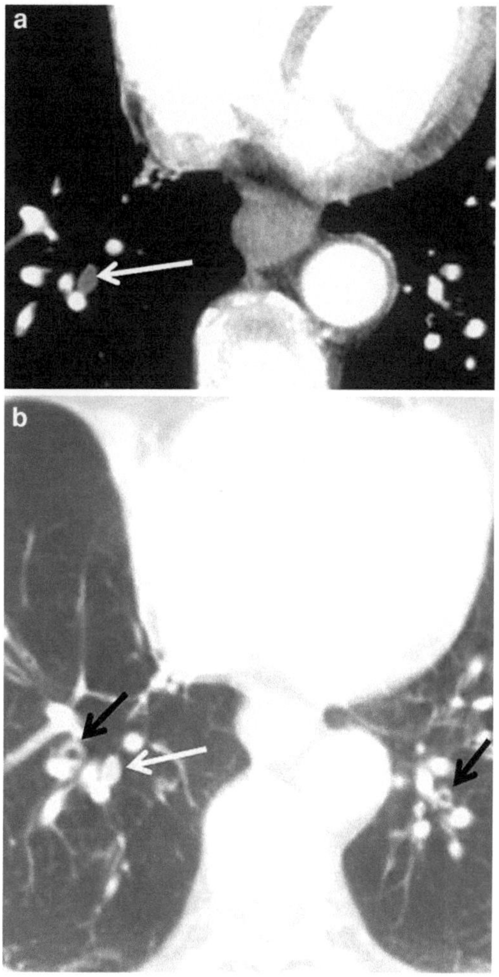

Fig. 7.12 Pitfall: mucus plug CT scan in mediastinal (**a**) and lung (**b**) windows shows a low attenuation mucus plug in a subsegmental right lower lobe bronchus (*thin arrows*). Normal enhancing subsegmental pulmonary arteries are adjacent to the mucus plug. Also note airway thickening (*black arrows in b*) involving subsegmental bronchi in both lower lobes

Transthoracic Echocardiography

Transthoracic echocardiography (TTE) lacks sufficient sensitivity or specificity to be used in diagnosis of PE on its own. From pooled data, the prevalence of right ventricular dysfunction (presence of ventricular wall motion abnormalities and dilation of the right ventricular cavity) in normotensive patients is approximately 30–40%

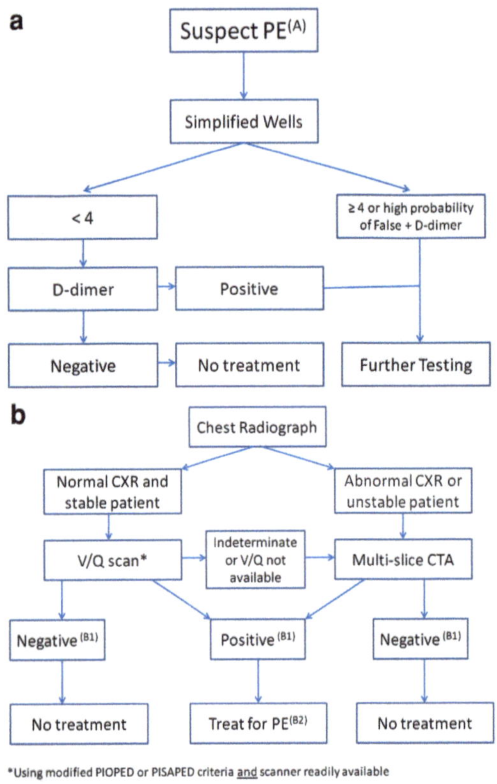

Fig. 7.13 Diagnostic algorithm for acute pulmonary embolism. **a** If signs/symptoms of DVT, leg ultrasound should be performed first. **b** (1) If test results are discordant with pre-test clinical probability of PE,clinical judgment is needed to review other possible options: V/Q scan or repeat CTA if CTA initially done; CTA if V/Q initially done; digital subtraction angiography in a center of expertise; serial lower extremity ultrasound. (2) If an isolated subsegmental PE is noted on multi-slice CTA, it is reasonable to have a risks/benefits discussion regarding treatment

[43]. Evidence of right ventricular dysfunction is more common in massive PE for which standard diagnostic methods have excellent sensitivity.

Summary/Future Directions

Adjuvant testing is most helpful in assessing the patient's pre-test probability of PE prior to more definitive testing. It may be helpful in prognosis, and as such, may affect decision-making for diagnostic testing. For example, for patients needing an expedited diagnosis (e.g. significant cardiopulmonary compromise and/or signs of right heart strain), clinicians may opt for CTA rather than V/Q.

Diagnostic Algorithms for Acute PE

A variety of algorithms have been proposed for the diagnosis of acute PE [26, 44, 45]. Many incorporate the use of a clinical decision tool and D-dimer to determine if further testing is necessary. The Christopher Study Investigators showed that an algorithm using the simplified Wells criteria, D-dimer, and CTA was effective in managing suspected PE [13].

We propose a two-tiered algorithm (see Fig. 7.13).

Figure 7.13a involves the use of Wells criteria (simplified) and D-dimer to capture patients with extremely low probability of PE that do not need further testing.

Figure 7.13b incorporates imaging. The technical expertise for each imaging modality must be taken into account when determining the appropriate algorithm at a given center. In addition, patient stability may dictate initial testing, as CTA is more conducive for the unstable patient needing rapid diagnosis.

Special Cases

Pregnancy

Pregnancy and the immediate postpartum period have been reported to carry up to a five-fold increase in VTE events [46]. The risks of radiation exposure to the fetus and maternal breasts present a significant challenge during pregnancy. Fetal radiation exposures of CTA versus V/Q scan are 0.1–0.7 and 0.9 mGy, respectively. Doses under 1 mGy are considered negligible [47]. Iodinated contrast from CTA does cross the placenta, and raises concern for effects on fetal thyroid tissue. However, a recent study showed that normal

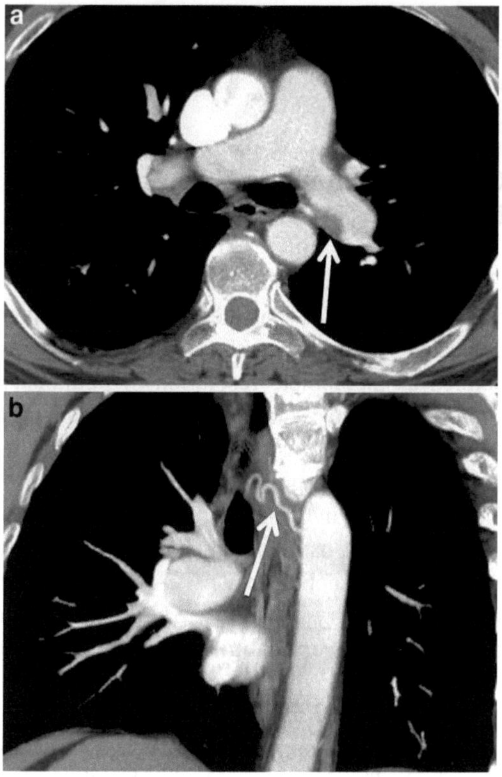

Fig. 7.14 Chronic pulmonary embolism with bronchial collaterals. **a** Contrast-enhanced CT scan shows an eccentric chronic clot in the left main pulmonary artery (*arrow*). **b** Coronal reconstructed CT image shows an enlarged, tortuous bronchial artery collateral (*arrow*)

thyroxine levels were present in all neonates of 344 pregnant women who had iodinated contrast for CTA [48]. A potential benefit of CTA is identification of an alternative diagnosis.

A recent retrospective study comparing CTA and V/Q scanning in pregnancy concluded that both modalities are comparable for PE diagnosis, but CTA had significantly more maternal radiation dose [49]. Maternal breast radiation dose for CTA versus V/Q scan are 10–30 and 0.3–0.5 mGy, respectively, which is a 30–100 fold increase in radiation for CTA. CTA was able to identify an alternative diagnosis in 12% of patients suspected of having PE.

Diagnostic Path for Pregnancy

A suggested algorithm for pregnant patients may start with D-dimer and a clinical assessment tool (e.g. Wells criteria), which may potentially rule out VTE. If there is still suspicion in a hemodynamically stable patient, duplex ultrasonography (if clinically suspected) can diagnose DVT, without ionizing radiation. If the ultrasound is negative or not warranted, chest radiography can potentially make an alternative diagnosis with minimal radiation.

If the radiograph is clear, V/Q scan is the recommended test of choice given the decreased maternal breast radiation exposure and equivalence in diagnostic accuracy as CTA. If the radiograph is not clear or a rapid diagnosis is needed, CTA could be used with a lower radiation protocol.

Renal Failure

Iodinated contrast may potentially cause acute kidney injury, particularly in patients with impaired renal function. Therefore, it is relatively contraindicated in patients with impaired renal function or renal failure. In PIOPED II, only 1 of 824 patients who had CTA developed renal failure with nonionic contrast, primarily because patients with abnormal serum creatinine were excluded from the study [25].

Diagnostic Pathway for Patients with Renal Failure

As with pregnancy, D-dimer with a clinical decision tool and the use of venous ultrasonography if there are signs of DVT can potentially avoid further testing. If no DVT is found, V/Q or perfusion-only scanning is the recommended test of choice if the chest radiograph is clear.

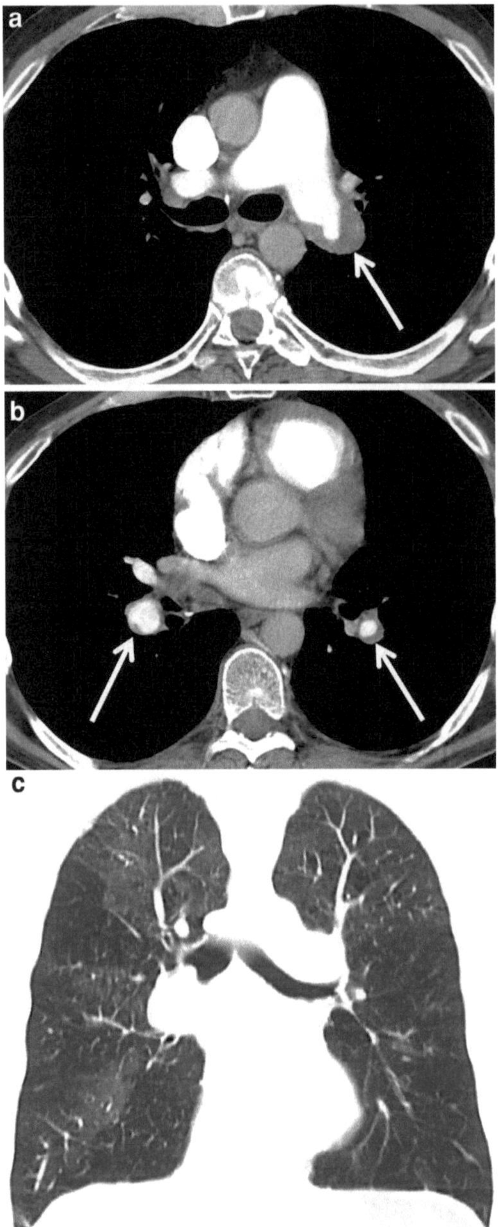

Fig. 7.15 Chronic pulmonary embolism with mosaic perfusion. **a** and **b** Contrast-enhanced CT images show eccentric chronic clot in the left main pulmonary artery (*arrow in a*) and eccentric clot in the right and left lower lobe pulmonary arteries (*arrows in b*). The main pulmonary artery is enlarged. **c** Coronal reformation in lung windows shows patchy areas of ground-glass opacity associated with relatively larger vessels. There are patchy areas of lucency (oligemia) associated with diminished vessel size. The oligemic areas represent decreased perfusion distal to the chronic pulmonary emboli

If creatinine is mildly elevated, clinical judgment should be used to determine if CTA is warranted.

Chronic Pulmonary Thromboembolic Disease

Chronic pulmonary thromboembolism will be reviewed here briefly, as there is another chapter dedicated to its discussion. Chronic PTE is defined as incomplete resolution of pulmonary emboli and may lead to the development of pulmonary hypertension (chronic thromboembolic-associated pulmonary hypertension—CTEPH). The incidence of CTEPH is likely underestimated, as many cases are diagnosed at autopsy, but is approximately 2–4% of patients who had a history of PE [50, 51]. Identification of chronic PE is critical given that CTEPH is a potentially reversible form of pulmonary hypertension with surgical intervention.

CTA features for chronic PE have been well-described. The intraluminal clot location of a chronic PE is usually eccentric and has an obtuse angle to the vessel (Figs. 7.13, 7.14). This differs from the appearance of acute PE, which is either central or eccentric with a sharp angle to the vessel. Vessel stenosis, post-stenotic dilation, webs, and bands are vascular findings seen in chronic PE. Enlarged collateral arteries (bronchial and intercostals) may be present and are not a feature seen in acute PE (Fig. 7.14). Lung parenchymal findings include mosaic perfusion, areas of pleural thickening, or scarring from areas of prior infarction (Fig. 7.14). Associated findings of enlargement of the main pulmonary artery and right ventricular wall hypertrophy are frequently present when there is associated pulmonary hypertension (Fig. 7.15).

Conclusion

Chest CTA has replaced pulmonary DSA and is now the gold standard for diagnosis of acute pulmonary embolism. Advances in CT technology have allowed for continued improved accuracy. Additionally, CT often reveals alternative diagnoses to explain the patient's clinical presentation. However, one challenge of CTA is its potential overuse. For this reason, when pulmonary embolism is a diagnostic consideration, chest radiography, a clinical decision tool, and possibly D-dimer should be used to identify low risk patients that do not need further testing. In addition, if the chest radiograph is normal, V/Q scan should be considered as the next imaging study to evaluate for pulmonary embolism.

References

1. Anderson FA Jr, Wheeler HB, Goldberg RJ, et al. A population-based perspective of the hospital incidence and case-fatality rates of deep vein thrombosis and pulmonary embolism: the Worcester DVT study. Arch Intern Med. 1991;151:933–8.
2. Silverstein MD, Heit JA, Mohr DN, Petterson TM, O'Fallon WM, Melton LJ 3rd. Trends in the incidence of deep vein thrombosis and pulmonary embolism: a 25-year population-based study. Arch Intern Med. 1998;158:585–93.
3. Dalen JE, Alpert JS. Natural history of pulmonary embolism. Prog Cardiovasc Dis. 1975;17(4):259–70.
4. Spencer FA, Emery C, Lessard D, et al. The Worcester venous thromboembolism study: a population-based study of the clinical epidemiology of venous thromboembolism. J Gen Intern Med. 2006;21:722–7.
5. Hirsh J, Hull RD, Raskob GE. Epidemiology and pathogenesis of venous thrombosis. J Am Coll Cardiol. 1986;8(6 Suppl B):104B–13B.
6. Alikhan R, Cohen AT, Combe S, et al. Risk factors for venous thromboembolism in hospitalized patients with acute medical illness: analysis of the MEDENOX Study. Arch Intern Med. 2004;164(9):963–8.
7. Anderson FA Jr, Spencer FA. Risk factors for venous thromboembolism. Circulation. 2003;107(23 Suppl 1): I9–26.
8. Stein PD, Beemath A, Matta F, et al. Clinical characteristics of patients with acute pulmonary embolism: data from PIOPED II. Am J Med. 2007;120(10):871–9.
9. West J, Goodacre S, Sampson F. The value of clinical features in the diagnosis of acute pulmonary embolism: systematic review and meta-analysis. QJM. 2007;100(12):763–9.
10. Stein PD, Henry JW. Clinical characteristics of patients with acute pulmonary embolism stratified according to their presenting syndromes. Chest. 1997;112(4):974–9.
11. Wells PS, Anderson DR, Rodger M, et al. Excluding pulmonary embolism at the bedside without diagnostic imaging: management of patients with suspected pulmonary embolism presenting to the emergency department by using a simple clinical model and d-dimer. Ann Intern Med. 2001;135(2):98–107.
12. Wolf SJ, McCubbin TR, Feldhaus KM, Faragher JP, Adcock DM. Prospective validation of Wells criteria in the evaluation of patients with suspected pulmonary embolism. Ann Emerg Med. 2004;44(5):503–10.
13. van Belle A, Büller HR, Huisman MV, et al. Effectiveness of managing suspected pulmonary embolism using an algorithm combining clinical probability, D-dimer testing, and computed tomography. JAMA. 2006;295(2):172–9.
14. Pasha SM, Klok FA, Snoep JD, et al. Safety of excluding acute pulmonary embolism based on an unlikely clinical probability by the Wells rule and normal D-dimer concentration: a meta-analysis. Thrombosis Res. 2010;125:e123–7.
15. Kline JA, Courtney DM, Kabrhel C, Moore CL, Smithline HA, Plewa MC, Richman PB, OÕNeil BJ, Nordenholz K. Prospective multicenter evaluation of the pulmonary embolism rule-out criteria. J Thromb Haemost. 2008;6:772–80.
16. Carrier M, Righini M, Djurabi RK, et al. VIDAS D-dimer in combination with clinical pre-test probability to rule out pulmonary embolism: a systematic review of management outcome studies. Thromb Haemost. 2009;101:886–92.
17. Brotman DJ, Segal JB, Jani JT, Petty BG, Kickler TS. Limitations of D-dimer testing in unselected inpatients with suspected venous thromboembolism. Am J Med. 2003;114:276–82.
18. Hirai LK, Takahashi JM, Yoon HC. A prospective evaluation of a quantitative D-dimer assay in the evaluation of acute pulmonary embolism. J Vasc Interv Radiol. 2007;18:970–4.
19. Elliott CG, Goldhaber SZ, Visani L, DeRosa M. Chest radiographs in acute pulmonary embolism: results from the International Cooperative Pulmonary Embolism Registry. Chest. 2000;118:33–8.
20. The PIOPED Investigators. Value of the ventilation/perfusion scan in acute pulmonary embolism: results of the prospective investigation of pulmonary embolism diagnosis (PIOPED). JAMA. 1990;263(20):2753–59.
21. Sostman HD, Miniati M, Gottschalk A, Matta F, Stein PD, Pistolesi M. Sensitivity and specificity of perfusion scintigraphy combined with chest radiography for acute pulmonary embolism in PIOPED II. J Nucl Med. 2008;49:1741–8.
22. Stein PD, Freeman LM, Sostman HD, et al. SPECT in acute pulmonary embolism. J Nucl Med. 2009;50:1999–2007.
23. Coxson HO, Baile EM, King GG, Mayo JR. Diagnosis of subsegmental pulmonary emboli: a

multi-center study using a porcine model. J Thorac Imaging. 2005;20:24–31.
24. Quinn MF, Lundell CJ, Klotz TA, et al. Reliability of selective pulmonary arteriography in the diagnosis of pulmonary embolism. AJR. 1987;149:469–71.
25. Stein PD, Fowler SE, Goodman LR, et al. Multidetector comuted tomography for acute pulmonary embolism. N Engl J Med. 2006;354:2317–27.
26. Stein PD, Woodard PK, Weg JG, et al. Diagnostic pathways in acute pulmonary embolism: recommendations of the PIOPED II investigators. Am J Med. 2006;119:1048–55.
27. Kuriakose J, Patel S. Acute pulmonary embolism. Radiol Clin N Am. 2010;48:31–50.
28. Pesavento R, de Conti G, Minotto I, et al. The value of 64-detector row computed tomography for the exclusion of pulmonary embolism. Thromb Haemost. 2011;105(5):901–7.
29. Coche E, Verschuren F, Keyeux A, et al. Diagnosis of acute pulmonary embolism in outpatients: comparison of thin-collimation multi–detector row spiral CT and planar ventilation-perfusion scintigraphy. Radiology. 2003;229:757–65.
30. Brunot S, Corneloup O, Latrabe V, Montaudon M, Laurent F. Reproducibility of multidetector spiral computed tomography in detection of subsegmental acute pulmonary embolism. Euro Radiol. 2005;15:2057–63.
31. Perrier A, Roy PM, Sanchez O, et al. Multidetector-row computed tomography in suspected pulmonary embolism. N Engl J Med. 2005;352:1760–8.
32. Eyer BA, Goodman LR, Washington L. Clinicians' response to radiologists' reports of isolated subsegmental pulmonary embolism or inconclusive interpretation of pulmonary embolism using MDCT. Am J Roentgenol. 2005;184:623–8.
33. Donato AA, Khoche S, Santora J, Wagner B. Clinical outcomes in patients with isolated subsegmental pulmonary emboli diagnosed by multidetector CT pulmonary angiography. Thrombosis Res. 2010;126:e266–70.
34. van der Meer RW, Pattynama PM, van Strijen MJ, et al. Right ventricular dysfunction and pulmonary obstruction index at helical CT: prediction of clinical outcome during 3-month follow-up in patients with acute pulmonary embolism. Radiology. 2005;235(3):798–803.
35. Lim KE, Chan CY, Chu PH, Hsu YY, Hsu WC. Right ventricular dysfunction secondary to acute massive pulmonary embolism detected by helical computed tomography pulmonary angiography. Clin Imaging. 2005;29(1):16–21.
36. Stein PD, Chenevert TL, Fowler SE, et al. Gadolinium-enhanced magnetic resonance angiography for pulmonary embolism: a multicenter prospective study (PIOPED III). Ann Intern Med. 2010;152(7):434–43, W142–3.
37. Hadizadeh DR, Gieseke J, Lohmaier SH, et al. Peripheral MR angiography with blood pool contrast agent: prospective intraindividual comparative study of high-spatial-resolution steady-state MR angiography versus standard-resolution first-pass MR angiography and DSA. Radiology. 2008;249(2):701–11.
38. Meyer T, Binder L, Hruska N, Luthe H, Buchwald AB. Cardiac troponin I elevation in acute pulmonary embolism is associated with right ventricular dysfunction. J Am Coll Cardiol. 2000;36(5):1632–6.
39. Pruszczyk P, Bochowicz A, Torbicki A, et al. Cardiac troponin T monitoring identifies high-risk group of normotensive patients with acute pulmonary embolism. Chest. 2003;123(6):1947–52.
40. Giannitsis E, Müller-Bardorff M, Kurowski V, et al. Independent prognostic value of cardiac troponin T in patients with confirmed pulmonary embolism. Circulation. 2000;102(2):211–7.
41. Ferrari E, et al. The ECG in pulmonary embolism. Chest. 1997;111:537–43.
42. Stein PD, et al. Clinical characteristics of patients with acute pulmonary embolism. Am J Cardio. 1991;68:1723–4.
43. Gibson NS, Sohne M, Buller HR. Prognostic value of echocardiography and spiral computed tomography in patients with pulmonary embolism. Curr Opin Pulm Med. 2005;11(5):380–4.
44. Roy PM, Colombet I, Durieux P, Chatellier G, Sors H, Meyer G. Systematic review and meta-analysis of strategies for the diagnosis of suspected pulmonary embolism. BMJ. 2005;331(7511):259.
45. Gandara E, Wells PS. Diagnosis: use of clinical probability algorithms. Clin Chest Med. 2010;31(4):629–39.
46. Prevention of venous thrombosis and pulmonary embolism. NIH consensus development. JAMA. 1986;256:744–9.
47. Hurwitz LM, Yoshizumi T, Reiman RE, et al. Radiation dose to the fetus from body MDCT during early gestation. Am J Roentgenol. 2006;186:871–6.
48. Bourjeily G, Chalhoub M, Phornphutkul C, Alleyne TC, Woodfield CA, Chen KK. Neonatal thyroid function: effect of a single exposure to iodinated contrast medium in utero. Radiology. 2010;256(3):744–50.
49. Revel MP, Cohen S, Sanchez O, et al. Pulmonary embolism during pregnancy: diagnosis with lung scintigraphy or CT angiography? Radiology. 2011;258(2):590–8.
50. Pengo V, Lensing AW, Prins MH, et al. Incidence of chronic thromboembolic pulmonary hypertension after pulmonary embolism. N Engl J Med. 2004;350:2257–64.
51. Becattini C, Agnelli G, Pesavento R, et al. Incidence of chronic thromboembolic pulmonary hypertension after a first episode of pulmonary embolism. Chest. 2006;130:172–5.

Non-Thrombotic Vascular Diseases of the Chest

8

Elena Peña, Carole Dennie, and George Chandy

Abstract

Non-thrombotic pulmonary vascular diseases may involve any portion of the pulmonary vascular tree from the main pulmonary artery through to the capillaries, venules, and central veins. They may be congenital or acquired. In this chapter, the typical presentation, important laboratory, as well as imaging findings of the more common or clinically significant entities are reviewed.

Keywords

Congenital pulmonary vascular disease • Acquired pulmonary vascular disease • Non-thrombotic pulmonary vascular disease • Pulmonary vasculitis • Pulmonary artery aneurysm

Congenital Anomalies of the Pulmonary Arteries

Left Pulmonary Artery Sling

Pulmonary sling occurs when the left pulmonary artery (LPA) arises from the posterior aspect of the right pulmonary artery (RPA) and courses between the trachea and esophagus to reach the left hilum [1]. There are two types. In Type I, the LPA is located above the carina abutting the distal trachea and proximal right mainstem bronchus. It compresses the adjacent airways resulting in air trapping and hyperinflation of the right lung [2, 3].

E. Peña
Department of Medical Imaging, Cardiac and Thoracic Imaging Sections, The Ottawa Hospital, Civic Campus, 1053 Carling Ave., Ottawa, ON K1Y4E9, Canada

C. Dennie (✉)
Department of Medical Imaging, Radiology and Medicine, University of Ottawa, 1053 Carling Avenue, Ottawa, ON, Canada
e-mail: cdennie@ottawahospital.on.ca

G. Chandy
Division of Respirology, Department of Medicine, Ottawa Heart Institute Pulmonary Hypertension Clinic, The Ottawa Hospital, 501 Smyth Road, Ottawa, ON K1H8L6, Canada

J. P. Kanne (ed.), *Clinically Oriented Pulmonary Imaging*, Respiratory Medicine, DOI: 10.1007/978-1-61779-542-8_8,

Type II is more common and associated with congenital tracheobronchial abnormalities [4]. The most important is a long tracheal stenosis associated with complete cartilaginous rings due to lack of development of the posterior membranous trachea [5–7]. Other associations include right pulmonary hypoplasia or agenesis with a small or absent RPA [8, 9]. This type is associated with a high mortality.

Clinical Features

Respiratory symptoms typically develop during infancy, and the severity depends on the presence of airway abnormalities. Symptoms may be accentuated by an acute respiratory infection [10]. Feeding difficulty may be another manifestation. Patients may also be asymptomatic [2, 10, 11].

Imaging Features

Contrast-enhanced CT and MRI can depict the vascular abnormality (see Fig. 8.1) and associated airway and pulmonary parenchymal findings in addition to assisting with surgical planning [2, 12–14].

Unilateral Proximal Interruption of the Pulmonary Artery

Proximal interruption of the right or left pulmonary artery is characterized by a blind ending artery at the hilum and systemic perfusion of the ipsilateral lung via aortopulmonary collaterals [15]. RPA interruption is more common and presents as an isolated abnormality whereas LPA interruption is associated with a right aortic arch and other congenital cardiovascular anomalies, most commonly tetralogy of Fallot.

Clinical Features

Repeated pulmonary infections, hemoptysis, and dyspnea are the most common symptoms [16]. In 10% of patients, hypertrophied collateral vessels rupture, causing hemoptysis [17]. Pulmonary hypertension is the leading prognostic determinant and affects approximately 19–25% of patients [16].

Imaging Features

Contrast-enhanced CT shows termination of the affected pulmonary artery within 1 cm of its origin (see Fig. 8.2a). Ipsilateral lung volume is decreased leading to ipsilateral mediastinal shift and elevation of the hemidiaphragm. There is hyperinflation of the contralateral lung. A serrated appearance of the pleura is commonly present due to the presence of prominent intercostal vessels (see Fig. 8.2b), and there are peripheral parenchymal linear opacities perpendicular to the pleura where systemic collaterals enter the lung from the chest wall (see Fig. 8.2c).

Pulmonary Arteriovenous Malformation

Pulmonary arteriovenous malformations (PAVM) are direct communications between a pulmonary artery and a pulmonary vein without an intervening capillary network. They can be isolated anomalies but in 60% are associated with hereditary hemorrhagic telangiectasia (HHT), also known as Osler-Weber-Rendu disease, an autosomal dominant condition presenting with epistaxis, mucocutaneous and visceral telangiectasia, and a family history of disease [18]. Up to 50% of patients with HHT have multiple lesions.

Clinical Features

Typical clinical features include hemoptysis, epistaxis, and dyspnea. PAVMs can cause a significant right-to-left shunt resulting in hypoxemia, stroke, and paradoxical emboli. They have a tendency to occur in the basilar regions of the lung resulting in symptoms of platypnea (increased shortness of breath when sitting or standing up) and orthodeoxia (increased hypoxemia when sitting or standing up). In the past, lesions were surgically resected, but percutaneous embolization is now the treatment of choice [19, 20].

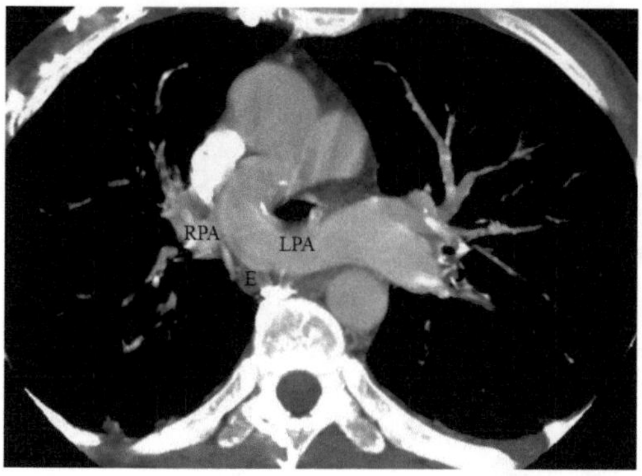

Fig. 8.1 Pulmonary artery sling in a 45-year-old man with recurrent pulmonary infections and sudden pleuritic chest pain. Contrast-enhanced axial maximum intensity projection (MIP) CT image shows an anomalous origin of the left pulmonary artery (LPA) from the right pulmonary artery (RPA) crossing between the trachea and esophagus (E) to the left hilum

Imaging Features

Contrast-enhanced thin-section CT is the most accurate noninvasive imaging modality to detect PAVMs. It demonstrates the size and number of lesions as well as the feeding artery and draining vein. Most PAVMs have a single feeding artery and draining vein (see Fig. 8.3a, b). CT plays an important role in treatment planning and post-treatment follow-up. A PAVM with a feeding artery greater than 3 mm generally requires treatment.

Acquired Diseases of the Pulmonary Arteries

Pulmonary Vasculitis

Pulmonary vasculitides are noninfectious inflammatory disorders that affect the pulmonary vessels, from the main pulmonary artery to the alveolar capillaries [21, 22]. Pulmonary vasculitides are challenging to diagnose because the signs and symptoms overlap those of infection, malignancy, and connective tissue disease [23, 24]. The combination of clinical presentation, laboratory

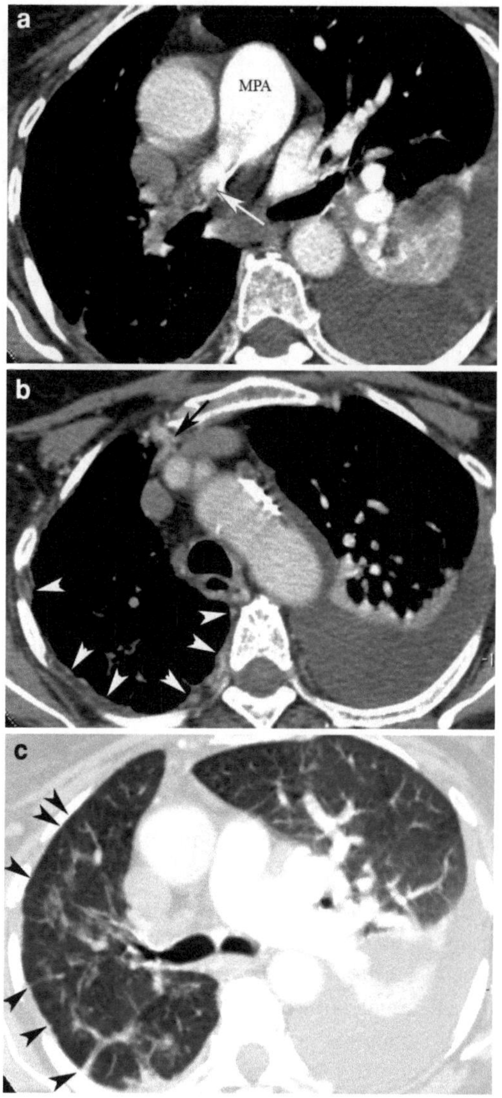

Fig. 8.2 Proximal interruption of the right pulmonary artery in a 53-year-old man with progressive shortness of breath. **a** Contrast-enhanced axial CT image shows abrupt termination of the proximal right pulmonary artery (*arrow*) and dilation of the main pulmonary artery (MPA). **b** Contrast-enhanced axial CT image of the same patient shows a serrated appearance of the right pleura as a result of dilated systemic collateral arteries (*arrowheads*). Enlargement of the right internal thoracic (mammary) artery (*arrow*) is also present. **c** Contrast-enhanced axial CT image (lung windows) in the same patient demonstrates loss of volume of the right hemithorax associated with multiple linear opacities (*arrowheads*) perpendicular to the pleural surface due to systemic collaterals entering the lung

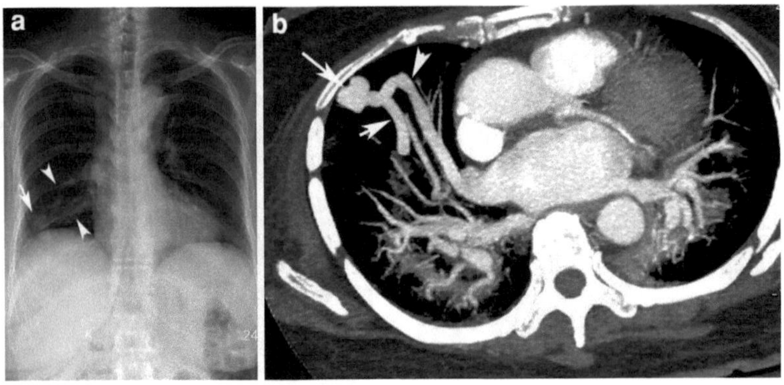

Fig. 8.3 Pulmonary arteriovenous malformation in a 72-year-old man with fever of unknown origin. **a** Chest radiograph shows a nodular opacity in the right lower lung zone (*arrow*) and two tubular structures (*arrowheads*) coursing from the nodule towards the right hilum. **b** Contrast-enhanced oblique MIP CT image demonstrates the enhancing nidus (*long arrow*) and a feeding artery arising from a dilated branch of the right middle lobe artery (*short arrow*) as well as a draining vessel into a branch of the right inferior pulmonary vein (*arrowhead*)

findings, and imaging characteristics can be highly suggestive of a specific diagnosis [25].

Clinical Features

Clinical symptoms and signs of pulmonary vasculitis are listed in Table 8.1 [21, 26].

Symptoms and signs suggestive of multi-organ involvement such as uveitis, skin rash, sinus congestion, shortness of breath, hemoptysis, and renal failure associated with constitutional symptoms as well as abnormal chest radiography should raise the possibility of vasculitis [21, 26].

The Chapel Hill classification of pulmonary vasculitis is based on the pathology, laboratory findings, and size of vessel involved. We review the most common vasculitides included in the Chapel Hill classification as well as some of the more common ones not yet included in the classification. The diseases are listed in Table 8.2 along with the size of the vessel affected [27, 28].

Laboratory Tests

ANCA tests are crucial in the work-up of patients with suspected pulmonary vasculitis.

Table 8.1 Signs and symptoms of pulmonary vasculitis [21, 26]

Hemoptysis
Glomerulonephritis
Deforming ulcerating upper airway lesions
Mononeuritis multiplex
Palpable purpura
Pulmonary renal syndrome (DAH and glomerulonephritis)
Diffuse alveolar hemorrhage (DAH)

ANCA-associated granulomatous vasculitides include Wegener granulomatosis, Churg–Strauss syndrome, and microscopic polyangiitis (MPA). This group of diseases share common clinical features, involvement of small vessels, and respond to immunosuppessant therapy [21].

Two indirect immunoflorescent staining patterns have been described: cytoplasmic ANCA (c-ANCA) and perinuclear ANCA (p-ANCA). c-ANCA has a sensitivity, specificity, and positive predictive value of 90–95, 90, and >90%, respectively, for ANCA-associated vasculitis [5].

A biopsy may be avoided in the presence of a positive c-ANCA in the proper clinical setting [21, 26]. In comparison, a positive p-ANCA

Table 8.2 Classification of vasculitis according to vessel size [27, 28]

Size of vessel and type of artery	Vasculitis
Large vessel vasculitis Elastic arteries (aorta and pulmonary artery and their main branches)	Behçet Hughes–Stovin Takayasu
Small vessel vasculitis Small arterioles, capillaries, venules Diagnosis requires involvement of capillaries and venules, such as purpura, glomerulonephritis, or pulmonary capillaritis	*ANCA-associated vasculitis*: Wegener granulomatosis Churg–Strauss syndrome Microscopic polyangiitis
	Non-associated ANCA vasculitis: Henoch–Schönlein purpura Goodpasture syndrome Vasculitis associated with collagen vascular disease (systemic lupus erythematosus, rheumatoid arthritis) Drug-induced vasculitis

(p-ANCA) provides only suggestive evidence of Churg–Strauss syndrome or MPA [29] as it may be positive in patients with Goodpasture syndrome, rheumatoid arthritis, infection, and inflammatory bowel disease [30–33].

Anti-glomerular basement membrane (anti-GBM) antibodies should also be sought in patients with suspected pulmonary vasculitis, particularly among those who have a combination of diffuse lung involvement on imaging and renal failure. The presence of these antibodies is indicative of Goodpasture syndrome [26].

Imaging Features

The imaging characteristics of vasculitis on CT depend on the type and size of vessel affected [27, 28]. A practical algorithmic approach to the diagnosis of pulmonary vasculitis is suggested and is shown in Fig. 8.4 [27].

Large Vessel Vasculitis

Large vessel vasculitides mainly affect the aorta and its largest branches. Pulmonary artery involvement occurs in about 15% of patients. They should be suspected in the presence of signs and symptoms of systemic arterial ischemia. The two main patterns of pulmonary artery involvement include pulmonary artery aneurysms and stenosis.

Behçet Disease

Behçet disease is a chronic systemic vasculitis predominantly affecting young men from the Far East to the Mediterranean Sea. The prevalence of pulmonary involvement is 8% [34]. It is the most common cause of pulmonary artery aneurysms [35].

Clinical Features

Patients typically present with oral and genital ulcers, uveitis, skin lesions, and arterial and venous occlusions and aneurysms. The most common presentation of pulmonary arterial aneurysms is hemoptysis [34, 36]. Rupture into a bronchus or the lung parenchyma is a major cause of death occurring in up to 50% of patients.

Imaging Features

Contrast-enhanced CT pulmonary angiographic manifestations include pulmonary arterial aneurysms and thromboses resulting in wedge-shaped airspace consolidation due to infarction or hemorrhage. Superior vena cava thrombosis accompanied by thrombosis of other mediastinal veins may also

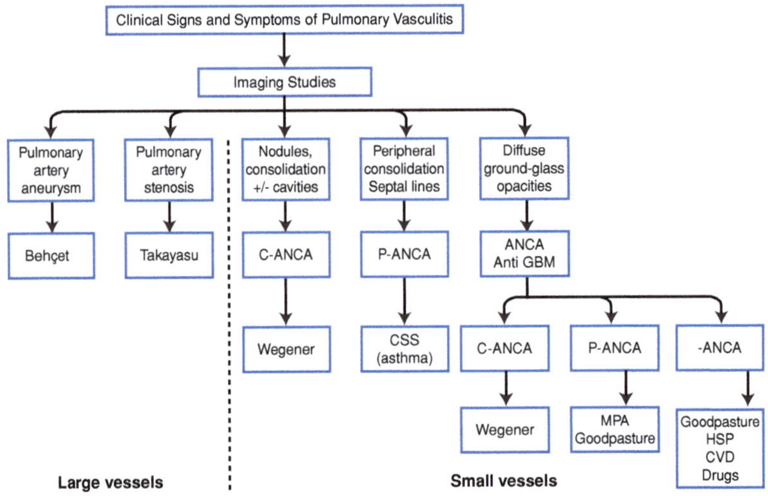

Fig. 8.4 Algorithmic Approach to Differential Diagnosis of Pulmonary Vasculitis [27]. *c-ANCA* cytoplasmic ANCA, *p-ANCA* perinuclear ANCA, *Anti GBM* Anti-glomerular basement membrane antibodies, *CSS* Churg–Strauss syndrome, *MPA* microscopic polyangiitis, *HSP* Henoch–Schönlein purpura, *CVC* collagen vascular disease. Adapted from Chung et al. [27]. Used by permission

occur [34, 35, 37]. Pulmonary artery aneurysms may be fusiform or saccular and are usually multiple, bilateral, and located in the lower lobes or hilar regions. They may be totally or partially thrombosed [38, 39] and resolve in up to 75% of patients receiving immunosupressant therapy [39, 40]. Behçet disease may also affect the aorta, causing aneurysms (see Fig. 8.5).

Takayasu Arteritis

Takayasu arteritis typically affects young women of Eastern Asian origin. The age at presentation varies between 10 and 40 years. It predominantly affects the thoracoabdominal aorta and its major branches. The estimated annual incidence is 0.12–0.26 cases per 100,000 [41]. Pulmonary involvement occurs in 15%, typically leading to stenosis of the affected arteries. Vascular involvement is characterized by an acute inflammatory and chronic fibrotic phase [42].

Clinical Features

Patients present with fever, myalgia, arthralgia, weight loss, and limb claudication. On physical examination, there may be systemic hypertension, diminished or absent pulses, vascular bruits, and discrepant blood pressure measurements.

Imaging Features

The findings on contrast-enhanced CT or MRI include concentric mural thickening of the aorta, its major branches, pulmonary arteries, and occasionally the coronary arteries. Arterial stenosis, occlusion, and aneurysm formation are also features (see Fig. 8.6a). The findings correlate with the phase of disease (see Fig. 8.6b) and are summarized in Table 8.3 [43, 44]. Pulmonary arterial involvement is characterized by stenosis or occlusion of segmental and subsegmental arteries (see Fig. 8.6c). This is usually associated with a mosaic attenuation pattern on lung windows.

Small Vessel Vasculitis

This category includes vasculitis involving arterioles, venules, and capillaries. The most common causes include:

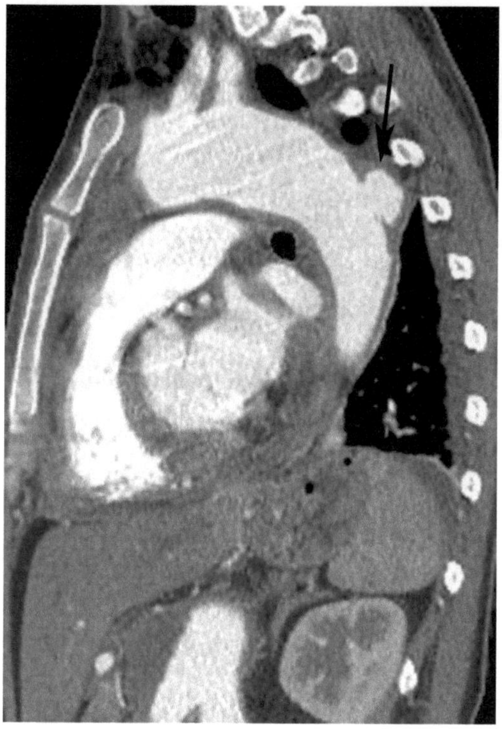

Fig. 8.5 Behçet disease in a 39-year-old female. Sagittal oblique MIP CT image depicts a saccular pseudoaneurysm of the proximal descending thoracic aorta (*arrow*)

1. ANCA-associated vasculitis (most common) such as Wegener granulomatosis, Churg–Strauss syndrome, and microscopic polyangiitis.
2. Vasculitis associated with diffuse alveolar hemorrhage (DAH) and not associated with ANCA such as Henoch–Schönlein purpura, Goodpasture syndrome, vasculitis associated with collagen vascular disease, and drug-induced vasculitis.

Wegener Granulomatosis

Wegener granulomatosis, now referred to as ANCA-associated necrotizing granulomatous vasculitis, is the most common form of ANCA-associated vasculitis. It is slightly more common in males than females, and most patients are Caucasian. It affects medium and small pulmonary vessels. c-ANCA is positive in >90% of patients who have the generalized form of disease and in 50% of patients with disease limited to the lungs [25].

Clinical Features

The clinical presentation can involve constitutional symptoms of weight loss, fever, and arthralgia in addition to the classic triad of ENT (ear, nose, throat), pulmonary, and renal involvement summarized in Table 8.4 [21, 26, 28].

Imaging Features

Nodules and Masses

The most common CT feature is multiple pulmonary nodules or masses (90%) (see Fig. 8.7). They are bilateral and most often subpleural [45]. They have no zonal predominance and vary in size between 2 and 10 cm. Nodules usually have a sharp outer margin and may be surrounded by ground-glass opacity due to hemorrhage [45, 46]. Cavitation develops in 50%, and the inner wall of the cavity is irregular with a spiculated outer margin [45, 47] (see Fig. 8.8). Rarely, the nodules may be centrilobular (10%) or have a tree-in-bud apperance.

Consolidation

Wedge-shaped, mass-like peripheral areas of consolidation occur in 50% of patients (see Figs. 8.9, 8.10). They are due to infarction or airway involvement [46, 48, 49].

Ground-glass Opacities

Diffuse ground-glass opacities occur in 20–30% of patients and are generally due to DAH secondary to necrotizing capillaritis (see Fig. 8.11) [45, 47].

Tracheobronchial Involvement

Bronchial wall thickening is present in 70% of patients [45]. The large airways are affected in 30% and manifest as tracheal wall thickening, stenosis, or both, usually 2–4 cm in length and most commonly in a subglottic location (see Fig. 8.12a, b) [22, 27, 40, 45, 50, 51].

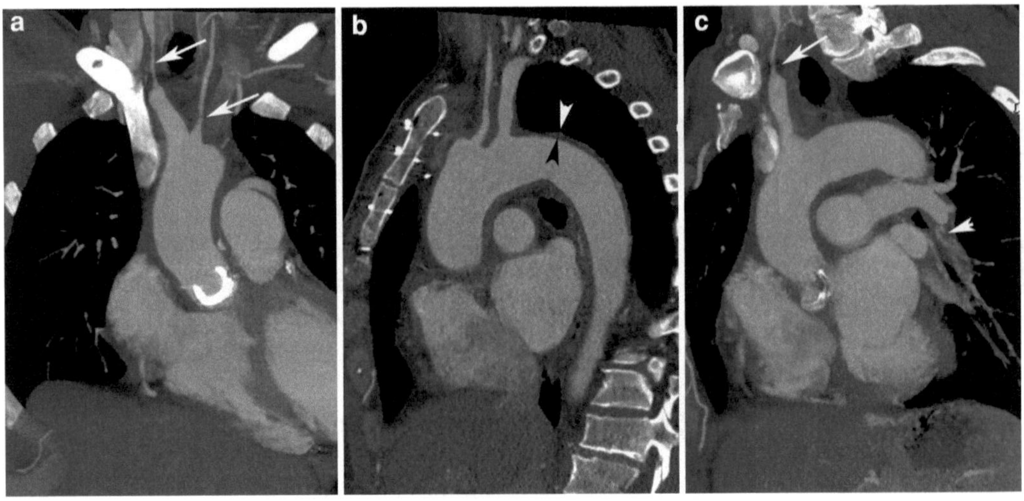

Fig. 8.6 Takayasu arteritis in a 46-year-old female with previous aortic valve replacement and coronary artery bypass graft surgery and vasculitis on pathological examination of the aorta. **a** Contrast-enhanced coronal oblique MIP CT image shows circumferential mural thickening and narrowing of the right and left common carotid arteries (*arrows*). **b** Contrast-enhanced sagittal oblique MIP CT image shows diffuse concentric mural thickening of the thoracic aorta (*arrowheads*) and supra-aortic vessels, in the acute inflammatory phase of the disease. **c** Contrast-enhanced sagittal oblique MIP CT image shows abrupt cutoff and narrowing of the left lower lobe pulmonary artery due to chronic obstruction (*short arrow*). Note the stenosis of the left carotid artery (*long arrow*)

Table 8.3 Morphological and functional imaging findings in Takayasu arteritis

Phase of disease	Morphologic findings on CT and MR	Functional imaging on CT, MR, and PET
Acute inflammatory	Concentric thickening of aortic wall +/− calcification	Delayed contrast enhancement on CT and MR FDG uptake
Chronic fibrotic	Stenosis, occlusion, post-stenotic dilation Calcification of aortic wall	Absence of delayed enhancement on CT and MR No FDG uptake

Table 8.4 Clinical triad in patients with Wegener granulomatosis

Upper airway involvement (nearly 100%)	Sinusitis Otitis Ulcerations Airway narrowing
Lower respiratory tract involvement (lung involvement 90%, tracheobronchial tree 10–50%)	Cough Chest pain Dyspnea Hemoptysis
Glomerulonephritis (80%)	Hematuria Proteinuria Azotemia

Differential Diagnosis

The main differential diagnoses are listed in Table 8.5. The presence of upper respiratory symptoms, laboratory findings indicative of glomerulonephritis, and positive serum c-ANCA help clinch the diagnosis [51].

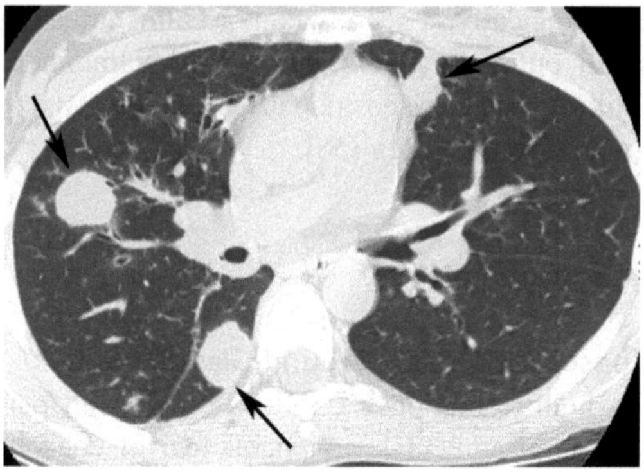

Fig. 8.7 Wegener granulomatosis. High-resolution CT image shows multiple bilateral well-circumscribed nodules (*arrows*)

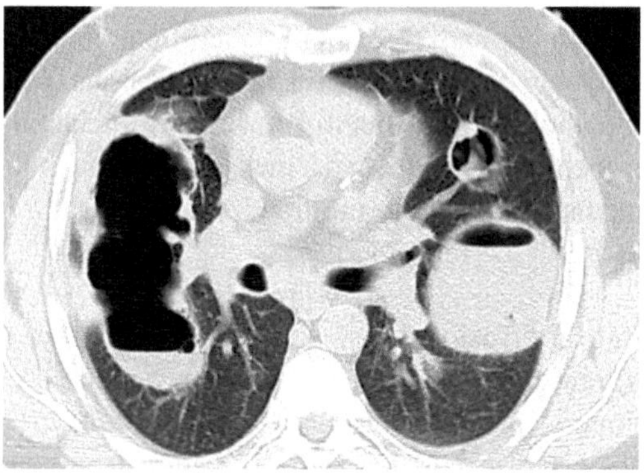

Fig. 8.8 Wegener granulomatosis. High-resolution CT image shows large bilateral cavitary nodules and masses containing air-fluid levels

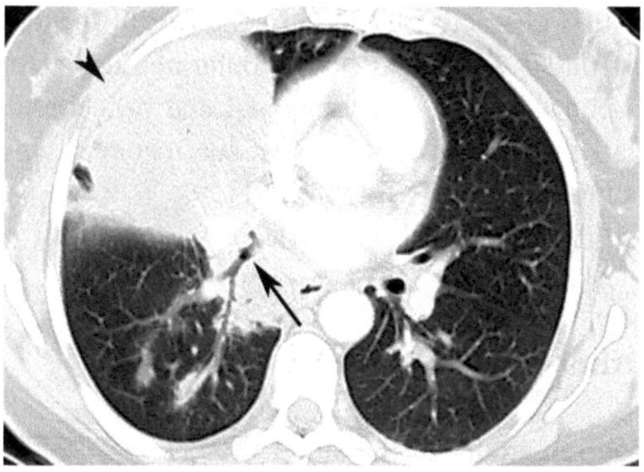

Fig. 8.9 Wegener granulomatosis. High-resolution CT image shows peribronchial consolidation (*arrow*) in the right lower lobe and "mass-like" consolidation (*arrowhead*) in the right middle lobe without air bronchograms

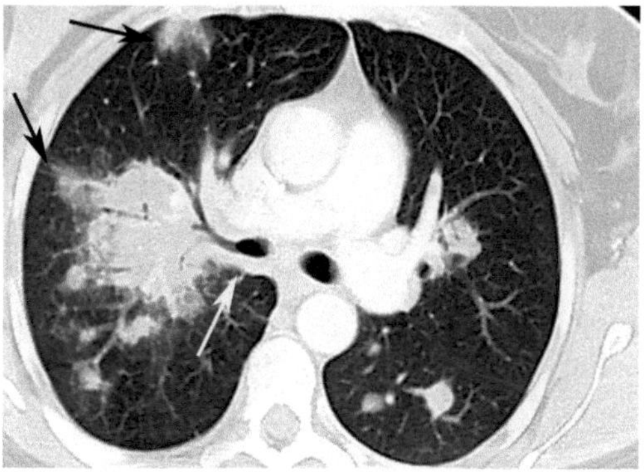

Fig. 8.10 Wegener granulomatosis. Contrast-enhanced axial CT image (lung window) demonstrates peribronchial consolidation in the right upper lobe and multiple nodules, some demonstrating a halo sign resulting from perilesional hemorrhage (*black arrows*). Note significant circumferential thickening of the right upper lobe bronchus (*white arrow*) as a sign of bronchial involvement

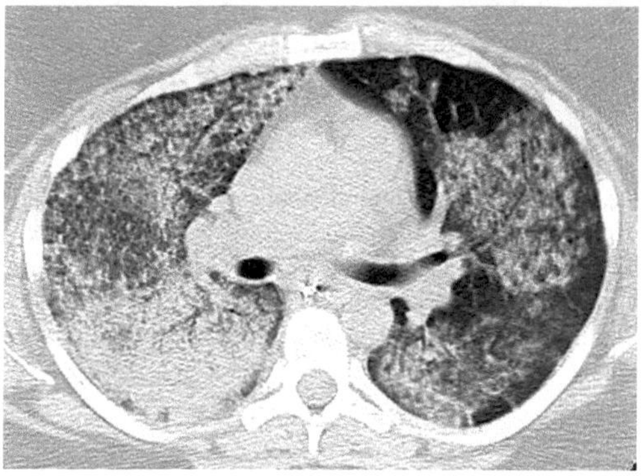

Fig. 8.11 Wegener granulomatosis in a 53-year-old male with recurrent pulmonary hemorrhage. High-resolution CT image shows extensive bilateral confluent ground-glass opacities and consolidation from diffuse alveolar hemorrhage

Churg–Strauss Syndrome

This disorder (which is also known as allergic granulomatosis and angiitis) is a multisystem disease of the small- and medium-sized arteries. The annual incidence is 1–3 cases per 100,000 [52]. The mean age at presentation is 38 years with men and women equally affected. The vast majority of patients are Caucasian (92–98%).

Clinical Features

The characteristic clinical triad is asthma, peripheral eosinophilia, and chronic rhinosinusitis

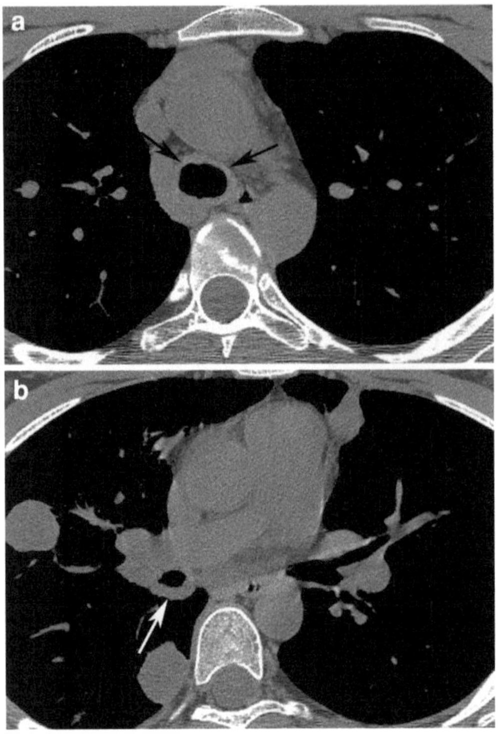

Fig. 8.12 Wegener granulomatosis. **a** High-resolution CT image (mediastinal window) shows circumferential thickening of the distal tracheal wall (*arrows*) at the level of the carina. **b** Marked thickening of the wall of the right intermediate bronchus (*arrow*) is shown

[26]. The diagnostic criteria for Churg–Strauss syndrome are outlined in Table 8.6 and have a sensitivity of 85% and specificity of 100% [53].

Asthma is a characteristic feature and typically develops nearly a decade prior to the diagnosis of Churg–Strauss syndrome. Peripheral neuropathy is present in 66–76% and rash in 51–70%. Renal involvement is less frequent compared to other small vessel vasculitides [54]. Cardiac involvement may develop in 13–47% and is the leading cause of mortality [55]. Cardiac manifestations include arrhythmias, angina, myocardial infarction, left ventricular failure, myocarditis, and pericarditis [56].

Serum p-ANCA is positive in 40–75% of cases and is helpful but not diagnostic in this disorder [57]. Surgical biopsy remains the gold standard for diagnosis and can be obtained from the lung, skin, or involved peripheral nerve. Pathologically, a necrotizing vasculitis affecting small pulmonary vessels and an inflammatory infiltrate rich in eosinophils with necrotizing granulomas are seen [58].

Imaging Features

Consolidation and Ground-Glass Opacities

On high-resolution CT (HRCT), transient, patchy, non-segmental, peripheral foci of consolidation, ground-glass opacities, or both are seen in 90% and are associated with bronchial wall thickening.

Nodules and Interlobular Septal Thickening

Small centrilobular nodules are present in 63% of patients and correspond to eosinophilic and lymphocytic infiltration in the bronchiolar wall at pathology [36]. Interlobular septal thickening is identified in 50% and may be due to septal edema, eosinophilic infiltration, and mild fibrosis [59] (see Fig. 8.13a, b).

Pleural Effusions

A total of 50% of patients develop unilateral or bilateral pleural effusions [22, 27, 40, 50, 51]. They may occur due to heart failure from cardiomyopathy or eosinophilic pleuritis [54, 59, 60].

Airway Involvement

The eosinophilic involvement of the bronchial wall is characterized by bronchial wall thickening on HRCT. Small centrilobular nodules, tree-in-bud opacities, and bronchial and bronchiolar wall thickening may also be due to underlying asthma (see Fig. 8.14) [59, 61].

Other Small Vessel Vasculitides

The remainder of the small vessels vasculitides share common HRCT features, specifically diffuse ground-glass opacities that may progress to consolidation due to DAH. They are associated with capillaritis at pathology. These diseases

Table 8.5 Imaging based differential diagnosis of Wegener granulomatosis

Bilateral subpleural cavitary nodules	Infection: septic embolism, necrotizing pneumonia, fungal infection, tuberculosis Neoplasm: metastases, lymphoma Organizing pneumonia
Peribronchovascular nodules or consolidation	Kaposi sarcoma

Table 8.6 Diagnostic criteria for Churg–Strauss syndrome [53]

Vasculitis at site of biopsy and at least four of following
Asthma
Blood eosinophilia
Mono- or polyneuropathy
Migratory pulmonary infiltrates
Sinus abnormalities
Extravascular eosinophils on biopsy specimen

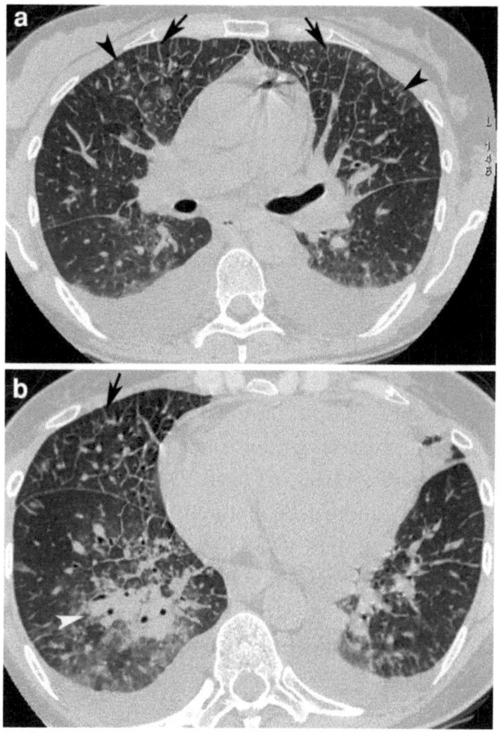

Fig. 8.13 Churg–Strauss syndrome in a 49-year-old female with pleuritic chest pain and hypoxia. **a** Axial unenhanced CT image (lung window) shows interlobular septal thickening (*arrows*), ill-defined centrilobular nodules (*arrowhead*), and small bilateral pleural effusions. **b** Axial CT image (lung window) shows right lower lobe peribronchial consolidation and peripheral ground-glass opacities surrounding the consolidation (*arrowhead*). There is also interlobular septal thickening in the right middle lobe (*arrow*)

include one of the ANCA-associated vasculitides (MPA) as well as Henoch–Schönlein purpura, Goodpasture syndrome, vasculitis associated with collagen vascular disease, and drug-induced vasculitis. Drugs such as crack cocaine may induce a pulmonary capillaritis leading to DAH. Entities causing DAH are classified into three groups and are summarized in Table 8.7 [21, 62, 63]. There are other rare vasculitides, but these are beyond the scope of this chapter.

Microscopic Polyangiitis

MPA is a systemic necrotizing vasculitis of small vessels without granulomatous inflammation. The annual incidence is about 0.36 cases per 100,000 [52]. It is the most common cause of pulmonary renal syndrome [64]. The mean age at presentation is 50 years, and the most common clinical manifestation is rapidly progressive glomerulonephritis (90%). Pulmonary involvement occurs in 25–50% [29, 65] and, in patients who develop lung disease, DAH due to capillaritis is the most common manifestation [21, 66]. p-ANCA is positive in 40–80% of patients.

Henoch–Schönlein Purpura

This is the most common childhood vasculitis. It is characterized by immune complex deposition in the skin and kidneys and presents with the classic triad of purpura, arthritis, and abdominal pain. Lung involvement is rare but more common in adults (see Fig. 8.15).

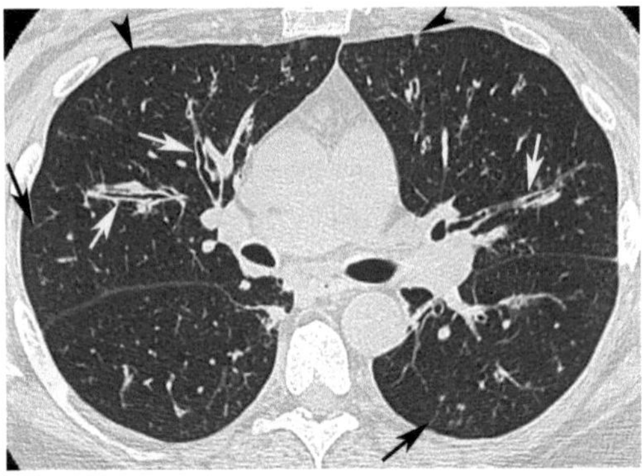

Fig. 8.14 Churg–Strauss syndrome. High-resolution CT image shows bronchial wall thickening (*white arrows*), centrilobular nodules (*arrowheads*), and interlobular septal thickening (*black arrows*)

Goodpasture Syndrome

This disease has a bimodal distribution with patients presenting between the ages of 20–30 years and 60–70 years. Males are affected slightly more frequently than females. The triad of circulating anti-GBM antibody (90%), DAH, and glomerulonephritis is typical. Presenting symptoms are usually respiratory in nature, with hemoptysis occurring in 80–95% of patients (see Fig. 8.16).

Systemic Lupus Erythematosus

Systemic lupus erythematosus (SLE) accounts for 50–70% of pulmonary vasculitides due to collagen vascular disease [67]. It is characterized by an immune complex mediated necrotizing vasculitis involving the arterioles and capillaries. DAH accounts for 22% of pulmonary complications in patients with SLE (see Fig. 8.17) [68].

Imaging Features of DAH

HRCT features include perihilar ground-glass opacities, patchy bilateral lung consolidation, or both [69]. The opacities may spare the apices and costophrenic angles and have a lower lung distribution in 25% [70]. Smooth interlobular septal thickening tends to develop within 2–3 days on a background of ground-glass opacities giving rise to the "crazy-paving pattern" due to hemorrhage resorption. Ill-defined centrilobular nodules may be present reflecting the presence of intra-alveolar macrophages [71]. Interstitial fibrosis may eventually appear with recurrent hemorrhage (see Fig. 8.18) [22, 27, 40, 50, 51, 72].

Pulmonary Artery Aneurysms and Pseudoaneurysms

Pulmonary aneurysms are defined as a focal dilation of the pulmonary artery. They are uncommon and may not only result from vasculitis but can also result from congenital and other acquired causes listed in Table 8.8 [73].

Clinical Features

Pulmonary artery aneurysms should be included in the differential diagnosis in patients who present with hemoptysis with or without hilar enlargement or focal parenchymal consolidation due to pulmonary hemorrhage on a chest radiograph. The mortality rate from pulmonary artery aneurysm rupture has been reported to be up to 100% [74], and, consequently, early diagnosis is crucial.

Imaging Features

Contrast-enhanced CT angiography confirms the presence, assesses the size and location of the aneurysm, and may be used to plan surgical or endovascular treatment.

Mycotic Aneurysms

These are caused by infection and are in fact pseudoaneurysms at pathology, consequently at greater risk of rupture. Bacteria are the most common cause, but fungi are occasionally responsible (see Fig. 8.19). Mycotic aneurysms

Table 8.7 Vasculitis associated with diffuse alveolar hemorrhage

ANCA-associated small vessel vasculitis	Wegener granulomatosis Churg–Strauss syndrome Microscopic polyangiitis
Immune complex mediated vasculitis	Goodpasture syndrome Systemic lupus erythematosus
Miscellaneous	Diffuse alveolar damage Drug reaction Coagulopathy Infection

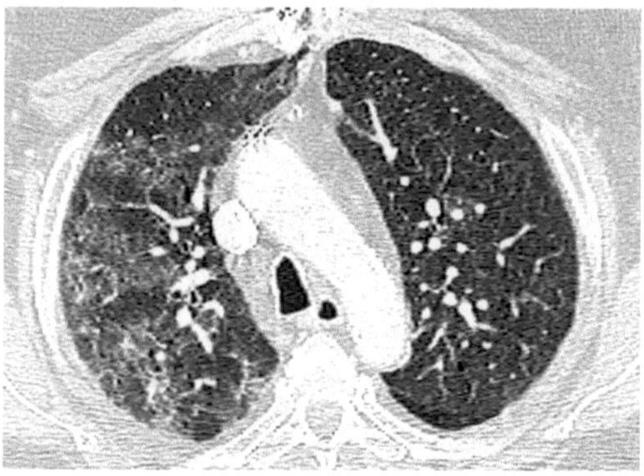

Fig. 8.15 Henoch–Schönlein purpura in a 74-year-old male with hemoptysis. High-resolution CT image shows bilateral ground-glass opacities in the upper lobes due to diffuse alveolar hemorrhage

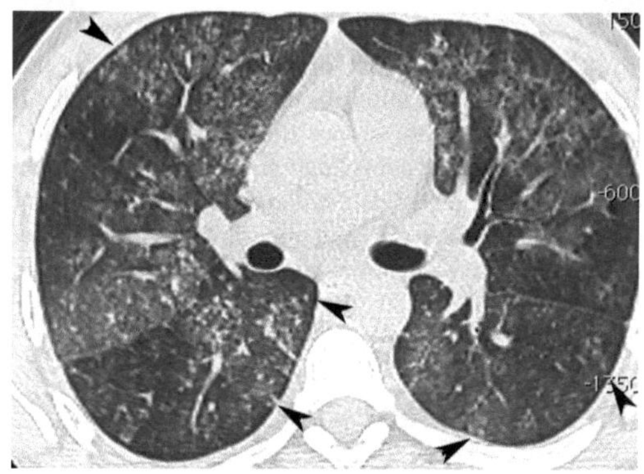

Fig. 8.16 Goodpasture syndrome in a 20-year-old male presenting with renal failure and shortness of breath. High-resolution CT image shows diffuse bilateral ground-glass opacities and poorly defined centrilobular nodules (*arrowheads*)

are usually seen in intravenous drug users and are often associated with infective endocarditis and septic embolism [75].

Rasmussen aneurysms are mycotic pseudoaneurysms that develop in the peripheral pulmonary arteries in the upper lobes secondary to tuberculosis.

Iatrogenic Aneurysms

Pulmonary artery catheters may cause pseudoaneurysms when they are positioned too distally in a pulmonary artery (see Fig. 8.20). Other iatrogenic causes include chest tube insertion, penetrating trauma, conventional angiography, surgical resection, or biopsy (see Fig. 8.21). Coil embolization is the preferred treatment [73].

Neoplasms

Primary lung cancer and metastases may erode into the pulmonary arteries resulting in pseudoaneurysm formation (see Fig. 8.22). Rarely, primary tumors arising from the pulmonary arteries, such as leiomyosarcoma and angiosarcoma, may cause focal expansion and aneurysmal dilation of the affected artery.

Fibrosing Mediastinitis

Fibrosing mediastinitis is a rare benign inflammatory condition characterized by progressive proliferation of dense fibrous tissue within the mediastinum [76]. The etiology remains unclear. Some postulate that it is due to a fibroinflammatory response to *Histoplasma capsulatum* antigens [76–80]. There are two types: focal and diffuse. Their characteristics are listed in Table 8.9 [80].

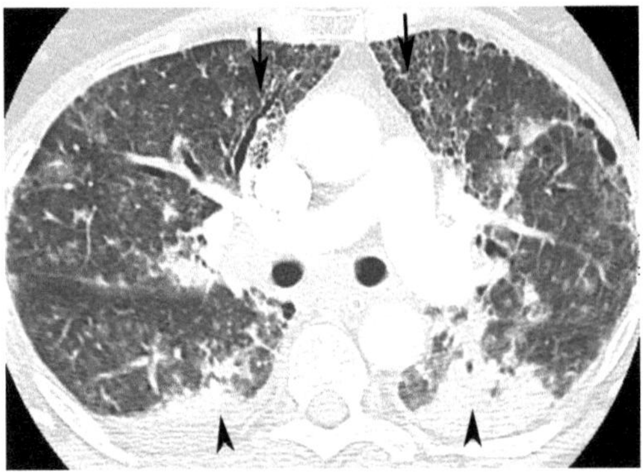

Fig. 8.17 Systemic lupus erythematosus (SLE) associated pulmonary vasculitis. Contrast-enhanced axial CT image (lung window) shows diffuse bilateral ground-glass opacities and consolidation (*arrowheads*) in the lower lobes due to alveolar hemorrhage. Note reticulation and bronchiectasis in the right upper lobe and lingula due to SLE associated interstitial pulmonary fibrosis (*arrows*)

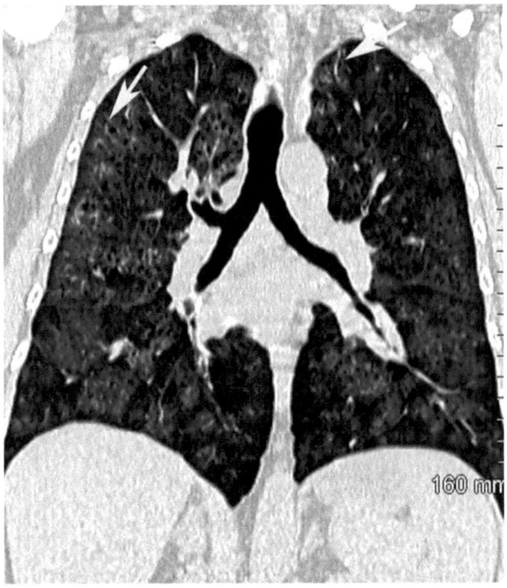

Fig. 8.18 Diffuse alveolar hemorrhage in a 33-year-old female crack cocaine abuser with a history of recurrent pulmonary hemorrhage. Coronal reformatted image from high-resolution CT shows bilateral ground-glass opacities on a background of reticulation (*arrows*) from pulmonary fibrosis secondary to recurrent pulmonary hemorrhage

Clinical Features

Fibrosing mediastinitis usually presents in young adults. Males and females are affected equally. Signs and symptoms are related to obstruction or compression of vital mediastinal structures [77, 81–85]. Systemic signs such as fever and weight loss are less often present [81, 85–88].

Imaging Features

A soft tissue mass that obliterates the normal mediastinal fat planes and encases and narrows adjacent structures is the most common CT and MR finding (see Figs. 8.23a, b, c; 8.24a, b) [89–91]. Contrast-enhanced CT depicts the extent, level, and length of vascular stenosis and may show collateral systemic vessels in the mediastinum and chest wall (see Fig. 8.25a, b). The mediastinal and pulmonary parenchymal CT features are listed in Table 8.10.

On MR, extensive regions of decreased signal intensity in the mediastinum on T2-weighted imaging may distinguish fibrosing mediastinitis from other infiltrative lesions of the mediastinum such as metastatic carcinoma and lymphoma, both of which typically have increased signal intensity [80]. Heterogeneous enhancement has also been reported after gadolinium administration. Phase contrast cine sequences may help quantify vascular stenosis.

Differential Diagnosis

Malignant infiltrative mediastinal lesions including lung carcinoma, metastatic carcinoma, lymphoma, mediastinal sarcoma, or mediastinal desmoid tumors need to be considered. In the presence of a calcified infiltrative mediastinal mass in a young patient from an endemic area for histoplasmosis, the most likely diagnosis is fibrosing mediastinitis. If the mass is non-calcified, biopsy and culture of the mass should be performed to exclude neoplasm. It is essential that the lesion be extensively biopsied to exclude malignancy, especially lymphoma. Surgical sampling is preferred to transthoracic needle biopsy [77, 80].

Table 8.8 Causes of congenital and acquired pulmonary aneurysms [73]

Congenital	Acquired
Deficiency of vessel wall	Pulmonary hypertension
Valvular and post-valvular stenosis	Vasculitis Behçet Hughes–Stovin syndrome
Increased flow due left to right shunt Patent ductus arteriosus, ventricular septal defect, atrial septal defect Sequelae of congenital heart disease repair (tetralogy of Fallot)	Mycotic aneurysms and pseudoaneurysms Bacterial (IV drug users) Fungal Tuberculous (Rasmussen)
	Neoplasm Iatrogenic causes Chest tube insertion Penetrating trauma Connective tissue abnormalities Marfan syndrome Ehlers–Danlos syndrome Cystic medial necrosis

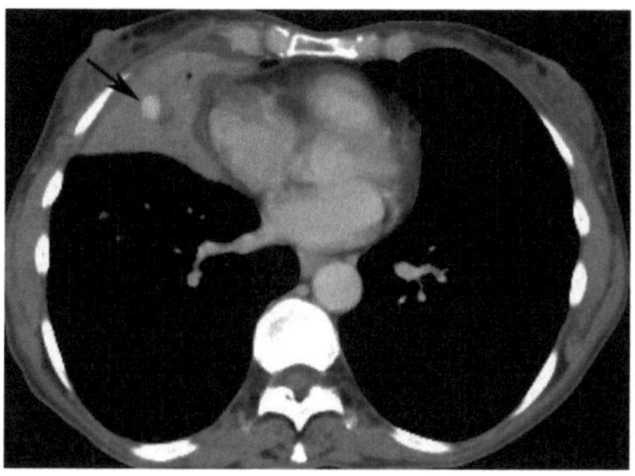

Fig. 8.19 Mycotic pseudoaneurysm in a 60-year-old female with right middle lobe pneumonia. Contrast-enhanced axial CT image shows a focal area of enhancement (*arrow*) within the right middle lobe consolidation corresponding to a mycotic pseudoan-eurysm

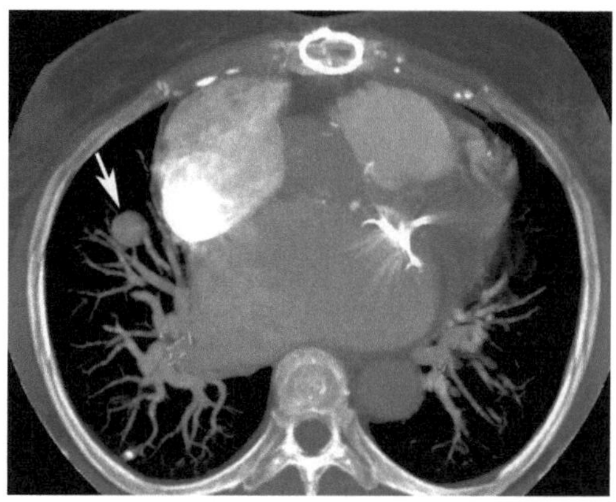

Fig. 8.20 Pseudoaneurysm of the pulmonary artery in a 75-year-old female with a recent aortic valve replacement and new lung nodule on chest radiography. Contrast-enhanced MIP axial CT image shows an enhancing nodule (*arrow*), consistent with a pseudoaneurysm involving a subsegmental branch of the right middle lobe artery as a result of pulmonary artery catheter injury shortly after surgery

Non-Thrombotic Pulmonary Embolism

Non-thrombotic pulmonary embolism is uncommon. However, some of the embolic material may have a typical imaging appearance.

Tumor Embolism/Intravascular Pulmonary Metastases

Tumor emboli occur when tumor fragments remain and grow within the pulmonary arteries. They may be microscopic or macroscopic. Tumor embolism is seen most commonly with cancer of the breast, stomach, kidney, and prostate, as well as hepatocellular carcinoma and choriocarcinoma.

Clinical Features

In patients with known malignancy, acute to subacute dyspnea and signs of pulmonary

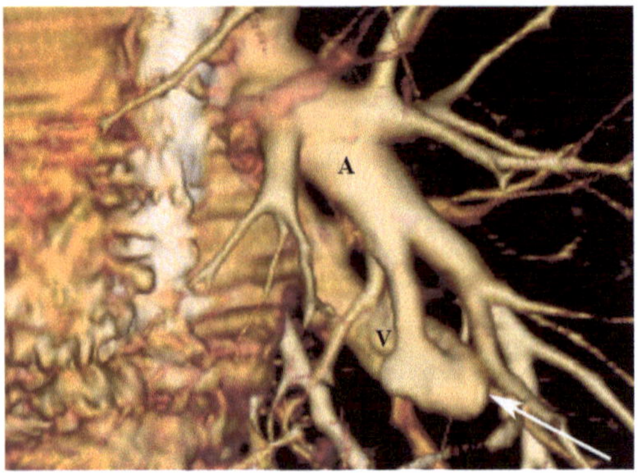

Fig. 8.21 Pulmonary arteriovenous fistula in a 53-year-old female after pulmonary wedge resection for coccidioidomyocis. Three-dimensional volume-rendered CT image, posterior view of the pulmonary vessels shows a fistula (*arrow*) between a subsegmental artery in the right lower lobe (A) and a branch of the right inferior pulmonary vein (V)

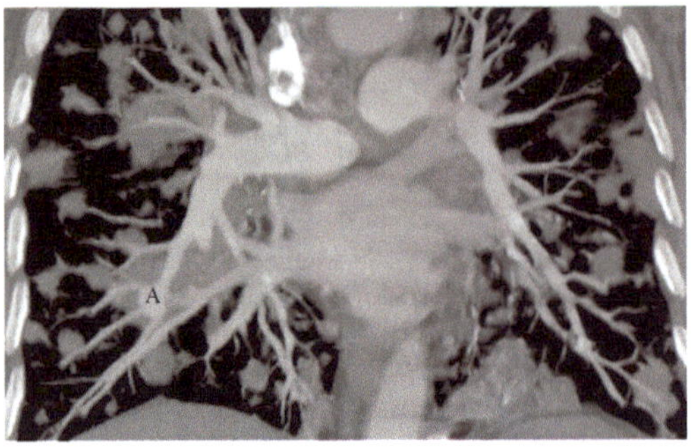

Fig. 8.22 A 70-year-old female with metastatic angiosarcoma of the face and neck. Contrast-enhanced coronal oblique MIP CT image shows a pseudoaneurysm (A) arising from a subsegmental branch of the right lower lobe artery. Note the multiple bilateral lung nodules

hypertension or cor pulmonale, tumor embolism should be considered as a potential cause. The most common symptom is subacute progressive dyspnea occurring in 57–100% of patients [92–94]. Pleuritic chest pain, cough, and hemoptysis are also frequent complaints [95]. Hypoxemia is invariable, and hypocapnia or an increased alveolar-arterial oxygen gradient may also be found [92].

Tumor embolism is clinically and radiologically indistinguishable from bland pulmonary thromboembolism and, in the vast majority, is discovered at autopsy [96]. The antemortem diagnosis is only made in 6% of patients [97].

Imaging Features

On contrast-enhanced CT pulmonary angiography, tumor embolism in the main, lobar, and segmental pulmonary arteries presents as filling defects that mimic acute or chronic pulmonary embolism. Tumor emboli in subsegmental arteries appear as multifocal vascular dilation and beading [98], most evident on lung windows (see Fig. 8.26). When arterioles in the center of the secondary pulmonary lobule are affected, a tree-in-bud pattern results [99]. On lung windows, peripheral wedge-shaped consolidation due to infarction or peripheral ground-glass opacities due to pulmonary hemorrhage may be present.

Septic Embolism

Septic embolism is defined as a thrombus containing microorganisms (bacteria, fungi, or parasites) embedded in fibrin that reaches the pulmonary arteries [100]. Predisposing factors are listed in Table 8.11 [101, 102].

Clinical Features

Febrile patients with cough, hemoptysis, and pulmonary opacities on imaging associated with an active extrapulmonary infection [103, 104] should be suspected of having septic emboli. Blood cultures, echocardiography, and CT are essential diagnostic tools [103].

Imaging Features

CT typically shows multiple 1–3 cm nodules in different stages of cavitation (see Fig. 8.27a). These have a lower zone predominance. A vessel leading to the nodule ("feeding vessel sign"), reflecting the hematogenous origin of the process may be identified [102, 105]. This is not a specific sign and may be found in

Table 8.9 Types of fibrosing mediastinitis and distinctive imaging characteristics

Type	CT findings	Etiology
Focal (82%)	Calcified mass (63%) in hilar, paratracheal, or subcarinal regions	Inflammatory reaction to *Histoplasma capsulatum* in susceptible population
Diffuse (18%)	Infiltrative non-calcified mass affecting multiple mediastinal compartments	Autoimmune/idiopathic disorder

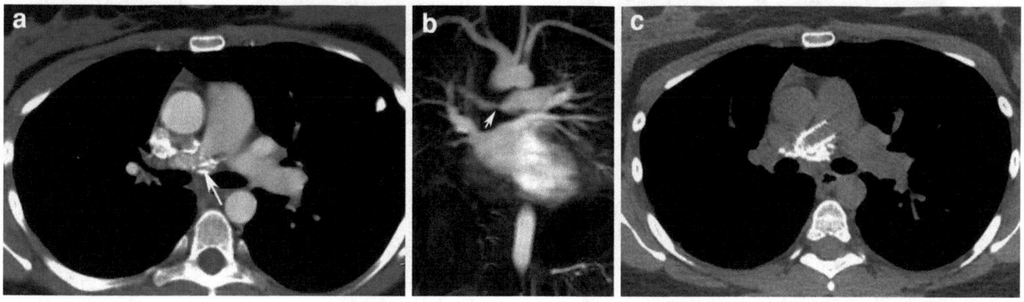

Fig. 8.23 Fibrosing mediastinitis associated with histoplasmosis in a 23-year-old female with pulmonary hypertension. **a** Contrast-enhanced CT image shows a calcified mass narrowing the right pulmonary artery (*arrow*). Note the dilated main pulmonary artery. **b** Coronal oblique MR angiogram of the pulmonary arteries shows significant stenosis of the right pulmonary artery (*arrow*) due to a markedly hypointense mediastinal process corresponding to calcification seen on CT. **c** Unenhanced axial CT image following therapy shows a metallic stent in the right pulmonary artery

hematogeneous metastases and bland pulmonary emboli. Nodules may also have a surrounding ground-glass halo ("halo sign") on lung windows, due to perilesional hemorrhage. This may also be seen in other hemorrhagic and non-hemorrhagic lesions [106, 107]. In a recent study [108], septic emboli due to gram-positive organisms were larger, more frequently had air bronchograms, and were more often cavitary than those due to gram-negative organisms while the "halo sign" and "feeding vessel sign" were more common with septic emboli due to gram-negative organisms.

Septic emboli occluding a pulmonary artery (see Fig. 8.27b) may present with wedge-shaped peripheral foci of consolidation with or without cavitation due to pulmonary infarction (see Fig. 8.28). Peripheral ground-glass opacities from pulmonary hemorrhage may also be present.

When infective endocarditis is present, valvular vegetations are only rarely identified on non-gated contrast-enhanced CT due to their small size and the presence of motion artifact. However, perivalvular abscesses are occasionally seen (see Fig. 8.27c). Due to its excellent spatial resolution, transesophageal echocardiography is the imaging modality of choice to detect valvular vegetations, abscesses, and leaflet perforations [109].

Air Embolism

Air embolism may occur in the arterial or venous circulation. In venous embolism, air enters the systemic venous circulation, traverses the right heart, and enters the pulmonary arterial circulation. It is usually iatrogenic.

In arterial embolism, air enters the pulmonary venous circulation and passes through the left heart and into the systemic arteries. The most important effects are on the heart, brain, and spinal cord.

The most common causes of venous and arterial air embolism are listed in Table 8.12 [110–112].

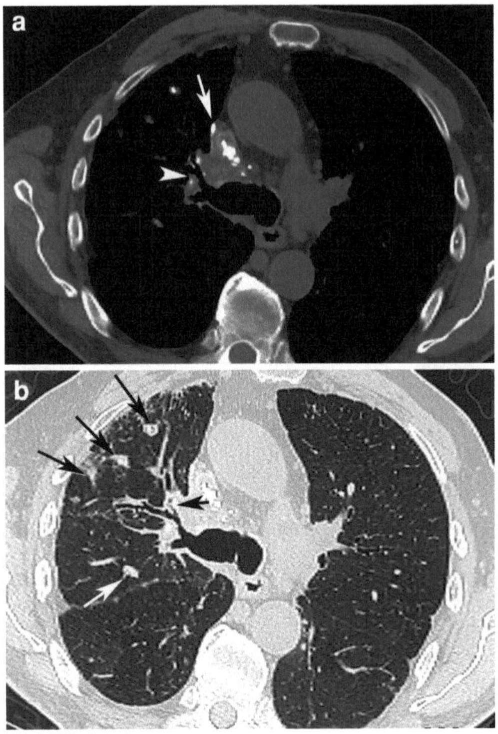

Fig. 8.24 Fibrosing mediastinitis in a 84-year-old male with shortness of breath. **a** Unenhanced CT image shows a calcified right hilar mass encasing the superior vena cava (*arrow*) and right upper lobe bronchus (*arrowhead*). **b** Unenhanced CT image (lung window) shows narrowing and distortion of the right upper lobe bronchus (*short arrow*). Also note the calcified nodules (*long arrows*) in right upper lobe due to prior histoplasmosis

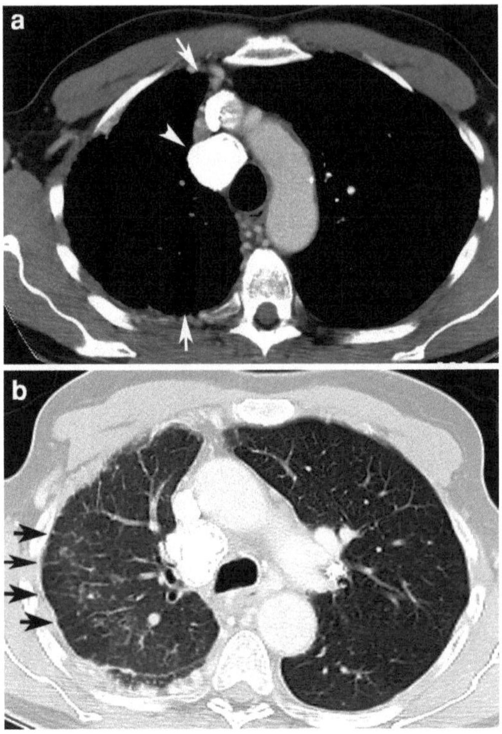

Fig. 8.25 Fibrosing mediastinitis in a 77-year-old male with a history of previous exposure histoplasmosis. **a** Contrast-enhanced CT image depicts multiple systemic collateral vessels along the pleural surface (*posterior arrow*) and a dilated right internal thoracic artery (*anterior arrow*). Note the calcified right paratracheal mass (*arrowhead*). **b** Contrast-enhanced CT image (lung window) shows multiple linear opacities perpendicular to the pleural surface (*arrows*) due to collateral vessels entering the lung

Clinical Features

Most patients with venous air embolism are asymptomatic. Arterial embolism has much more serious consequences. Signs and symptoms include: headache, seizures, coma, paresthesias, paralysis, arrhythmias, and cardiac arrest [110, 111].

Imaging Features

Small amounts of air may be seen in the systemic veins, right side of the heart, or main pulmonary artery on CT in the case of venous embolism. In arterial embolism, air may be identified in the left-sided cardiac chambers, coronary arteries (see Fig. 8.29), and systemic arteries including those of the brain [113].

Talc and Other Foreign Body Embolism

Embolism of talc, starch, and cellulose occurs when intravenous drug users inject crushed oral preparations of amphetamines or other drugs (methadone hydrochloride, hydromorphone hydrochloride, pentazocine) [114]. These drugs contain talc, cornstarch, and cellulose as insoluble fillers. The insoluble particles become trapped in the pulmonary arterioles and capillaries, causing thrombosis and vascular occlusion. They migrate through the vessel wall into the interstitium where they induce inflammation, a foreign body giant cell granulomatous

Table 8.10 CT features of fibrosing mediastinitis depending on affected mediastinal structure

Mediastinal findings	Parenchymal findings
Pulmonary vein stenosis or obstruction	Ground-glass opacities and interlobular septal thickening (hemorrhage)
Arterial or venous obstruction	Wedge-shaped peripheral opacities without air bronchograms (pulmonary infarcts)
Airway stenosis or obstruction	Recurrent atelectasis or pneumonia
Proximal pulmonary artery stenosis or obstruction	Dilation of pulmonary artery and right ventricle (pulmonary hypertension)

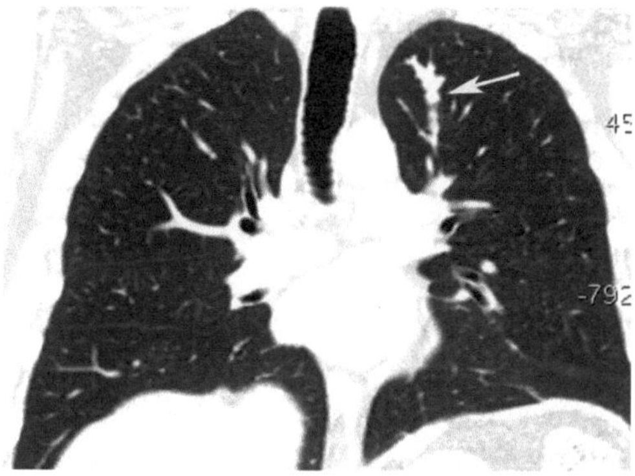

Fig. 8.26 Tumor embolism in a 40-year-old male with a history of chordoma. Coronal reformatted image (lung window) shows dilation and beading of a subsegmental artery (*arrow*) in the left upper lobe

reaction, and fibrosis [115]. Panacinar emphysema may also develop [116].

Clinical Features

Most patients are asymptomatic, although progressive dyspnea, persistent cough, non-specific chest pain, and occasionally anorexia, fever, and night sweats may occur [117]. Cor pulmonale as a result of pulmonary hypertension may eventually ensue.

Talc deposits may be visualized in retinal blood vessels on physical examination [118]. Pulmonary function tests show slight to moderate hypoxemia and reduction in carbon monoxide diffusion. Definitive diagnosis requires histological examination of the lung, usually achieved at autopsy [119]. Transbronchial or open lung biopsy specimens show macrophages with intracellular talc crystals [117]. These are irregular and birefringent under polarized light.

Table 8.11 Predisposing factors for septic embolism

Tricuspid valve endocarditis +/− history of intravenous drug abuse
Septic thrombophlebitis
Alcoholism
Skin infection
Immunologic deficiency (lymphoma)
Indwelling catheters or pacemaker wires

Imaging Features

On HRCT, several small nodular and reticular opacities are seen throughout the lungs [120] (see Fig. 8.30). There may be a fine granular pattern, ground-glass opacities, or both [121, 122]. The nodules tend to coalesce over time and form dense foci of consolidation that resemble progressive massive fibrosis. Areas of high attenuation in the foci of consolidation correspond to the presence of talc. Dilation of the central pulmonary arteries and right cardiac chambers may be present due to pulmonary hypertension.

When methylphenidate is the injected material, the CT findings characteristically show panlobular emphysema involving the lower lung zones without evidence of bullae [121, 123].

Fat Embolism

The term fat embolism (FE) refers to the liberation of fat into the systemic circulation. Fat embolism syndrome (FES) comprises a triad of respiratory distress, mental status changes, and a

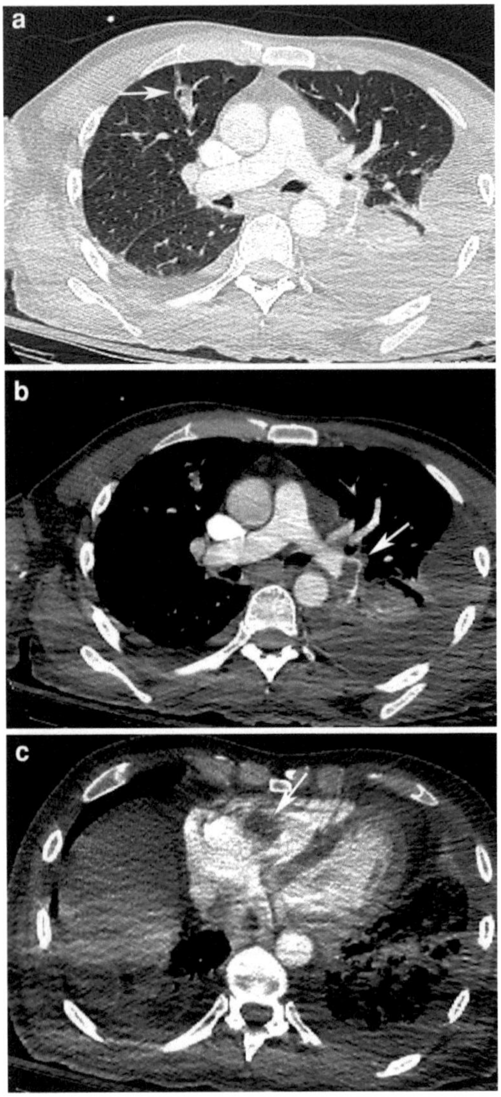

Fig. 8.27 Septic embolism in a 40-year-old intravenous drug abuser. **a** Contrast-enhanced CT image (lung window) shows a cavitary nodule (*arrow*) in the right upper lobe. **b** Contrast-enhanced CT image shows a filling defect in the left lower lobe artery (*arrow*). Note the loculated left pleural effusion due to empyema. **c** Contrast-enhanced CT image shows a nodular filling defect in the tricuspid valve region representing a vegetation (*arrow*)

petechial rash [124]. FE is an infrequent complication of fractures [125] seen in only 1–3% of simple long bone fractures, but in more severe trauma, the incidence may be as high as 10–20% [126–128].

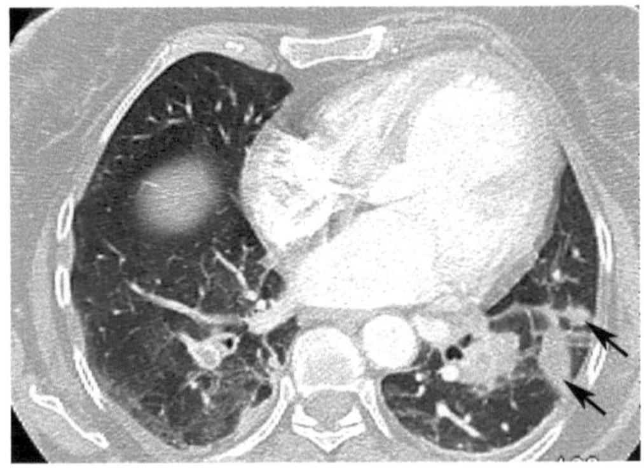

Fig. 8.28 Septic pulmonary embolism in a 32-year-old patient with history of intravenous drug abuse. Contrast-enhanced CT image (lung window) shows subpleural opacities (*arrows*) reflecting pulmonary infarcts

Clinical Features

The major signs are respiratory distress, confusion, restlessness, stupor, delirium, seizures, and coma unrelated to head injury and a petechial rash on the anterior surface of the neck and thorax developing 2 to 3 days following trauma [129]. In the setting of trauma, FE and traumatic lung contusion should be distinguished from each other. Lung contusion is evident immediately following trauma whereas FE is delayed for 12–24 h.

Imaging Features

CT shows bilateral patchy or diffuse ground-glass opacities with a predominant peripheral distribution, confluent areas of consolidation, and centrilobular nodules along interlobular septa and interlobar fissures. A crazy-paving pattern may be present. Abnormalities slowly improve within one week. In contrast, lung contusion tends to be unilateral or asymmetric and begins to resolve within 24 h.

Amniotic Fluid Embolism

Amniotic fluid embolism (AE) is a rare complication of pregnancy. Small amounts of amniotic fluid enter the maternal circulation

Table 8.12 Causes of venous and arterial air embolism

Venous embolism		Arterial embolism	
Iatrogenic	Non iatrogenic	Iatrogenic	Non iatrogenic
Surgery Insertion and maintenance of intravenous catheters Diagnostic or therapeutic air injection Barotrauma secondary to positive pressure ventilation Transthoracic needle biopsy Contrast administration material for CT (23%)	SCUBA diving	Penetrating thoracic trauma (iatrogenic or accidental) Transthoracic needle biopsy and thoracentesis Open heart surgery	SCUBA diving

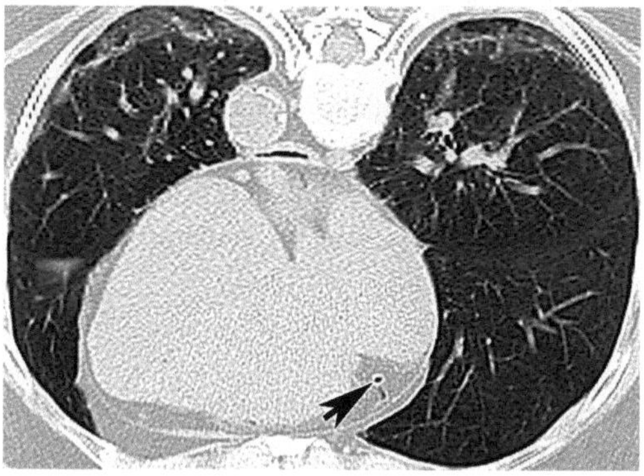

Fig. 8.29 Air embolism in a 60-year-old male unresponsive immediately post CT-guided lung biopsy. Unenhanced CT image shows gas within the right coronary artery (*arrow*)

during normal labor but large amounts may be pumped into the venous circulation by uterine contractions when there is disruption of the uterine wall associated with rupture of the amniotic membranes. This may cause pulmonary vascular obstruction by squamous cells, mucin, and hair fragments. Left ventricular dysfunction as a result of acute pulmonary hypertension may occur leading to acute pulmonary edema. An immunologic reaction similar to anaphylaxis may also develop [130].

Clinical Features

The symptoms usually begin during the immediate postpartum period although some have reported onset during labor and cesarean section [131]. Clinical manifestations include a sudden onset of cardiovascular collapse, cyanosis, and hemorrhage or disseminated intravascular coagulopathy. In less severe cases, progressive dyspnea is the major complaint [132]. Diagnosis is confirmed when squamous cells, mucin, and hair fragments are identified in pulmonary capillary blood collected through a pulmonary artery catheter [133]. Amniotic cells detected in bronchoalveolar lavage (BAL) fluid also support the diagnosis [134].

Imaging Features

Bilateral airspace consolidation indistinguishable from pulmonary edema from another cause [135] is the main CT imaging abnormality. The differential diagnosis is massive pulmonary hemorrhage and aspiration.

Consolidation may persist or resolve within a few days. Cardiac enlargement may also be seen secondary to pulmonary hypertension and cor pulmonale with or without left ventricular failure.

Primary Pulmonary Artery Sarcoma

Pulmonary artery sarcomas (PAS) are rare tumors. The most common histologic types are undifferentiated sarcoma, leiomyosarcoma, and malignant fibrous histiocytoma [136, 137].

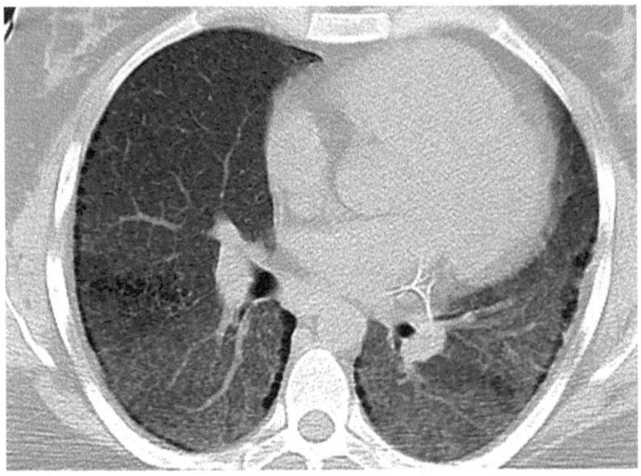

Fig. 8.30 Talc embolism in a 35-year-old female intravenous drug abuser. High-resolution CT image depicts a fine granular pattern throughout both lungs and diffuse ground-glass opacities

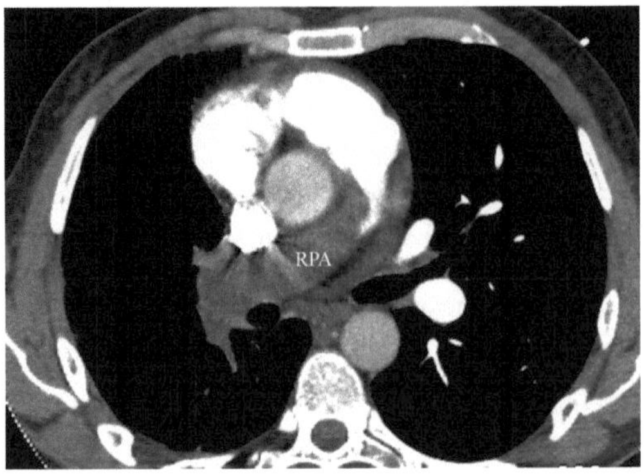

Fig. 8.31 Pulmonary artery sarcoma in a 47-year-old male. Contrast-enhanced axial CT image depicts a lobulated filling defect occluding the right pulmonary artery (RPA)

Clinical Features

PAS presents with nonspecific symptoms, which include dyspnea (73%), chest pain (45%), cough (42%), and hemoptysis (24%). Symptoms may mimic acute pulmonary embolism [136], congenital pulmonary artery stenosis, fibrosing mediastinitis, or lung cancer. Patients may also present with pulmonary hypertension [138].

PAS should be suspected in patients with large pulmonary emboli, constitutional symptoms, a unilateral filling defect, and "emboli" refractory to anticoagulation [139, 140].

Imaging Features

On contrast-enhanced CT pulmonary angiography, the most common manifestations are intra-arterial filling defects mimicking acute or chronic thromboemboli. The most specific findings are filling defects occupying the entire lumen of the main or proximal right or left pulmonary artery [138, 141, 142] (see Fig. 8.31), expansion of the involved artery, and extraluminal extension. Delayed contrast-enhanced CT or gadolinium-enhanced MR imaging and FDG/PET are useful to distinguish PAS from bland emboli. PAS shows delayed enhancement, whereas non-vascularized thrombus does not enhance [136, 143]. PAS may also show increased uptake on FDG/PET [144, 145].

Pulmonary parenchymal findings on CT also include a mosaic attenuation pattern (43%) [141], foci of peripheral consolidation abutting the pleura (71%), parenchymal bands (43%), and subpleural nodules (14%) [136]. The lung is the most common site of metastatic disease [138].

Diseases of the Capillaries and Venules

Pulmonary Veno-Occlusive Disease and Pulmonary Capillary Hemangiomatosis

Pulmonary veno-occlusive disease (PVOD) and pulmonary capillary hemangiomatosis (PCH) are rare disorders with limited epidemiologic data in the scientific literature. In the Dana Point classification of pulmonary hypertension, they form subgroup 1' of pulmonary arterial hypertension (PAH) [146]. PVOD and PCH may be separate entities or may be at different ends of the spectrum of a single disorder. Both diseases are felt to be idiopathic but are associated with many conditions listed in Table 8.13 of which systemic sclerosis is the most common [147–155].

Pathologically, PVOD is characterized by intimal fibrosis of interlobular veins and venules leading to venous obstruction and interlobular septal edema [156, 157], whereas PCH is

Table 8.13 Entities associated with PVOD and PCH

PVOD	PCH
Systemic lupus erythematosus	Systemic lupus erythematosus
Systemic sclerosis	Systemic sclerosis
HIV	Takayasu arteritis
Rheumatoid arthritis	Kartagener syndrome
Langerhans cell histiocytosis	Hypertrophic cardiomyopathy
Stem cell transplantation	

characterized by the proliferation of capillary channels within alveolar walls eventually causing venous compression and occlusion [158–160]. The pathologic changes in both diseases lead to chronically increased capillary hydrostatic pressure and subsequent PAH [160].

Clinical Features

Patients typically present with signs and symptoms of pulmonary hypertension including an insidious onset of dyspnea and fatigue. Occasionally, hemoptysis is a feature. Age at presentation varies between 7 and 70 years with most patients presenting between the ages of 20 and 40 years. One-third of patients with PVOD are children. In adults with PVOD, men are more frequently affected. Findings of pulmonary arterial hypertension, pulmonary edema on imaging studies, and a normal pulmonary artery occlusion pressure at right heart catheterization are very suggestive of PVOD, but many patients do not have the classic findings. Investigators have also found a lower DLCO, arterial oxygen saturation by pulse oximetry during a 6 min walk test, and resting paO2 in patients with PVOD compared to other patients with PAH. Occult hemorrhage on BAL is also more frequent in PVOD [154].

Prognosis is uniformly poor for both diseases with a median survival of 2–3 years. Careful work-up is necessary in order exclude PVOD/PCH as the use of vasodilator therapy increases perfusion of the capillary bed with no possibility of increasing venous outflow, possibly leading to severe and occasionally fatal pulmonary edema.

Although the definitive diagnosis of PVOD and PCH is histological, open lung biopsy is a high-risk procedure in these patients. Hence a noninvasive diagnostic approach is preferable [161–164].

Imaging Features

On CT and MR, cardiac and pulmonary arterial signs of pulmonary hypertension are present. The left cardiac chambers are normal [155, 162, 165–169].

The most specific signs of PVOD on HRCT include diffuse, smooth interlobular septal thickening, ground-glass opacities, and mediastinal lymphadenopathy (see Fig. 8.32) [154, 155, 162, 168]. Pleural effusions are more common in PVOD than PCH. Montani et al. [154] showed that the presence of two or three imaging findings including lymph node enlargement, interlobular septal thickening, and centrilobular nodules had a sensitivity of 75% and specificity of 84.6% for detecting PVOD, but the absence or presence of only one of these imaging features could not reliably exclude it.

On HRCT, PCH is more commonly associated with poorly defined centrilobular ground-glass nodules than PVOD (see Fig. 8.33a, b).

However, there is significant overlap in the imaging findings of both disease entities. It is, therefore, perhaps more important to distinguish them from other forms of PAH than from each other due to their poor prognoses and possible adverse reaction to vasodilator agents. The presence of septal thickening, ground-glass centrilobular nodules, or both should alert the clinician to the possibility of these diagnoses. If other noninvasive tests also raise the possibility of PVOD/PCH, earlier referral for transplantation should be considered.

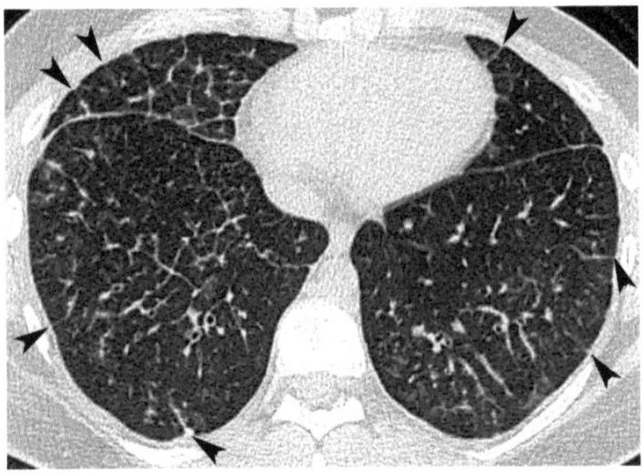

Fig. 8.32 Pulmonary veno-occlusive disease in a 24-year-old male. High-resolution CT image shows smooth interlobular septal thickening (*arrowheads*) and diffuse ground-glass nodules. Courtesy of Dr. Tan-Lucien Mohammed (Cleveland, OH)

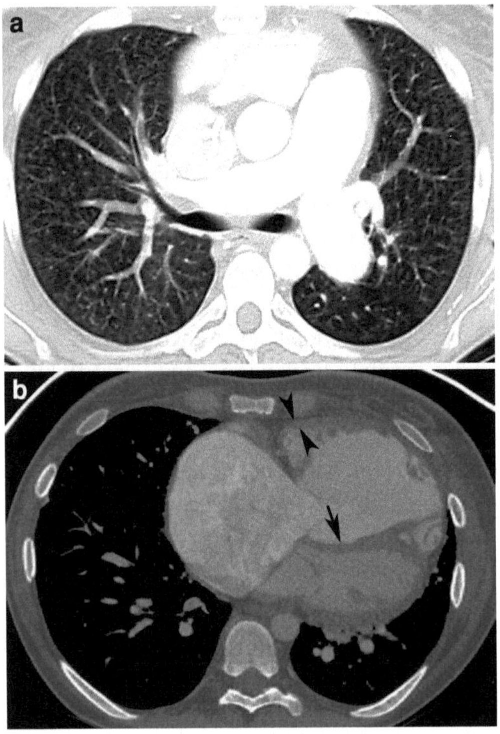

Fig. 8.33 Pulmonary capillary hemangiomatosis in a 30-year-old female with pulmonary hypertension. **a** Axial MIP CT image shows diffuse centrilobular nodules without interlobular septal thickening. **b** Contrast-enhanced axial CT image shows marked dilation of the right atrium and ventricle. There is right ventricular hypertrophy (*arrowheads*) and bowing of the interventricular septum towards the left (*arrows*) due to pulmonary hypertension

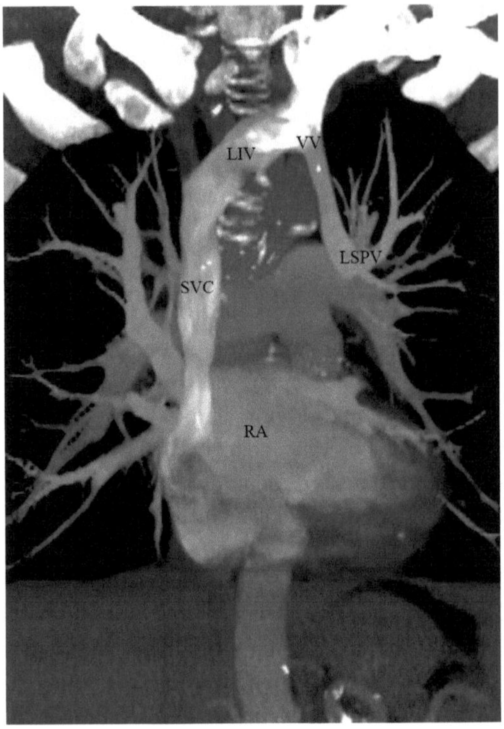

Fig. 8.34 Partial anomalous pulmonary venous return from the left superior pulmonary vein (LSPV) to a vertical vein (VV). Coronal MIP CT image shows anomalous drainage of the LSPV into a vertical vein draining into the left innominate vein (LIV) and then the SVC

Congenital Anomalies of the Pulmonary Veins

Partial Anomalous Pulmonary Venous Return

Partial anomalous pulmonary venous return (PAPVR) is defined by abnormal drainage of one or more pulmonary veins directly into the systemic venous circulation resulting in a left-to-right shunt. Pulmonary veins can drain into the right atrium or one of its tributaries. Patients are usually asymptomatic.

There are two main subtypes of PAPVR: partial anomalous venous drainage (PAPVD) and partial anomalous pulmonary venous connection (PAPVC).

PAPVD is an anomalous vein draining into the left atrium related to an intracardiac anomaly or defect such as sinus venous defect or malposition of the septum primum. When malpositioning of the septum primum is present, leftward shift of the posterior aspect of the septum results in drainage of the right pulmonary veins into the right atrium. Heterotaxy syndrome and polysplenia are usually associated [170, 171].

In PAPVC, the anomalous vein drains into a systemic vein proximal to the right atrium. The most common type is the left superior pulmonary vein draining into the left brachiocephalic vein. A vertical vein courses superolateral to the aortic arch towards the left brachiocephalic vein (see Fig. 8.34). This type of PAPVR is not associated with congenital heart disease. On the right, PAPVC of the right superior pulmonary vein (RSPV) draining into the low superior vena cava or the superior cavoatrial junction is the most common (see Fig. 8.35a). A sinus venous defect is associated with anomalous drainage of the RSPV in 82% of patients [172] (see Fig. 8.35b). When a sinus venous defect is present, the wall that separates the RSPV from the SVC is not present or is unroofed, resulting in the RSPV draining into the SVC or right atrium. Cardiovascular symptoms are present when the shunt is hemodynamically significant, in which case surgical correction is indicated.

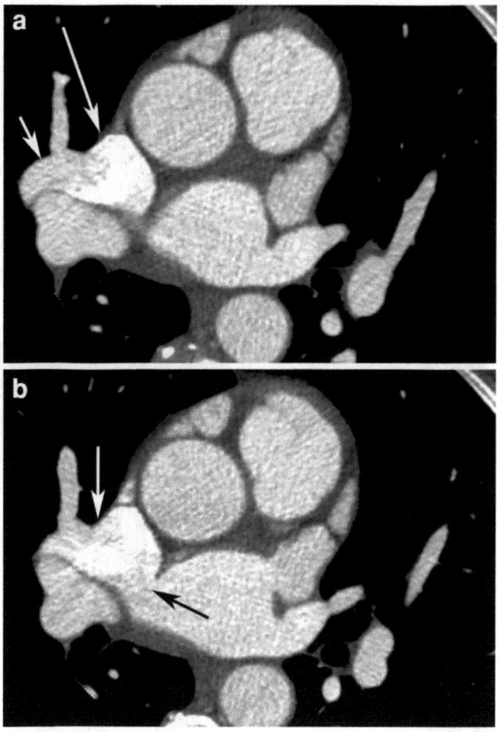

Fig. 8.35 Partial anomalous pulmonary venous return and sinus venosus defect. **a** Contrast-enhanced CT image shows a vessel (*short arrow*) from the right upper lobe draining into the posterolateral aspect of the superior vena cava (SVC) (*long arrow*). **b** Contrast-enhanced CT image in the same patient shows communication between the atria through a sinus venosus defect (*black arrow*). Note a second anomalous draining vein from the anterior segment of the right upper lobe into the SVC (*white arrow*)

Scimitar Syndrome

Scimitar syndrome, also known as venolobar or hypogenetic lung syndrome, is a variant of PAPVC. It occurs almost invariably on the right and is characterized by PAPVC of part of the right lung or the entire right lung into the inferior vena cava or another systemic vein. It is associated with right lung and pulmonary artery hypoplasia, dextrocardia, and Bochdalek hernia. The need for surgical correction depends on the spectrum of associated congenital anomalies [173].

Imaging Features

On contrast-enhanced CT or MR imaging, the anomalous pulmonary veins in PAPVD, PAPVC, and scimitar syndrome are well-depicted (see Fig. 8.36a, b). Coronal reformations on CT (see Fig. 8.36c) and coronal acquisitions on MR angiography are especially useful to outline the course of the anomalous vein. Cine MR can also assess any associated intracardiac abnormalities, and phase contrast imaging can provide an estimate of the degree of left-to-right shunting. In scimitar syndrome, the draining vein courses inferomedially, parallel to the right atrium towards the hemidiaphragm and IVC, with the characteristic appearance of a scimitar or Turkish sword. RPA hypoplasia and systemic collateral supply to the right lung can also be imaged (see Fig. 8.36d).

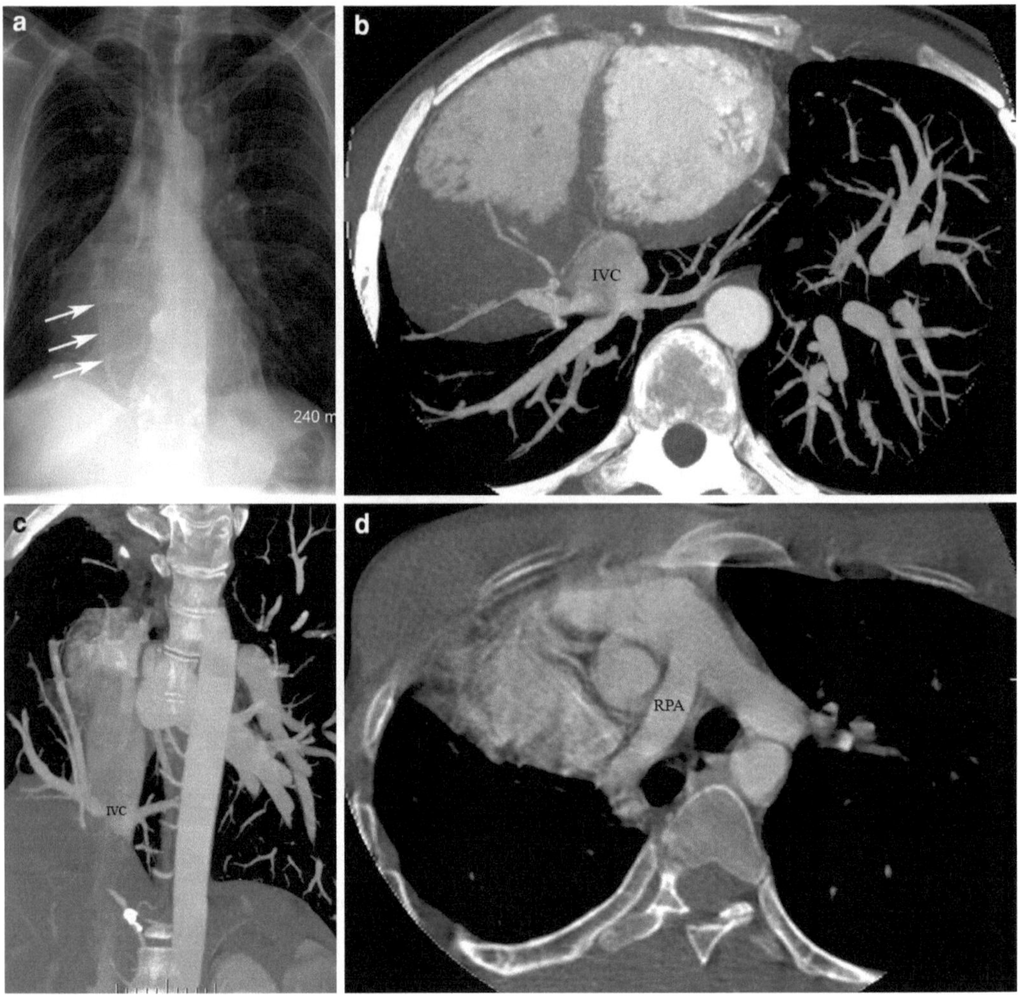

Fig. 8.36 Scimitar syndrome. **a** Chest radiograph shows a large tubular opacity (*arrows*) coursing towards the right cardiophrenic angle. **b** Axial MIP CT image demonstrates multiple right pulmonary veins draining into the inferior vena cava (IVC). **c** Coronal MIP CT image in the same patient shows several pulmonary veins (*arrows*) draining into the IVC. **d** Contrast-enhanced axial CT image shows a small right pulmonary artery (RPA) and volume loss of the right lung with displacement of mediastinal structures towards the right

Acquired Diseases of the Pulmonary Veins

Post Radiofrequency Catheter Ablation Pulmonary Vein Stenosis

Atrial fibrillation (AF) is the most common supraventricular arrhythmia. The myocardium of the left atrium extends for a variable length into the pulmonary veins. Over 90% of ectopic beats initiating AF arise from the pulmonary vein ostia [174]. Radiofrequency catheter ablation (RFCA) of the left atrium within 5 mm of the pulmonary vein (PV) ostia is performed to isolate these electrical foci and is a treatment offered for isolated AF. Symptomatic complications are uncommon. PV stenosis has been reported in 40–100% of patients [175]. Only 11% of patients develop severe stenosis, and, in one study, only 3% of patients

Table 8.14 Complications associated with radiofrequency catheter ablation of pulmonary veins

Pulmonary vein stenosis, dissection, or occlusion
Perforation of pulmonary vein or left atrium
Atrio-esophageal fistula
Hematoma
Veno-occlusive disease
Venous infarction
Pulmonary hypertension
Fibrosing mediastinitis
Pleural or pericardial effusion or hemopericardium
Transient atrial septal defect
Stroke
Hemothorax

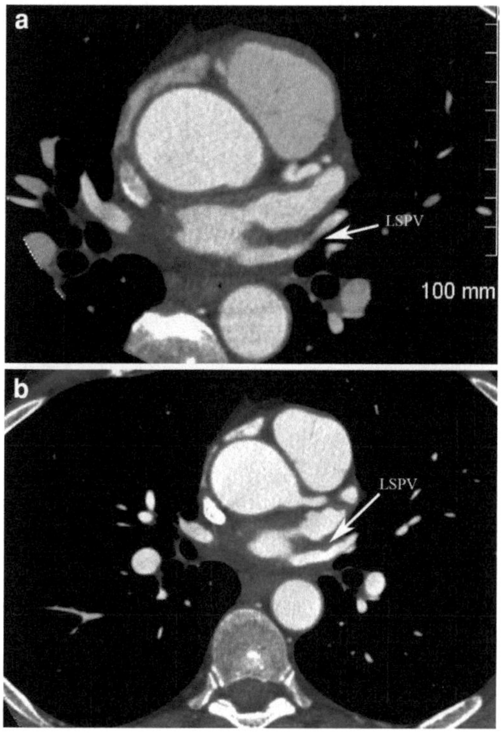

Fig. 8.37 Radiofrequency ablation induced pulmonary vein stenosis in a 62-year-old male 1 year following radiofrequency catheter ablation (RFCA) for atrial fibrillation. **a** Contrast-enhanced axial CT image shows focal narrowing of the left superior pulmonary vein (LSPV) (*arrow*). **b** Contrast-enhanced axial CT shows a normal left superior pulmonary vein (LSPV) prior to RFCA (*arrow*)

with 65% luminal stenosis were symptomatic [176].

Clinical Features

Patients may present with dyspnea on exertion. PV stenosis may be treated successfully with angioplasty with or without stenting [177].

Imaging Features

MDCTA is the modality of choice to delineate the anatomy of the PV before RFCA and to image post-procedural complications which are listed in Table 8.14 [171, 178].

Minimal PV stenosis is common following ablation, but significant stenosis may cause focal ground-glass opacities and thickening of the interlobular septa in the affected lobe on lung windows due to focal venous hypertension and edema [179]. It may lead to pulmonary vein thrombosis (see Fig. 8.37a, b) [175].

References

1. Siripornpitak S, Reddy GP, Schwitter J, Higgins CB. Pulmonary artery sling: anatomical and functional evaluation by MRI. J Comput Assist Tomogr. 1997;21(5):766–8.
2. Lee KH, Yoon CS, Choe KO, et al. Use of imaging for assessing anatomical relationships of tracheobronchial anomalies associated with left pulmonary artery sling. Pediatr Radiol. 2001;31(4):269–78.
3. Newman B. Congenital bronchopulmonary foregut malformations: concepts and controversies. Pediatr Radiol. 2006;36(8):773–91.
4. Zylak CJ, Eyler WR, Spizarny DL, Stone CH. Developmental lung anomalies in the adult: radiologic-pathologic correlation. Radiographics. 2002;22 Spec No:S25–43.
5. Rosenberg BF, Tantiwongse T, Wittenborg MH. Anomalous course of left pulmonary artery with respiratory obstruction. Radiology. 1956;67(3):339–45.
6. Newman B, Meza MP, Towbin RB, Nido PD. Left pulmonary artery sling: diagnosis and delineation of associated tracheobronchial anomalies with MR. Pediatr Radiol. 1996;26(9):661–8.
7. Berdon WE, Baker DH, Wung JT, et al. Complete cartilage-ring tracheal stenosis associated with anomalous left pulmonary artery: the ring-sling complex. Radiology. 1984;152(1):57–64.

8. Chen SJ, Lee WJ, Lin MT, et al. Left pulmonary artery sling complex: computed tomography and hypothesis of embryogenesis. Ann Thorac Surg. 2007;84(5):1645–50.
9. Newman B, Gondor M. MR evaluation of right pulmonary agenesis and vascular airway compression in pediatric patients. Am J Roentgenol. 1997;168(1):55–8.
10. Collins RT II, Weinberg PM, Ewing S, Fogel M. Images in cardiovascular medicine: pulmonary artery sling in an asymptomatic 15-year-old boy. Circulation. 2008;117(18):2403–6.
11. Ganesh V, Hoey ET, Gopalan D. Pulmonary artery sling: an unexpected finding on cardiac multidetector CT. Postgrad Med J. 2009;85(1001):128.
12. Kagadis GC, Panagiotopoulou EC, Priftis KN, Vaos G, Nikiforidis GC, Anthracopoulos MB. Preoperative evaluation of the trachea in a child with pulmonary artery sling using 3-dimensional computed tomographic imaging and virtual bronchoscopy. J Pediatr Surg. 2007;42(5):E9–13.
13. du Plessis AM, Andronikou S, Goussaard P. Bridging bronchus and sling left pulmonary artery: a rare entity demonstrated by coronal CT with 3D rendering display and minimal-intensity projections. Pediatr Radiol. 2008;38(9):1024–6.
14. Baden W, Schaefer J, Kumpf M, et al. Comparison of imaging techniques in the diagnosis of bridging bronchus. Eur Respir. 2008;31(5):1125–31.
15. Kieffer SA, Amplatz K, Anderson RC, Lillehei CW. Proximal interruption of a pulmonary artery. Am J Roentgenol Radium Ther Nucl Med. 1965;95(3): 592–7.
16. Bouros D, Pare P, Panagou P, Tsintiris K, Siafakas N. The varied manifestation of pulmonary artery agenesis in adulthood. Chest. 1995;108(3):670–6.
17. Rene M, Sans J, Dominguez J, Sancho C, Valldeperas J. Unilateral pulmonary artery agenesis presenting with hemoptysis: treatment by embolization of systemic collaterals. Cardiovasc Intervent Radiol. 1995;18(4):251–4.
18. Jaskolka J, Wu L, Chan RP, Faughnan ME. Imaging of hereditary hemorrhagic telangiectasia. Am J Roentgenol. 2004;183(2):307–14.
19. Abdel Aal AK, Hamed MF, Biosca RF, Saddekni S, Raghuram K. Occlusion time for Amplatzer vascular plug in the management of pulmonary arteriovenous malformations. Am J Roentgenol. 2009;192(3):793–9.
20. Gupta P, Mordin C, Curtis J, Hughes JM, Shovlin CL, Jackson JE. Pulmonary arteriovenous malformations: effect of embolization on right-to-left shunt, hypoxemia, and exercise tolerance in 66 patients. Am J Roentgenol. 2002;179(2):347–55.
21. Brown KK. Pulmonary vasculitis. Proc Am Thorac Soc. 2006;3(1):48–57.
22. Hansell DM. Small-vessel diseases of the lung: CT-pathologic correlates. Radiology. 2002;225(3): 639–53.
23. Travis WD, Colby TV, Lombard C, Carpenter HA. A clinicopathologic study of 34 cases of diffuse pulmonary hemorrhage with lung biopsy confirmation. Am J Surg Pathol. 1990;14(12): 1112–25.
24. Watts RA, Lane SE, Bentham G, Scott DG. Epidemiology of systemic vasculitis: a ten-year study in the United Kingdom. Arthritis Rheum. 2000;43(2):414–9.
25. Hagen EC, Daha MR, Hermans J, et al. Diagnostic value of standardized assays for anti-neutrophil cytoplasmic antibodies in idiopathic systemic vasculitis: EC/BCR project for ANCA assay standardization. Kidney Int. 1998;53(3):743–53.
26. Frankel SK, Cosgrove GP, Fischer A, Meehan RT, Brown KK. Update in the diagnosis and management of pulmonary vasculitis. Chest. 2006;129(2): 452–65.
27. Chung MP, Yi CA, Lee HY, Han J, Lee KS. Imaging of pulmonary vasculitis. Radiology. 2010;255(2):322–41.
28. Jennette JC, Falk RJ, Andrassy K, et al. Nomenclature of systemic vasculitides: proposal of an international consensus conference. Arthritis Rheum. 1994;37(2):187–92.
29. Guillevin L, Durand-Gasselin B, Cevallos R, et al. Microscopic polyangiitis: clinical and laboratory findings in eighty-five patients. Arthritis Rheum. 1999;42(3):421–30.
30. Mulder AH, Horst G, van Leeuwen MA, Limburg PC, Kallenberg CG. Antineutrophil cytoplasmic antibodies in rheumatoid arthritis: characterization and clinical correlations. Arthritis Rheum. 1993;36(8):1054–60.
31. Schnabel A, Csernok E, Isenberg DA, Mrowka C, Gross WL. Antineutrophil cytoplasmic antibodies in systemic lupus erythematosus: prevalence, specificities, and clinical significance. Arthritis Rheum. 1995;38(5):633–7.
32. Cojocaru M, Cojocaru IM, Iacob SA. Prevalence of anti-neutrophil cytoplasmic antibodies in patients with chronic hepatitis C infection associated mixed cryoglobulinemia. Rom J Intern Med. 2006;44(4):427–31.
33. Zholudev A, Zurakowski D, Young W, Leichtner A, Bousvaros A. Serologic testing with ANCA, ASCA, and anti-OmpC in children and young adults with Crohn's disease and ulcerative colitis: diagnostic value and correlation with disease phenotype. Am J Gastroenterol. 2004;99(11):2235–41.
34. Erkan F, Gul A, Tasali E. Pulmonary manifestations of Behcet's disease. Thorax. 2001;56(7):572–8.
35. Hiller N, Lieberman S, Chajek-Shaul T, Bar-Ziv J, Shaham D. Thoracic manifestations of Behcet disease at CT. Radiographics. 2004;24(3):801–8.
36. Hamuryudan V, Yurdakul S, Moral F, et al. Pulmonary arterial aneurysms in Behcet's syndrome: a report of 24 cases. Br J Rheumatol. 1994;33(1):48–51.

37. Uzun O, Akpolat T, Erkan L. Pulmonary vasculitis in Behcet disease: a cumulative analysis. Chest. 2005;127(6):2243–53.
38. Chae EJ, Do KH, Seo JB, et al. Radiologic and clinical findings of Behcet disease: comprehensive review of multisystemic involvement. Radiographics. 2008;28(5):e31.
39. Tunaci M, Ozkorkmaz B, Tunaci A, Gul A, Engin G, Acunas B. CT findings of pulmonary artery aneurysms during treatment for Behcet's disease. Am J Roentgenol. 1999;172(3):729–33.
40. Marten K, Schnyder P, Schirg E, Prokop M, Rummeny EJ, Engelke C. Pattern-based differential diagnosis in pulmonary vasculitis using volumetric CT. Am J Roentgenol. 2005;184(3):720–33.
41. Seko Y. Giant cell and Takayasu arteritis. Curr Opin Rheumatol. 2007;19(1):39–43.
42. Gotway MB, Araoz PA, Macedo TA, et al. Imaging findings in Takayasu's arteritis. Am J Roentgenol. 2005;184(6):1945–50.
43. Choe YH, Han BK, Koh EM, Kim DK, Do YS, Lee WR. Takayasu's arteritis: assessment of disease activity with contrast-enhanced MR imaging. Am J Roentgenol. 2000;175(2):505–11.
44. Schmidt WA, Blockmans D. Use of ultrasonography and positron emission tomography in the diagnosis and assessment of large-vessel vasculitis. Curr Opin Rheumatol. 2005;17(1):9–15.
45. Lee KS, Kim TS, Fujimoto K, et al. Thoracic manifestation of Wegener's granulomatosis: CT findings in 30 patients. Eur Radiol. 2003;13(1):43–51.
46. Komocsi A, Reuter M, Heller M, Murakozi H, Gross WL, Schnabel A. Active disease and residual damage in treated Wegener's granulomatosis: an observational study using pulmonary high-resolution computed tomography. Eur Radiol. 2003;13(1):36–42.
47. Lohrmann C, Uhl M, Kotter E, Burger D, Ghanem N, Langer M. Pulmonary manifestations of Wegener granulomatosis: CT findings in 57 patients and a review of the literature. Eur J Radiol. 2005;53(3):471–7.
48. Ananthakrishnan L, Sharma N, Kanne JP. Wegener's granulomatosis in the chest: high-resolution CT findings. Am J Roentgenol. 2009;192(3):676–82.
49. Franks TJ, Koss MN. Pulmonary capillaritis. Curr Opin Pulm Med. 2000;6(5):430–5.
50. Mayberry JP, Primack SL, Muller NL. Thoracic manifestations of systemic autoimmune diseases: radiographic and high-resolution CT findings. Radiographics. 2000;20(6):1623–35.
51. Castaner E, Alguersuari A, Gallardo X, et al. When to suspect pulmonary vasculitis: radiologic and clinical clues. Radiographics. 2010;30(1):33–53.
52. Bosch X, Guilabert A, Espinosa G, Mirapeix E. Treatment of antineutrophil cytoplasmic antibody associated vasculitis: a systematic review. JAMA. 2007;298(6):655–69.
53. Keogh KA, Specks U. Churg–Strauss syndrome. Semin Respir Crit Care Med. 2006;27(2):148–57.
54. Choi YH, Im JG, Han BK, Kim JH, Lee KY, Myoung NH. Thoracic manifestation of Churg–Strauss syndrome: radiologic and clinical findings. Chest. 2000;117(1):117–24.
55. Keogh KA, Specks U. Churg–Strauss syndrome: clinical presentation, antineutrophil cytoplasmic antibodies, and leukotriene receptor antagonists. Am J Med. 2003;115(4):284–90.
56. Solans R, Bosch JA, Perez-Bocanegra C, et al. Churg–Strauss syndrome: outcome and long-term follow-up of 32 patients. Rheumatology. 2001;40(7):763–71.
57. Silva CI, Muller NL. Churg–Strauss syndrome: imaging of the chest. Philladelphia: Saunders-Elsevier; 2008. p. 821–7.
58. Katzenstein AL. Diagnostic features and differential diagnosis of Churg–Strauss syndrome in the lung: a review. Am J Clin Pathol. 2000;114(5):767–72.
59. Silva CI, Muller NL, Fujimoto K, Johkoh T, Ajzen SA, Churg A. Churg–Strauss syndrome: high resolution CT and pathologic findings. J Thorac Imaging. 2005;20(2):74–80.
60. Johkoh T, Muller NL, Akira M, et al. Eosinophilic lung diseases: diagnostic accuracy of thin-section CT in 111 patients. Radiology. 2000;216(3):773–80.
61. Kim YK, Lee KS, Chung MP, et al. Pulmonary involvement in Churg–Strauss syndrome: an analysis of CT, clinical, and pathologic findings. Eur Radiol. 2007;17(12):3157–65.
62. Ioachimescu OC, Sieber S, Kotch A. Idiopathic pulmonary haemosiderosis revisited. Eur Respir. 2004;24(1):162–70.
63. Green RJ, Ruoss SJ, Kraft SA, Duncan SR, Berry GJ, Raffin TA. Pulmonary capillaritis and alveolar hemorrhage: update on diagnosis and management. Chest. 1996;110(5):1305–16.
64. Niles JL, Bottinger EP, Saurina GR, et al. The syndrome of lung hemorrhage and nephritis is usually an ANCA-associated condition. Arch Intern Med. 1996;156(4):440–5.
65. Jennette JC, Falk RJ. Small-vessel vasculitis. N Engl J Med. 1997;337(21):1512–23.
66. Akikusa B, Sato T, Ogawa M, Ueda S, Kondo Y. Necrotizing alveolar capillaritis in autopsy cases of microscopic polyangiitis: incidence, histo-pathogenesis, and relationship with systemic vasculitis. Arch Pathol Lab Med. 1997;121(2):144–9.
67. Kim JS, Lee KS, Koh EM, Kim SY, Chung MP, Han J. Thoracic involvement of systemic lupus erythematosus: clinical, pathologic, and radiologic findings. J Comput Assist Tomogr. 2000;24(1):9–18.
68. Kim EA, Lee KS, Johkoh T, et al. Interstitial lung diseases associated with collagen vascular diseases: radiologic and histopathologic findings. Radiographics. 2002;22 Spec No:S151–65.

69. Primack SL, Miller RR, Muller NL. Diffuse pulmonary hemorrhage: clinical, pathologic, and imaging features. Am J Roentgenol. 1995;164(2): 295–300.
70. Lauque D, Cadranel J, Lazor R, et al. Microscopic polyangiitis with alveolar hemorrhage: a study of 29 cases and review of the literature: Groupe d'Etudes et de Recherche sur les Maladies "Orphelines" Pulmonaires (GERM"O"P). Medicine (Baltimore). 2000;79(4):222–33.
71. Cheah FK, Sheppard MN, Hansell DM. Computed tomography of diffuse pulmonary haemorrhage with pathological correlation. Clin Radiol. 1993;48(2):89–93.
72. Eschun GM, Mink SN, Sharma S. Pulmonary interstitial fibrosis as a presenting manifestation in perinuclear antineutrophilic cytoplasmic antibody microscopic polyangiitis. Chest. 2003;123(1): 297–301.
73. Nguyen ET, Silva CI, Seely JM, Chong S, Lee KS, Muller NL. Pulmonary artery aneurysms and pseudoaneurysms in adults: findings at CT and radiography. Am J Roentgenol. 2007;188(2): W126–34.
74. DeLima LG, Wynands JE, Bourke ME, Walley VM. Catheter-induced pulmonary artery false aneurysm and rupture: case report and review. J Cardiothorac Vasc Anesth. 1994;8(1):70–5.
75. Fraser RS, Muller NL, Colman N, Pare PD. Pulmonary hypertension and edema. In: Muller NL, Colman N, Pare PD, editors. Diagnosis of diseases of the chest. Philladelpia: Saunders; 1999. p. 1935–7.
76. Loyd JE, Tillman BF, Atkinson JB, Des Prez RM. Mediastinal fibrosis complicating histoplasmosis. Medicine (Baltimore). 1988;67(5):295–310.
77. Lloyd JE, Tillman BF, Atkinson JB, Des Prez RM. Mediastinal fibrosis complicating histoplasmosis. Medicine (Baltimore). 1988;67:295–310.
78. Goodwin RA, Nickell JA, Des Prez RM. Mediastinal fibrosis complicating healed primary histoplasmosis and tuberculosis. Medicine (Baltimore). 1972;51(3):227–46.
79. Peebles RS, Carpenter CT, Dupont WD, Loyd JE. Mediastinal fibrosis is associated with human leukocyte antigen-A2. Chest. 2000;117(2):482–5.
80. Rossi SE, McAdams HP, Rosado-de-Christenson ML, Franks TJ, Galvin JR. Fibrosing mediastinitis. Radiographics. 2001;21(3):737–57.
81. Mole TM, Glover J, Sheppard MN. Sclerosing mediastinitis: a report on 18 cases. Thorax. 1995;50(3):280–3.
82. Hanley PC, Shub C, Lie JT. Constrictive pericarditis associated with combined idiopathic retroperitoneal and mediastinal fibrosis. Mayo Clin Proc. 1984;59(5):300–4.
83. Kalweit G, Huwer H, Straub U, Gams E. Mediastinal compression syndromes due to idiopathic fibrosing mediastinitis—report of three cases and review of the literature. Thorac Cardiovasc Surg. 1996;44(2):105–9.
84. Cochrane A, Warren R, Mullerworth M, Manolas E. Fibrosing mediastinitis with coronary artery involvement. Ann Thorac Surg. 1991;51(4):652–4.
85. Flieder DB, Suster S, Moran CA. Idiopathic fibroinflammatory (fibrosing/sclerosing) lesions of the mediastinum: a study of 30 cases with emphasis on morphologic heterogeneity. Mod Pathol. 1999;12(3):257–64.
86. Mathisen DJ, Grillo HC. Clinical manifestation of mediastinal fibrosis and histoplasmosis. Ann Thorac Surg. 1992;54(6):1053–57; discussion 1057–58.
87. Urschel HC Jr, Razzuk MA, Netto GJ, Disiere J, Chung SY. Sclerosing mediastinitis: improved management with histoplasmosis titer and ketoconazole. Ann Thorac Surg. 1990;50(2):215–21.
88. Sherrick AD, Brown LR, Harms GF, Myers JL. The radiographic findings of fibrosing mediastinitis. Chest. 1994;106(2):484–9.
89. Farmer DW, Moore E, Amparo E, Webb WR, Gamsu G, Higgins CB. Calcific fibrosing mediastinitis: demonstration of pulmonary vascular obstruction by magnetic resonance imaging. Am J Roentgenol. 1984;143(6):1189–91.
90. Rodriguez E, Soler R, Pombo F, Requejo I, Montero C. Fibrosing mediastinitis: CT and MR findings. Clin Radiol. 1998;53(12):907–10.
91. Weinstein JB, Aronberg DJ, Sagel SS. CT of fibrosing mediastinitis: findings and their utility. Am J Roentgenol. 1983;141(2):247–51.
92. Chan CK, Hutcheon MA, Hyland RH, Smith GJ, Patterson BJ, Matthay RA. Pulmonary tumor embolism: a critical review of clinical, imaging, and hemodynamic features. J Thorac Imaging. 1987;2(4):4–14.
93. Kane RD, Hawkins HK, Miller JA, Noce PS. Microscopic pulmonary tumor emboli associated with dyspnea. Cancer. 1975;36(4):1473–82.
94. Roberts KE, Hamele-Bena D, Saqi A, Stein CA, Cole RP. Pulmonary tumor embolism: a review of the literature. Am J Med. 2003;115(3):228–32.
95. Rossi SE, Goodman PC, Franquet T. Non-thrombotic pulmonary emboli. Am J Roentgenol. 2000;174(6):1499–508.
96. Jakel J, Ramaswamy A, Kohler U, Barth PJ. Massive pulmonary tumor microembolism from a hepatocellular carcinoma. Pathol Res Pract. 2006;202(5):395–9.
97. Brock SJ, Fuller C, Iveson TJ. Pulmonary tumour emboli: a difficult ante-mortem diagnosis. Clin Oncol. 2000;12(1):56–7.
98. Shepard JA, Moore EH, Templeton PA, McLoud TC. Pulmonary intravascular tumor emboli: dilated and beaded peripheral pulmonary arteries at CT. Radiology. 1993;187(3):797–801.
99. Tack D, Nollevaux MC, Gevenois PA. Tree-in-bud pattern in neoplastic pulmonary emboli. Am J Roentgenol. 2001;176(6):1421–2.

100. Fred HL, Harle TS. Septic pulmonary embolism. Am Fam Phys/GP. 1970;1(5):81–7.
101. Roberts WC, Buchbinder NA. Right-sided valvular infective endocarditis: a clinicopathologic study of twelve necropsy patients. Am J Med. 1972;53(1): 7–19.
102. Huang RM, Naidich DP, Lubat E, Schinella R, Garay SM, McCauley DI. Septic pulmonary emboli: CT-radiographic correlation. Am J Roentgenol. 1989;153(1):41–5.
103. Cook RJ, Ashton RW, Aughenbaugh GL, Ryu JH. Septic pulmonary embolism: presenting features and clinical course of 14 patients. Chest. 2005;128(1):162–6.
104. MacMillan JC, Milstein SH, Samson PC. Clinical spectrum of septic pulmonary embolism and infarction. J Thorac Cardiovasc Surg. 1978;75(5): 670–9.
105. Kuhlman JE, Fishman EK, Teigen C. Pulmonary septic emboli: diagnosis with CT. Radiology. 1990;174(1):211–3.
106. Kuhlman JE, Fishman EK, Siegelman SS. Invasive pulmonary aspergillosis in acute leukemia: characteristic findings on CT, the CT halo sign, and the role of CT in early diagnosis. Radiology. 1985;157(3):611–4.
107. Kim Y, Lee KS, Jung KJ, Han J, Kim JS, Suh JS. Halo sign on high resolution CT: findings in spectrum of pulmonary diseases with pathologic correlation. J Comput Assist Tomogr. 1999;23(4):622–6.
108. Kwon WJ, Jeong YJ, Kim KI, et al. Computed tomographic features of pulmonary septic emboli: comparison of causative microorganisms. J Comput Assist Tomogr. 2007;31(3):390–4.
109. Mylonakis E, Calderwood SB. Infective endocarditis in adults. N Engl J Med. 2001;345(18): 1318–30.
110. Kizer KW, Goodman PC. Radiographic manifestations of venous air embolism. Radiology. 1982; 144(1):35–9.
111. Orebaugh SL. Venous air embolism: clinical and experimental considerations. Crit Care Med. 1992;20(8):1169–77.
112. Gallagher TJ. Scuba diving accidents: decompression sickness, air embolism. J Fla Med Assoc. 1997;84(7):446–51.
113. Woodring JH, Fried AM. Nonfatal venous air embolism after contrast-enhanced CT. Radiology. 1988;167(2):405–7.
114. Hill AD, Toner ME, FitzGerald MX. Talc lung in a drug abuser. Ir J Med Sci. 1990;159(5):147–8.
115. Bendeck SE, Leung AN, Berry GJ, Daniel D, Ruoss SJ. Cellulose granulomatosis presenting as centrilobular nodules: CT and histologic findings. Am J Roentgenol. 2001;177(5):1151–3.
116. Schmidt RA, Glenny RW, Godwin JD, Hampson NB, Cantino ME, Reichenbach DD. Panlobular emphysema in young intravenous Ritalin abusers. Am Rev Respir Dis. 1991;143(3):649–56.
117. Jorens PG, Van Marck E, Snoeckx A, Parizel PM. Nonthrombotic pulmonary embolism. Eur Respir. 2009;34(2):452–74.
118. Nan DN, Fernandez-Ayala M, Iglesias L, Garcia-Palomo D, Parra JA, Farinas MC. Talc granulomatosis: a differential diagnosis of interstitial lung disease in HIV patients. Chest. 2000;118(1): 258–60.
119. Fields TA, McCall SJ, Reams BD, Roggli VL, Palmer SM, Howell DN. Pulmonary embolization of microcrystalline cellulose in a lung transplant recipient. J Heart Lung Transplant Off Public Int Soc Heart Transplant. 2005;24(5):624–7.
120. Diaz-Ruiz MJ, Gallardo X, Castaner E, Mata JM, Catala J, Ferreres JC. Cellulose granulomatosis of the lungs. Eur Radiol. 1999;9(6):1203–4.
121. Ward S, Heyneman LE, Reittner P, Kazerooni EA, Godwin JD, Muller NL. Talcosis associated with IV abuse of oral medications: CT findings. Am J Roentgenol. 2000;174(3):789–93.
122. Demeter S, Raymond GS, Puttagunta L, Barrie JR. Residents' corner: answer to case of the month #66: intravenous pulmonary talcosis with complicating massive fibrosis. Can Assoc Radiol J. 1999;50(6):413–15.
123. Stern EJ, Frank MS, Schmutz JF, Glenny RW, Schmidt RA, Godwin JD. Panlobular pulmonary emphysema caused by i.v. injection of methylphenidate (Ritalin): findings on chest radiographs and CT scans. Am J Roentgenol. 1994; 162(3):555–60.
124. Parisi DM, Koval K, Egol K. Fat embolism syndrome. Am J Orthop. 2002;31(9):507–12.
125. Koessler MJ, Fabiani R, Hamer H, Pitto RP. The clinical relevance of embolic events detected by transesophageal echocardiography during cemented total hip arthroplasty: a randomized clinical trial. Anesth Analg. 2001;92(1):49–55.
126. King MB, Harmon KR. Unusual forms of pulmonary embolism. Clin Chest Med. 1994;15(3): 561–80.
127. Dudney TM, Elliott CG. Pulmonary embolism from amniotic fluid, fat, and air. Prog Cardiovasc Dis. 1994;36(6):447–74.
128. Richards RR. Fat embolism syndrome. Can J Surg. 1997;40(5):334–9.
129. Muller NL, Fraser RS, Colman NC, Pare PD. Radiologic diagnosis of diseases of the chest. 1st ed. Philladelpia: Saunders; 2001.
130. Davies S. Amniotic fluid embolus: a review of the literature. Can J Anaesth. 2001;48(1):88–98.
131. Clark SL. New concepts of amniotic fluid embolism: a review. Obstet Gynecol Surv. 1990;45(6):360–8.
132. Clark SL, Hankins GD, Dudley DA, Dildy GA, Porter TF. Amniotic fluid embolism: analysis of the national registry. Am J Obstet Gynecol. 1995;172(4 Part 1):1158–67; discussion 1159–67.
133. Karetzky M, Ramirez M. Acute respiratory failure in pregnancy: an analysis of 19 cases. Medicine (Baltimore). 1998;77(1):41–9.

134. Pluymakers C, De Weerdt A, Jacquemyn Y, Colpaert C, Van de Poel E, Jorens PG. Amniotic fluid embolism after surgical trauma: two case reports and review of the literature. Resuscitation. 2007;72(2):324–32.
135. Fidler JL, Patz EF Jr, Ravin CE. Cardiopulmonary complications of pregnancy: radiographic findings. Am J Roentgenol. 1993;161(5):937–42.
136. Yi CA, Lee KS, Choe YH, Han D, Kwon OJ, Kim S. Computed tomography in pulmonary artery sarcoma: distinguishing features from pulmonary embolic disease. J Comput Assist Tomogr. 2004;28(1):34–9.
137. Cox JE, Chiles C, Aquino SL, Savage P, Oaks T. Pulmonary artery sarcomas: a review of clinical and radiologic features. J Comput Assist Tomogr. 1997;21(5):750–5.
138. Baker PB, Goodwin RA. Pulmonary artery sarcomas: a review and report of a case. Arch Pathol Lab Med. 1985;109(1):35–9.
139. Olsson HE, Spitzer RM, Erston WF. Primary and secondary pulmonary artery neoplasia mimicking acute pulmonary embolism. Radiology. 1976; 118(1):49–53.
140. Blackmon SH, Rice DC, Correa AM, et al. Management of primary pulmonary artery sarcomas. Ann Thorac Surg. 2009;87(3):977–84.
141. Dennie CJ, Veinot JP, McCormack DG, Rubens FD. Intimal sarcoma of the pulmonary arteries seen as a mosaic pattern of lung attenuation on high-resolution CT. Am J Roentgenol. 2002; 178(5):1208–10.
142. Smith WS, Lesar MS, Travis WD, et al. MR and CT findings in pulmonary artery sarcoma. J Comput Assist Tomogr. 1989;13(5):906–9.
143. Weinreb JC, Davis SD, Berkmen YM, Isom W, Naidich DP. Pulmonary artery sarcoma: evaluation using Gd-DTPA. J Comput Assist Tomogr. 1990;14(4):647–9.
144. Thurer RL, Thorsen A, Parker JA, Karp DD. FDG imaging of a pulmonary artery sarcoma. Ann Thorac Surg. 2000;70(4):1414–5.
145. Chong S, Kim TS, Kim BT, Cho EY, Kim J. Pulmonary artery sarcoma mimicking pulmonary thromboembolism: integrated FDG PET/CT. Am J Roentgenol. 2007;188(6):1691–3.
146. Simonneau G, Galie N, Rubin LJ, et al. Clinical classification of pulmonary hypertension. J Am Coll Cardiol. 2004;43(12 Suppl S):5S–12S.
147. Leinonen H, Pohjola-Sintonen S, Krogerus L. Pulmonary veno-occlusive disease. Acta Med Scand. 1987;221(3):307–10.
148. Morassut PA, Walley VM, Smith CD. Pulmonary veno-occlusive disease and the CREST variant of scleroderma. Can J Cardiol. 1992;8(10):1055–8.
149. Veeraraghavan S, Koss MN, Sharma OP. Pulmonary veno-occlusive disease. Curr Opin Pulm Med. 1999;5(5):310–3.
150. Kishida Y, Kanai Y, Kuramochi S, Hosoda Y. Pulmonary venoocclusive disease in a patient with systemic lupus erythematosus. J Rheumatol. 1993;20(12):2161–2.
151. Hourseau M, Capron F, Nunes H, Godmer P, Martin A, Kambouchner M. Pulmonary veno-occlusive disease in a patient with HIV infection: a case report with autopsy findings. Ann Pathol. 2002;22(6):472–5.
152. Hamada K, Teramoto S, Narita N, Yamada E, Teramoto K, Kobzik L. Pulmonary veno-occlusive disease in pulmonary Langerhans' cell granulomatosis. Eur Respir. 2000;15(2):421–3.
153. Johnson SR, Patsios D, Hwang DM, Granton JT. Pulmonary veno-occlusive disease and scleroderma associated pulmonary hypertension. J Rheumatol. 2006;33(11):2347–50.
154. Montani D, Achouh L, Dorfmuller P, et al. Pulmonary veno-occlusive disease: clinical, functional, radiologic, and hemodynamic characteristics and outcome of 24 cases confirmed by histology. Medicine (Baltimore). 2008;87(4):220–33.
155. Holcomb BW Jr, Loyd JE, Ely EW, Johnson J, Robbins IM. Pulmonary veno-occlusive disease: a case series and new observations. Chest. 2000; 118(6):1671–9.
156. Pietra GG, Capron F, Stewart S, et al. Pathologic assessment of vasculopathies in pulmonary hypertension. J Am Coll Cardiol. 2004;43(12 Suppl S):25S–32S.
157. Lantuejoul S, Sheppard MN, Corrin B, Burke MM, Nicholson AG. Pulmonary veno-occlusive disease and pulmonary capillary hemangiomatosis: a clinicopathologic study of 35 cases. Am J Surg Pathol. 2006;30(7):850–7.
158. Wagenvoort CA, Beetstra A, Spijker J. Capillary haemangiomatosis of the lungs. Histopathology. 1978;2(6):401–6.
159. Tron V, Magee F, Wright JL, Colby T, Churg A. Pulmonary capillary hemangiomatosis. Hum Pathol. 1986;17(11):1144–50.
160. Eltorky MA, Headley AS, Winer-Muram H, Garrett HE Jr, Griffin JP. Pulmonary capillary hemangiomatosis: a clinicopathologic review. Ann Thorac Surg. 1994;57(3):772–6.
161. Rabiller A, Jais X, Hamid A, et al. Occult alveolar haemorrhage in pulmonary veno-occlusive disease. Eur Respir. 2006;27(1):108–13.
162. Resten A, Maitre S, Humbert M, et al. Pulmonary hypertension: CT of the chest in pulmonary venoocclusive disease. Am J Roentgenol. 2004; 183(1):65–70.
163. Rambihar VS, Fallen EL, Cairns JA. Pulmonary veno-occlusive disease: antemortem diagnosis from roentgenographic and hemodynamic findings. Can Med Assoc J. 1979;120(12):1519–22.
164. Montani D, O'Callaghan DS, Savale L, et al. Pulmonary veno-occlusive disease: recent progress and current challenges. Respir Med. 2010;104(Suppl 1):S23–32.
165. Valdes L, Gonzalez-Juanatey JR, Alvarez D, et al. Diagnosis of pulmonary veno-occlusive disease:

new criteria for biopsy. Respir Med. 1998;92(7): 979–83.
166. Cassart M, Gevenois PA, Kramer M, et al. Pulmonary venoocclusive disease: CT findings before and after single-lung transplantation. Am J Roentgenol. 1993;160(4):759–60.
167. Swensen SJ, Tashjian JH, Myers JL, et al. Pulmonary venoocclusive disease: CT findings in eight patients. Am J Roentgenol. 1996;167(4):937–40.
168. Dufour B, Maitre S, Humbert M, Capron F, Simonneau G, Musset D. High-resolution CT of the chest in four patients with pulmonary capillary hemangiomatosis or pulmonary venoocclusive disease. Am J Roentgenol. 1998;171(5):1321–4.
169. Resten A, Maitre S, Musset D. CT imaging of peripheral pulmonary vessel disease. Eur Radiol. 2005;15(10):2045–56.
170. Van Praagh S, Carrera ME, Sanders S, Mayer JE Jr, Van Praagh R. Partial or total direct pulmonary venous drainage to right atrium due to malposition of septum primum: anatomic and echocardiographic findings and surgical treatment: a study based on 36 cases. Chest. 1995;107(6):1488–98.
171. Rajiah P, Kanne JP. Computed tomography of pulmonary venous variants and anomalies. J Cardiovasc Comput Tomogr. 2010;4(3):155–63.
172. Gustafson RA, Warden HE, Murray GF, Hill RC, Rozar GE. Partial anomalous pulmonary venous connection to the right side of the heart. J thorac cardiovasc surg. 1989;98(5 Part 2):861–8.
173. Woodring JH, Howard TA, Kanga JF. Congenital pulmonary venolobar syndrome revisited. Radiographics. 1994;14(2):349–69.
174. Shah DC, Haissaguerre M, Jais P. Toward a mechanism-based understanding of atrial fibrillation. J Cardiovasc Electrophysiol. 2001; 12(5):600–1.
175. Ravenel JG, McAdams HP. Pulmonary venous infarction after radiofrequency ablation for atrial fibrillation. Am J Roentgenol. 2002;178(3): 664–6.
176. Scharf C, Sneider M, Case I, et al. Anatomy of the pulmonary veins in patients with atrial fibrillation and effects of segmental ostial ablation analyzed by computed tomography. J Cardiovasc Electrophysiol. 2003;14(2):150–5.
177. Robbins IM, Colvin EV, Doyle TP, et al. Pulmonary vein stenosis after catheter ablation of atrial fibrillation. Circulation. 1998;98(17): 1769–75.
178. Lacomis JM, Wigginton W, Fuhrman C, Schwartzman D, Armfield DR, Pealer KM. Multidetector row CT of the left atrium and pulmonary veins before radio-frequency catheter ablation for atrial fibrillation. Radiographics. 2003;23 Spec No:S35–48; discussion S48–50.
179. Thakur RK, Klein GJ, Yee R, Zardini M. Embolic complications after radiofrequency catheter ablation. Am J Cardiol. 1994;74(3):278–9.

Imaging of Pulmonary Hypertension

9

Mark L. Schiebler, James Runo, Leif Jensen,
and Christopher J. François

Abstract

Pulmonary hypertension (PH) is a silent disease with many causes that comes to clinical attention late in its course. There are indirect features of PH found on noninvasive imaging studies, but the diagnosis of this disease and its therapeutic management still require right heart catheterization with pressure measurements of the pulmonary artery. In general, with chronic PH, the main pulmonary artery is enlarged, there is tapering of the peripheral pulmonary arteries, there is decreased vessel compliance from muscular hypertrophy of the arterial walls, and there is reduced pulmonary blood flow. This is accompanied by changes in the right heart including right ventricular (RV) hypertrophy, RV enlargement, RV dysfunction, and tricuspid regurgitation. In the acute setting, such as with massive pulmonary emboli, the abrupt change in pulmonary arterial pressure has a dramatic effect on right heart contractility. The peak velocity of the tricuspid regurgitation jet, as measured by echocardiography or MRI, is loosely correlated with pulmonary arterial pressure. Untreated PH results in a rapid clinical decline with death frequently occurring within 3 years of diagnosis. Even with treatment, the mean survival time is still less than 4 years.

M. L. Schiebler (✉) · C. J. François
Department of Radiology,
University of Wisconsin School of Medicine
and Public Health, 600 Highland Avenue,
Madison, WI 53792, USA
e-mail: mschiebler@uwhealth.org

J. Runo
Department of Pulmonary and Critical Care Medicine,
University of Wisconsin School of Medicine and
Public Health, 5252 MFCB, 1685 Highland Avenue,
Madison, WI 53705-2281, USA

L. Jensen
Diagnostic Radiology, E3/366 Clinical Science Center,
University of Wisconsin–Madison,
600 Highland Avenue, Madison,
WI 53792-3252, USA

J. P. Kanne (ed.), *Clinically Oriented Pulmonary Imaging*,
Respiratory Medicine, DOI: 10.1007/978-1-61779-542-8_9,

Keywords
Pulmonary hypertension · Pulmonary arterial hypertension · Chronic thromboembolic pulmonary hypertension · Eisenmenger syndrome · Computed tomographic angiography · Magnetic resonance angiography · Right heart catheterization

Introduction

Fortunately, within the spectrum of all the diseases of the chest which the clinician can expect to encounter, pulmonary hypertension (PH) is a relatively rare phenomenon. While the extremely common disorder of systemic arterial hypertension (SAH) is known as the "silent killer", one could give the moniker of the "invisible silent killer" to PH. The clinician and patient have the opportunity to screen for SAH with a simple blood pressure cuff. Unfortunately, there is no simple screening test to detect PH early in its course. The analogy to SAH is apt: just as the retinal vessels show pruning and amputation of the capillary bed in longstanding SAH, one can imagine the unsuspecting secondary lobule of the lung trying to survive through the ravages of hypertensive-induced smooth muscle hypertrophic narrowing of its feeding pulmonary arterioles. While there are many secondary lobules that must be similarly affected by this process before dyspnea sets in, there is no "turning back of the clock" once this disease manifests itself in the vascular bed of the lung [1]. Thus the lessons learned from SAH, a disease that leads to end stage arteriolar sclerosis in all the end organs of the body, encapsulates many of the issues the clinician must deal with while treating patients with symptomatic PH where irreversible end organ damage has usually already occurred to the pulmonary circulation by the time of presentation.

Definition

PH is a diagnosis that is invasively established by right heart catheterization. The three current criteria by which this diagnosis can be made are as follows [2–4]:

1. Mean pulmonary artery pressure (mPAP) of >25 mmHg at rest
2. Pulmonary capillary wedge pressure (PCWP) <15 mmHg, or
3. Pulmonary vascular resistance (PVR) of >3 Wood units [1, 5].

Typically, at rest, the right heart is not able to generate systolic PAP >40 mmHg acutely [6]. Thus, any mPAP of >40 mmHg implies chronic PH. The severity level of this condition is categorized by the amount of mPAP at rest: Severe >50 mmHg, Moderate = 30–50 mmHg, and Mild <30 mmHg.

The Dana Point 2009 Classification system makes subtle distinction between pulmonary arterial hypertension (PAH) and pulmonary hypertension (PH). They refer to PAH as the best descriptor for this disease in categories 1 (PAH) and 1′ pulmonary veno-occlusive disease (PVOD) and/or pulmonary capillary hemangiomatosis (PCH); while the term pulmonary hypertension (PH) is reserved for categories 2–5 (see Table 9.1). For the purposes of this publication, we combine these two entities (PAH & PH) under the moniker of PH for simplification, as the distinction between PAH and PH in this classification scheme has a more semantic origin than physiologic meaning.

Epidemiology

The number of de novo cases of pulmonary PH that come to the attention of clinicians pales in comparison to the frequency of COPD, asthma, pneumonia, lung cancer, or pulmonary embolism. It is quite likely that the prevalence of this disease is vastly underestimated in both developed countries and even more so for developing countries [7]. The frequency of occurrence of PH is difficult to measure as it is a silent disease until late in its course when most of the patients have severe functional and hemodynamic problems [8]. It is estimated that there are more than 100,000 persons in the USA with this disease [9], with one estimate as high as 1:2,000 individuals [10]. A separate study showed about 26 cases/million in the Scottish Isles [11]. In the French registry, there were 15.0 cases/million adult inhabitants [8]. PH is one of the few vascular diseases that occurs more commonly in females than in males (1.7:1) [12]. Recently this figure has been updated for the United States in the REVEAL study showing that PH involves females 80% of the time [13]. This disorder has also been linked to genetic mutations and thus can be inherited [14, 15].

While some causes of PH are amenable to either medical or surgical treatment (chronic thromboembolic pulmonary hypertension (CTEPH) and left-to-right congenital shunts), PH frequently leads to premature death. In the USA over the 20-year reporting period of 1980–2000, the number of deaths and hospitalizations attributable to PH have increased [16]. The clinical features most predictive of survival are the 6-min walking test, the New York Heart Association class, and the mixed venous oxygen saturation level [17]. In the French registry data of 674 PH patients the relative frequency of diseases causing PH was shown to be: 39.2% idiopathic, 15.3% connective tissue diseases, 11.3% congenital heart disease, 10.4% portal hypertension, 9.5% anorexigen [8, 18], and 6.2% HIV assiociated [8]. Historically, without treatment, the estimated mean survival after diagnosis is 2.8 years [12, 19]. For untreated PH, the estimated 3-year survival rate from a 1991 study was approximately 41%. In one study of long-term continuous intravenous prostacyclin therapy, 3-year survival increased to approximately 63% [20]. The mean treated survival time is now reported to be 3.6 years [12].

Clinical Presentation

Patients usually present to medical attention with shortness of breath about 2 years after the onset of symptoms [12]. Historically, the time from symptom onset to diagnosis showed an average delay of 2 years with a mean age of disease onset of 36 years (±15 years) [12]. Recent US data continues to show a delay in diagnosis from symptom onset to diagnosis of 2.8 years; however, now the average age at diagnosis is much older (50.1 years) [13]. Echocardiography at the time of presentation typically yields rather advanced disease with the presence of right ventricular hypertrophy (87%), tricuspid regurgitation, and elevated right atrial pressures. The clinical presentation is quite variable with the following frequency of findings found: dyspnea (60%), positive antinuclear antibody (29%), syncope (13%), fatigue (19%), and Raynaud's phenomenon (10%) [12].

Clinical Classification System

The categorization of this disorder has been changed many times. The most current is the Dana Point (2009) Classification [3] (Table 9.1). The aim of this model is to shift from a strictly causative to a treatment-based scheme that sorts the diseases that cause PH into similar pathophysiologic mechanisms, clinical symptoms, and treatment options. This classification system for PH has been revised quite frequently and will likely undergo further revision as new information becomes available.

Simple Fluid Mechanical Model for the Understanding of the Causes of PH

There are many causes of PH. In fact, the list of potential etiologies can be a bit challenging to

Table 9.1 Updated clinical classification of PH (Dana Point 2009) [3]

1.	Pulmonary arterial hypertension (PAH)		
		1.1 Idiopathic PAH	
		1.2 Heritable	
			1.2.1 BMPR2
			1.2.2 ALK1, endoglin (with or without hereditary hemorrhagic telangiectasia)
			1.2.3 Unknown
		1.3 Drug- and toxin-induced	
		1.4 Associated with	
			1.4.1 Connective tissue diseases
			1.4.2 HIV infection
			1.4.3 Portal hypertension
			1.4.4 Congenital heart diseases
			1.4.5 Schistosomiasis
			1.4.6 Chronic hemolytic anemia
		1.5 Persistent pulmonary hypertension of the newborn	
1'.	Pulmonary veno-occlusive disease (PVOD) and/or pulmonary capillary hemangiomatosis (PCH)		
2.	Pulmonary hypertension owing to left heart disease		
		2.1 Systolic dysfunction	
		2.2 Diastolic dysfunction	
		2.3 Valvular disease	
3.	Pulmonary hypertension owing to lung diseases and/or hypoxia		
		3.1 Chronic obstructive pulmonary disease	
		3.2 Interstitial lung disease	
		3.3 Other pulmonary diseases with mixed restrictive and obstructive pattern	

(continued)

Table 9.1 (continued)

		3.4 Sleep-disordered breathing
		3.5 Alveolar hypoventilation disorders
		3.6 Chronic exposure to high altitude
		3.7 Developmental abnormalities
4.	Chronic thromboembolic pulmonary hypertension (CTEPH)	
5.	Pulmonary hypertension with unclear multifactorial mechanisms	
		5.1 Hematologic disorders: myeloproliferative disorders, splenectomy
		5.2 Systemic disorders: sarcoidosis, pulmonary Langerhans cell histiocytosis: lymphangioleiomyomatosis, neurofibromatosis, vasculitis
		5.3 Metabolic disorders: glycogen storage disease, Gaucher disease, thyroid disorders
		5.4 Others: tumoral obstruction, fibrosing mediastinitis, chronic renal failure on dialysis

recall at a moment's notice even for those individuals with a nearly photographic memory. Instead, we present here a simple heuristic device shown in Fig. 9.1 that uses a fluid mechanical model to help the reader organize the many disorders that can cause PH. Just like a large dam constructed on a river for the generation of hydroelectric power creates a reservoir upstream, any impediment to the vascular flow from the pulmonary arterial system through the lungs and then onto the aorta can eventually lead to PH. Depending on the amount of preload [21] or location of the obstruction of the vessels involved, clinical presentation and imaging findings will vary appropriately.

Pathophysiology and Histology of both Acute and Chronic PH

Interestingly enough, we have all had a period of PH in our lives. The miracle of the first breath in a newborn child is accompanied by a profound transition of the pulmonary arterial system from a high-pressure state to a much lower pressure as the alveoli fill with air and the remaining amniotic fluid is resorbed. With air filling the alveoli, the pulmonary vascular bed is rapidly converted into a low resistance state. In the normal infant this lowered pulmonary vascular resistance is immediately accompanied by an

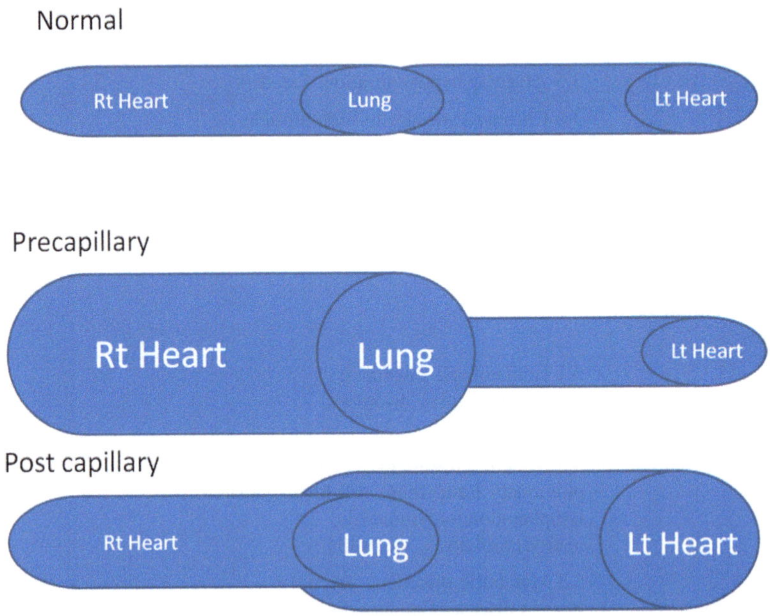

Fig. 9.1 Simplified fluid mechanics model for the basic understanding of PH. *Normal physiology* the Qp (pulmonary blood flow) matches the Qs (systemic blood flow), thus the amount of blood flow entering the lungs is nearly equal to the amount leaving the aorta. *Pre capillary PH* there is a problem in getting either normal flow or normal volume to the last order arteriole proximal to the alveolus. There are many causes for this. This may result from longstanding volume overload from a left-to-right shunt. This could be a consequence of lung disease. Whatever the cause, the result is the same; there is back pressure that reverberates retrograde into the pulmonary arterial system. Over time, this pressure will typically cause right ventricular hypertrophy. *Post-capillary PH* in this scenario, there is a limitation to the oxygenated blood's egress from the alveolus into the pulmonary vein. This can be created by limiting the outflow at any location from the small venules, as in pulmonary veno-occlusive disease, all the way to the proximal ascending aorta

important cascade of physiological changes: (1) a marked decrease in pulmonary artery pressure, (2) decreased flow from the pulmonary artery to the aorta via the patent ductus arteriosis (PDA), (3) closure of the foramen ovale, and (4) a tenfold increase in blood flow to the lung parenchyma and the pulmonary veins [22]. Of note is the fact that for the normal fetus, the PDA acts as a pressure relief valve for the right heart, protecting it from the high-pressure circuit of the lungs. This feature of in utero physiology is of key importance, as the right ventricle is only designed to pump blood at low pressures. The placement and design of the right ventricle has given rise to the tongue-in-cheek moniker of the "piggyback ventricle."

Understanding the histology of the small and large pulmonary arteries and how they adapt to increasing pulmonary arterial pressure is instructive [23]. The smaller pulmonary arteries (1.0–0.001 mm) are responsible for the largest pressure drop in PH. These small vessels have walls consisting of smooth muscle that hypertrophies with chronic PH. This finding is similar to the kidney and the arteriolar sclerosis occurring in SAH. In contrast, the larger pulmonary arteries (40.0–1.1 mm) have walls that primarily consist of elastin fibers rather than smooth muscle cells. This organization is similar to the histology of the normal aorta. These vessels are normally very flexible and show a dynamic change in caliber (also known as vessel compliance) during the cardiac cycle in response to the stroke volume from the right ventricle. These vessels get larger during systolic flow and decrease in size during diastole. These larger pulmonary arteries are also the site of maximal dilation with PH. This feature is one of the major imaging findings that can be

Table 9.2 Summary of the primary causes and treament issues in PH

Primary causes of precapillary PH
Idiopathic pulmonary fibrosis
CTEPH
Left-to-right shunts
Primary causes of post-capillary PH
Left ventricular failure/atrial fibrillation
Mitral valve disease
Mediastinal fibrosis
Left atrial mass (myxoma)
PVOD (rare)
Key points in the treatment of PH
CTEPH is under diagnosed and may complicate acute pulmonary embolism
Vasodilator therapy will aggravate CHF in post-capillary PH
Prostacyclin therapy in PVOD can be fatal as the Qp is lowered from peripheral arterial dilation and the attendant drop in pulmonary arterial pressure
Proximal lamellar clot found in CTEPH can be removed with thromboembolectomy

found in patients with PH (Table 9.2). Table 9.3 enumerates the imaging findings that can be seen with acute PH. With chronic PH, these larger vessels enlarge and become less compliant because of smooth muscle proliferation with or without neointimal formation. In situ thrombosis may also occur, no doubt aggravated by slower flow in these vessels resulting from increase in pulmonary vascular resistance (Fig. 9.2). With longstanding left-to-right shunts as a cause for PH, atherosclerosis may develop in the larger pulmonary arteries (Fig. 9.3).

Acute PH

The most common cause of acute PH is related to pulmonary emboli. In addition, hypoxia in and of itself can lead to vasoconstriction in the pulmonary arterial bed. As this resistance is elevated, there is a decrease in pulmonary blood flow and an increase in the pulmonary artery pressure. This situation can occur with massive pulmonary embolism. This acutely elevated pulmonary artery pressure, depending on its severity, can result in acute right heart strain [24], and rapid right ventricular enlargement (RVE) ensues without hypertrophy. This is a key finding at imaging and reflects the fact that the compensatory mechanism of muscular hypertrophy in the RV has not yet had time to develop. Table 9.3 shows the imaging findings that can be associated with acute PH.

Sleep Apnea

Chronic hypoxia at night related to sleep apnea can also lead to PH. This is a more insidious cause and can be treated with a continuous pulmonary airway pressure (CPAP) mask at night after documentation with a sleep study (Fig. 9.4). Sometimes this diagnosis can be suggested from a chest radiograph when a large PA is associated with a large body habitus and limited inspiratory excursion. However, these findings can be seen in normal individuals who are simply hypoventilated resulting in crowding at the level of the vascular pedicle leading to a false appearance of PA enlargement.

Table 9.3 Comparative analysis of currently available diagnostic imaging tests and angioinvasive interventions for the evaluation of *acute* pulmonary arterial hypertension

Structure	Findings	CXR	NC CT	CTA	MRI	TTE	V/Q scan	PA gram	Rt Ht cath
IVC	Nl IVC	++		+	++	++		++++	++++
Azygos vein	Nl Az vein	++	S	U	P	I	N	E	
RA	Nl RA	+	++	++	++++	+++		++	++
Interatrial septum	Bowing		+	++	++++	+++			
PFO	Open PFO			+	++	+++			
TV	TR				++++	++++		++	++
RV	Nl RV thickness		++	++	++++	++			+
	Enlarged RV	+	++	++	++++	+++		++	++
	Abnl RV motion			+	++++	+++		++	++
	Abnl RV minor axis		++	+++	++++	+++			
IV septum	Septal bounce		+	++	++++	++++			
PV valve	PR (±)				++++	+++		++	++
PA	PAP >25 mmHg at rest							++++	++++
	Acute PE	+	+	++++	+++	+++	+++	++++	+++
PA branches	Acute emboli	+		++++	+++	++	++++	++++	++++
Precapillary obstruction	Acute microvasculature emboli			+	++	++	++++	+	+
Post-capillary obstruction	Severe LV infarction	+	+	++	++++	+++			+

Abbreviations TTE trans-thoracic echocardiography, *Az* azygos, *CVP* central venous pressure, *PAs* pulmonary arteries, *PAP* pulmonary artery pressure, *PT* pulmonary trunk, *Ca++* calcification, *Rt Ht* cath–right heart catheterization, *CTEPH* chronic thromboembolic pulmonary hypertension, *CVP* central venous pressure

Cor Pulmonale from Chronic PH

A common cause of death in patients with chronic PH is right heart failure (cor pulmonale). There are two basic physiologic situations we will discuss. One is related to simple pressure overload, and the second is related to volume overload secondarily leading to a pressure overload situation. Right ventricular (RV) failure results from response to the chronic afterload induced by PH. Over time, this chronic afterload induces right ventricular hypertrophy (RVH). Table 9.4 enumerates the imaging findings that can be found in chronic PH with early cor pulmonale. While in the short term the RV is able to cope with this pressure head, failure ultimately occurs, as the RV is no longer able to keep up with the demand for pulmonary circulation. When this happens, there is an uncoupling between the pulmonary blood flow (Qp) and systemic outflow (Qs) that is subjectively experienced as dyspnea.

In the setting of left-to-right shunts at the atrial (atrial septal defects) or ventricular level (ventricular septal defects), the RV primarily adapts to this increase in volume by dilation first. For a while, the pulmonary vascular bed adapts by increasing its capacitance through enlargement of the large pulmonary vessels. However this response only lasts so long and the chronic volume overload leads to an increase in pressure seen by the small arterioles, which in turn, respond by their only method of adaptation: irreversible smooth muscle hypertrophy. This feeds back into the larger pulmonary

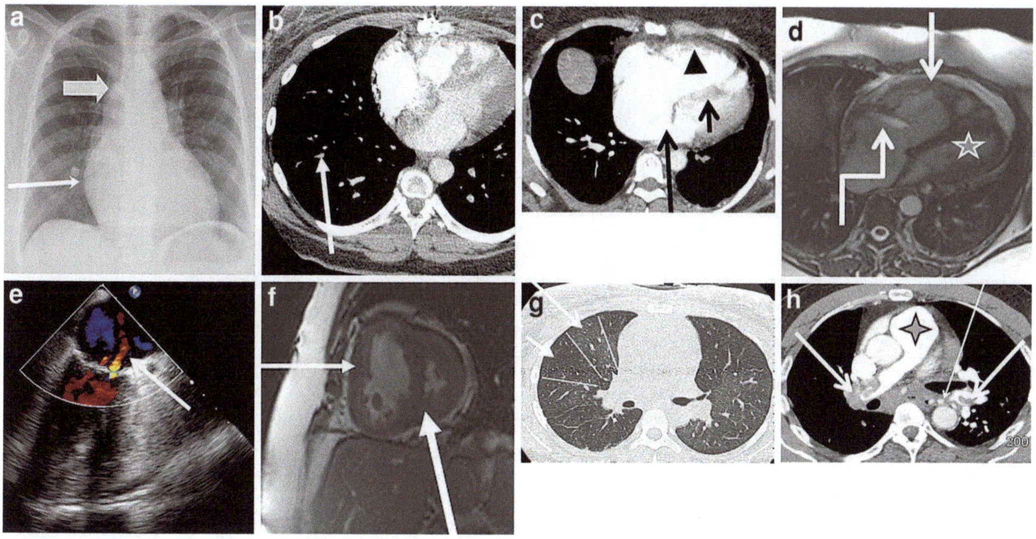

Fig. 9.2 **a** Chronic thromboembolic pulmonary hypertension (CTEPH). PA chest radiograph shows enlarged pulmonary arteries with peripheral pruning, right atrial enlargement (*thin arrow*), and azygos vein enlargement (*thick arrow*) indicative of elevated central venous pressures. **b** Chronic thromboembolic pulmonary hypertension (CTEPH). CTA with subsegmental embolus (*arrow*). **c** Chronic thromboembolic pulmonary hypertension (CTEPH). CTA with right ventricular hypertrophy (*arrowhead*), septal straightening (*short arrow*) and atrial septal aneurysm (*long arrow*). **d** Chronic thromboembolic pulmonary hypertension (CTEPH). Four-chamber MR SSFP showing tricuspid regurgitation jet (*jagged arrow*), right ventricular hypertrophy (*straight arrow*), right atrial enlargement, interventricular septum straightening, and a small left ventricular chamber (*star*). **e** CTEPH Transesophageal echocardiography (TEE) of tricuspid regurgitation (*arrow*). **f** CTEPH Short axis cardiac SSFP MRI showing septal bowing (*thick arrow*) and right ventricular hypertrophy (thin arrow). **g** Chronic thromboembolic pulmonary hypertension (CTEPH). Unenhanced CT showing with wedge shaped areas of mosaic perfusion (separated by *white lines*) secondary to multiple chronic thromboemboli. *Small arrow* shows a region of diminished perfusion and *large arrow* shows a region of increased perfusion. Note that this pattern can be seen with air trapping as well. To separate air trapping from diminished perfusion, imaging at end expiration is useful. This is due to the fact that the regions of air trapping will be of exaggerated lower attenuation at end expiration while the regions related to diminished vascularity from vascular insufficiency will normalize in their attenuation values. **h** End stage CTEPH. CTA showing eccentric chronic wall thrombi (*thick arrows*), an enlarged pulmonary trunk (*star*), and bronchial arterial enlargement (*thin arrow*)

arteries and further complicates the volume overload by an increased pulmonary arterial pressure, which in turn, creates further stress on the RV because of this increase in afterload along with the problem of increased volume from the left-to-right shunt. The RV is poorly adapted to cope with increasing pressure and is even less able to deal with an increase in volume. These two stresses together overwhelm the RV's ability to adapt, and it begins to fail. At this point, patients begin to present with dyspnea, systemic and peripheral venous congestion, or both. The progressive loss of pulmonary blood flow results in the inability to fully oxygenate enough blood in the systemic blood flow to keep up with the baseline metabolic rate, ultimately leading to death. These patients experience profound shortness of breath as this disorder speeds to its morbid conclusion.

Chronically, as PH progresses with less blood returning from the lungs, cardiac output and coronary perfusion suffer accordingly. As this vicious cycle of flow disturbance continues to rebalance, tissue perfusion also suffers. In the end stages of advanced cor pulmonale, the extent of central venous hypertension leads to organs filling with interstitial fluid, which in turn acts to increase the tissue perfusion pressure

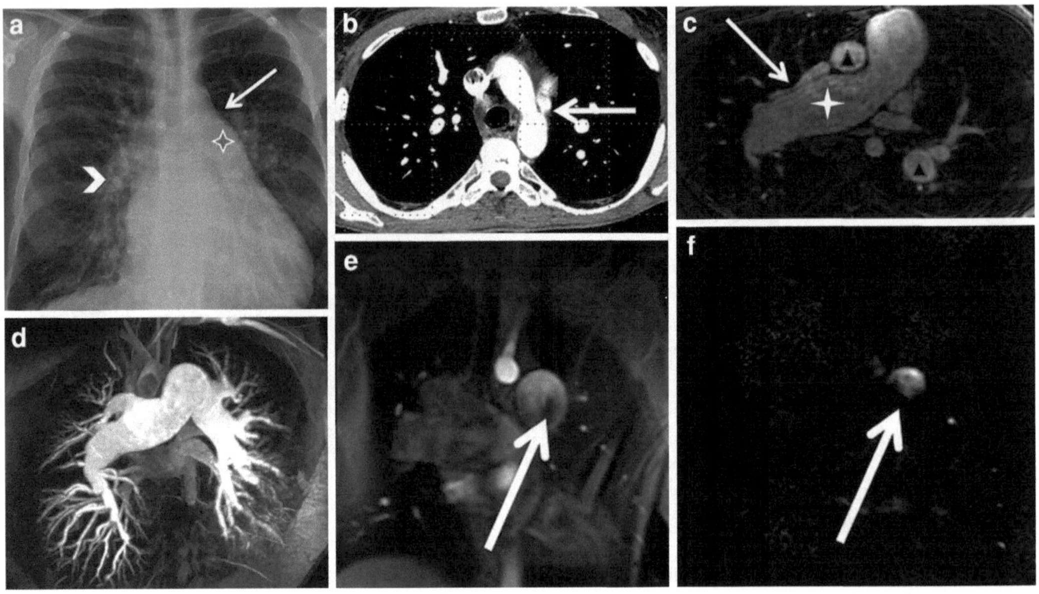

Fig. 9.3 PH secondary to patent ductus arteriosis. **a** PA radiograph shows straightening of the aortopulmonary window (*arrow*) indicative of the persistent ductus, enlarged pulmonary trunk (*star*), overcirculation vascularity with enlargement of the interlobar artery (*arrow head*), with associated PH suggested by pruning of the arteries in the periphery of the lung. **b** CTA showing the ductus origin (*arrow*) from the inferior margin of the aortic arch. **c:** Eisenmenger syndrome from partial anomalous pulmonary venous return with a large ASD. **c** Reformatted axial image from a 17 s breath hold volume MRA scan of the chest showing the anomalous pulmonary venous connection of the right upper lobe pulmonary vein (*arrow*) to the superior vena cava. Note the enormously dilated right main pulmonary artery (*star*) and the diminutive aorta (*triangles*). **d** Eisenmenger syndrome from partial anomalous pulmonary venous return. **d** MRA thick slab maximum intensity projection (MIP) showing massively enlarged pulmonary arteries with peripheral pruning. **e, f** Eisenmenger syndrome from partial anomalous pulmonary venous return. **e** Phase contrast magnitude and complex difference image (**f**) at the same location showing flow reversal in the left main pulmonary artery during systole (*arrows*)

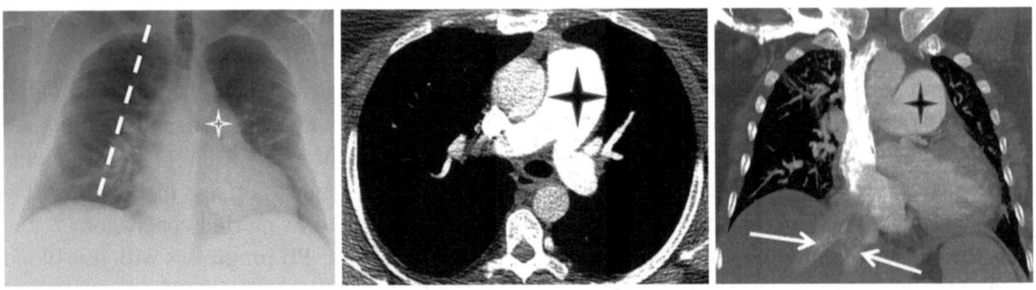

Fig. 9.4 **a** PH from sleep apnea: PA radiograph shows morbid obesity with the patient's soft tissues spilling off of the lateral aspects of the digital image and an enlarged pulmonary artery (*star*) with peripheral arterial vessel pruning seen as a lack of vascularity (lateral to the *dashed white line*). These findings are radiographically consistent with a Pickwickian body habitus and chronic CO_2 retention and can be associated with significant left ventricular diastolic dysfunction. **b** PH from sleep apnea: CTA shows abundant subcutaneous fat and an enlarged pulmonary trunk (*star*). **c** PH from sleep apnea: Coronal MIP from CTA shows massive pulmonary trunk enlargement (*star*) and contiguous contrast reflux into the hepatic veins (*arrows*), which is an indirect sign of elevated central venous pressures

Table 9.4 Comparative analysis of diagnostic imaging tests and angioinvasive interventions for the evaluation of *chronic severe pulmonary arterial hypertension with early cor pulmonale*

Structure	Findings	CXR	NC CT	CTA	MRI	TTE	V/Q scan	PA gram	Rt Ht cath
IVC	Large IVC	++		+	++	++		++++	++++
Azygos vein	Large Az vein on upright cxr	++	S	U	P	I	N	E	
RA	Enlarged RA	+	++	++	++++	+++		++	++
Interatrial septum	Bowing		+	++	++++	+++			
PFO	Open PFO			+	++	+++			
TV	TR				++++	++++		++	++
RV	RVH		++	++	++++	++			+
	Enlarged RV	+	++	++	++++	+++		++	++
	Abnl RV motion			+	++++	+++		++	++
	Abnl RV minor axis		++	+++	++++	+++			
IV septum	*D* shape		+	++	++++	++++			
PV	PR (±)				++++	+++		++	++
PA	Enlarged PT	++	++++	++++	++++	+++			
	Wall Ca++ of PT	+	++++	+++				++	++
	Ca++ chronic PE	+	++++	++		+		++	+
	PAP >25 mmHg at rest							++++	++++
PA branches	Enlarged interlobar arteries	++	++++	++++	++++			+++	+++
	Pruning of PAs	+++	+++	+++	+++			++++	
Capillary obstruction	Microvasculature Emboli (CTEPH)						++++	+	
	Mitral valve disease	+	++	++	+++	++++			+
	Left ventricular failure	+	++	++	++++	+++			+

Abbreviations TTE trans-thoracic echocardography, *Az* azygos, *CVP* central venous pressure, *PAs* pulmonary arteries, *PAP* pulmonary artery pressure, *PT* pulmonary trunk, *Ca++* calcification, *Rt Ht Cath* right heart catheterization, *CTEPH* chronic thromboembolic pulmonary hypertension

needed to supply encapsulated organs with arterial blood. This becomes part of the attendant death spiral in this disorder.

Treatment

Treatments for PH aim to limit further insult to the pulmonary arterial system from the offending cause and decrease RV afterload by modulation of peripheral pulmonary arterial resistance [25–27]. For preload shunt lesions such as ASD, VSD, PDA, and partial anomalous pulmonary venous return (PAPVR), surgery can be a life-saving intervention or at least help in limiting further volume–pressure overload damage to the pulmonary arterial circuit. For non-surgical causes and idiopathic PH, vasodilator medical therapy is now available and helps to relax the pulmonary arteriolar smooth muscles and thereby decrease PH. Sildenafil is a phosphodiesterase inhibitor that prevents the breakdown of a downstream mediator of nitric oxide (NO), allowing for pulmonary artery vessel wall dilation and, thus, results in a decrease in mPAP. Calcium channel blockers can also be used in the presence of acute vasoreactivity. The exact choice of which medical regimen to use is made during right heart catheterization and determined by the severity of the right heart failure as assessed by the following hemodynamic parameters: right atrial pressure, cardiac output, mixed venous saturation, and pulmonary vascular resistance.

Imaging Findings

Chest Radiography

The pressure within the pulmonary arterial system cannot be determined by any imaging test. Therein lays the "Achilles heel" of trying to use these studies for the initial diagnosis of this disease. However, there are important chest radiographic findings that can suggest the possibility of PH when imaging is performed at total lung capacity (TLC) or closely approximated to that degree of maximal voluntary inspiratory effort. Many chest radiographic interpretations are overzealous in describing cardiopulmonary system findings on exams that have limited degree of inspiration. These findings frequently "disappear" when good quality exams are performed. For example, overdiagnosis of pulmonary venous hypertension by chest radiography is often a consequence of hypoventilation and not true disease. Please note that interpreting pulmonary vascularity from a supine radiograph is also fraught with problems and should not be performed. This is due to the fact that in the supine position systemic venous return increases, the azygos vein is normally distended, and lung volumes tend to be lower causing crowding of the perihilar structures.

For the patient presenting with shortness of breath, the chest radiograph is usually the first imaging study performed. There are six major categories of pulmonary vascularity that can be discerned from the chest radiograph: (1) normal, (2) undercirculation (right-to-left shunts), (3) overcirculation (left-to-right shunts), (4) systemic vascularity (bronchial arterial supply to lungs associated with pulmonary atresia), (5) pulmonary venous hypertension, and (6) PH. The distinction between normal and abnormal pulmonary vascularity is usually straightforward. In the clinical setting of new-onset dyspnea or chronic dyspnea, a patient can certainly have a normal chest radiograph and still have PH. The primary purpose of the chest radiograph is to help evaluate for the common causes of dyspnea. The diagnosis of PH is usually made only after excluding all of the more common diseases that result in dyspnea. For example, in younger patients, a pneumonia or pulmonary embolism as a cause of dyspnea is likely to be more common than PH; while for older individuals, congestive heart failure is a much more common cause of dyspnea than PH. Almost all of the other causes of dyspnea are more common than a new diagnosis of PH. In summary, the notion of PH as a cause for a patient's dyspnea is often arrived at as a diagnosis of exclusion after all of the common causes have been ruled out.

The most common radiographic finding of PH is a normal or near normal chest radiograph. This is to be expected from a disease of the small vessels of the lung (arterial or venous) that, only late in its course, impacts the larger pulmonary arteries. As clinical symptoms progress, some of the findings that may become apparent radiographically include enlargement of the pulmonary trunk and interlobar arteries, but these are not commonly appreciated until clinical symptoms are significant. There are many conditions that can also lead to an enlarged pulmonary trunk and these are shown in Table 9.5. Knowing that PH is a clinically silent disease and that imaging is not able to measure pulmonary arterial pressure, perhaps we should ask the following question, "What are the radiographic findings seen on chest radiography that relate to PH?" There are two general categories of answers to this question. The first relates to the physiological changes of PH within the cardiovascular system and the second relates to the amount of time these changes have had to work their way into the morphological features visible on the chest radiograph.

The toughest interpretive radiographic challenge for diagnosis is PH with normal lung parenchyma. The key finding in this instance is an

Table 9.5 Differential diagnosis of pulmonary trunk enlargement

Idiopathic enlargement of the pulmonary trunk	
Overcirculation vascularity	PDA
	ASD
	VSD
	PAPVR
Partial absence of the pericardium	
Pulmonary valve disease	Absent pulmonary valve
	Regurgitation
	Stenosis
Pulmonary hypertension	
Aneurysm	Vasculitis (Beçhet disease)
	Mycotic
	Traumatic pseudoaneurysm
Intravascular tumor	Metastatic
	Primary

unexplained enlargement of the pulmonary trunk. The patient may or may not be dyspneic. The interlobar pulmonary arteries can also be enlarged. The upper limit of size for the right interlobar pulmonary artery is 17 mm; measurements larger than this are commonly associated with PH, left-to-right shunt vascularity, or both [28]. While the differential diagnosis for pulmonary trunk enlargement includes a number of entities that need to be excluded, the radiologist and clinician should consider that PH may be present (Table 9.5). Although uncommon, with longstanding PH, pulmonary trunk calcification may be apparent, reflecting atherosclerosis.

With abnormal lung parenchyma (Figs. 9.5 and 9.6), the diagnosis of PH is more easily thought of, and thus it is easier to consider searching for its common radiographic signs. The commonly seen chest radiographic findings of PH include: enlargement of the pulmonary trunk, enlargement of the interlobar pulmonary artery, and pruning of the pulmonary arterial tree with lack of normal vascularity in the periphery of the lung. Associated emphysema or pulmonary fibrosis may be present. The right atrium may be enlarged, and the retrosternal area on the lateral view may be filled in as the right ventricular outflow tract enlarges [29]. Unfortunately, many of these findings are subtle on the chest radiograph and are frequently overlooked, further adding to the delay in diagnosis.

In the situation of excess preload to the RV related to a left-to-right shunt, Qp/Qs will be abnormally high with more pulmonary blood flow than aortic blood flow. These shunts are typically repaired if Qp/Qs exceeds 1.5:1. The hallmark of left-to-right shunting on chest radiography is overcirculation vascularity as shown by enlargement of the pulmonary arterial system and pulmonary trunk (Fig. 9.3). The larger the shunt, the earlier patients are likely to become symptomatic. In late adulthood, smaller shunts such as ASD and PDA may be detected during routine imaging as an occult congenital heart lesion. Longstanding shunts can damage the pulmonary arterial system and lead to severe pulmonary hypertension where the PA pressures exceed systemic pressures and shunt reversal occurs. This is also known as Eisenmenger syndrome (Fig. 11.3).

In the 1–35% of patients with a patent foramen ovale, flow across the interatrial septum from right to left can occur whenever the right atrial pressure exceeds the left atrial pressure. This is particularly problematic in the setting of severe pulmonary embolism associated with acute PH where small emboli may squeeze

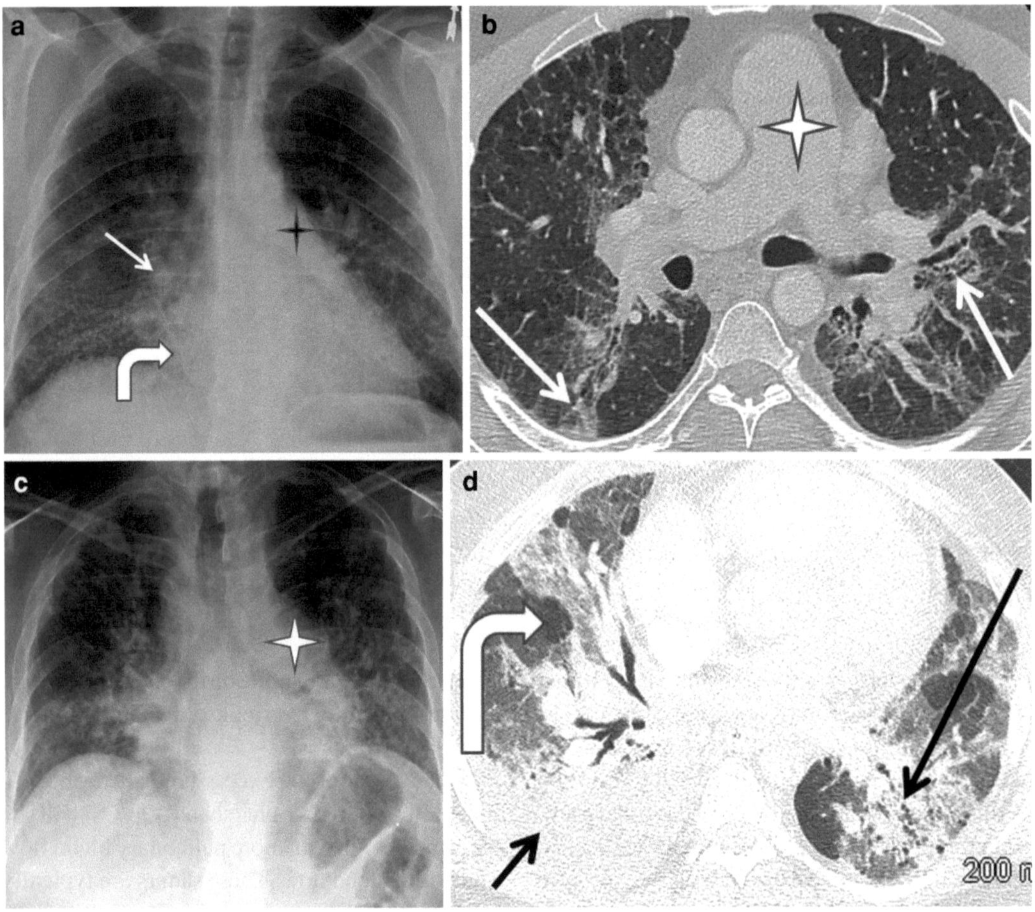

Fig. 9.5 **a** Chronic hypersensitivity pneumonitis with PH. PA radiograph shows an enlarged pulmonary trunk (*star*), an enlarged interlobar artery (*arrow*), an enlarged right atrial border (*curved arrow*), and basilar predominant fibrosis. **b** Chronic hypersensitivity pneumonitis with massive enlargement of the pulmonary trunk (*star*) and pulmonary fibrosis (*arrows*). **c** PH from severe chronic hypersensitivity pneumonitis. More severe case of chronic hypersensitivity pneumonitis (Farmer's lung) with end stage pulmonary fibrosis and PH with PA radiograph that shows basilar fibrosis and an enlarged pulmonary trunk (*star*). **d** PH from severe chronic hypersensitivity pneumonitis (Farmer's lung): HRCT image shows right pleural effusion (*short arrow*), pulmonary fibrosis (*long arrow*) and air trapping (*curved arrow*)

through this communication to gain access to the systemic circulation.

Nuclear Medicine Ventilation–Perfusion Scan

Ventilation–perfusion (V/Q) scanning is central for the diagnosis of CTEPH and is considered to be the most reliable test for showing the multiple subsegmental V/Q mismatches found in this disorder [30].

PH related to congenital heart disease with Eisenmenger syndrome can also be identified on V/Q scanning when ^{99m}Tc-macroaggregated albumin (MAA) accumulates in organs other than the lung [31]. This phenomenon occurs when particles of MAA, which are usually trapped in the small capillaries of the lung, bypass this filter through the right-to-left shunt to enter the systemic circulation. The degree of right-to-left shunting can be easily determined as well by determining the percentage uptake by

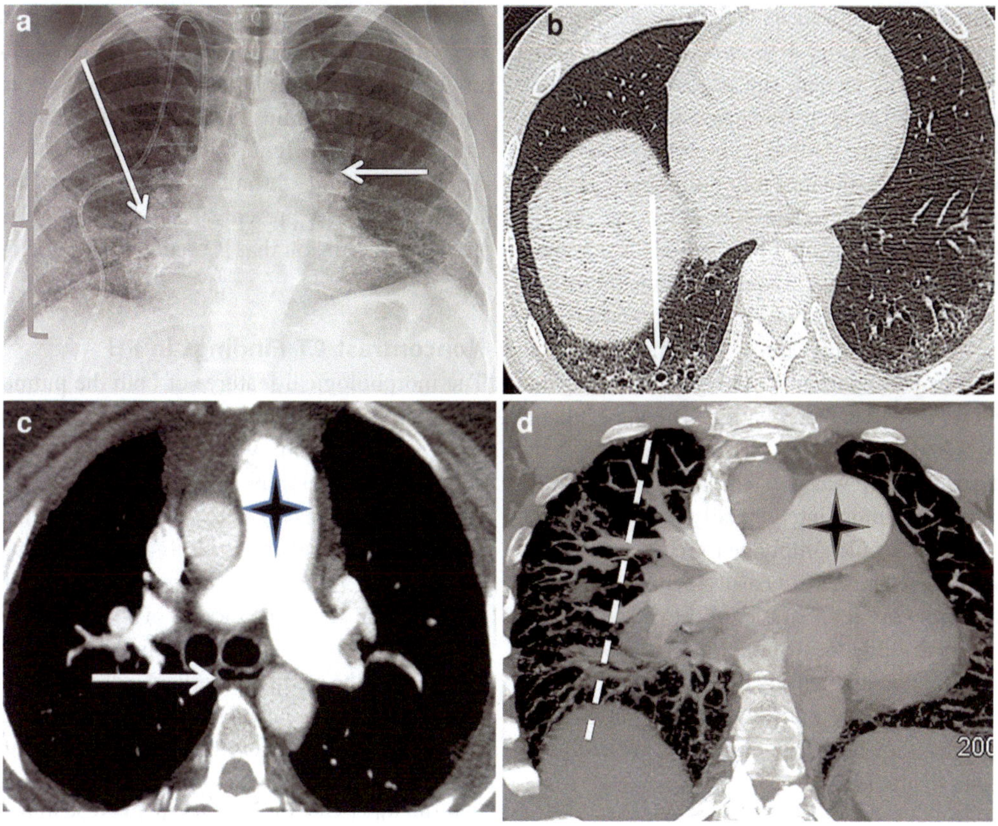

Fig. 9.6 Systemic sclerosis as a cause of PH. **a** PA radiograph shows basilar fibrosis (*bracket*) and enlarged pulmonary arteries (*arrows*). **b** HRCT image shows a nonspecific interstitial pneumonia (NSIP) pattern of basilar fibrosis characterized by ground-glass opacity, reticulation, and traction bronchiectasis (*arrow*). **c** Systemic sclerosis as a cause of PH. Esophageal dilation (*arrow*) with enlarged pulmonary trunk (*star*). **d** Systemic sclerosis as a cause of PH. CTA Paddle wheel thick slab MIP showing pulmonary trunk enlargement (*star*) with peripheral pruning of the small pulmonary arteries beyond the *dashed white line*

the lung versus the other organs such as the brain. Furthermore, the degree of intrapulmonic shunting in hepatopulmonary syndrome can be determined using this method as well [32].

Echocardiography

The use of transthoracic echocardiography (TTE) is the mainstay of noninvasive imaging for PH. Specifically, the use of Doppler ultrasound to estimate the degree of pulmonary arterial pressure using the gradient across the jet of tricuspid regurgitation (TR) is central to the diagnosis and management of this disease (Fig. 9.5). Other findings of chronic PH found at echocardiography that are related to disease prognosis are: (1) right atrial enlargement, (2) reduced tricuspid annular plane systolic excursion (TAPSE), and (3) pericardial effusion [4, 33]. In acute PH (typically secondary to massive pulmonary embolism) McConnell's sign [34] can be found, wherein the rapid change in pressure and Laplace's law conspire to limit the contractility of the free wall of the RV adjacent to the tricuspid valve plane where the ventricle is the largest in its short axis [35]. There is in fact paradoxical motion at this location in the RV as it strains against a sudden change in pulmonary arterial circuit afterload.

To obtain a noninvasive estimate of the PAP, two methodological assumptions are used by echocardiographers. First, the modified Bernoulli equation is employed to determine the pressure gradient (PG) ($PG = 4\ V^2$, where V^2 is the TR jet velocity), and second, the pressure in the right atrium (RAP) needs to be estimated as well. These assumptions are problematic. One issue with noninvasive estimates of pulmonary arterial pressure (PAP) as determined by the TR jet velocity method using TTE methods is that there is a significant error associated with these estimates. Fisher et al. [36] have recently showed that the 95% confidence limits for this error were found to be about ±40 mmHg when compared with right heart catheterization. The same authors also found that for 48% of cases, the error in the estimate of PAP was greater than 10 mmHg [36].

Perhaps a more intellectually honest appraisal of this data would simply be to recognize that all noninvasive pressure measurements are fraught with error. In fact, Galie et al. [4] have recently published guidelines that suggest that echocardiographic assessment of PH should be confined to the probability of the fact that PH may be present rather than a confirmation or exclusion of this diagnosis.

Imaging Findings of RV Strain

The mechanism for all of the imaging findings of PH that can be appreciated in the RV noninvasively is related to fact that the right ventricle is struggling to contract against a pressure overload [34]. There are three direct findings of right heart strain that can be observed: (1) free wall dyskinesia seen at the site of the free wall next to the atrioventricular groove where the free wall is the farthest from the intraventricular septum ("McConnell's Sign" at echocardiography) [2, 34, 35], (2) Straightening of the interventricular septum at CT or MR scanning, or (3) Bowing of the interventricular septum from right ventricle toward the left ventricle at systole indicating pulmonary arterial pressures that are greater than systemic pressures (Figs. 9.2, 9.5 and 9.6). There is also an indirect finding of right ventricular strain and that is the jet of TR. The velocity of this TR jet increases proportionally with the severity of PH [36]. In addition, the secondary signs of right ventricular decompensation with PH can be found in the ventricular free wall thickness and the degree of dilation of the right ventricle as reflected in an increase in the minor and major axes and increased RV strain [37]. The differences in thickness of the right ventricular free wall are dependent on the chronicity of the PH and how much volume is present. There may also be a pericardial effusion that is seen with chronic PH.

Noncontrast CT Findings in PH

The morphological features of both the pulmonary arterial system and the lung parenchyma are well demonstrated with routine noncontrast computed tomography (CT). Many studies have shown a relationship between main pulmonary artery enlargement and PH [38–41]. Enlargement of the main pulmonary artery is a sign of PH [38, 39]. Tan et al. [40] showed in 36 patients with parenchymal lung disease and nine normal individuals that the mean CT-derived measurement of main pulmonary arterial diameter is 3.6 cm (±0.6 cm) for patients with mPAP >20 mmHg and 2.7 cm (±0.2 cm) in normals. They found that the most specific finding of PH was to combine the measurement of PA diameter of >2.9 cm with the presence of three out of five lobes having a segmental pulmonary artery-to-bronchus ratio of >1:1 (100% specific) [40]. Sanal et al. [41] in their analysis of acute moderate or severe (≥50 mmHg) PH of 190 patients with acute pulmonary embolism showed a main pulmonary measurement of 2.9 cm to be abnormal (sensitivity 0.87, specificity 0.89). Their data were not corrected for sex, race, or body surface area [41]. Devaraj et al. have recently shown that the right and left pulmonary artery diameters exceeding 1.8 cm are the best predictor of mortality in patients with bronchiectasis as these CT findings are considered to be a biomarker for PH [42]. In their series of 55 patients being evaluated for lung transplantation, Haimovici et al. [39] found that the best correlation between the mean pulmonary artery pressures for CT-derived measurement of the pulmonary vessels was related to the combined main PA and left PA cross-sectional area corrected for body surface area (BSA). Edwards showed that using 10 mm thick

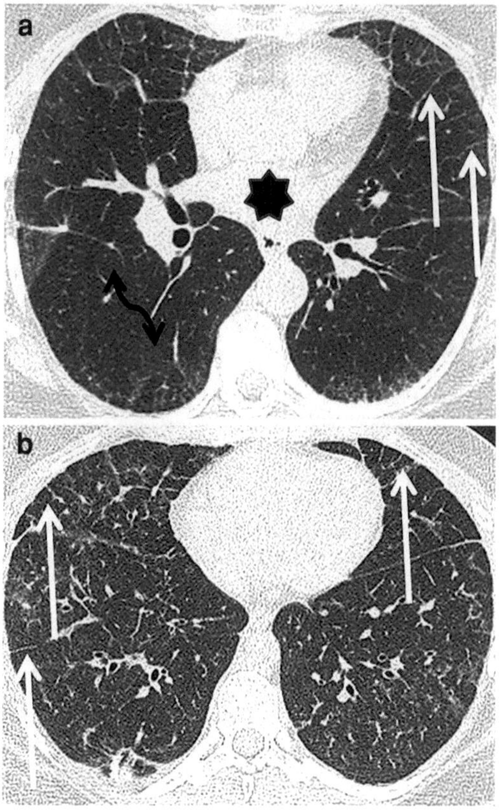

Fig. 9.7 **a, b** Pulmonary veno-occlusive disease (PVOD) as a cause of PH: (A–B) HRCT images show the characteristic findings of PVOD including interlobular septal thickening (*arrows*), normal left atrial size (*star*), and parenchymal oligemia (*curved arrow*). This is also associated with pulmonary arterial enlargement (*not shown*). (Case courtesy of Jeffrey Kanne, M.D., Madison, W.)

non-gated axial CT images, a main PA diameter of >3.32 cm obtained at the level of the bifurcation showed a sensitivity of 58% and a specificity of 95% for the presence of PH in their retrospectively analyzed cohort of 100 normal and 12 patients with PH of >20 mmHg [43]. In the setting of acute respiratory distress syndrome (ARDS), Beiderlinden et al. [44] reported on 103 patients that had CT and right heart catheterization performed. In their series, a main pulmonary artery diameter of ≥2.9 cm was only modestly helpful in the prediction of PH (sensitivity of 0.54, specificity of 0.63). Some authors have proposed using the ratio of the pulmonary artery diameter to the aortic diameter as a proxy for pulmonary arterial enlargement [45]. However, the utility of this ratio is limited by the great deal of variability in aortic size independent of pulmonary arterial pressures. While many studies have attempted to determine how useful size measurements of the pulmonary arteries are on non-gated CT scans, to date the results are clearly not sensitive or specific for PH.

CT can be very helpful in the diagnosis of a rare but clinically important cause of PH, pulmonary veno-occlusive disease (PVOD) [15, 46, 47]. The imaging findings on CT that help distinguish PVOD from the other more common causes of PH include patchy ground-glass opacities (GGO), poorly defined centrilobular nodules in a random lung zonal distribution, smooth interlobular septal thickening, and lymphadenopathy [46] as these features are not typical of precapillary causes of PH (Fig. 9.7). This imaging diagnosis is of critical importance to these (PVOD) patients because administration of vasodilators can be fatal [46].

Intrapulmonary shunts at the capillary level are occult on CT. Nuclear medicine studies are the most useful tests for that disorder. Patients with hepatopulmonary syndrome may have abnormal CT scans. Vessels extending to the lung periphery may be apparent. Secondary findings of portal venous hypertension such as ascites, esophageal varicies, and hepatic cirrhosis may be apparent (Fig. 9.8).

CT Angiography of PH

An important cause of PH is CTEPH [48–51]. Diagnosis of this disorder can be made on CT angiography (CTA) but it is more commonly established with V/Q scanning (Fig. 9.2) [48]. CTA findings of chronic pulmonary thromboembolic disease include eccentric or circumferential thrombus, calcified thrombus, bands, and webs. Findings that suggest associated pulmonary hypertension include central pulmonary artery enlargement and tortuousity, pulmonary arterial atherosclerotic calcification, RV enlargement and hypertrophy, and bronchial artery hypertrophy.

The lungs are often heterogeneous with areas of high attenuation (ground-glass opacity) and enlarged pulmonary arteries and areas of low attenuation with small pulmonary arteries, a pattern referred to as "mosaic perfusion". Individually, many of these findings are not specific for CTEPH; however, coexistence of multiple of these findings should raise the question of CTEPH [52].

Cardiac gating is important in pulmonary arterial measurements as it limits the amount of motion from vessel compliance and cardiac bulk translational motion during scan acquisition, reducing error. Post-processing of gated CT volumes allows for facile measurement of any vessel in its true cross sectional (short axis). Contrast enhanced imaging provides distinction between vessel lumen and vessel wall. Lin et al. [53] determined normal double oblique short axis measurements for the right heart from 103 asymptomatic individuals. While their data were not corrected for BSA, sex, or race, it showed the end diastolic double oblique short axis for main pulmonary artery diameter to have a range of 1.89–3.03 cm (±2 S.D) [53].

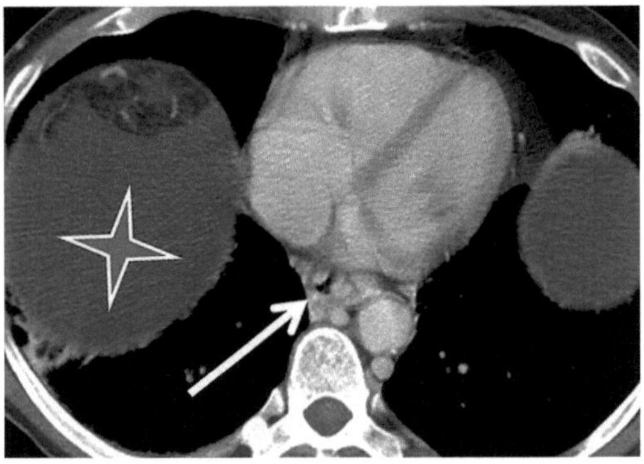

Fig. 9.8 Portopulmonary PH: CT shows the ravages of hepatic cirrhosis with ascites (*star*) and esophageal varicies (*arrow*). The typical pulmonary findings of PH on CT are not seen until late in this disease. The accompanying hypoalbuminemia may lead to volume overload, third spacing, and right heart failure. Pulmonary hypertension occurs in up to 16% patients referred for liver transplantation [57]

Magnetic Resonance Imaging of PH

Magnetic resonance imaging (MRI) and magnetic resonance angiography (MRA) are frequently used as adjuncts to standard imaging tests for PH. While MRI is *less expensive*, a more accurate, and a more reproducible test than echocardiography for assessment of right heart function and valvular regurgitation; echocardiography remains firmly entrenched as the mainstay for PH diagnosis prior to right heart catheterization. This referral pattern favoring echocardiography may be related to the familiarity and convenience of this method, as echocardiography can be performed acutely at the bedside.

MRI and MRA play important roles in the presurgical evaluation of shunt lesions that can cause PH. MRI and MRA can easily depict both extrapulmonic shunts and intracardiac shunts. Phase contrast MRA methods can be used to quantify shunt volume, jet velocity, and direction. Standard balanced steady-state free precession (bSSFP) methods are now routinely used for non-contrast MRI functional assessment of effects of the shunt on the heart. Using most current MRI systems, cardiac gated short axis bSSFP images of the left ventricle and axial cardiac gated SSFP images of the right ventricle can be obtained. Using these stacked time resolved data sets and a standalone workstation with software for cardiac function and flow analysis, the pertinent cardiac metrics of right ventricular stroke volume, right ventricular ejection fraction (RVEF), tricuspid and pulmonic valvular regurgitation jet velocity, and tricuspid and pulmonic valvular regurgitant volume can be calculated (Table 9.6). MRI methods are now considered to be the most accurate of the non-invasive methods for quantification of cardiac function and valvular regurgitation.

MRA techniques have also been used to study CTEPH [54]. MRA is similar to CTA in showing the detail of the central pulmonary arteries and can also show subsegmental vessels as well using parallel imaging and breath holding techniques. Ghio et al. [55] have shown that the

Table 9.6 Information routinely available from cardiac MRI for treatment planning and follow-up in patients with PH

Flow and velocity quantification (phase contrast)	
Tricuspid valve	Inflow amount
	Regurgitation amount
	Max/min velocity
Pulmonic valve	Inflow amount
	Regurgitation amount
	Max/min velocity
Right and left PA	Net flow
	Max/min velocity
Morphological quantification (steady-state free procession)	
Right atrium	
	Size
	Shunt location (ASD,PFO)
	RA thrombi
Right ventricle	
	End diastolic volume
	End systolic volume
	Stroke volume
	End diastolic volume index
	End systolic volume index
	Minor and major axis
	RV thrombi
	Shunt locations
Pulmonary veins	
	PAPVR
Left atrium	
	Shunt locations
	LA thrombi
Left ventricle	
	End diastolic volume
	End systolic volume
	Stroke volume
	End diastolic volume index
	End systolic volume index
	Minor and major axis
	Shunt locations

combination of elevated mPAP and diminished RVEF portends a very poor prognosis, while patients with PH and preserved RVEF have a significantly better survival. Sanz et al. [56] showed that delayed contrast enhancement (DCE) in the myocardium is common in PH and the degree of DCE at septal insertions in cases of PH has been found to be dependent on the severity of the disease.

In summary, the use of MRI in the setting of PH can be a helpful adjunct to the currently available tests of right heart catheterization, transthoracic echocardiography, V/Q scanning, and pulmonary function tests, as it is the best test for the analysis of RVEF, which is a biomarker for survival in this disease.

References

1. McLaughlin VV, Archer SL, Badesch DB, Barst RJ, Farber HW, Lindner JR, Mathier MA, McGoon MD, Park MH, Rosenson RS, Rubin LJ, Tapson VF, Varga J, Harrington RA, Anderson JL, Bates ER, Bridges CR, Eisenberg MJ, Ferrari VA, Grines CL, Hlatky MA, Jacobs AK, Kaul S, Lichtenberg RC, Moliterno DJ, Mukherjee D, Pohost GM, Schofield RS, Shubrooks SJ, Stein JH, Tracy CM, Weitz HH, Wesley DJ. ACCF/AHA 2009 expert consensus document on pulmonary hypertension: a report of the American College of Cardiology Foundation Task force on expert consensus documents and the American Heart Association: developed in collaboration with the American College of Chest Physicians, American Thoracic Society, Inc., and the Pulmonary Hypertension Association. Circulation. 2009;119:2250–94.
2. Champion HC, Michelakis ED, Hassoun PM. Comprehensive invasive and noninvasive approach to the right ventricle-pulmonary circulation unit: state of the art and clinical and research implications. Circulation. 2009;120:992–1007.
3. Simonneau G, Robbins IM, Beghetti M, Channick RN, Delcroix M, Denton CP, Elliott CG, Gaine SP, Gladwin MT, Jing ZC, Krowka MJ, Langleben D, Nakanishi N, Souza R. Updated clinical classification of pulmonary hypertension. J Am Coll Cardiol. 2009;54:S43–54.
4. Galie N, Hoeper MM, Humbert M, Torbicki A, Vachiery JL, Barbera JA, Beghetti M, Corris P, Gaine S, Gibbs JS, Gomez-Sanchez MA, Jondeau G, Klepetko W, Opitz C, Peacock A, Rubin L, Zellweger M, Simonneau G. Guidelines for the diagnosis and treatment of pulmonary hypertension: the task force for the Diagnosis and Treatment of Pulmonary Hypertension of the European Society of Cardiology (ESC) and the European Respiratory Society (ERS), endorsed by the International Society of Heart and Lung Transplantation (ISHLT). Eur Heart J. 2009;30:2493–537.
5. McLaughlin VV, Archer SL, Badesch DB, Barst RJ, Farber HW, Lindner JR, Mathier MA, McGoon MD, Park MH, Rosenson RS, Rubin LJ, Tapson VF, Varga J. ACCF/AHA 2009 expert consensus document on pulmonary hypertension a report of the American College of Cardiology Foundation Task Force on Expert Consensus Documents and the American Heart Association developed in collaboration with the American College of Chest Physicians; American Thoracic Society, Inc.; and the Pulmonary Hypertension Association. J Am Coll Cardiol. 2009;53:1573–619.
6. Chin KM, Kim NH, Rubin LJ. The right ventricle in pulmonary hypertension. Coron Artery Dis. 2005;16: 13–8.
7. Humbert M. The burden of pulmonary hypertension. Eur Respir J. 2007;30:1–2.
8. Humbert M, Sitbon O, Chaouat A, Bertocchi M, Habib G, Gressin V, Yaici A, Weitzenblum E, Cordier JF, Chabot F, Dromer C, Pison C, Reynaud-Gaubert M, Haloun A, Laurent M, Hachulla E, Simonneau G. Pulmonary arterial hypertension in France: results from a national registry. Am J Respir Crit Care Med. 2006;173:1023–30.
9. Thenappan T, Shah SJ, Rich S, Gomberg-Maitland M. A USA-based registry for pulmonary arterial hypertension: 1982–2006. Eur Respir J. 2007;30:1103–10.
10. Le Pavec J, Humbert M. Reference centers for rare respiratory diseases. Presse Med. 2007;36:933–5.
11. Peacock AJ, Murphy NF, McMurray JJ, Caballero L, Stewart S. An epidemiological study of pulmonary arterial hypertension. Eur Respir J. 2007;30:104–9.
12. Rich S, Dantzker DR, Ayres SM, Bergofsky EH, Brundage BH, Detre KM, Fishman AP, Goldring RM, Groves BM, Koerner SK, et al. Primary pulmonary hypertension. A national prospective study. Ann Intern Med. 1987;107:216–23.
13. Badesch DB, Raskob GE, Elliott CG, Krichman AM, Farber HW, Frost AE, Barst RJ, Benza RL, Liou TG, Turner M, Giles S, Feldkircher K, Miller DP, McGoon MD. Pulmonary arterial hypertension: baseline characteristics from the REVEAL Registry. Chest. 2010;137:376–87.
14. Sztrymf B, Yaici A, Girerd B, Humbert M. Genes and pulmonary arterial hypertension. Respiration. 2007;74:123–32.
15. Runo JR, Vnencak-Jones CL, Prince M, Loyd JE, Wheeler L, Robbins IM, Lane KB, Newman JH, Johnson J, Nichols WC, Phillips JA 3rd. Pulmonary veno-occlusive disease caused by an inherited mutation in bone morphogenetic protein receptor II. Am J Respir Crit Care Med. 2003;167:889–94.
16. Hyduk A, Croft JB, Ayala C, Zheng K, Zheng ZJ, Mensah GA. Pulmonary hypertension surveillance–United States, 1980–2002. MMWR Surveill Summ. 2005;54:1–28.
17. Stricker H, Domenighetti G, Popov W, Speich R, Nicod L, Aubert JD, Soler M. Severe pulmonary hypertension: data from the Swiss Registry. Swiss Med Wkly. 2001;131:346–50.

18. Souza R, Humbert M, Sztrymf B, Jais X, Yaici A, Le Pavec J, Parent F, Herve P, Soubrier F, Sitbon O, Simonneau G. Pulmonary arterial hypertension associated with fenfluramine exposure: report of 109 cases. Eur Respir J. 2008;31:343–8.
19. D'Alonzo GE, Barst RJ, Ayres SM, Bergofsky EH, Brundage BH, Detre KM, Fishman AP, Goldring RM, Groves BM, Kernis JT, et al. Survival in patients with primary pulmonary hypertension. Results from a national prospective registry. Ann Intern Med. 1991; 115:343–9.
20. Barst RJ, Langleben D, Frost A, Horn EM, Oudiz R, Shapiro S, McLaughlin V, Hill N, Tapson VF, Robbins IM, Zwicke D, Duncan B, Dixon RA, Frumkin LR. Sitaxsentan therapy for pulmonary arterial hypertension. Am J Respir Crit Care Med. 2004;169:441–7.
21. Beghetti M, Galie N. Eisenmenger syndrome a clinical perspective in a new therapeutic era of pulmonary arterial hypertension. J Am Coll Cardiol. 2009;53:733–40.
22. Musewe NN, Poppe D, Smallhorn JF, Hellman J, Whyte H, Smith B, Freedom RM. Doppler echocardiographic measurement of pulmonary artery pressure from ductal Doppler velocities in the newborn. J Am Coll Cardiol. 1990;15:446–56.
23. Runo JR, Loyd JE. Primary pulmonary hypertension. Lancet. 2003;361:1533–44.
24. Hui-li G. The management of acute pulmonary arterial hypertension. Cardiovasc Ther. 2011;29:153–75.
25. Galie N, Seeger W, Naeije R, Simonneau G, Rubin LJ. Comparative analysis of clinical trials and evidence-based treatment algorithm in pulmonary arterial hypertension. J Am Coll Cardiol. 2004;43:81S–8S.
26. Doyle RL, McCrory D, Channick RN, Simonneau G, Conte J. Surgical treatments/interventions for pulmonary arterial hypertension: ACCP evidence-based clinical practice guidelines. Chest. 2004;126:63S–71S.
27. Badesch DB, Abman SH, Ahearn GS, Barst RJ, McCrory DC, Simonneau G, McLaughlin VV. Medical therapy for pulmonary arterial hypertension: ACCP evidence-based clinical practice guidelines. Chest. 2004;126:35S–62S.
28. Bush A, Gray H, Denison DM. Diagnosis of pulmonary hypertension from radiographic estimates of pulmonary arterial size. Thorax. 1988;43:127–31.
29. Sleeper JC, Orgain ES, Mc IH. Primary pulmonary hypertension. Review of clinical features and pathologic physiology with a report of pulmonary hemodynamics derived from repeated catheterization. Circulation. 1962;26:1358–69.
30. Tunariu N, Gibbs SJ, Win Z, Gin-Sing W, Graham A, Gishen P, Al-Nahhas A. Ventilation–perfusion scintigraphy is more sensitive than multidetector CTPA in detecting chronic thromboembolic pulmonary disease as a treatable cause of pulmonary hypertension. J Nucl Med. 2007;48:680–4.
31. Kume N, Suga K, Uchisako H, Matsui M, Shimizu K, Matsunaga N. Abnormal extrapulmonary accumulation of 99 mTc-MAA during lung perfusion scanning. Ann Nucl Med. 1995;9:179–84.
32. Krowka MJ, Wiseman GA, Burnett OL, Spivey JR, Therneau T, Porayko MK, Wiesner RH. Hepatopulmonary syndrome: a prospective study of relationships between severity of liver disease, PaO(2) response to 100% oxygen, and brain uptake after (99m)Tc MAA lung scanning. Chest. 2000;118:615–24.
33. Habib G, Torbicki A. The role of echocardiography in the diagnosis and management of patients with pulmonary hypertension. Eur Respir Rev. 2010;19:288–99.
34. McConnell MV, Solomon SD, Rayan ME, Come PC, Goldhaber SZ, Lee RT. Regional right ventricular dysfunction detected by echocardiography in acute pulmonary embolism. Am J Cardiol. 1996;78:469–73.
35. Sosland RP, Gupta K. Images in cardiovascular medicine: McConnell's Sign. Circulation. 2008;118: e517–8.
36. Fisher MR, Forfia PR, Chamera E, Housten-Harris T, Champion HC, Girgis RE, Corretti MC, Hassoun PM. Accuracy of Doppler echocardiography in the hemodynamic assessment of pulmonary hypertension. Am J Respir Crit Care Med. 2009;179:615–21.
37. Cho EJ, Jiamsripong P, Calleja AM, Alharthi MS, McMahon EM, Khandheria BK, Belohlavek M. Right ventricular free wall circumferential strain reflects graded elevation in acute right ventricular afterload. Am J Physiol Heart Circ Physiol. 2009;296:H413–20.
38. Kuriyama K, Gamsu G, Stern RG, Cann CE, Herfkens RJ, Brundage BH. CT-determined pulmonary artery diameters in predicting pulmonary hypertension. Invest Radiol. 1984;19:16–22.
39. Haimovici JB, Trotman-Dickenson B, Halpern EF, Dec GW, Ginns LC, Shepard JA, McLoud TC. Relationship between pulmonary artery diameter at computed tomography and pulmonary artery pressures at right-sided heart catheterization. Massachusetts General Hospital Lung Transplantation Program. Acad Radiol. 1997;4:327–34.
40. Tan RT, Kuzo R, Goodman LR, Siegel R, Haasler GB, Presberg KW. Utility of CT scan evaluation for predicting pulmonary hypertension in patients with parenchymal lung disease. Medical College of Wisconsin Lung Transplant Group. Chest. 1998;113:1250–6.
41. Sanal S, Aronow WS, Ravipati G, Maguire GP, Belkin RN, Lehrman SG. Prediction of moderate or severe pulmonary hypertension by main pulmonary artery diameter and main pulmonary artery diameter/ascending aorta diameter in pulmonary embolism. Cardiol Rev. 2006;14:213–4.
42. Devaraj A, Wells AU, Meister MG, Loebinger MR, Wilson R, Hansell DM. Pulmonary hypertension in patients with bronchiectasis: prognostic significance of CT signs. Am J Roentgenol. 2011;196:1300–4.

43. Edwards PD, Bull RK, Coulden R. CT measurement of main pulmonary artery diameter. Br J Radiol. 1998;71:1018–20.
44. Beiderlinden M, Kuehl H, Boes T, Peters J. Prevalence of pulmonary hypertension associated with severe acute respiratory distress syndrome: predictive value of computed tomography. Intensive Care Med. 2006;32:852–7.
45. Ng CS, Wells AU, Padley SP. A CT sign of chronic pulmonary arterial hypertension: the ratio of main pulmonary artery to aortic diameter. J Thorac Imaging. 1999;14:270–8.
46. Resten A, Maitre S, Humbert M, Rabiller A, Sitbon O, Capron F, Simonneau G, Musset D. Pulmonary hypertension: CT of the chest in pulmonary venoocclusive disease. Am J Roentgenol. 2004;183:65–70.
47. Swensen SJ, Tashjian JH, Myers JL, Engeler CE, Patz EF, Edwards WD, Douglas WW. Pulmonary venoocclusive disease: CT findings in eight patients. Am J Roentgenol. 1996;167:937–40.
48. Dartevelle P, Fadel E, Mussot S, Chapelier A, Herve P, de Perrot M, Cerrina J, Ladurie FL, Lehouerou D, Humbert M, Sitbon O, Simonneau G. Chronic thromboembolic pulmonary hypertension. Eur Respir J. 2004;23:637–48.
49. McNeil K, Dunning J. Chronic thromboembolic pulmonary hypertension (CTEPH). Heart. 2007;93:1152–8.
50. Lang IM. Chronic thromboembolic pulmonary hypertension (CTEPH). Dtsch Med Wochenschr. 2008;133(Suppl 6):S206–8.
51. Seyfarth HJ, Halank M, Wilkens H, Schafers HJ, Ewert R, Riedel M, Schuster E, Pankau H, Hammerschmidt S, Wirtz H. Standard PAH therapy improves long term survival in CTEPH patients. Clin Res Cardiol. 2010;99:553–6.
52. Castaner E, Gallardo X, Ballesteros E, Andreu M, Pallardo Y, Mata JM, Riera L. CT diagnosis of chronic pulmonary thromboembolism. Radiographics. 2009;29:31–50. discussion 50–3.
53. Lin FY, Devereux RB, Roman MJ, Meng J, Jow VM, Simprini L, Jacobs A, Weinsaft JW, Shaw LJ, Berman DS, Callister TQ, Min JK. The right sided great vessels by cardiac multidetector computed tomography: normative reference values among healthy adults free of cardiopulmonary disease, hypertension, and obesity. Acad Radiol. 2009;16:981–7.
54. Oberholzer K, Romaneehsen B, Kunz P, Kramm T, Thelen M, Kreitner KF. Contrast-enhanced 3D MR angiography of the pulmonary arteries with integrated parallel acquisition technique (iPAT) in patients with chronic-thromboembolic pulmonary hypertension CTEPH-sagittal or coronal acquisition? Rofo. 2004;176:605–9.
55. Ghio S, Gavazzi A, Campana C, Inserra C, Klersy C, Sebastiani R, Arbustini E, Recusani F, Tavazzi L. Independent and additive prognostic value of right ventricular systolic function and pulmonary artery pressure in patients with chronic heart failure. J Am Coll Cardiol. 2001;37:183–8.
56. Sanz J, Dellegrottaglie S, Kariisa M, Sulica R, Poon M, O'Donnell TP, Mehta D, Fuster V, Rajagopalan S. Prevalence and correlates of septal delayed contrast enhancement in patients with pulmonary hypertension. Am J Cardiol. 2007;100:731–5.
57. Hoeper MM, Krowka MJ, Strassburg CP. Portopulmonary hypertension and hepatopulmonary syndrome. Lancet. 2004;363:1461–8.

Obstructive Pulmonary Diseases

10

Megan Saettele, Timothy Saettele, and Jonathan Chung

Abstract

Obstructive lung diseases represent a growing burden to society. Chest radiography and computed tomography (CT) have historically been the main imaging resources used to evaluate these disorders. While much information can be learned from conventional studies, more advanced imaging modalities like high resolution CT, synchrotron radiation CT, hyperpolarized helium-3 magnetic resonance imaging, and optical coherence tomography allow greater structural and functional characterization of the lungs and airways. Improvements in these technologies will allow patients to be classified according to disease phenotype, and potentially benefit from more specific treatment of their disease.

Keywords

COPD · Asthma · Chronic bronchitis · Emphysema · Radiograph · CT · MRI · High resolution CT · Synchrotron radiation CT · Hyperpolarized helium-3 magnetic resonance imaging · Optical coherence tomography

Introduction

It is currently estimated that 24 million people in the United States have chronic obstructive pulmonary disease (COPD), but only half have been diagnosed. By 2020, COPD is projected to be the third leading cause of death in the United States [1]. Likewise, the costs of asthma to society are substantial. Diagnosis of obstructive pulmonary diseases may not always be straightforward. While pulmonary function testing (PFT) has long been the diagnostic tool for functional evaluation, new imaging technology allows earlier diagnosis and physiologic assessment of obstructive pulmonary diseases. This information

M. Saettele (✉)
Department of Radiology,
University of Missouri-Kansas City,
4401 Wornall Road,
Kansas City, MO 64111, USA
e-mail: saettelem@umkc.edu

T. Saettele
Department of Pulmonary/Critical Care,
University of Missouri-Kansas City,
2301 Holmes Street,
Kansas City, MO 64108, USA

J. Chung
Institute of Advanced Biomedical Imaging,
National Jewish Health, 1400 Jackson St, Denver,
CO 80206, USA

J. P. Kanne (ed.), *Clinically Oriented Pulmonary Imaging*,
Respiratory Medicine, DOI: 10.1007/978-1-61779-542-8_10,

can further direct therapy [1] and may result in improved outcomes.

Imaging of obstructive pulmonary diseases has significantly advanced over the last 20 years. Prior to the advent of computed tomography (CT) and high-resolution computed tomography (HRCT), chest radiography was the standard for detecting parenchymal changes in COPD and asthma. Chest radiography still remains the initial imaging assessment, despite being neither sensitive nor specific. Radiographic images are easily obtained, inexpensive, and require minimal radiation exposure. Their use is mainly to aid in exclusion of other diagnoses, including pneumonia, cancer, congestive heart failure, pleural effusion, and pneumothorax [2]. This is primarily because chest radiography poorly depicts subtle damage to small airways or lung parenchyma, as many imaging manifestations are not recognized until the disease process has reached an advanced stage. Chest radiographs are suggested in the acute evaluation of adults with obstructive pulmonary disease who fulfill one or more of the following criteria: those who have a clinical diagnosis of chronic obstructive pulmonary disease, a history of recent fever, clinical or electrocardiographic evidence of heart disease, a history of intravenous drug abuse, seizures, immunosuppression, evidence of other lung disease, or prior thoracic surgery [3].

With the development of CT and HRCT technology, radiologists can now diagnose early and even preclinical obstructive pulmonary processes. Further advancements in pulmonary imaging (including synchrotron radiation CT, hyperpolarized helium-3 magnetic resonance imaging (^{3}He), and optical coherence tomography) are bringing new technology to the forefront of evaluation of obstructive pulmonary diseases, including asthma, emphysema, and chronic bronchitis.

When interpreting images in patients with obstructive lung diseases, it is important to understand the anatomy relevant to these processes. The secondary pulmonary lobule is the smallest unit of lung structure bordered by connective tissue septa that can also be identified on HRCT images. Three primary components account for visualization and appropriate characterization of parenchymal abnormalities: the interlobular septa, centrilobular structures, and lobular parenchyma and acini [4]. Interlobular septa contain pulmonary veins and lymphatics and surround the secondary pulmonary lobule. They are best visualized in the lung periphery and bases where there is a higher concentration of lymphatics. Centrilobular structures are centrally located within the secondary pulmonary lobule and consist of intralobular arteries, bronchiolar branches, lymphatics, and connective tissue. Lobular parenchyma consists of alveoli and capillary beds that surround the centrilobular structures [4]. Recognition of these anatomical structures allows one to form an educated differential diagnosis when interpreting HRCT.

Asthma

Asthma is a chronic syndrome of the airways characterized by inflammation, bronchial hyper-responsiveness, and airflow obstruction [5]. It is common, with a prevalence of 5–10% in the general population [6]. Although asthma can occur at any age, most patients are symptomatic by age five. Risk factors include premature birth, maternal cigarette smoking during pregnancy, exposure to inhaled tobacco smoke and other pollutants, childhood lower respiratory tract viral infections, obesity, and low socioeconomic status [5]. Genetics are also involved with several gene mutations linked to asthma. Asthma runs in families and affects races disproportionally. Signs and symptoms vary between affected individuals, but generally include recurrent episodes of wheezing, breathlessness, chest tightness, and coughing. Symptoms can be intermittent or persistent, and range in severity from mild to severe.

Inflammation is at the heart of the disorder. Mast cells, eosinophils, T lymphocytes, macrophages, and neutrophils are found in the airway walls of asthmatics [7]. The inflammatory products of these cells induce the changes of obstruction and hyper-responsiveness.

Acute exposure to inhaled allergens or irritants may trigger an IgE-mediated release of histamine, tryptase, leukotrienes, and prostaglandins from mast cells. These products induce bronchoconstriction, which usually reverses spontaneously or with bronchodilator treatment. Aspirin and nonsteroidal anti-inflammatory drugs (NSAIDS) may also induce bronchoconstriction in some individuals. Other triggers may include exercise, cold air, and stress, although it is not entirely clear whether the same mechanisms are involved.

In addition to bronchoconstriction, other factors may limit airflow when persistent inflammation is present, including airway edema and the formation of mucus plugs [8]. Chronic inflammation can induce permanent structural airway changes, termed remodeling. These changes include smooth muscle hypertrophy and hyperplasia, mucus gland hyperplasia, subepithelial fibrosis, thickening of the sub-basement membrane, and blood vessel proliferation and dilation. As airway remodeling advances, airflow obstruction may not be fully reversible. This represents one etiology of chronic obstructive pulmonary disease (COPD), described below.

The clinical presentation of asthma is quite variable, and different phenotypes have been described [9]. There is clearly a subset of patients with an atopic component, in which IgE-mediated allergic responses to aeroallergens are the major pathways leading to bronchoconstriction. These patients often present in childhood and have other allergic conditions, including atopic dermatitis, seasonal allergic rhinitis, and allergic conjunctivitis. They usually have positive results to allergen skin tests. Other patients display airway hyper-responsiveness without atopy as a major feature. Patients who present in adulthood are more likely to fall into this category. Some patients are more prone to exacerbations than others. Exacerbations are periods of acute or subacute symptoms with measurable decreases in airflow, often triggered by aeroallergens or respiratory infections. Other disease phenotypes are currently being identified and refined.

Spirometry in asthmatics is also variable. People with intermittent symptoms may have normal values at baseline and develop obstruction during bronchoconstriction, characterized by forced expiratory volume in one second (FEV_1) to forced vital capacity (FVC) ratios less than 0.70, mainly due to decreases in FEV_1. The obstruction in these patients is typically reversible, and FEV_1 may normalize following bronchodilator treatment. Patients with persistent symptoms or exacerbation may not show full reversibility following inhaled bronchodilator therapy, especially when airway remodeling is present. More extensive pulmonary function testing may show increases in total lung capacity (TLC) and residual volume (RV) in these patients, indicating air trapping.

Radiographic evaluation in asthma, while nonspecific, may show bronchial wall thickening. This is typically more evident on the lateral view in the central aspect of the lungs where the larger airways are concentrated. Pulmonary hyperinflation may also result depicted as depression of the diaphragm, flattening of the normal diaphragmatic curvature, and an increase in retrosternal space [10]. Hyperinflation is not commonly seen, however, unless underlying emphysema is also present [11]. Given the young age of many patients at diagnosis, it is important to limit unnecessary radiologic evaluation so as to reduce the total lifetime radiation exposure. Children are inherently more sensitive to radiation than adults and have more time to express radiation-induced cell damage [12]. Radiographic evaluation at regular intervals is not indicated and should be limited to patients presenting with atypical features or if concern for complications exists [11].

Recent studies have identified CT as a useful modality for evaluating airway wall thickness and air trapping (Fig. 10.1). These features correlate with severity of airflow obstruction and increased hospitalizations, respectively. Three-dimensional multidetector CT (MDCT) technology has been used to correlate airway wall thickness measured on CT with airway epithelial thickness measured on endobronchial biopsy specimens, indicating that patients with more severe asthma generally have increased wall thickness [13]. HRCT can also be employed

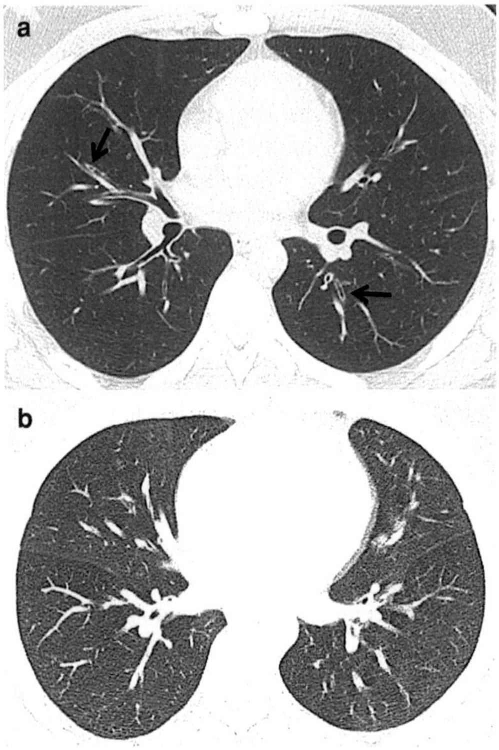

Fig. 10.1 Asthma. **a** HRCT image shows moderate bronchial wall thickening (*arrows*). **b** Axial static expiratory CT shows diffuse hyperlucency of the lower lobes indicative of air trapping

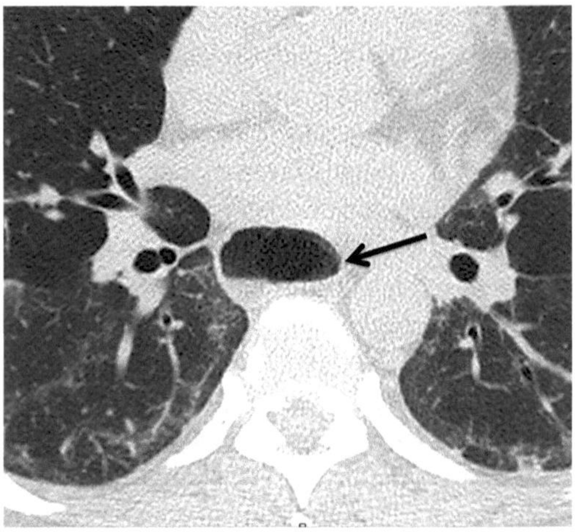

Fig. 10.2 Esophageal dysmotility in systemic sclerosis. HRCT image shows marked esophageal dilation with an air-fluid level (*arrow*), indicative of esophageal dysmotility; ground-glass opacity and reticulation in the lower lobes represent associated nonspecific interstitial pneumonia. Patients with esophageal dysmotility are at increased risk for aspiration and exacerbation of asthma symptoms

to assess the degree of air trapping. Patients with greater than 9.66% of lung tissue with less than −850 Hounsfield units (HU) on CT are classified as having an air trapping phenotype [14]. These patients have increased numbers of hospitalizations, ICU visits, and requirement for mechanical ventilation [14].

CT imaging of patients with asthma is not routinely undertaken but may be useful in evaluating associated disease processes like gastroesophageal reflux disease (GERD), esophageal dysmotility, and rhinosinusitis. Sinus CT is commonly performed to assess the extent of mucosal alterations in rhinosinusitis. Esophageal dysmotility increases patients' risk for aspiration, which may exacerbate asthma symptoms and can manifest on CT as dilation of the esophagus or retained esophageal fluid (Fig. 10.2). Recognition of subtle findings of GERD, such as distal esophageal thickening (Fig. 10.3), may alter patient management. Imaging findings associated with rhinosinusitis and GERD can identify patients who may benefit from additional therapy. When these associated disease processes are treated, patients often experience symptomatic improvement in their asthma.

Another common CT finding in asthma patients is bronchiectasis (Fig. 10.4) [15], defined as irreversible dilation of a bronchus such that the bronchial diameter is larger than the internal diameter of the adjacent pulmonary artery. Bronchiectasis is associated with mucus retention and higher rates of infection. Lynch et al. reported 77 versus 59% and Park et al. reported 31 versus 7% of asthma patients who met CT criteria for bronchial dilation compared to normal subjects, respectively [16, 17]. Studies have suggested that asthma is more severe in individuals with higher degrees of bronchiectasis detected on MDCT [18]. Given that bronchi may transiently dilate in response to acute pulmonary disease, erroneous diagnosis of bronchiectasis in patients with acute pneumonia or aspiration should be avoided.

Complications of asthma can be subdivided into acute and chronic. Acute complications

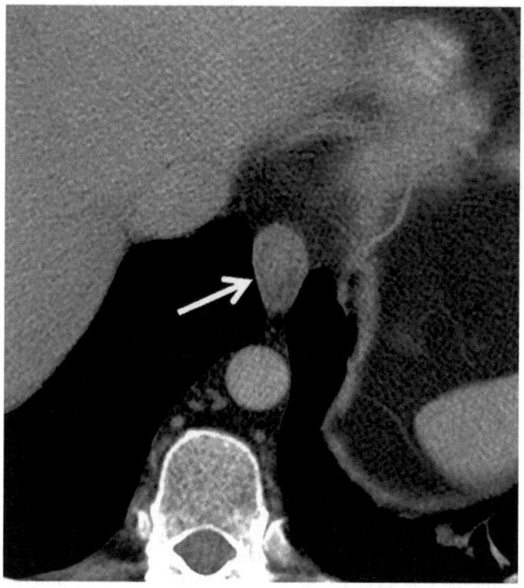

Fig. 10.3 Gastroesophageal reflux disease. CT image demonstrates distal esophageal thickening (*arrow*) likely reflecting reflux related esophageal changes

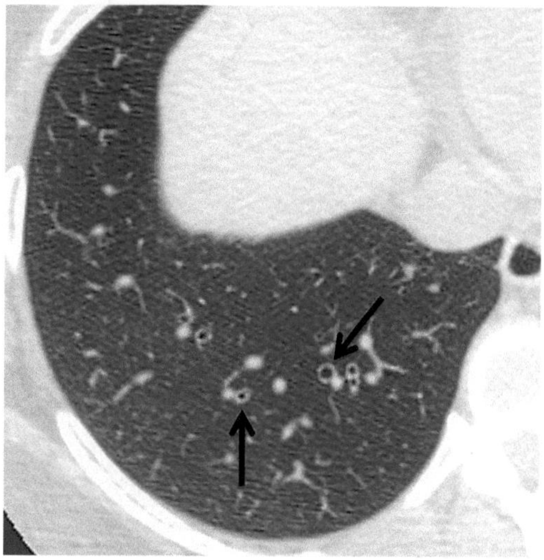

Fig. 10.4 Bronchiectasis in asthma. HRCT image shows dilated bronchi (*arrows*) greater in diameter than the adjacent pulmonary arteries. Bronchi are also thickened, consistent with large airways disease from asthma

include pneumothorax, pneumomediastinum, mucus impaction with or without atelectasis, and pneumonia [11]. Chronic comorbidities include allergic bronchopulmonary aspergillosis (ABPA), chronic eosinophilic pneumonia (CEP), and Churg-Strauss vasculitis [11]. ABPA is a hypersensitivity reaction to fungus, usually *Aspergillus fumigatus*, that colonizes the airways and results in asthma that is more difficult to control [19]. It complicates a small percentage of cases of steroid-dependent asthma. Key CT features include central and upper lung predominant varicose or cylindrical bronchiectasis, mucoid impaction, and centrilobular nodules (Fig. 10.5) [11]. Evaluation for ABPA is complicated by the fact that central upper lobe predominant cylindrical bronchiectasis may also be seen in patients with asthma without concurrent ABPA. Bronchiectasis in most cases of asthma without concomitant ABPA is mild while bronchiectasis in cases of ABPA tends to be moderate-to-severe.

Chronic eosinophilic pneumonia presents in middle age with symptoms of subacute weight loss, night sweats, low grade fevers, cough, and dyspnea [20]. It follows the development of asthma in most patients, but sometimes may present concurrently with asthma symptoms. Although peripheral eosinophilia is usually modest, high levels are found in bronchoalveolar lavage fluid. It may be suggested by subacute to chronic upper lobe predominant patchy airspace opacities on chest radiography. A peripheral or reverse "bat wing" distribution of opacities, often called the radiographic negative of pulmonary edema, may be present. This pattern may not be fully recognized until CT imaging is performed [11]. HRCT mirrors the peripheral predominant pattern of pulmonary opacities on radiography (Fig. 10.6). Over time, a migratory or fleeting pattern of pulmonary consolidation and ground-glass opacity may be present. Organizing pneumonia is often difficult to distinguish from CEP on imaging; however, the relative absence of eosinophilia and usual absence of asthma in the latter diagnosis is often helpful in distinguishing these two entities. CEP may resolve with a centripetal pattern. That is, pulmonary consolidation may preferentially decrease along its outer margins, sometimes leading to a "wisp of smoke" pattern on HRCT.

Churg-Strauss vasculitis is a rare granulomatous vasculitis often associated with eosinophilia that occurs in patients with asthma. It can affect any organ system, but the lungs are nearly

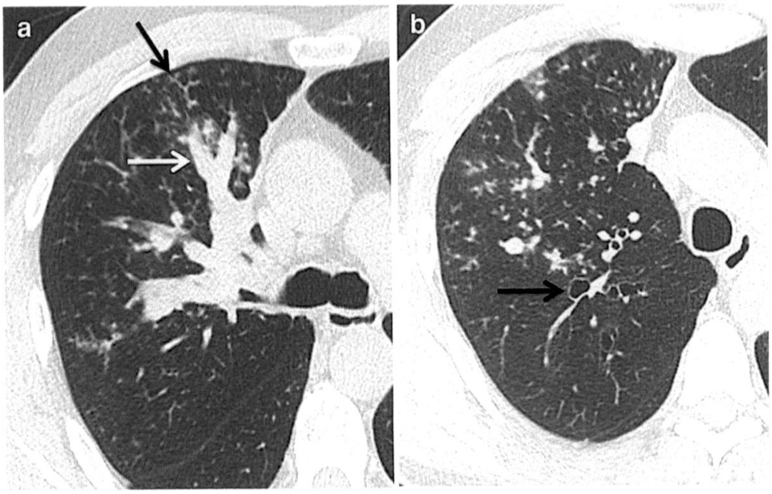

Fig. 10.5 Allergic bronchopulmonary aspergillosis. **a** CT image shows mucus plugging (*white arrow*) in centrally bronchiectatic airways and tree-in-bud nodules (*black arrow*). **b** CT shows central bronchiectasis (*arrow*); the airways are enlarged relative to the adjacent pulmonary artery. Centrilobular nodularity and mucous plugging are also present

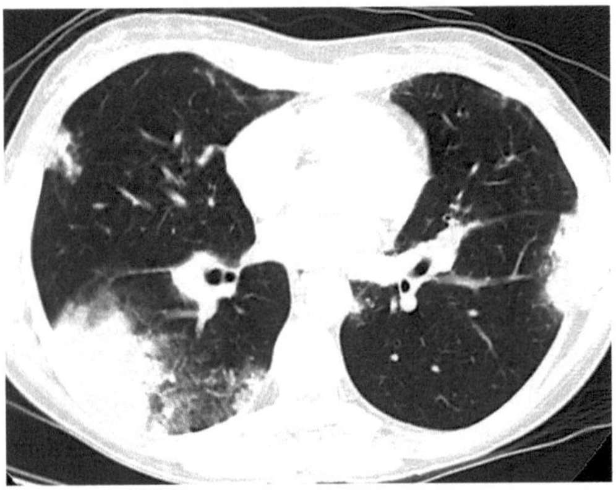

Fig. 10.6 Chronic eosinophilic pneumonia. CT image shows peripheral mass-like consolidation. This appearance is nonspecific and may be seen in multifocal pneumonia, pulmonary infarcts, cryptogenic organizing pneumonia, or eosinophilic pneumonia. A history of asthma can help suggest the diagnosis

always involved [11]. Imaging findings are non specific, but may include patchy, migratory consolidation and/or ground glass opacities (Fig. 10.7). Thickening of the airway walls and interlobular septa can occur, presumably related to eosinophilic infiltration. Cardiac involvement may lead to signs of left-sided heart failure including pulmonary edema, pleural effusions, and pericardial effusion. Effusions, in addition, may be eosinophilic. Identifying extrapulmonary involvement in a patient with a typical presentation is key to suggesting a diagnosis.

Mimickers of asthma are also important to keep in mind. Clinically, the most common condition misdiagnosed as asthma is vocal cord dysfunction [21]. It may be mistaken for asthma because of inspiratory or expiratory stridor heard in patients with this disorder. It may be suspected when a patient has a history inconsistent with asthma, intermittent hoarseness of voice, pulmonary function testing that does not show obstruction, and when imaging studies fail to reveal bronchial wall abnormalities. Laryngoscopy is the gold standard for diagnosis.

Clinically significant inspiratory stridor from obstructive tracheal or carinal lesions can also be mistakenly attributed to asthma. Common causes of focal tracheal airway narrowing include benign and malignant tracheal neoplasms, post-intubation tracheal stenosis (Fig. 10.8), and vascular rings [11]. More diffuse tracheal narrowing may be seen in sarcoidosis, Wegener granulomatosis, amyloidosis (Fig. 10.9), relapsing polychondritis, and tracheobronchopathia osteo-

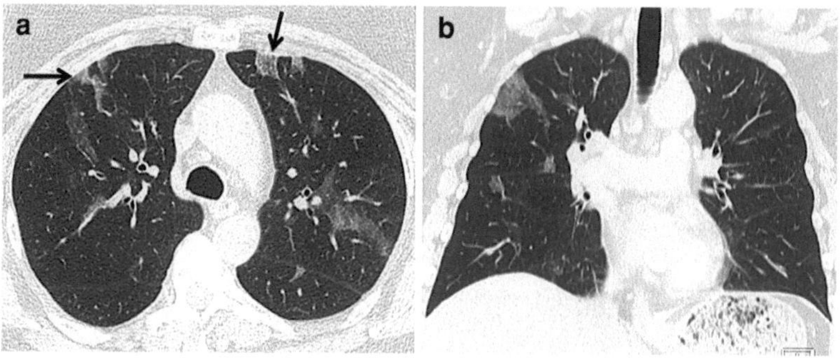

Fig. 10.7 Churg-Strauss vasculitis. Axial (**a**) and coronal (**b**) CT images show patchy ground-glass opacities (*arrows*) both centrally and peripherally within the lungs

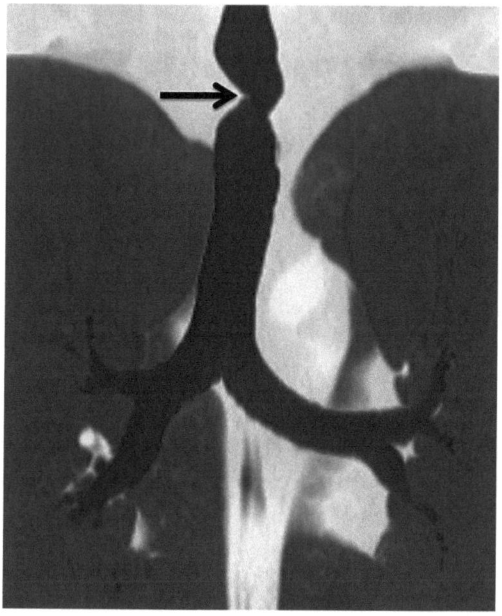

Fig. 10.8 Focal tracheal narrowing from tracheostomy. Coronal minimum intensity projection (MinIP) shows focal superior tracheal narrowing

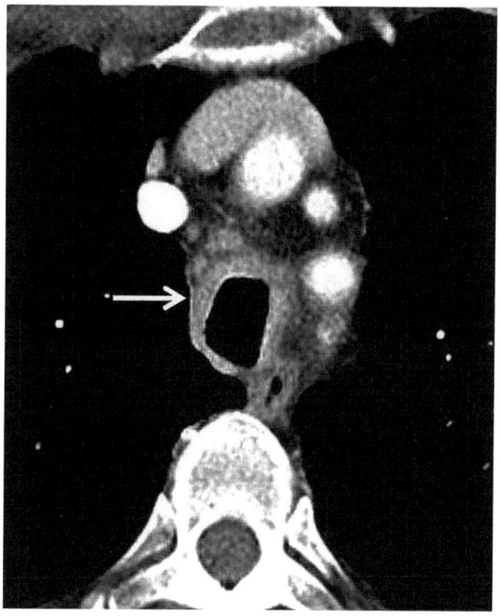

Fig. 10.9 Tracheal amyloidosis. Contrast-enhanced CT image shows circumferential thickening (*arrow*) of the trachea causing subtle tracheal narrowing. Though the imaging findings in this case are not specific, the circumferential involvement would be inconsistent with relapsing polychondritis or tracheobronchopathia osteochondroplastica

chondroplastica [11]. These lesions are amenable to imaging and may be apparent on either the frontal or lateral chest radiograph as narrowing of the trachea or carina. CT is much more sensitive to tracheal diseases compared to radiography given its vastly superior spatial and contrast resolutions. CT permits further characterization of obstructing lesions and delineation of mediastinal anatomy for surgical planning.

Other clinical mimickers of asthma include bronchiolitis obliterans (BO), sarcoidosis, hypersensitivity pneumonitis, and tracheobronchomalacia (TBM). Patients with BO present with obstructive symptoms that are not reversed with bronchodilators. Bronchial wall thickening, bronchial dilation, expiratory air trapping, and

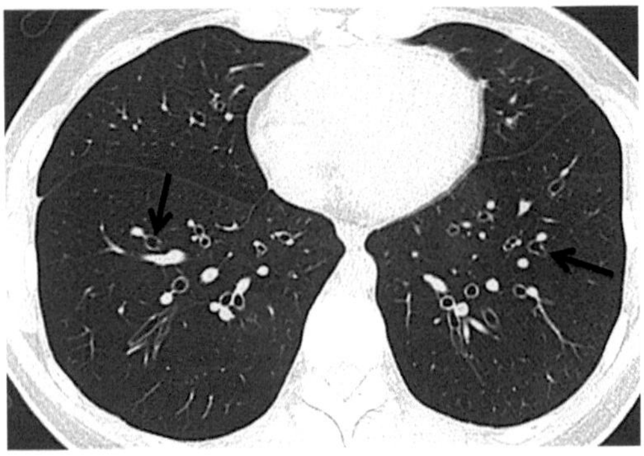

Fig. 10.10 Obliterative bronchiolitis. CT image during expiration shows diffuse air-trapping and diffuse cylindrical bronchiectasis (*arrows*) in this patient with obliterative bronchiolitis from collagen vascular disease

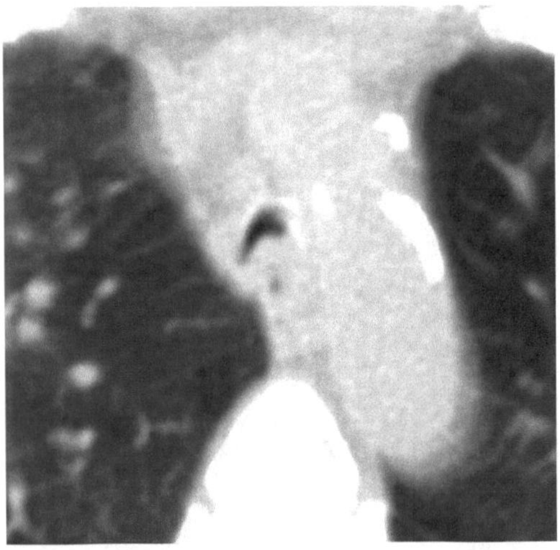

Fig. 10.11 Tracheobronchomalacia. Dynamic expiratory CT shows severe collapse of the trachea, nearly occluding the tracheal lumen, essentially diagnostic of tracheomalacia

decreased attenuation during inspiration are seen in both BO and asthma on CT [22]. Inspiratory mosaic attenuation and lobular areas of air trapping favor a diagnosis of obliterative bronchiolitis (Fig. 10.10). However, a small subset of BO patients with diffuse air trapping may be indistinguishable on imaging from patients with asthma [11]. Sarcoidosis may be favored by demographic features and extrapulmonary involvement, while hypersensitivity pneumonitis may be suggested by exposure history. Imaging features of sarcoidosis include symmetric mediastinal and hilar lymphadenopathy with or without upper lobe predominant perilymphatic nodules. Hypersensitivity pneumonitis manifests on HRCT as lobular areas of air trapping and ground-glass opacity (classically centrilobular in location) [23]. In both chronic sarcoidosis and chronic hypersensitivity pneumonitis, pulmonary fibrosis may develop and is often upper lung preponderant. TBM has been defined as greater than 50% collapse of the trachea or main bronchi during static or dynamic expiration (Fig. 10.11) [24]. However, current evidence suggests substantial overlap between normal and abnormal patients as even asymptomatic normal patients may demonstrate a high degree of large airways collapse [25].

Chronic Obstructive Pulmonary Disease

COPD is characterized by chronic airflow obstruction in the setting of small airways disease and parenchymal destruction [26]. It is the result of an inflammatory response caused by inhalation of noxious particles or gases, usually cigarette smoke, but also products of combustion like burning wood or biomass fuels and air pollution. COPD is extremely common. Prevalence of at least moderate disease is estimated at 10% in adults over 40 years and increases significantly with age [27, 28]. Historically, men have been affected more than women, but recently rates of disease are becoming equal between the sexes [29]. In the U.S., the death rate is higher for men than women, although more women than men currently die from the disease [30]. COPD is currently the sixth leading cause of death worldwide [31].

Genetic and environmental factors are involved in development of the disease. Smoking is a risk factor, and increasing pack-years smoked correlates with more advanced disease [27]. Other risk factors include childhood respiratory infections, low socioeconomic status, and chronic exposure to fumes of combustible products, occupational dusts and chemicals, and indoor and outdoor air pollution. Airflow obstruction is more common in siblings of those with severe COPD [32]. Alpha-1 antitrypsin (AAT) deficiency, a rare autosomal dominant disorder resulting in early emphysema, is the most well-known genetic cause of COPD. There are likely multiple other genetic variants that predispose to airflow obstruction and disease development, and research is ongoing in this area [33].

The natural history of COPD is an accelerated decrease in lung function over time. Normal aging results in a gradual decline of FEV_1, whereas patients with COPD who continue to smoke have decline at an accelerated rate. When the offending agent is removed, the rate of FEV_1 decline reverts back to normal [34]. Typical symptoms of COPD include the insidious onset of progressive exertional dyspnea, chronic cough, and chronic sputum production. In a person with these symptoms who has risk factors for the disease, spirometry is used to confirm the diagnosis. The spirometric hallmark is the finding of airflow obstruction that is not fully reversible, typically a post-bronchodilator FEV_1/FVC ratio less than 0.70. Spirometry, along with patient symptoms, aids in assessment of disease severity.

COPD is a heterogeneous disease. Clinical presentations among patients may be substantially different. COPD has classically been described as an overlap of emphysema and chronic bronchitis. Chronic uncontrolled asthma may also be included when it results in obstruction that is not completely reversible. Historically, patients were classified as having emphysematous type with predominant symptoms of exertional dyspnea or bronchial type with predominant symptoms of cough and sputum production. This classification has fallen out of favor because clinical distinctions have not been shown to correlate with pathologic findings [35]. It is known that a broad spectrum of disease phenotypes exists. There are multiple different diseases that result in chronic, irreversible airflow obstruction, and these may respond to differing therapies. Although spirometry is useful in diagnosis, it does not often distinguish the etiology of disease. Current research is focusing on the correlation between genetic variants and thoracic imaging findings, including varying degrees of air trapping, emphysema, and airway wall thickening, to determine subtypes of COPD and related susceptibility genes [36]. Imaging findings may prove to be the best predictor of disease phenotype and help guide therapy [37].

Emphysema

Emphysema refers to destruction of the acinus, the unit of lung structure distal to the terminal bronchiole. Inflammation is central to its development. Inflammatory cells are recruited to sites of irritant exposure, and their products cause injury to normal tissue. In addition, an imbalance between proteinases and anti-proteinases may develop, favoring destruction of elastic fibers and alveolar attachments. Loss of lung elasticity leads to increased compliance and higher lung volumes. The overall result of these processes is enlargement and destruction of the airspaces. With alveolar loss there is inherently less surface area for gas exchange, and hypoxia and hypercapnia are not uncommon in later stages of disease. Moreover, healthy lung parenchyma helps maintain adjacent airway patency through wall attachments that tether the airways open [38]. Emphysematous lung tissue loses its ability to support adjacent airways, which can lead to airway collapse and resultant air trapping.

Pulmonary function testing reflects these abnormalities. In addition to airflow obstruction, increases in RV, TLC, and functional residual capacity (FRC) are manifestations of air trapping and decreased elastic recoil. Reduced diffusing capacity of carbon monoxide (DLCO) is an indication of dysfunctional gas exchange from loss of alveolar surface area.

Pathologically, emphysema is a group of diseases that show irreversible alveolar septal destruction and enlargement of airspaces distal to the terminal bronchiole [39]. Four histologic patterns have been described and correlate with

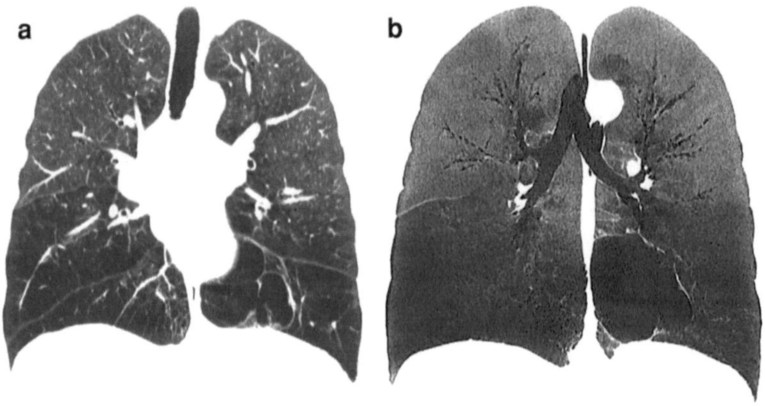

Fig. 10.12 Panlobular emphysema. **a** Coronal CT image shows diffuse decreased attenuation in the lung bases highly suggestive of panlobular emphysema in this patient with alpha-1-antitrypsin deficiency. **b** Coronal MinIP accentuates the relative diffuse basilar low attenuation

the anatomic location of septal destruction on imaging. Panlobular emphysema (PLE) involves the entire acinus. That is, the alveoli enlarge and become indistinct from the alveolar ducts and respiratory bronchioles, making the acini appear uniform. It most commonly affects the lower lobes of the lung (Fig. 10.12). It is the common pathologic finding in AAT deficiency. Patients with AAT deficiency typically do not manifest panlobular emphysematous changes prior to age 30. However, any person with emphysema younger than age 45 or without a smoking history should be screened for this disorder. Other rare causes of lower lung panlobular emphysema include "Ritalin® lung" (from IV injection of crushed methylphenidate tablets) and hypocomplementemic urticarial vasculitis syndrome. In contrast, centrilobular emphysema (CLE) is characterized by enlargement and destruction of the respiratory bronchioles, leaving more distal alveolar ducts and sacs unaffected until late in the disease [40]. It is predominantly found in an upper lobe and posterior distribution and is the type of emphysema most associated with smoking (Fig. 10.13) [41]. Paraseptal emphysema (PSE) describes enlargement and destruction of alveolar ducts and sacs adjacent to the pleura, along lobular septa, and along larger airways and blood vessels (Fig. 10.14). The distinguishing feature from CLE is that PSE spares the respiratory bronchioles [42]. It may be associated with fibrosis between the enlarged airspaces and can be found concurrently with CLE. Paracicatricial emphysema consists of enlargement and destruction of airspaces adjacent to scarring (Fig. 10.15) [39]. It can affect any part of the acinus.

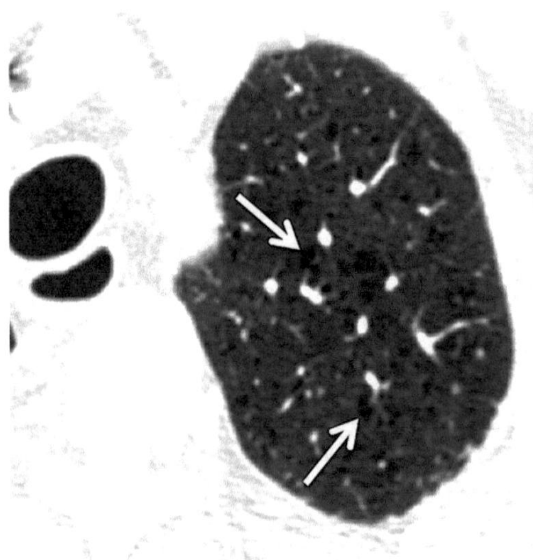

Fig. 10.13 Centrilobular emphysema. CT image shows focal centrilobular lucencies (*arrows*) without discernable walls in the left upper lobe essentially diagnostic of centrilobular emphysema

Radiologic evaluation of emphysema begins with the chest radiograph. Imaging findings that help support the diagnosis include lung

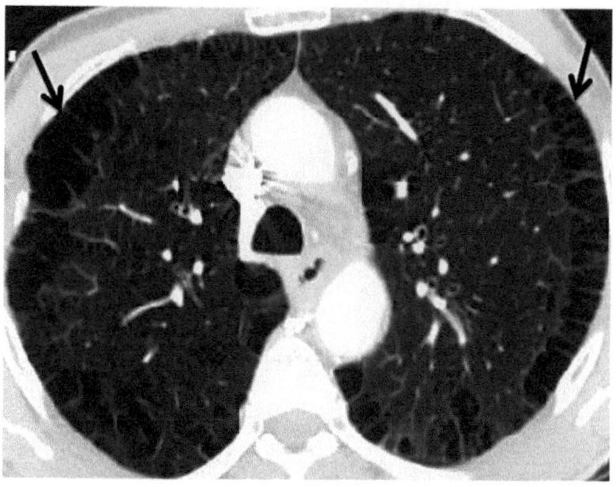

Fig. 10.14 Paraseptal emphysema. CT image shows subpleural cystic spaces (*arrows*) typical of paraseptal emphysema. In contradistinction to honeycombing, the cystic spaces in this case do not stack on *top* of one another and appear to coalesce with adjacent cysts

hyperinflation, loss of pulmonary vascular markings and the normal vascular branching pattern, bronchial wall thickening, and large focal lucencies with thin walls, indicative of bullae (Fig. 10.16) [39]. It is nearly impossible to distinguish the different types of emphysema on chest radiography alone. However, if a concurrent disease process fills the surrounding airspaces, such as edema, hemorrhage, or consolidation, these findings may bring out the anatomical location and definition of the small emphysematous spaces. For example, small lucencies seen within pneumonia may represent centrilobular emphysema.

Conventional CT improves depiction of extent, type, and anatomic distribution of emphysema while even greater qualitative assessment is provided with HRCT [43]. Thin section contiguous images, typically acquired at 1–1.25 mm, can detect early subclinical emphysema. Post-processing techniques, like minimum intensity projection images, can help to further qualify morphologic patterns of emphysema.

HRCT is 88% sensitive, 90% specific, and 89% accurate in the diagnosis of CLE [44]. Randomly distributed centrilobular low-attenuation spaces (below-950 HU) with imperceptible septal walls are suggestive of CLE [41]. Upper and posterior lung parenchyma is affected most often, particularly in heavy smokers. Pruning and distortion of the pulmonary vascular bed, which can occur in all forms of emphysema, can be seen on CT as arborization and loss of the normal vascular pattern, as well as bowing of remaining vessels about the emphysematous spaces [41].

HRCT is 48% sensitive, 97% specific, and 89% accurate at detecting PLE [44]. Its low sensitivity is likely attributable to the loss of juxtaposition of normal lung and emphysematous spaces. In contrast to CLE, the lung destruction primarily involves the lower lungs. Other CT findings include panlobular low-attenuation spaces with imperceptible septal walls, loss of vessel caliber, and decrease in vessel attenuation [39, 43]. Patients with AAT deficiency may also have associated bronchial wall thickening or bronchiectasis [45].

PSE has a characteristic appearance on CT. Imaging shows dilated, rectangular distal airspaces which share adjoining walls in a subpleural or peripheral location within the upper lung zones [39]. PSE has been implicated in causing spontaneous pneumothorax, particularly in tall, young, thin males. It can also progress to bullous emphysema. It is important to note that there is a higher incidence of lung cancer adjacent to bullae, and therefore it is important to analyze bullae appearances, as changes in size, shape, and wall thickness may indicate malignancy [1].

Paracicatricial emphysema occurs around areas of parenchymal scarring. This is most often seen in conditions that cause lung scarring, such as tuberculosis, silicosis, sarcoidosis, paracoccidioidomycosis, and adenocarcinoma

In addition to distinguishing emphysema subtypes, CT, specifically micro-CT and volumetric CT, has been used to identify and quantify the degree of proximal airway and terminal bronchiole destruction in COPD. Patients with fewer proximal airways and greater terminal bronchiole destruction have been shown to have more severe emphysematous disease [46, 47]. Diaz et al. assessed the relationship between central airway count and emphysema burden in a subset of smokers and found that subjects with greater than or equal to 25% emphysema had a

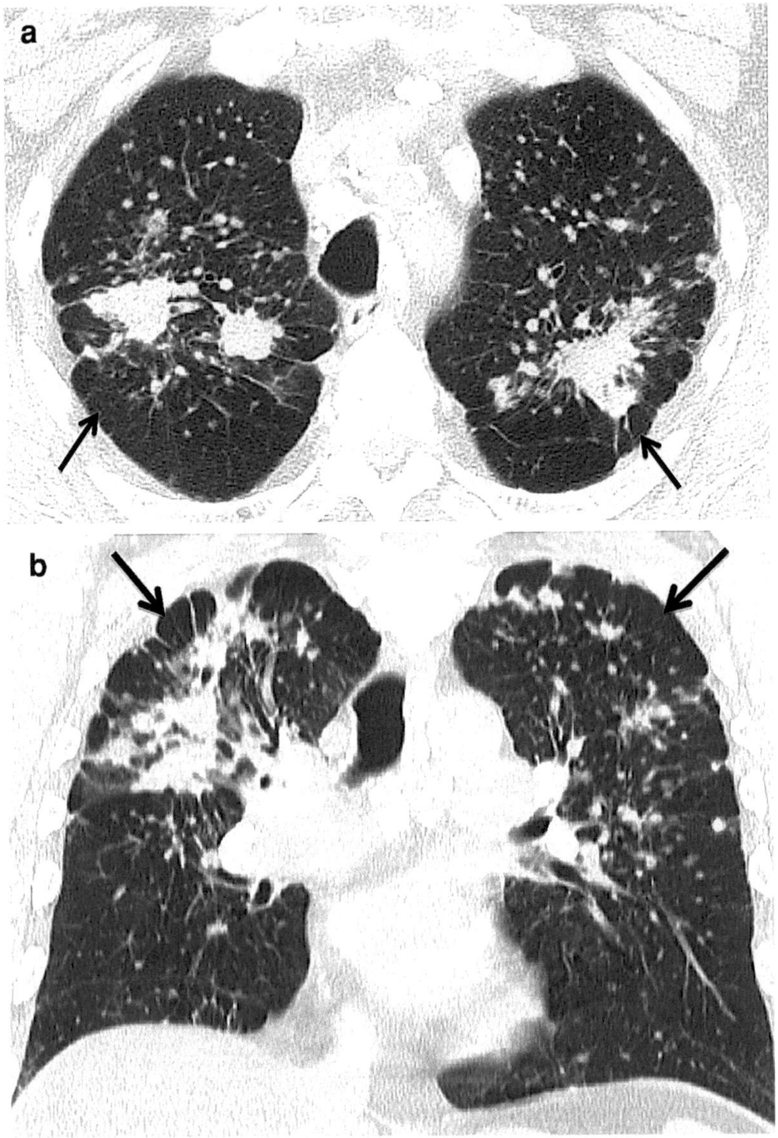

Fig. 10.15 Paracicatricial emphysema in complicated silicosis. Axial (**a**) and coronal (**b**) images from chest CT show progressive massive fibrosis in the upper lobes with associated centrilobular nodularity in this patient with complicated silicosis. There are peripheral areas of decreased lung attenuation (*arrows*) consistent with paracicatricial emphysema

statistically significant lower total airway count than subjects with less than 25% emphysema. In addition, they further showed that total airway count on CT has a direct association with lower predicted FEV_1 and DLCO [48]. Another recent study showed CT extent of emphysema to be helpful in prediction of mortality in COPD [49].

While CT is useful in diagnosing and monitoring emphysema patients, it can also be used for presurgical planning and post-surgical imaging of lung volume reduction surgery (LVRS), a viable option for a subset of patients with severe emphysema. The National Emphysema Treatment Trial (NETT), a randomized controlled trial of 1,218 patients with

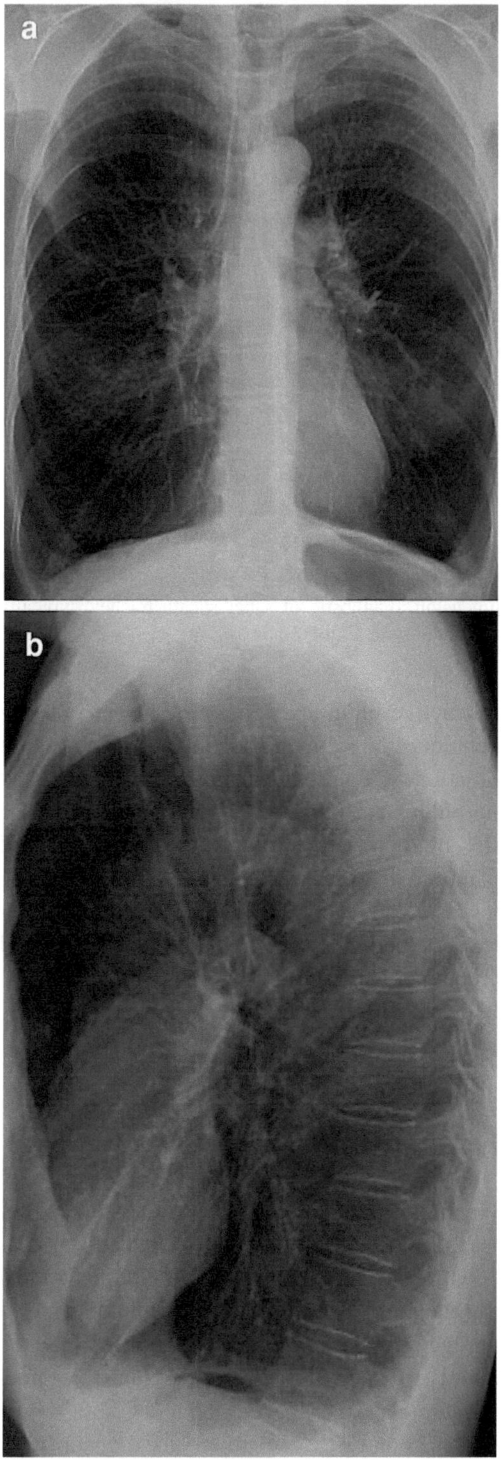

◄ **Fig. 10.16** Panlobular emphysema on radiography. PA (**a**) and lateral (**b**) chest radiographs show hyperinflation of the lungs suggested by flattening of the diaphragm and increased size of the retrosternal space. There is also relative paucity of lung markings at the lung bases, consistent with basilar predominant panlobular emphysema

emphysema, showed that LVRS was most beneficial in a subgroup of subjects with low exercise capacity and upper lobe predominant emphysema [50].

Chronic Bronchitis

Chronic bronchitis is defined as sputum production and cough on most days over at least 3 months for two consecutive years, when other causes have been ruled out. It is a result of chronic exposure to cigarette smoke or other inhaled irritants that cause airway epithelial injury. There is typically an infiltration of CD8+ T cells, neutrophils, and macrophages in the airway walls [51]. Chronic inflammation of the small airways leads to remodeling, characterized by squamous and mucus metaplasia of the airway epithelium, smooth muscle hypertrophy, and fibrosis of the airway wall [52]. Goblet and mucus cells increase in number and size. There is an increase in mucus secretion and the composition of airway mucus is altered. In addition, loss of cilia, ciliary dysfunction, and increased smooth muscle and connective tissue may be found in the airways [39]. This process leads to obstruction with luminal occlusion caused by mucus [53], airway narrowing [54], and alteration of the surface tension of the airway [55].

Chronic bronchitis is a clinical diagnosis, with radiographs only providing supportive evidence. Chest radiography is an early step in evaluation, although it may be unrevealing. Nonspecific radiographic features that may suggest the diagnosis include bronchial wall thickening, tram

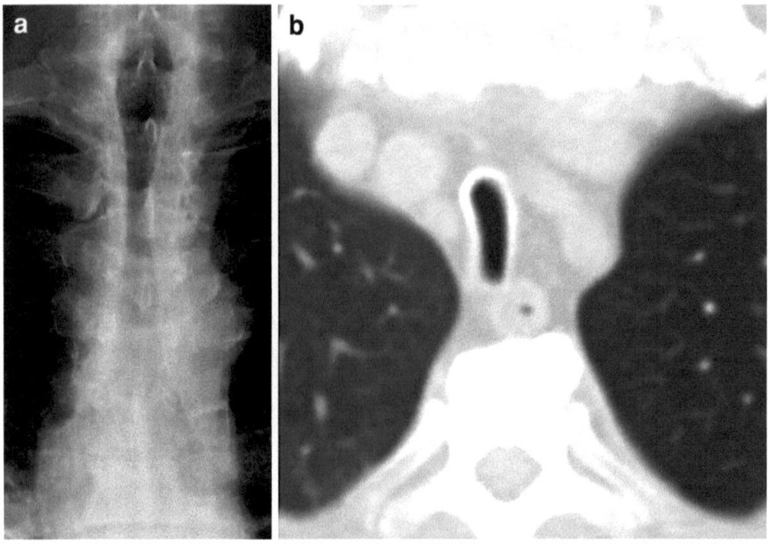

Fig. 10.17 Saber sheath trachea. **a** Magnified image from a PA chest radiograph shows narrowing of the trachea. **b** CT image shows decreased lateral tracheal dimension and increased anterior–posterior tracheal dimension, diagnostic of saber sheath trachea, typically associated with COPD

tracking, interstitial thickening, hyperinflation, and tortuous pulmonary arteries. In addition, saber sheath tracheal (increased AP diameter of the tracheal) deformation may also raise the possibility of chronic bronchitis, due to its strong association (Fig. 10.17). Chest CT and HRCT evaluation may better depict airway inflammation, seen as bronchial wall thickening and centrilobular opacities. However, these findings are nonspecific. Many patients with chronic bronchitis also concomitantly have features of centrilobular emphysema on CT [56]. Acute exacerbations of chronic bronchitis, characterized by periods of worsening dyspnea, cough, and sputum production, are often attributable to infections.

New Technology in Imaging of Obstructive Pulmonary Diseases

New, innovative technology may change the way obstructive pulmonary diseases are diagnosed, evaluated, and treated. In the future, therapy will be directed at "subsets" or "phenotypes" of patients. While MDCT has been the primary imaging modality for evaluation of obstructive pulmonary diseases, newer imaging techniques offer unique advantages. Synchrotron radiation CT provides both functional and morphological information. Hyperpolarized ^{3}He MR offers improved temporal resolution and quantitative measurements of functional lung tissue. Lastly, optical coherence tomography delivers depth-resolved 3D imaging of small structures, including airways less than 2 mm in diameter.

Synchrotron Radiation CT

Synchrotron radiation CT is a technique pioneered by Bayat et al. that uses inhaled xenon as a contrast agent to image both lung function and morphology. The complicated technique uses a K-edge subtraction method to image only the contrast dispersed within the lungs without measurement of adjacent bone or soft tissue. Xenon contrast can then be quantifiably measured, allowing for assessment of regional ventilation [57]. Limitations to its utilization include high radiation exposure, limited availability of Synchrotron radiation sources, and the requirement for the x-ray beam plane to remain stationary, which mandates coordinated automated movement of the patient for image acquisition [58].

Hyperpolarized ^{3}He MR

Hyperpolarized helium 3 (^{3}He) MR imaging, although currently FDA approved for investigational use only, has the potential to become widely utilized and approved for clinical applications. ^{3}He MR entails optical pumping of helium into airways and imaging its dispersion [59]. Diffusion-weighted images are obtained to calculate the apparent diffusion coefficient (ADC) of helium, which is a measurement of airspace size. It allows evaluation of the spatial and temporal distribution of ventilation, as compared to Synchrotron radiation CT, which evaluates spatial ventilation only. Airspace size and regional oxygen partial pressure are also able to be determined [60]. The ADC coefficient of helium is increased in larger, more damaged alveoli as the emphysematous alveolar spaces allow greater distribution of helium [59]. Evaluation of the ADC of helium distribution may also offer insight into early obstructive lung disease. Smokers without emphysema by CT imaging showed heterogeneous distribution of helium, while nonsmokers had homogeneous dispersal. This suggests the possibility of detecting presymptomatic declining lung function and emphysematous changes [61]. Patients with asthma often demonstrate more ventilation defects than their normal counterparts on ^{3}He MR lung ventilation imaging [62]. Furthermore, ^{3}He MR lung ventilation imaging both predicts and correlates with spirometric asthma severity, including decreased FEV_1/FVC and DLCO measurements [63]. Although still investigational, ^{3}He is considered relatively safe, lacks ionizing radiation, and has been shown to have no serious adverse effects on patients. It also can be utilized in patients with varying lung function (including normal subjects, smokers, and patients with obstructive disease) [60]. Individuals can also be assessed over time, allowing for monitoring of therapeutic response [63]. Limitations to current use include availability of ^{3}He [11]. Alternative options exist, including the use of pure oxygen for ventilation imaging. However, in patients with obstructive pulmonary disease, administration of high concentrations of oxygen should be cautioned, as respiratory depression can ensue [64].

Optical Coherence Tomography

Optical coherence tomography (OCT) has been used since the early 1990s to evaluate the retina and coronary arteries [65]. Improvements in technology and resolution have allowed utilization in thoracic imaging. OCT uses an endobronchial fiber-optic probe to emit near-infrared light. A detector collects reflected and back scattered signals and generates an image with resolution approaching 5–15 nm [66]. This micro resolution has been useful in evaluation of endoluminal lesions, with studies suggesting the ability to distinguish among neoplasia, carcinoma in situ, metaplasia, and dysplasia [67]. It can also provide microscopic information about the mural remodeling of the airways in COPD patients. As the site of obstruction is primarily based within the peripheral airways, particularly of the 11th and 12th generation [68], OCT can provide increased spatial resolution and more accurate measurements within these minute structures [66, 69] The increased sensitivity also allows for more accurate monitoring of disease progression [69].

References

1. Ferrara A. Chronic obstructive pulmonary disease. Radiol Technol. 2011;82(3):245–63.
2. Celli BR, MacNee W. Standards for the diagnosis and treatment of patients with COPD: a summary of the ATS/ERS position paper. Eur Respir J. 2004; 23(6):932–46.

3. Tsai TW, Gallagher EJ, Lombardi G, Gennis P, Carter W. Guidelines for the selective ordering of admission chest radiography in adult obstructive airway disease. Ann Emerg Med. 1993;22(12):1854–8.
4. Webb WR. Thin-section CT of the secondary pulmonary lobule: anatomy and the image–the 2004 Fleischner lecture. Radiology. 2006;239(2): 322–38.
5. From the Expert Panel Report 3 (EPR3): Guidelines for the Diagnosis and Management of Asthma, National Heart Lung and Blood Institute. 2007. http://www.nhlbi.nih.gov/guidelines/asthma/asthgdln.htm. Accessed 15 May 2011.
6. Centers for Disease Control and Prevention. 2007 National Health Interview Survey Data. Table 4-1 Current Asthma Prevalence Percents by Age, United States: National Health Interview Survey, 2007. Atlanta, GA: U.S. Department of Health and Human Services, CDC. 2010. http://www.cdc.gov/asthma/nhis/07/table4-1.htm. Accessed 15 May 2011.
7. Busse WW, Lemanske RF Jr. Asthma. N Engl J Med. 2001;344(5):350–62.
8. Holgate ST, Polosa R. The mechanisms, diagnosis, and management of severe asthma in adults. Lancet. 2006;368(9537):780–93.
9. Haldar P, Pavord ID, Shaw DE, et al. Cluster analysis and clinical asthma phenotypes. Am J Respir Crit Care Med. 2008;178(3):218–24.
10. Gibson GJ. Pulmonary hyperinflation a clinical overview. Eur Respir J. 1996;9(12):2640–9.
11. Woods AQ, Lynch DA. Asthma: an imaging update. Radiol Clin North Am. 2009;47(2):317–29.
12. Charles MW. Studies of mortality of atomic bomb survivors. Report 13: Solid cancer and noncancer disease mortality: 1950–1997. J Radiol Prot. 2003; 23(4):457–9.
13. Aysola RS, Hoffman EA, Gierada D, et al. Airway remodeling measured by multidetector CT is increased in severe asthma and correlates with pathology. Chest. 2008;134(6):1183–91.
14. Busacker A, Newell JD Jr, Keefe T, et al. A multivariate analysis of risk factors for the air-trapping asthmatic phenotype as measured by quantitative CT analysis. Chest. 2009;135(1):48–56.
15. Paganin F, Seneterre E, Chanez P, et al. Computed tomography of the lungs in asthma: influence of disease severity and etiology. Am J Respir Crit Care Med. 1996;153(1):110–4.
16. Lynch DA, Newell JD, Tschomper BA, Cink TM, Newman LS, Bethel R. Uncomplicated asthma in adults: comparison of CT appearance of the lungs in asthmatic and healthy subjects. Radiology. 1993;188(3):829–33.
17. Park CS, Muller NL, Worthy SA, Kim JS, Awadh N, Fitzgerald M. Airway obstruction in asthmatic and healthy individuals: inspiratory and expiratory thin-section CT findings. Radiology. 1997;203(2):361–7.
18. Takemura M, Niimi A, Minakuchi M, et al. Bronchial dilatation in asthma: relation to clinical and sputum indices. Chest. 2004;125(4):1352–8.
19. Greenberger PA. Allergic bronchopulmonary aspergillosis. J Allergy Clin Immunol. 2002;110(5): 685–92.
20. Alam M, Burki NK. Chronic eosinophilic pneumonia: a review. South Med J. 2007;100(1):49–53.
21. Hicks M, Brugman SM, Katial R. Vocal cord dysfunction/paradoxical vocal fold motion. Prim Care. 2008;35(1):81–103. vii.
22. Jensen SP, Lynch DA, Brown KK, Wenzel SE, Newell JD. High-resolution CT features of severe asthma and bronchiolitis obliterans. Clin Radiol. 2002;57(12):1078–85.
23. Silva CI, Churg A, Muller NL. Hypersensitivity pneumonitis: spectrum of high-resolution CT and pathologic findings. AJR Am J Roentgenol. 2007;188(2):334–44.
24. Lee EY, Litmanovich D, Boiselle PM. Multidetector CT evaluation of tracheobronchomalacia. Radiol Clin North Am. 2009;47(2):261–9.
25. Boiselle PM, O'Donnell CR, Bankier AA, et al. Tracheal collapsibility in healthy volunteers during forced expiration: assessment with multidetector CT. Radiology. 2009;252(1):255–62.
26. From the Global Strategy for the Diagnosis, Management and Prevention of COPD, Global Initiative for Chronic Obstructive Lung Disease (GOLD). 2010. http://www.goldcopd.org. Accessed 15 May 2011.
27. Buist AS, McBurnie MA, Vollmer WM, et al. International variation in the prevalence of COPD (the BOLD Study): a population-based prevalence study. Lancet. 2007;370(9589):741–50.
28. Menezes AM, Perez-Padilla R, Jardim JR, et al. Chronic obstructive pulmonary disease in five Latin American cities (the PLATINO study): a prevalence study. Lancet. 2005;366(9500):1875–81.
29. Mannino DM, Buist AS. Global burden of COPD: risk factors, prevalence, and future trends. Lancet. 2007;370(9589):765–73.
30. Centers for Disease Control and Prevention. MMWR weekly: Deaths from Chronic Obstructive Pulmonary Disease - United States, 2000–2005. (2008). http://www.cdc.gov/mmwr/preview/mmwrhtml/mm5745a4.htm. Accessed 15 May 2011.
31. Murray CJ, Lopez AD. Alternative projections of mortality and disability by cause 1990–2020: global burden of disease study. Lancet. 1997;349(9064): 1498–504.
32. McCloskey SC, Patel BD, Hinchliffe SJ, Reid ED, Wareham NJ, Lomas DA. Siblings of patients with severe chronic obstructive pulmonary disease have a significant risk of airflow obstruction. Am J Respir Crit Care Med. 2001;164(8 Pt 1):1419–24.
33. Silverman EK, Palmer LJ, Mosley JD, et al. Genomewide linkage analysis of quantitative spirometric phenotypes in severe early-onset chronic obstructive pulmonary disease. Am J Hum Genet. 2002;70(5):1229–39.
34. Fletcher C, Peto R. The natural history of chronic airflow obstruction. Br Med J. 1977;1(6077):1645–8.

35. Thurlbeck W, Henderson J, Fraser F, Bates D. Chronic obstructive lung disease. A comparison between clinical, roentgenologic, functional and morphologic criteria in chronic bronchitis, emphysema, asthma and bronchiectasis. J Occup Med. 1970;12(12):533.
36. Regan EA, Hokanson JE, Murphy JR, et al. Genetic epidemiology of COPD (COPDGene) study design. COPD. 2010;7(1):32–43.
37. Hansen B. Finding phenotypes. ACR Bull. 2011; 66(4):23.
38. Saetta M, Ghezzo H, Kim WD, et al. Loss of alveolar attachments in smokers. A morphometric correlate of lung function impairment. Am Rev Respir Dis. 1985;132(4):894–900.
39. Pipavath SN, Schmidt RA, Takasugi JE, Godwin JD. Chronic obstructive pulmonary disease: radiology-pathology correlation. J Thorac Imaging. 2009;24(3): 171–80.
40. Leopold JG, Gough J. The centrilobular form of hypertrophic emphysema and its relation to chronic bronchitis. Thorax. 1957;12(3):219–35.
41. Foster WL Jr, Pratt PC, Roggli VL, Godwin JD, Halvorsen RA Jr, Putman CE. Centrilobular emphysema: CT-pathologic correlation. Radiology. 1986;159(1):27–32.
42. Wright JL. Chronic airflow obstruction. In: Churg AM, Myers JL, Talezar HD, et al, editors. Thurlbeck's Pathology of the Lung. New York: Thieme; 2005.
43. Thurlbeck WM, Muller NL. Emphysema: definition, imaging, and quantification. AJR Am J Roentgenol. 1994;163(5):1017–25.
44. Copley SJ, Wells AU, Muller NL, et al. Thin-section CT in obstructive pulmonary disease: discriminatory value. Radiology. 2002;223(3):812–9.
45. King MA, Stone JA, Diaz PT, Mueller CF, Becker WJ, Gadek JE. Alpha 1-antitrypsin deficiency: evaluation of bronchiectasis with CT. Radiology. 1996;199(1):137–41.
46. Kim WD, Ling SH, Coxson HO, et al. The association between small airway obstruction and emphysema phenotypes in COPD. Chest. 2007; 131(5):1372–8.
47. Hogg JC, McDonough JE, Sanchez PG, et al. Micro-computed tomography measurements of peripheral lung pathology in chronic obstructive pulmonary disease. Proc Am Thorac Soc. 2009;6(6):546–9.
48. Diaz AA, Valim C, Yamashiro T, et al. Airway count and emphysema assessed by chest CT imaging predicts clinical outcome in smokers. Chest. 2010;138(4):880–7.
49. Haruna A, Muro S, Nakano Y, et al. CT scan findings of emphysema predict mortality in COPD. Chest. 2010;138(3):635–40.
50. Naunheim KS, Wood DE, Mohsenifar Z, et al. Long-term follow-up of patients receiving lung-volume-reduction surgery versus medical therapy for severe emphysema by the National Emphysema Treatment Trial Research Group. Ann Thorac Surg. 2006;82(2):431–43.
51. Cosio MG, Majo J. Inflammation of the airways and lung parenchyma in COPD: role of T cells. Chest. 2002;121(5 Suppl):160S–5S.
52. Kim V, Rogers TJ, Criner GJ. New concepts in the pathobiology of chronic obstructive pulmonary disease. Proc Am Thorac Soc. 2008;5(4):478–85.
53. Hogg JC, Chu F, Utokaparch S, et al. The nature of small-airway obstruction in chronic obstructive pulmonary disease. N Engl J Med. 2004;350(26): 2645–53.
54. James AL, Wenzel S. Clinical relevance of airway remodelling in airway diseases. Eur Respir J. 2007;30(1):134–55.
55. Macklem PT, Proctor DF, Hogg JC. The stability of peripheral airways. Respir Physiol. 1970;8(2): 191–203.
56. Webb WR. Radiology of obstructive pulmonary disease. AJR Am J Roentgenol. 1997;169(3):637–47.
57. Bayat S, Le Duc G, Porra L, et al. Quantitative functional lung imaging with synchrotron radiation using inhaled xenon as contrast agent. Phys Med Biol. 2001;46(12):3287–99.
58. Bayat S, Porra L, Suhonen H, et al. Imaging of lung function using synchrotron radiation computed tomography: what's new? Eur J Radiol. 2008;68(3 Suppl):S78–83.
59. Tino G, Ware LB, Moss M. Clinical year in Review IV: chronic obstructive pulmonary disease, nonpulmonary critical care, diagnostic imaging, and mycobacterial disease. Proc Am Thorac Soc. 2007;4(6):494–8.
60. Lutey BA, Lefrak SS, Woods JC, et al. Hyperpolarized ^{3}He MR imaging: physiologic monitoring observations and safety considerations in 100 consecutive subjects. Radiology. 2008;248(2): 655–61.
61. Fain SB, Panth SR, Evans MD, et al. Early emphysematous changes in asymptomatic smokers: detection with ^{3}He MR imaging. Radiology. 2006; 239(3):875–83.
62. Altes TA, Powers PL, Knight-Scott J, et al. Hyperpolarized ^{3}He MR lung ventilation imaging in asthmatics: preliminary findings. J Magn Reson Imaging. 2001;13(3):378–84.
63. de Lange EE, Altes TA, Patrie JT, et al. Evaluation of asthma with hyperpolarized helium-3 MRI: correlation with clinical severity and spirometry. Chest. 2006;130(4):1055–62.
64. Ley-Zaporozhan J, Kauczor HU. Imaging of airways: chronic obstructive pulmonary disease. Radiol Clin North Am. 2009;47(2):331–42.
65. Huang D, Swanson EA, Lin CP, et al. Optical coherence tomography. Science. 1991;254(5035):1178–81.
66. Coxson HO, Quiney B, Sin DD, et al. Airway wall thickness assessed using computed tomography and optical coherence tomography. Am J Respir Crit Care Med. 2008;177(11):1201–6.

67. Newton RC, Kemp SV, Shah PL, et al. Progress toward optical biopsy: bringing the microscope to the patient. Lung. 2011;189(2):111–9.
68. Kikawada M, Ichinose Y, Miyamoto D, Minemura K, Takasaki M, Toyama K. Peripheral airway findings in chronic obstructive pulmonary disease using an ultrathin bronchoscope. Eur Respir J. 2000;15(1):105–8.
69. Washko GR. Diagnostic imaging in COPD. Semin Respir Crit Care Med. 2010;31(3):276–85.

Imaging of Airway Disease

11

Shailaja J. Hayden and Sudhakar N. J. Pipavath

Abstract

Airway diseases are broadly classified into those affecting the trachea, the bronchi, and the bronchioles. This chapter will discuss imaging of diseases affecting the airway with relevance to clinical care providers. Elaborate tables and figures in this chapter provide a simplistic overview of approach to imaging the trachea, bronchi, and the bronchioles.

Keywords

High-resolution computed tomography (HRCT) · Tracheomalacia · Bronchiectasis · Bronchiolitis · Tree-in-bud pattern

Introduction

The human airway consists of the trachea, bronchi, bronchioles, and alveolar ducts and sacs. The classic Weibel model of airway anatomy describes 23 generations of airways from trachea to alveoli, created by symmetric dichotomous branching [1]. Although this model is valuable for its simplicity, in reality there is considerably more asymmetry and variability. Conceptually, airways can be divided into three categories:

- Conducting zone, consisting of the bronchi and membranous bronchioles, down to terminal bronchioles; these airways are not involved in gas exchange.
- Transitional zone, consisting of respiratory bronchioles, which have both gas-exchanging and non-gas-exchanging epithelium.
- Gas exchange zone, consisting of alveolar ducts, alveolar sacs, and alveoli. By definition, bronchi have cartilage in their walls and bronchioles do not. Airway diseases are often divided into diseases of the trachea, large airway disease, and small airways disease.

Diseases of the Trachea

The trachea extends from the inferior aspect of the cricoid cartilage to the carina, generally 10–12 cm in the adult. Its anterior aspect is

S. J. Hayden
Division of Pulmonary and Critical Care Medicine, University of Washington, 7101 Roosevelt Way NE #304, Seattle, WA 98115, USA
e-mail: sathys@uw.edu

S. N. J. Pipavath (✉)
Department of Radiology, University of Washington, 1959 NE Pacific Street #357115, Seattle, WA 98195, USA
e-mail: snjp@uw.edu

J. P. Kanne (ed.), *Clinically Oriented Pulmonary Imaging*, Respiratory Medicine, DOI: 10.1007/978-1-61779-542-8_11,

Table 11.1 Etiologies of tracheal narrowing

Tracheal stenosis Congenital Acquired
Tracheomalacia
Saber-sheath trachea
Tracheal tumors
Granulomatous infection
Wegener granulomatosis
Amyloidosis
Tracheobronchopathia osteochondroplastica
Relapsing polychondritis
Airway burns

supported by 18–22 semicircular cartilaginous rings; the posterior trachea is membranous. Tracheal diseases can be divided into complex congenital anomalies such as tracheoesophageal fistula, disorders that cause tracheal narrowing (see Table 11.1), or those which cause tracheal enlargement. Several selected diseases will be discussed further here.

Tracheal Stenosis

Congenital tracheal stenosis is often the result of ring-shaped cartilage (rather than the normal horseshoe shape). Acquired tracheal stenosis is usually a complication of tracheostomy (at the site of the stoma) or endotracheal intubation (most commonly subglottic in location). Clinical manifestations include dyspnea, difficulty clearing secretions, recurrent pneumonia, and respiratory failure. Physical exam may reveal stridor and monophonic wheezing. There may be flattening of both the inspiratory and expiratory limbs of a flow-volume curve. In acute post-intubation stenosis, radiographs may show tracheal narrowing, and CT often shows abnormal soft tissue internal to a normal appearing outer tracheal wall. Chronic stenosis causes fibrosis and deformity of the tracheal cartilage with a characteristic hourglass shape. It may be apparent on chest radiography (Fig. 11.1) but is best shown on a coronal reformatted CT. Bronchoscopy is often used to confirm the diagnosis. Management is individualized based on anatomy and etiology of stenosis; options include rigid or balloon dilation, laser therapy, airway stenting, or surgical resection (for stenotic segments less than 4 cm in length).

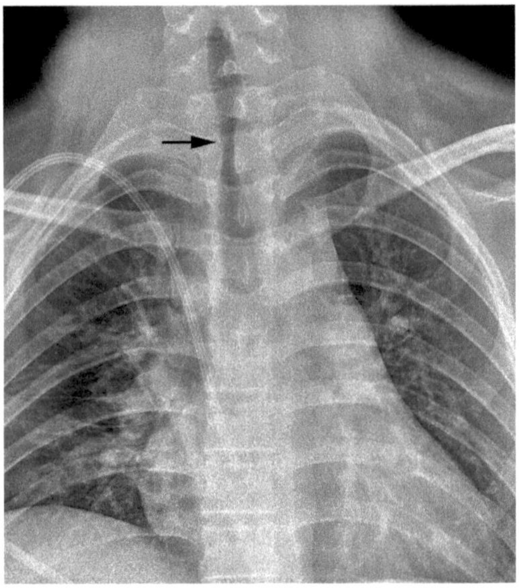

Fig. 11.1 Posteroanterior radiograph of the chest shows narrowing of the sub-glottic tracheal lumen (*arrow*)

Tracheomalacia

Tracheomalacia is defined as weakness of the tracheal wall, causing exaggerated narrowing during expiration, which can be congenital or acquired. Causes of acquired tracheomalacia include tracheostomy or endotracheal intubation, chest trauma or surgery, chronic compression as from a mediastinal goiter, relapsing polychondritis, emphysema, or recurrent infection. CT is accurate for diagnosis, but bronchoscopy remains the reference standard. The criteria are the same for both diagnostic modalities: excessive collapsibility, sometimes resembling the facial expression of frown (Fig. 11.2), and narrowing of the lumen by more than 50% during expiration. However, several studies [2] have

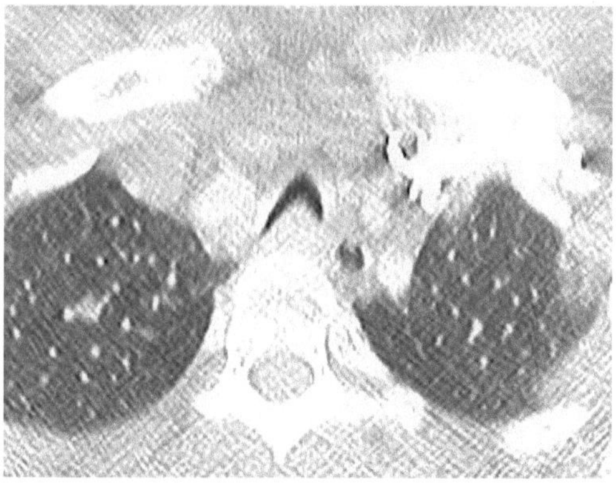

Fig. 11.2 CT image in expiratory phase shows excessive collapsibility of the trachea with narrowed tracheal lumen, anteriorly drawn posterior tracheal membrane and loss of normal convexity of the arch of the tracheal cartilage, resembling a frown on a face

shown more than 50% collapsibility in normal healthy volunteers, and, based on these findings, the authors recommend a conservative threshold of 70% decrease in luminal area to diagnose tracheomalacia by CT. A dynamic CT during active expiration or suspended inspiratory and expiratory CT showing reduction in lumen is valuable in the diagnosis of tracheomalacia (Fig. 11.3).

Saber-Sheath Trachea

Saber-sheath trachea is a common abnormality associated with chronic obstructive pulmonary disease. It is defined by coronal narrowing and sagittal widening of the intrathoracic trachea, with normal caliber of the cervical trachea. It is apparent on chest radiography, CT, and bronchoscopy, all of which show the characteristic coronal narrowing and sagittal widening of the trachea.

Tracheal Neoplasms

The overwhelming majority of malignant tracheal obstruction is from metastatic disease, with lung, laryngeal, and esophageal cancers being the most common etiologies. Primary tracheal tumors are uncommon [3]. The most frequently reported is squamous cell carcinoma, followed by adenoid cystic carcinoma. Even more rare neoplasms include carcinoid tumors, mucoepidermoid carcinoma, non-squamous carcinoma, small cell carcinoma, large cell carcinoma, adenocarcinoma, and sarcoma. Early diagnosis is difficult, as symptoms are often subtle and non specific (e.g., cough and dyspnea). Chest radiographs are not sensitive for smaller tumors. CT scan is excellent for identifying the presence of tumor and extent of direct or hematogenous spread. CT features that indicate a malignant tracheal process include nodular thickening, thickening greater than 2 cm, and endoluminal extension and infiltration of the surrounding soft tissues and organs (Fig. 11.4).

Amyloidosis

Respiratory tract amyloidosis is rare. AL amyloid accounts for 63–80% of cases. It can affect the larynx, tracheobronchial tree, or pulmonary parenchyma, with tracheobronchial disease being the most common [4]. Patients may be asymptomatic or may present with dyspnea, stridor, or even respiratory failure. Chest radiographs are often normal. CT may show airway wall thickening or irregularity, luminal narrowing, and sometimes calcification. Airway wall thickening can be circumferential, which indicates involvement of the posterior tracheal membrane (Fig. 11.5), or it can be focal, nodular, or plaque like. Diagnosis is made by bronchoscopy with biopsy; specimens show characteristic staining with Congo red dye and apple green birefringence under a polarized microscope.

Tracheobronchopathia Osteochondroplastica

This rare disorder of unknown cause is characterized by cartilaginous and osseous nodules

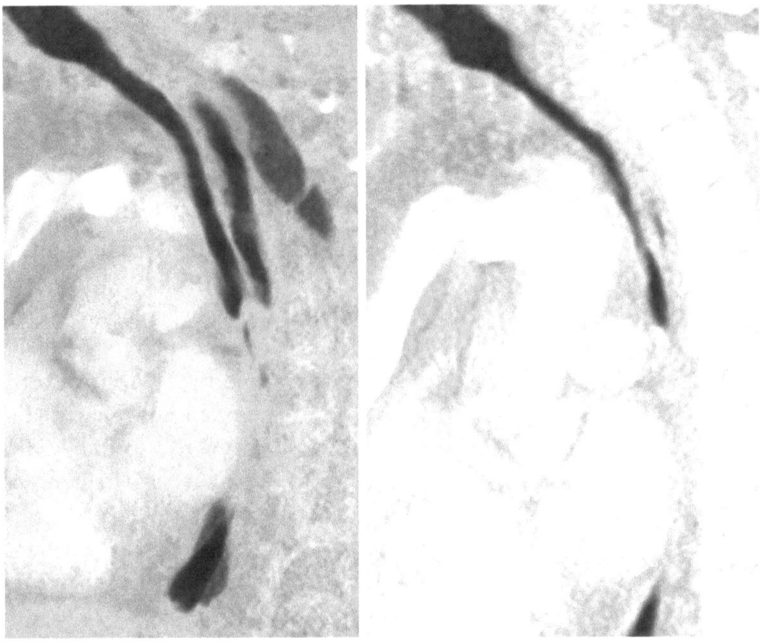

Fig. 11.3 Sagittal minimum intensity projection (MinIP) images show diminished AP diameter on inspiratory, **a** image and further collapse on expiratory image, **b** indicating tracheomalacia

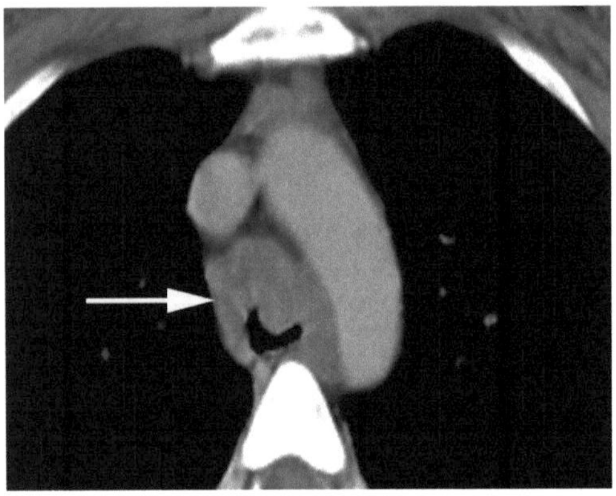

Fig. 11.4 Adenoidcystic carcinoma of the trachea. Contrast-enhanced CT image shows circumferential mass and nodular thickening (*arrow*)

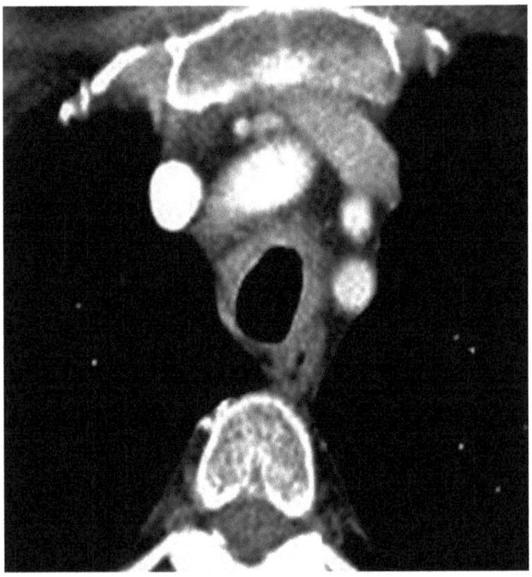

Fig. 11.5 Tracheal amyloidosis. Contrast-enhanced CT image shows smooth circumferential thickening of the trachea including the posterior tracheal membrane

within the submucosa of the trachea or bronchi. Patients are typically asymptomatic, although some may experience dyspnea, cough, or wheezing. Chest radiographs or CT show irregular nodular thickening and calcification, with sparing of the posterior tracheal membrane (Fig. 11.6). The disease progresses slowly and usually needs no specific treatment.

Relapsing Polychondritis

This systemic inflammatory disorder is characterized by auricular, nasal, or respiratory tract

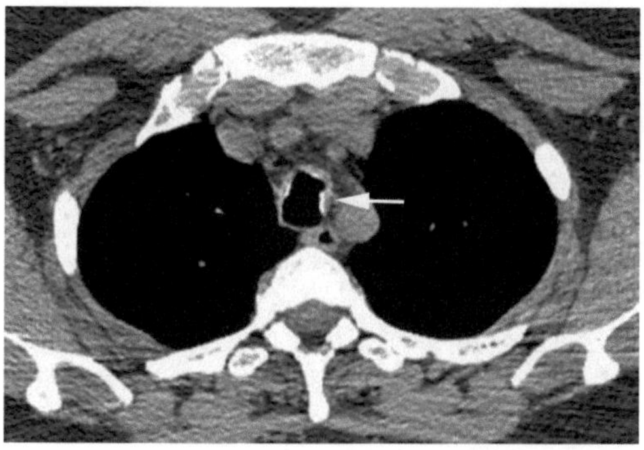

Fig. 11.6 Tracheobronchopathia osteochondroplastica (TBO). Transverse CT image shows calcified nodular thickening (*arrow*) sparing the posterior tracheal membrane

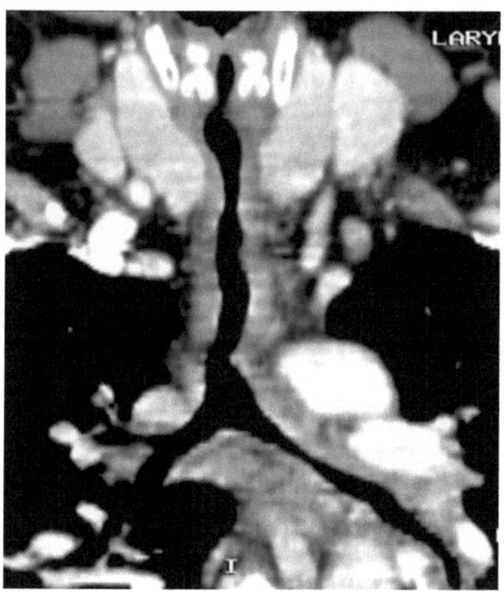

Fig. 11.7 Relapsing polychondritis. Coronal reformatted CT image shows diffuse thickening of the trachea and bronchi with smooth long segment luminal narrowing

chondritis, ocular inflammation, cochlear or vestibular dysfunction, and polyarthritis. Patients should be screened for involvement of large airways, as prompt treatment with corticosteroids (often in combination with other immunosuppressive agents) may prevent irreversible damage and life-threatening tracheobronchomalacia. Chest radiography may show narrowing of the trachea. CT findings include thickening of anterior and lateral tracheal walls and luminal narrowing (Fig. 11.7), especially on expiratory images. It characteristically spares the posterior tracheal membrane.

Mounier–Kuhn Syndrome

This congenital disorder is usually diagnosed in adulthood. Connective tissue weakness causes tracheobronchomegaly, frequently in conjunction with central bronchiectasis and tracheomalacia. Patients may be symptomatic or may present with recurrent respiratory infections and chronic cough. Diagnosis is made by CT, showing tracheal diameter greater than 3 cm, right main bronchus wider than 2.4 cm, and left main bronchus wider than 2.3 cm.

Wegener Granulomatosis

Airway involvement may affect up to 23% of patients with Wegener granulomatosis, a pulmonary-renal syndrome with vasculitis. CT is the imaging test of choice. The subglottic region is the most common location of airway involvement. Adjacent vocal cords may be involved and should be included in imaging of a patient with Wegener granulomatosis. CT findings include short segment circumferential mucosal thickening, ulceration, irregularity, and luminal stenosis (Fig. 11.8). Tracheal ring calcification is sometimes seen. Bronchial stenosis may be associated with distal consolidation or atelectasis.

Tracheal Infections

The trachea is rarely affected by infections in immunocompetent individuals. Tuberculosis (TB) and *Klebsiella rhinoscleromatis* are two such infections. TB typically causes thickening, enhancement, and irregular narrowing in active stages, and can heal with concentric stenosis or irregular wall thickening in late stages. TB favors the distal trachea and left main bronchus.

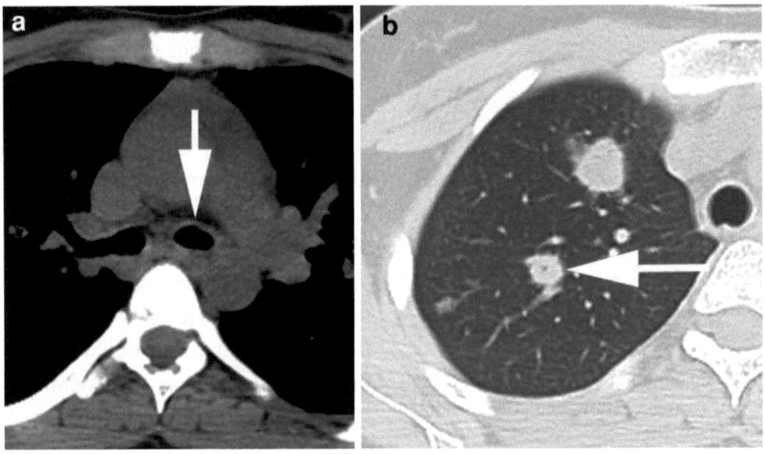

Fig. 11.8 Wegener granulomatosis. **a** Unenhanced CT image shows left main bronchial wall thickening (*arrow*). **b** The lung window shows two right upper lobe nodules with early cavitation in one of them (*arrow*)

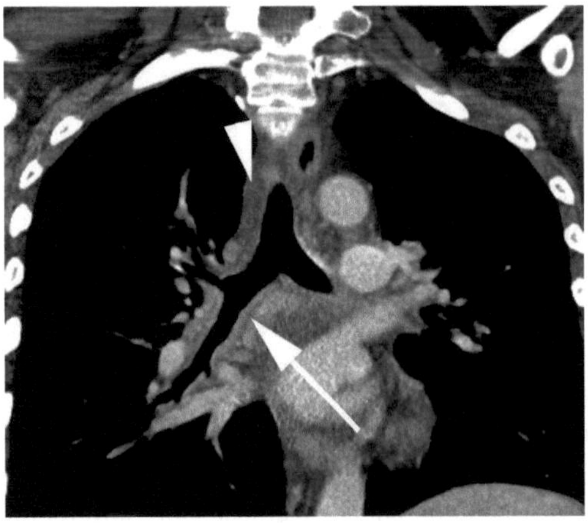

Fig. 11.9 Aspergillus fumigatus tracheobronchitis in blood stem cell transplant recipient. Coronal reformatted contrast-enhanced CT image shows diffuse smooth tracheobronchial thickening (*arrow*) with shaggy appearance of the surrounding mediastinal fat (*arrowhead*)

Associated pulmonary disease is useful in suggesting the diagnosis. Rhinoscleroma, an infection occurring primarily in tropical areas, shows diffuse nodular thickening and favors the distal trachea and proximal bronchi. This infection may heal with stricture and stenosis. Immunosuppressed individuals can develop diffuse tracheitis or tracheobronchitis (Fig. 11.9). *Aspergillus fumigatus* and herpes simplex virus (HSV) infections are commonly implicated in the immunosuppressed.

Bronchial Diseases

Bronchiectasis

Bronchiectasis is defined as irreversible pathologic dilation (or ectasia) of the cartilage-containing airways (bronchi). It is the final common pathway of a variety of underlying diseases that cause repeated episodes of airway infection and inflammation [5]. A vicious cycle ensues, in which the injured airway is more vulnerable to infection, and recurrent infections lead to further airway damage. *Traction bronchiectasis* occurs when airways are widened due to surrounding lung fibrosis; traction bronchiectasis is not true bronchiectasis.

Bronchiectasis is classified based on severity and morphology into three types, which can coexist in the same patient:

1. Cylindrical bronchiectasis is the least severe form. Bronchial dilation is uniform with smooth wall thickening.
2. Varicose bronchiectasis appears as bronchial dilation between narrowed segments,

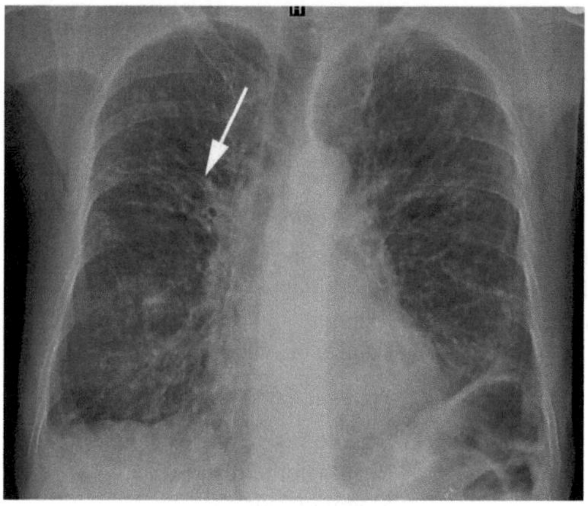

Fig. 11.10 Cystic fibrosis. Posteroanterior radiograph of the chest shows central and upper lung predominant bronchiectasis with tram tracking (*arrow*) from non-tapering thickened bronchial walls indicating cylindrical bronchiectasis

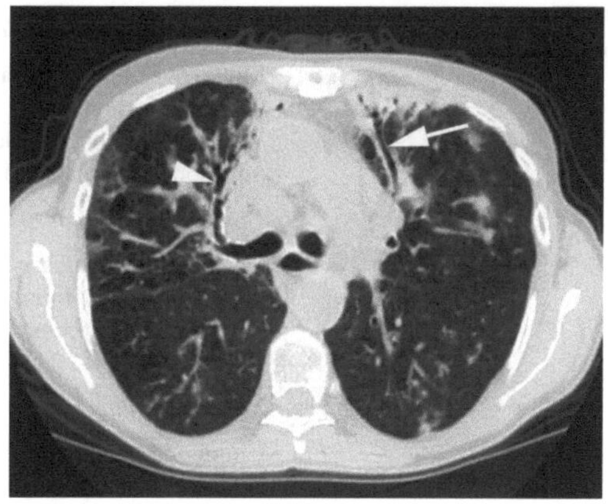

Fig. 11.11 Bronchiectasis. Unenhanced CT image shows a non-tapering dilated bronchus (*arrow*) indicating cylindrical bronchiectasis in the left upper lobe. Right upper lobe also shows bronchiectasis with an appearance akin to a "chain of black pearls" (*arrowhead*) indicating varicose bronchiectasis

Table 11.2 Identification of bronchiectasis by CT

1. Presence of one or more bronchi whose internal diameter exceeds that of the adjacent pulmonary artery branch (the "signet-ring sign")
2. Lack of normal bronchial tapering
3. Abnormal bronchial contours
4. Visibility of bronchi within 1 cm of the pleura

creating a beaded appearance, described as a "chain of black pearls".

3. Cystic or saccular bronchiectasis is the most severe form, with dilated bronchi that terminate in thick walled cysts.

Clinical manifestations of bronchiectasis can vary widely in severity, and include chronic cough, often with copious sputum production, dyspnea, hemoptysis, and constitutional symptoms such as fatigue and weight loss [6].

Pulmonary function testing generally reveals airflow obstruction, although patients with mild localized disease may have normal spirometry.

Chest radiographs may be abnormal in over 80% of patients with bronchiectasis [7], but these findings are generally nonspecific. Parallel line opacities called "tram tracks" (Fig. 11.10), or thick-walled bronchi in cross-section called ring opacities, which may also occur in other diseases, such as asthma and chronic bronchitis, are typically described on chest radiographs. Mucoid impaction may be seen as a tubular opacity ("finger-in-glove") or a branching structure ("hand-in-glove"). Cystic lesions, sometimes with air–fluid levels, may be seen in cystic bronchiectasis. Dilated bronchi are difficult to recognize on radiographs, but may be seen when a bronchus in cross-section appears larger than the adjacent artery, known as the "signet-ring sign." This becomes more apparent in severe disease.

The diagnostic study of choice is volumetric high-resolution chest CT (HRCT) [8]. Bronchial dilation can be recognized on HRCT (Fig. 11.11) by the presence of one or more bronchi whose internal diameter exceeds that of the adjacent pulmonary artery branch (the "signet-ring sign"); the lack of normal bronchial tapering, abnormal bronchial contours, or identification of bronchi within 1 cm of the pleura (Table 11.2) [9]. Common but nonspecific findings on HRCT include bronchial wall

Table 11.3 Etiologies of bronchiectasis

Congenital structural defect	*Cystic fibrosis and related disorders*
Moünier-Kuhn syndrome (congenital tracheobronchomegaly) Williams-Campbell syndrome (congenital tracheobronchomalacia)	Cystic fibrosis Young syndrome
Proximal airway obstruction	*Local immunologic reactions*
Usually implies a chronic component to the obstruction; e.g., foreign body, carcinoid tumor, fibrous stricture, broncholithiasis	Allergic bronchopulmonary aspergillosis Asthma Lung transplant rejection
Pulmonary infections	*Systemic inflammatory disorders*
Childhood pneumonias Adulthood necrotizing pneumonia Mycobacterial infection	Sarcoidosis Rheumatoid arthritis Sjögren syndrome Inflammatory bowel disease Relapsing polychondritis
Inhalational injury	*Miscellaneous*
Chronic or recurrent aspiration events Inhalation of gaseous toxin Thermal injury	Yellow nail syndrome Alpha-1 antitrypsin anomalies Idiopathic
Impaired host defense Hypogammaglobulinemia Primary ciliary dyskinesia HIV infection	

thickening; mucus- or fluid- filled bronchi; evidence of comorbid small airways disease, such as air-trapping; and evidence of bronchiolar inflammation, such as "tree-in-bud" opacities. Dilated bronchial arteries may also be seen in those with long standing bronchiectasis or bronchial inflammation.

The causes of bronchiectasis can be divided into several major categories, as described in Table 11.3. To distinguish these causes, the clinician should start by considering patient demographics and associated symptoms. There are some imaging characteristics that can direct suspicion of certain etiologies (Table 11.4). Despite extensive evaluation, the etiology remains unknown in over half of adult patients, and is classified as idiopathic.

Congenital Structural Defect

Mounier–Kuhn syndrome (congenital tracheobronchomegaly) is identified by central bronchiectasis and tracheal dilatation (>3 cm in diameter) on CT. Findings in Williams–Campbell syndrome (congenital tracheobronchomalacia) are characteristic with bronchiectasis affecting the 4–6th order bronchi (Fig. 11.12) and bronchomalacia.

Proximal Airway Obstruction

Focal bronchiectasis occurs due to chronic obstruction, such as with a foreign body, carcinoid tumor, fibrous stricture, or broncholithiasis. Most of these can be readily diagnosed with CT. If the cause is not apparent on imaging, bronchoscopy with airway inspection can be diagnostic.

Infection

Childhood pneumonia, adulthood necrotizing pneumonia, or mycobacterial infection can cause bronchiectasis. Tuberculosis classically causes unilateral upper lobe bronchiectasis (Fig. 11.13), whereas non-tuberculous mycobacterial infection often favors the right middle lobe and lingula (Fig. 11.14).

Table 11.4 Radiologic features that suggest a specific etiology of bronchiectasis

Focal bronchiectasis	Airway obstruction; congenital bronchial atresia
Central bronchiectasis	ABPA; CF; TB; Mounier–Kuhn syndrome; Williams–Campbell syndrome
Central bronchiectasis and tracheal dilatation	Diagnostic of Mounier–Kuhn syndrome
Bilateral upper lobe bronchiectasis	CF; ABPA
Unilateral upper lobe bronchiectasis	TB
Lower lobe bronchiectasis	Recurrent pulmonary infections; immunologic deficiency; PCD; Young syndrome; Mounier–Kuhn syndrome; chronic or recurrent aspiration events
Bronchiectasis of RML and lingula	*Mycobacterium avium* complex
Parenchymal abnormalities	RA (variety of abnormalities, including interstitial pneumonia organizing pneumonia, and rheumatoid nodules); ABPA (consolidation, frequently involving the upper lobes); traction bronchiectasis (adjacent fibrosis, no bronchial wall thickening)
Mucoid impaction	Frequently seen in ABPA and CF; less common in asthma
Situs inversus	Kartagener syndrome (subset of PCD)
Pleural effusion	Yellow nail syndrome (present in 36% of reported patients); RA (uncommon)
Ballooning of central bronchi on inspiration and collapse on expiration	Williams-Campbell syndrome

Abbreviation: *ABPA* = allergic bronchopulmonary aspergillosis, *CF* = cystic fibrosis, *PCD* = primary ciliary dyskinesia, *RA* = rheumatoid arthritis, *TB* = tuberculosis

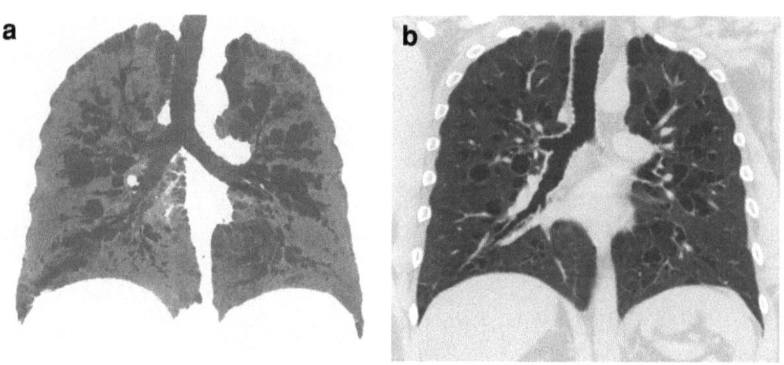

Fig. 11.12 Williams–Campbell syndrome. CT MinIP (**a**) and coronal reformat (**b**) images show bronchiectasis affecting the 4–6th order bronchi only, a characteristic appearance

Inhalational Injury

This category includes chronic or recurrent aspiration events, inhalation of gaseous toxin, and thermal injury. Even in patients without symptoms of choking while eating or drinking, a swallow study may be diagnostic of silent aspiration.

Impaired Host Defenses

Hypogammaglobulinemia is readily diagnosed via quantitative immunoglobulin levels. Primary ciliary dyskinesia (PCD) can be identified with high-speed video microscopy or electron microscopy of a nasal ciliated epithelium biopsy. Both typically cause lower lobe

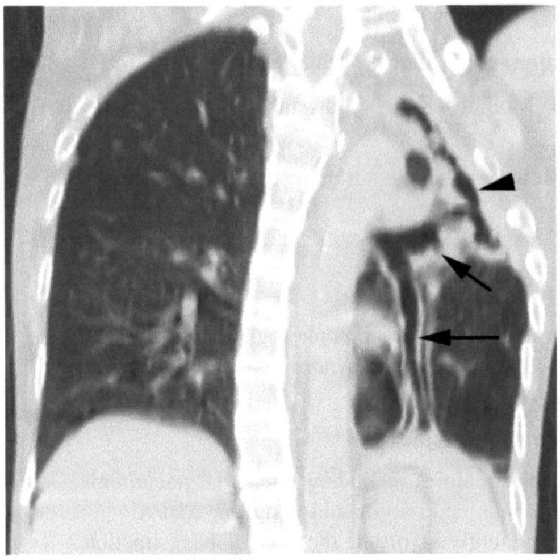

Fig. 11.13 Tuberculosis. Coronal reformatted CT shows destroyed left upper lobe with cavitation (*arrowhead*) and left upper lobe and lower lobe bronchiectasis (*arrow*)

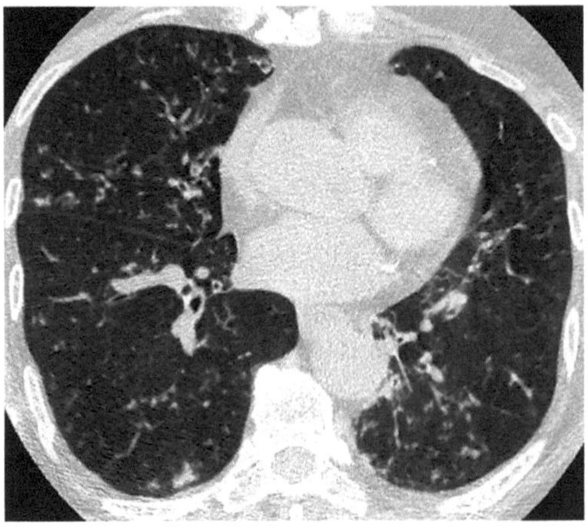

Fig. 11.14 *Mycobacterium avium* complex (MAC) infection. HRCT image shows patchy centrilobular nodularity and mild bronchiectasis involving the right middle lobe and both the lower lobes

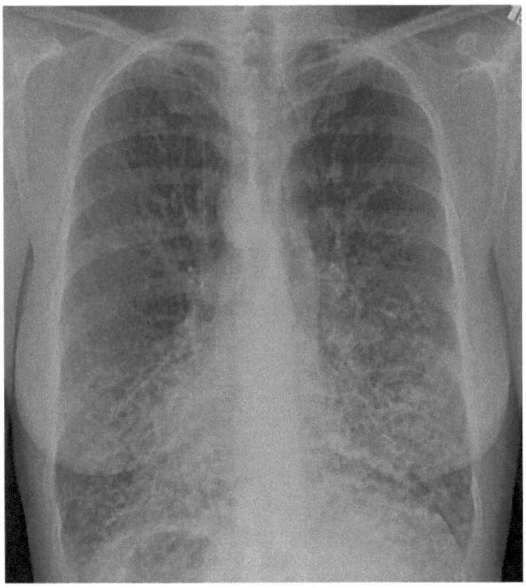

Fig. 11.15 Kartagener syndrome. PA chest radiograph shows lower lung predominant cystic bronchiectasis and situs inversus as indicated by dextrocardia and the gastric bubble on the right

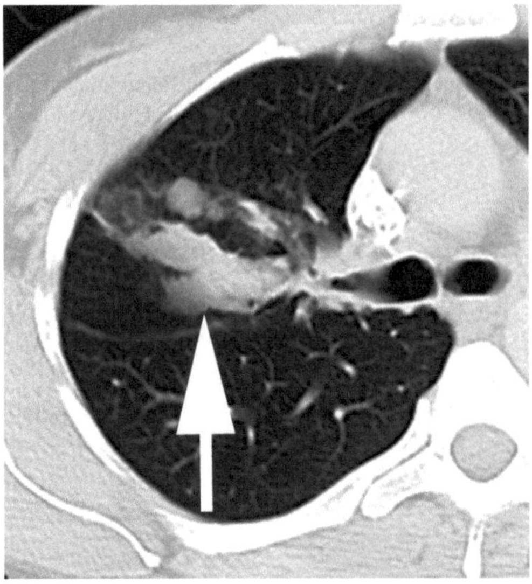

Fig. 11.16 Allergic bronchopulmonary aspergillosis (ABPA). Right upper lobe central bronchiectasis with mucus plugging—a "finger-in-glove" appearance seen on chest CT

bronchiectasis. Situs inversus, sinus disease, and bronchiectasis form the triad of Kartagener syndrome, a subset of PCD (Fig. 11.15). HIV infection is also associated with bronchiectasis.

Cystic Fibrosis and Related Disorders

Cystic fibrosis (CF) causes central and bilateral upper lobe bronchiectasis, often associated with

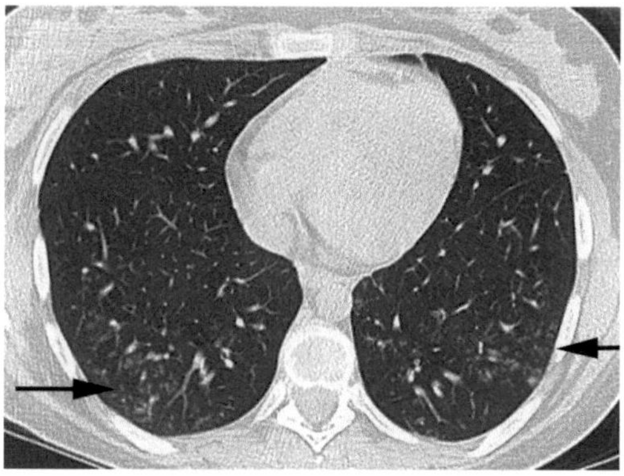

Fig. 11.17 Viral bronchiolitis. HRCT image shows patchy centrilobular nodules (*arrows*) in the lower lobes

mucoid impaction (Fig. 11.10). It is diagnosed via sweat chloride test, gene mutation analysis, or, in specialized centers, nasal transepithelial potential difference.

Local Immunologic Reactions

This category includes asthma, allergic bronchopulmonary aspergillosis (ABPA), and lung transplant rejection. ABPA, like CF, usually causes central and bilateral upper lobe bronchiectasis, often with mucoid impaction—sometimes described as a finger in glove appearance (Fig. 11.16) on a chest radiograph. Diagnostic criteria for ABPA have been well-described, and include a history of asthma, peripheral eosinophilia, skin test reactivity to *Aspergillus* antigens, precipitating serum antibodies to *A. fumigatus*, elevated levels of total IgE and IgE specific to *A. fumigatus,* and the radiographic findings of central bronchiectasis and/or fleeting pulmonary opacities.

Systemic Inflammatory Disorders

Sarcoidosis, rheumatoid arthritis, Sjögren syndrome, inflammatory bowel disease, and relapsing polychondritis can all cause bronchiectasis. Rheumatoid arthritis also causes a variety of other pulmonary abnormalities, including interstitial pneumonia, organizing pneumonia, and rheumatoid nodules. Diagnosis of these disorders is made thorough combined clinical evaluation, autoantibodies, and biopsy of affected tissue.

Miscellaneous Diagnoses

This category includes yellow nail syndrome, an abnormality of the lymphatic system resulting in discolored nails, lymphedema, airway disease, and various forms of pleuropulmonary disease; and alpha-1 antitrypsin deficiency, which typically causes panacinar emphysema, but can also cause bronchiectasis.

Small Airways Diseases

Bronchiolitis

Bronchiolitis is characterized by inflammation of small airways that are less than 2 mm in diameter and do not contain cartilage in their walls (bronchioles). Clinical manifestations include cough, wheezing, dyspnea, and airflow obstruction. Idiopathic cases tend to have more insidious onset of symptoms. The terminology is confusing, as bronchiolitis can be classified by etiology, histopathology, or radiographic appearance [10]. Histologic classifications are inconsistent in the literature, but commonly include *cellular bronchiolitis*, with subtypes of *infectious bronchiolitis, diffuse panbronchiolitis* and *follicular bronchiolitis*; *constrictive bronchiolitis* (also known as *obliterative bronchiolitis)*; *respiratory bronchiolitis* (due to cigarette smoke and *mineral dust-associated airway disease*) [11]. Most of these histologic patterns are not specific for a distinctive etiology. Bronchiolitis obliterans with organizing pneumonia (BOOP) is an interstitial pneumonia, and should not be confused with constrictive bronchiolitis (obliterative bronchiolitis or bronchiolitis obliterans)—a form of bronchiolitis. The term BOOP has been discarded for the more apt "cryptogenic organizing pneumonia" (COP).

The chest radiograph can be normal in bronchiolitis. Patients with Swyer-James-Macleod syndrome, a form of constrictive bronchiolitis, can show unilateral or asymmetric hyperinflation of the entire lung or lobe on a chest radiograph. CT is superior to radiography for evaluating known or

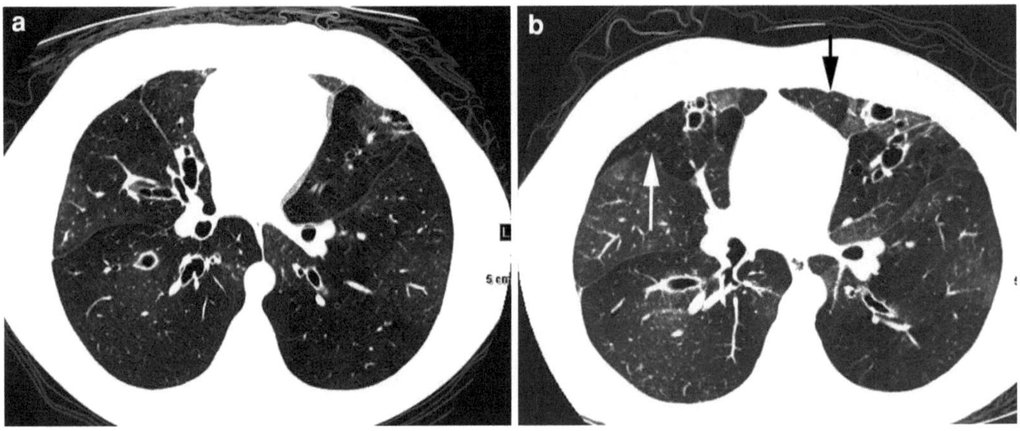

Fig. 11.18 Constrictive bronchiolitis presumably the sequela of acute respiratory distress syndrome. A. Inspiratory unenhanced CT shows a mosaic pattern of attenuation. Mild cylindrical bronchiectasis is also present. B. Corresponding image in expiration shows accentuation of difference in attenuation (*arrows*) indicating air trapping

suspected small airway disease. Normal bronchioles are typically not visible at CT. Inflammation causes them to become visible, appearing as centrilobular nodules that may have a V- or Y- shaped branching pattern sometimes giving a "tree-in-bud" pattern—a direct CT feature. Air trapping, an indirect CT feature, is best identified on dynamic or suspended expiratory CT scans [12]. Mosaic attenuation can be caused by air trapping or primary pulmonary vascular disease. Showing accentuation of difference in CT attenuation between the abnormal and normal lung on expiratory scans indicates air trapping. Diminution of attenuation difference on expiratory CT generally indicates pulmonary vascular disease related to differential lung perfusion. Cellular or inflammatory bronchiolitis often has direct CT features: centrilobular nodules, "tree-in-bud" pattern; and air trapping (an indirect CT feature) is seen inconsistently (Fig. 11.17). Constrictive bronchiolitis, on the other hand, has air trapping as the dominant feature, and centrilobular nodularity is an inconsistent feature (Fig. 11.18).

In infants and children, bronchiolitis is common and is usually caused by viral infection, especially by respiratory syncytial virus. In adults, it can be seen in the setting of infection, commonly from viruses or mycoplasma, or chronic infection with mycobacteria. Inhalational injury from cigarette smoke, nitrogen dioxide, diacetyl, or mineral dusts including iron oxide, aluminum, silica, or coal can cause bronchiolitis. Bronchiolitis can also result from a drug reaction or be associated with autoimmune disease or blood stem cell or solid organ transplantation (see Table 11.5). The distribution of radiographic abnormalities can be an important clue to etiology as detailed in Table 11.6.

Asthma

Asthma is characterized by reversible airflow obstruction, airway inflammation, and bronchial hyperresponsiveness. Classic clinical manifestations are episodic cough, wheezing, and dyspnea. The diagnosis is made by clinical evaluation and pulmonary function tests, and imaging studies are not routinely performed. Minimizing radiation exposure is especially important in the pediatric asthma population. Indications for imaging include concern for an alternate or comorbid diagnosis and evaluation for complications of asthma, such as pneumothorax, pneumomediastinum, or pneumonia.

Table 11.5 Classification, causes, imaging features and differential diagnosis of small airway disease [12]

Category	Type based on imaging or pathologic pattern	Prototype cause and other causes	Imaging features (HRCT)	Differential diagnosis
Inflammatory				
–	Infectious	Viruses, *Mycoplasma*, mycobacteria	Centrilobular nodules, tree-in-bud pattern, bronchial wall thickening, ground-glass abnormality in a patchy distribution	Hypersensitivity pneumonitis, aspiration (in lower lung distribution)
	Respiratory bronchiolitis	Cigarette smoking	Centrilobular nodules and patchy ground-glass opacities in an upper lung distribution	Hypersensitivity pneumonitis, pulmonary neovascularity in Eisenmenger syndrome
	Follicular bronchiolitis	Rheumatoid arthritis and Sjögren syndrome	Lower lung dominant centrilobular and peribronchiolar nodules, bronchiolectasis and bronchiectasis	Asian panbronchiolitis, immunodeficiency syndromes, infectious bronchiolitis
	Asian panbronchiolitis	Idiopathic, relatively exclusive in patients of Asian origin	Lower lung bronchiectasis, bronchiolectasis, centrilobular nodules	Follicular bronchiolitis, immunodeficiency syndromes, and infectious bronchiolitis
Fibrotic bronchiolitis				
–	Constrictive or obliterative bronchiolitis	Postinfectious, Swyer-James-Macleod syndrome, toxic fume inhalation	Patchy air trapping, bronchiectasis, and bronchiolectasis	Differential perfusion from pulmonary hypertension
	Obliterative bronchiolitis in postlung or hematopoietic stem cell transplant population	Postlung transplantation, chronic graft-versus-host disease	Lower lung dominant mosaic attenuation and air trapping with diminished vascularity	Postinfectious obliterative bronchiolitis

Radiographic studies are valuable in diagnosing allergic bronchopulmonary aspergillosis and Churg-Strauss vasculitis, both of which occur in asthmatics. Imaging studies may be helpful in identifying diseases that mimic asthma clinically, such as tracheal or carinal obstruction, hypersensitivity pneumonitis, bronchiolitis obliterans, tracheomalacia, bronchomalacia, eosinophilic pneumonia, and aspiration. Another common mimic, vocal cord dysfunction, can only be diagnosed at laryngoscopy.

The features of asthma on a chest radiograph are non specific and include bronchial wall thickening and hyperinflation. Chest CT may show additional findings including airway wall thickening, expiratory air trapping, and cylindrical bronchiectasis. However, these are nonspecific [13].

Table 11.6 Etiologies of bronchiolitis

Infectious
Acute infection with viruses, mycoplasma, other bacteria
Chronic infection with mycobacteria
Inhalational injury
Cigarette smoke
Nitrogen dioxide (silo fillers)
Diacetyl exposure (popcorn factory)
Mineral dusts
Drug induced reaction
Busulfan
Free-base cocaine
Gold
Penicillamine
Others
After organ transplantation
Post lung transplant
Post hematopoietic stem cell transplantation
Associated with other diseases
Rheumatoid arthritis
Sjogren syndrome
Dermatomyositis
Systemic lupus erythematosus
Inflammatory bowel disease
Idiopathic

Table 11.7 Appropriate imaging studies by suspected diagnosis

Tracheal disease	Start with radiograph, may proceed to chest CT
Bronchiectasis	Diagnostic study of choice is the thin section, high resolution, non-contrast chest CT, with 1–1.5 mm thick images taken every 10 mm, including inspiratory and expiratory scans
Bronchiolitis	When diagnosis is clear by history and exam (e.g., acute infectious bronchiolitis after viral prodrome), chest CT is most useful diagnostically
Asthma	No imaging needed unless there is concern for an alternate or comorbid diagnosis such as ABPA or for complications of asthma, such as pneumothorax or pneumonia

In summary, CT is the diagnostic imaging study of choice in patients with known or suspected airways disease (see Table 11.7). Expiratory imaging is important in suspected tracheobronchomalacia or small airways disease. Iodinated contrast material is generally only required for imaging patients with airway tumors.

References

1. Albertine KH. Anatomy of the lungs. In: Mason RJ, Broaddus VC, Martin T, King Jr. T, Schraufnagel D, Murray JF, Nadel JA, editors. Murray and Nadel's textbook of respiratory medicine. 5th ed. Philadelphia: Elsevier; 2010. p. 3–25.
2. Stern EJ, Graham CM, Webb WR, et al. Normal trachea during forced expiration: dynamic CT measurements. Radiology. 1993;187(1):27–31.
3. Gaissert HA, Burns J. The compromised airway: tumors, strictures, and tracheomalacia. Surg Clin North Am. 2010;90(5):1065–89.
4. Ozyigit LP, et al. Isolated laryngo-tracheal amyloidosis presenting as a refractory asthma and longstanding hoarseness. J Asthma. 2009;46(3):314–7.
5. Iseman MD, Chan ED. Bronchiectasis. In: Mason RJ, Broaddus VC, Martin T, King Jr. T, Schraufnagel D, Murray JF, Nadel JA, editors. Murray and Nadel's textbook of respiratory medicine. 5th ed. Philadelphia: Elsevier; 2010. p. 1023–46.
6. O'Donnell AE. Bronchiectasis. Chest. 2008;134(4): 815–23.
7. van der Bruggen-Bogaarts BA, et al. Screening for bronchiectasis: A comparative study between chest radiography and high-resolution CT. Chest. 1996; 109(3):608–11.
8. Javidan-Nejad C, Bhalla S. Bronchiectasis. Radiol Clin North Am. 2009;47(2):289–306.
9. Webb WR. Airway disease: bronchiectasis, chronic bronchitis, and bronchiolitis. In: Webb WR, Higgins CB, editors. Thoracic imaging. Philadelphia: Lippincott Williams & Wilkins; 2005. p. 527–52.
10. Allen TC. Pathology of small airways disease. Arch Pathol Lab Med. 2010;134(5):702–18.
11. Kang EY, et al. Bronchiolitis: classification, computed tomographic and histopathologic features, and radiologic approach. J Comput Assist Tomogr. 2009;33(1):32–41.
12. Pipavath S, Stern EJ. Imaging of small airway disease (SAD). Radiol Clin North Am. 2009;47(2): 307–16.
13. Woods AQ, Lynch DA. Asthma: an imaging update. Radiol Clin North Am. 2009;47(2):317–29.

Idiopathic Interstitial Pneumonias

12

Paul J. Lee and Jeffrey P. Kanne

Abstract

The idiopathic interstitial pneumonias are a distinct group of clinicopathologic entities. High-resolution computed tomography (HRCT) plays a critical role in the evaluation and management of patients. In the appropriate clinical setting, characteristic HRCT findings may be diagnostic, obviating the need for open lung biopsy. In more challenging or complicated cases, consensus among the clinician, radiologist, and pathologist may be required. This chapter describes and depicts the characteristic HRCT features of usual interstitial pneumonia, nonspecific interstitial pneumonia, cryptogenic organizing pneumonia, respiratory bronchiolitis, respiratory bronchiolitis associated interstitial lung disease, desquamative interstitial pneumonia, and lymphoid interstitial pneumonia.

Keywords

Interstitial lung disease (ILD) · High-resolution computed tomography (HRCT) · Usual interstitial pneumonia (UIP) · Nonspecific interstitial pneumonia (NSIP) · Cryptogenic organizing pneumonia (COP) · Respiratory bronchiolitis (RB) · Respiratory bronchiolitis–interstitial lung disease (RB-ILD) · Desquamative interstitial pneumonia (DIP) · Lymphoid interstitial pneumonia (LIP)

Introduction

Over 200 causes of interstitial lung disease have been described. Environmental and occupational exposures, systemic diseases, and genetic causes can all result in a variety of interstitial lung diseases. The idiopathic interstitial pneumonias (IIP) refer to a group of distinct clinicopathologic entities without known causes [1]. Classification of IIP has undergone several iterations as understanding of these entities evolves [2–4].

P. J. Lee (✉)
Department of Radiology, University of Wisconsin School of Medicine and Public Health, 600 Highland Avenue, Madison, WI 53792-3252, USA
e-mail: plee2@uwhealth.org

J. P. Kanne
Department of Radiology, University of Wisconsin School of Medicine and Public Health, 600 Highland Avenue, Madison, WI 53705, USA
e-mail: jkanne@uwhealth.org

J. P. Kanne (ed.), *Clinically Oriented Pulmonary Imaging*, Respiratory Medicine, DOI: 10.1007/978-1-61779-542-8_12,

The most common IIP is idiopathic pulmonary fibrosis (IPF), which accounts for approximately 40% of all idiopathic interstitial lung disease [5]. While idiopathic forms do exist, the other IIPs more commonly result from exposures, such as tobacco smoke or connective tissue disease.

High-resolution computed tomography (HRCT) plays a key role in assessing the patient with known or suspected interstitial lung disease. While the primary function of HRCT is to distinguish patients with usual interstitial pneumonia (UIP), which is associated with IPF, from those without UIP, HRCT findings can often suggest other causes of diffuse lung disease. Although surgical biopsy is advocated in patients with suspected IIP who do not have a definite UIP pattern on HRCT, consensus between clinicians and radiologists with expertise in interstitial lung disease may suffice to establish a diagnosis.

Usual Interstitial Pneumonia

IPF is uncommon with an incidence of 6.8–16.3 per 100,000 persons in the USA [6]. Men are affected twice as often as women, and the incidence increases with increasing age. While the exact cause of IPF remains unknown, environmental factors such as occupational dusts and fumes [7], cigarette smoke [8], and Epstein-Barr virus infection [9] may be contributory. Prognosis remains poor with fewer than 50% of patients surviving 5 years following diagnosis [10].

IPF is characterized histologically by UIP. The UIP pattern on HRCT consists of reticular opacities, traction bronchiectasis, and architectural distortion in a patchy subpleural and bibasilar distribution (Fig. 12.1) [11, 12]. These findings may be asymmetric but not unilateral. Honeycombing is a critical component of a confident, radiologic diagnosis of UIP (Figs. 12.2, 12.3). Honeycombing consists of clustered cystic spaces stacked upon a subpleural base. These cystic spaces have well-defined walls and typically range from 3 to 10 mm in size but may extend up to 2.5 cm in diameter [1, 5, 13]. Centrilobular and paraseptal emphysema may coexist with CT findings of UIP and should not be mistaken for honeycombing (Fig. 12.4) [8, 14–18]. Mild mediastinal lymphadenopathy is also common, typically involving the right paratracheal and subcarinal stations. The degree of lymphadenopathy typically correlates with the extent of parenchymal reticulation, although short axis lymph node measurements rarely exceed 1.5–2.0 cm in the absence of another superimposed cause [19, 20]. Ground-glass opacities can be associated with areas of fibrosis and may even represent regions of fibrosis. However, ground-glass opacities should account for a relatively minor component of parenchymal abnormality.

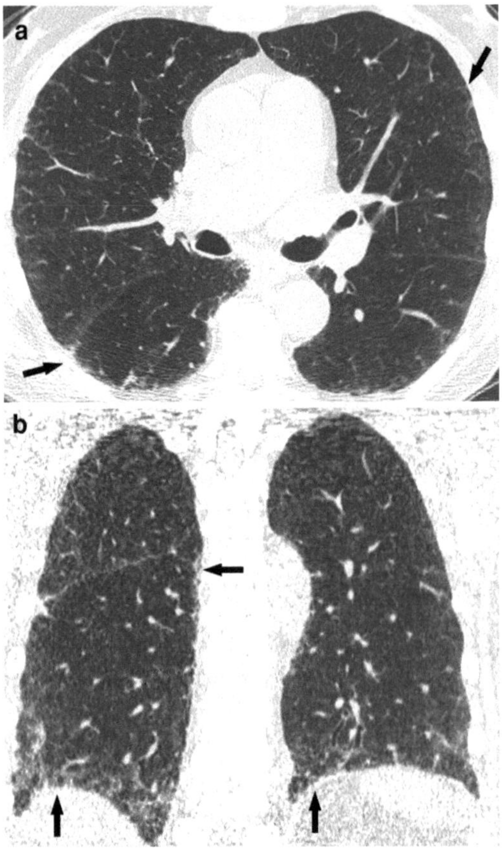

Fig. 12.1 Usual interstitial pneumonia. Transverse (**a**) and coronal reformatted (**b**) low-dose HRCT images show subpleural and basal reticulation (*arrows*)

Studies have shown that the positive predictive value of a confident CT diagnosis of UIP by expert pulmonary radiologists ranges from 90 to

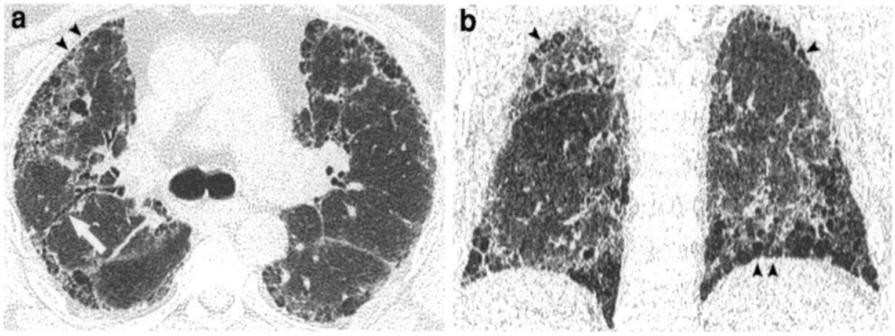

Fig. 12.2 Usual interstitial pneumonia. Transverse (**a**) and coronal reformatted (**b**) low-dose HRCT images show subpleural and basal predominant reticulation with subpleural honeycombing (*arrowheads*)

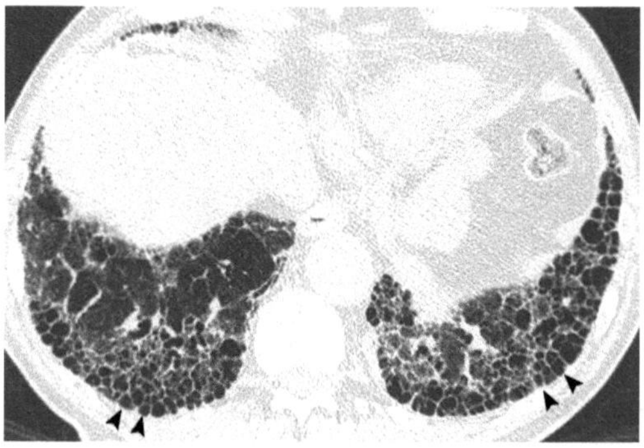

Fig. 12.3 Usual interstitial pneumonia. Transverse HRCT image shows extensive, symmetric honeycombing (*arrowheads*) in the lung bases

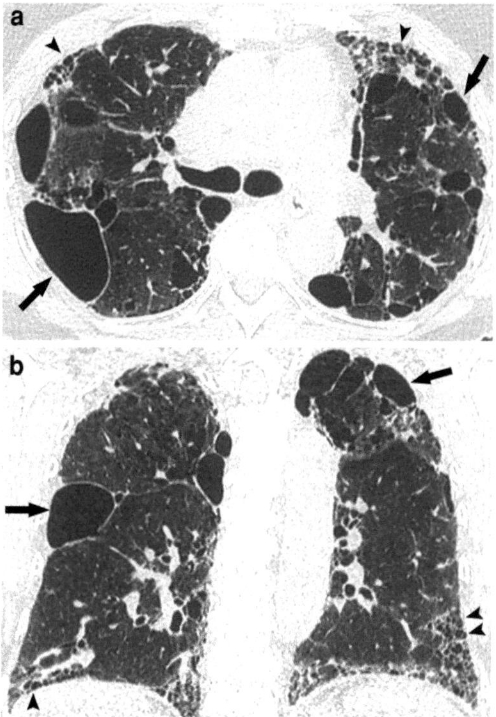

Fig. 12.4 Combined pulmonary fibrosis and emphysema. Transverse (**a**) and coronal reformatted (**b**) HRCT images show upper lobe predominant bullous emphysema (*arrows*) and basal predominant subpleural honeycombing (*arrowheads*)

100%. However, these studies also show that a confidant diagnosis is not made in 25–50% of histologically proven cases of UIP [21–27]. Silva et al. demonstrated that the findings of basal honeycombing, the absence of subpleural sparing, and the absence of centrilobular nodules best distinguish UIP from chronic hypersensitivity pneumonitis and nonspecific interstitial pneumonia (NSIP) [28]. CT findings that should suggest alternative etiologies include micronodules; air trapping; non-honeycomb cysts; consolidation; a peribronchovascular distribution of fibrosis, and significant pleural calcifications, plaques, or effusion [5].

Complications associated with IPF include acute exacerbation (Fig. 12.5), pulmonary hypertension [29–31], pulmonary thromboembolism, coronary artery disease, bronchogenic carcinoma (Fig. 12.6), pneumothorax (Fig. 12.7), pneumomediastinum, and infection. Opportunistic organisms in this setting include *Mycobacteria*, *Pneumocystis jiroveci*, and *Aspergillus* species [32, 33]. Acute exacerbation occurs in approximately 5–10% of patients on an annual basis. Associated CT findings include new ground-glass opacities and consolidation in a peripheral, diffuse, or multifocal random

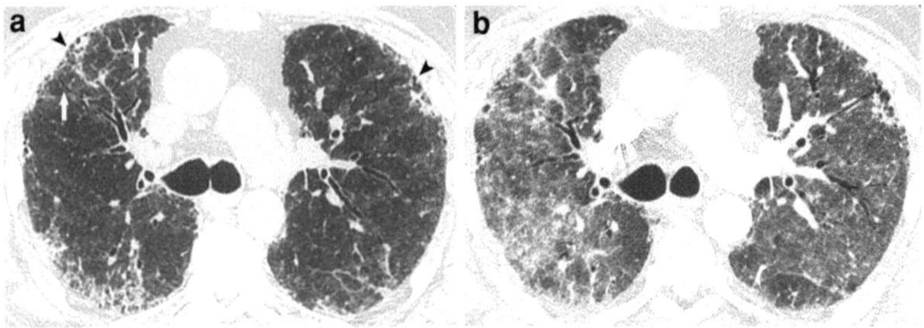

Fig. 12.5 Acute exacerbation of UIP. **a** HRCT image shows subpleural predominant reticulation with mild traction bronchiectasis (*arrows*) and bronchiolectasis (*arrowheads*). A small amount of ground-glass opacity is present. **b** HRCT 9 days later shows development of extensive ground-glass opacity

distribution (Fig. 12.8). It is unclear whether these acute exacerbations represent rapid advancement of the primary disease or superimposed infection, infarction, or other pathology difficult to separate from the primary process [34–39]. Pulmonary hypertension is commonly associated with IPF, although CT-derived vascular measurements may be of limited predictive value [40]. Bronchogenic carcinoma (Fig. 12.9) develops in approximately 10–15% of those with relatively longstanding IPF and usually manifests as new focal consolidation or nodule in a region of severe fibrosis [41]. The appropriate role of routine screening for these complications has not been defined [5].

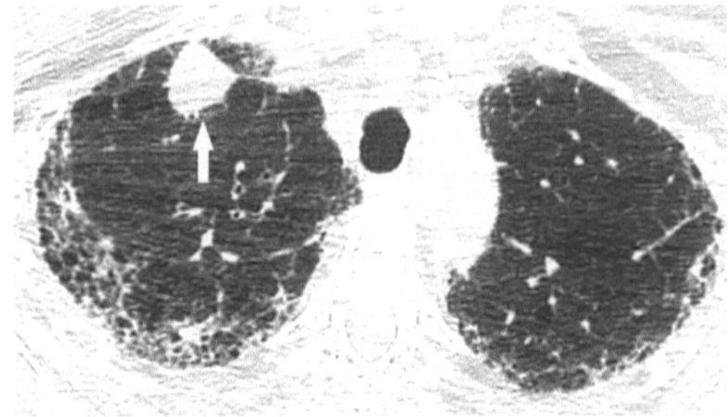

Fig. 12.6 UIP with bronchogenic carcinoma. HRCT image shows a large nodule (*arrow*) on a background of subpleural reticulation and honeycombing. Transthoracic needle biopsy showed non-small cell lung carcinoma

Nonspecific Interstitial Pneumonia

Nonspecific interstitial pneumonia (NSIP) was first used to classify patients with interstitial lung disease and surgical biopsies not fitting into any well-defined histologic pattern [3]. Currently, idiopathic NSIP is recognized as a distinct clinicopathologic entity associated with a better prognosis than IPF. Patients with idiopathic NSIP tend to be lifetime non-smoking females of Asian ethnicity [42]. However, NSIP is most commonly associated with connective tissue disease such as systemic sclerosis or may be the sequela of a drug reaction.

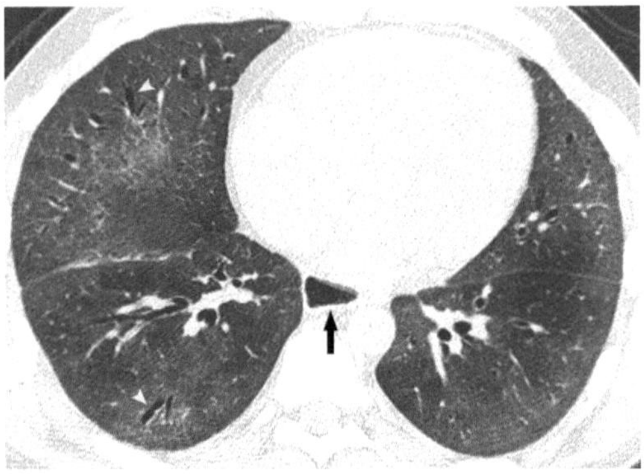

Fig. 12.7 NSIP associated with systemic sclerosis. HRCT image shows extensive ground-glass opacity. There is mild bronchial dilation (*arrowheads*). Note the patulous and fluid-filled esophagus (*arrow*)

While the HRCT findings of NSIP have proven to be more variable than was initially suggested [43–46], the majority of cases have ground-glass opacities and findings of fibrosis including fine reticulation, traction bronchiectasis, and volume loss in a symmetric mid to lower lung distribution (Figs. 12.7, 12.8) [47, 48]. The severity and distribution of these parenchymal abnormalities are more uniform than in UIP.

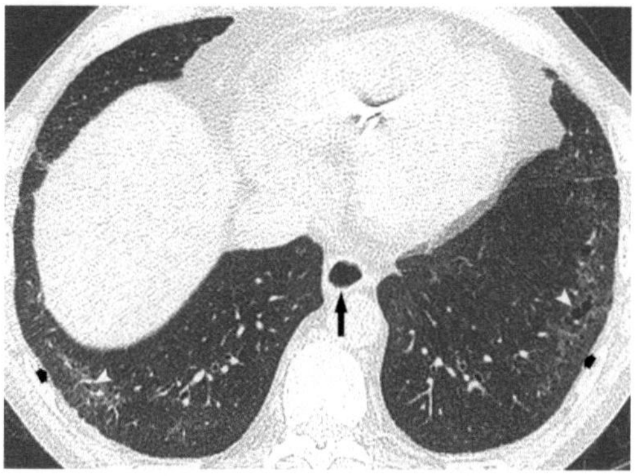

Fig. 12.8 NSIP associated with mixed connective tissue disease. HRCT image shows mild ground-glass opacity and reticulation in the lower lobes associated with mild traction bronchiectasis (*arrowheads*). Note the patulous esophagus (*thin arrow*). Mild subpleural sparing is evident (*wide arrows*)

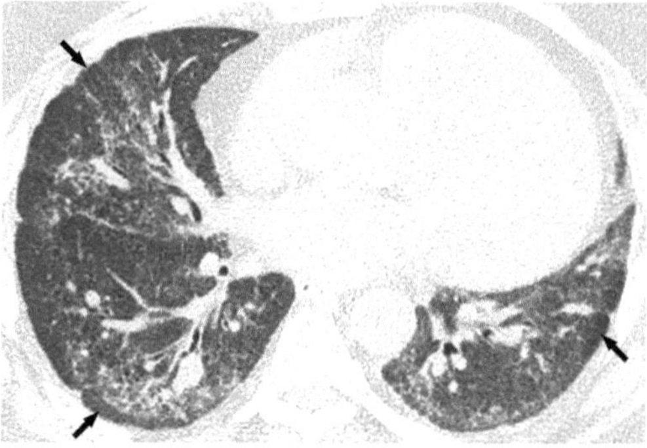

Fig. 12.9 NSIP associated with undefined connective tissue disease. HRCT image shows ground-glass opacity with reticulation in the lower lungs. Note the rim of relative subpleural sparing (*arrows*)

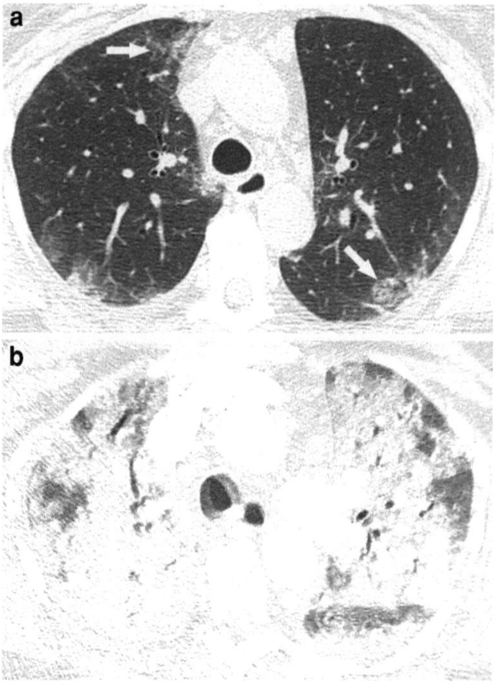

Fig. 12.10 Acute exacerbation of NSIP. **a** HRCT image shows multiple foci of peripheral ground-glass opacity (*arrows*). **b** HRCT image one month later shows extensive consolidation in both lungs. The patient presented with acute hypoxia and dyspnea

Distribution along the axial plane may be peripheral, peribronchovascular, or diffuse. When present and in the appropriate setting, a thin rim of subpleural sparing is a rather specific finding for NSIP and should heighten diagnostic confidence (Fig. 12.9) [43]. As with IPF, mild mediastinal lymphadenopathy is common, particularly at the right paratracheal and subcarinal stations, and correlates with the degree of parenchymal involvement. Given the high association of NSIP with underlying collagen vascular diseases and other disorders, associated abnormalities may be sought on available imaging studies.

Although NSIP is characterized by two histologic subtypes, cellular and fibrotic, there are generally no imaging features to reliably distinguish between the two. As would be expected, reticulation is more commonly seen with fibrotic subtype, although the cellular subtype may also demonstrate fine reticulation. In our experience, a posterior basilar and anterior apical distribution of reticulation, when present in the appropriate setting, is relatively specific for the fibrotic subtype. However, with regard to the extent of ground-glass opacity, consolidation, or traction bronchiectasis, there is no reliable separation in CT findings between the two subtypes [10, 49–51].

Additional findings on HRCT tend to be nonspecific or should suggest alternative etiologies. Relatively mild honeycombing may be seen in NSIP, but significant honeycombing is more commonly associated with a histologic diagnosis of UIP. The reported prevalence of consolidation in NSIP varies widely and may often represent superimposed infection or organizing pneumonia [10, 44, 48, 49, 51–57]. New consolidation or ground-glass opacities in an acutely ill patient with NSIP may represent an acute exacerbation (Fig. 12.10). While such exacerbations occur less commonly than in patients with IPF, the annual incidence of NSIP acute exacerbations may approach 5% [58]. With appropriate treatment, some findings of NSIP may be reversible on follow-up examination [59].

Cryptogenic Organizing Pneumonia

Organizing pneumonia (OP) refers to the histologic pattern described as polypoid plugs of loose organizing connective tissue within the alveoli. This pattern may be idiopathic but is more commonly associated with one of numerous underlying etiologies, including connective tissue disease and drug reaction. Formerly termed bronchiolitis obliterans organizing pneumonia (BOOP), cryptogenic OP (COP) refers to an idiopathic clinical syndrome characterized by organizing pneumonia. The newer terminology reflects the primary histologic features while avoiding confusion with small airways disease (bronchiolitis). Patients with COP are often initially diagnosed with community acquired pneumonia, and further workup is often pursued after failure of antibiotic treatment.

Characteristic HRCT findings of OP include unilateral or, more commonly, bilateral, patchy areas of consolidation, characteristically involving the lower lobes. Consolidation is present on HRCT in at least 90% of patients and follows a subpleural or peribronchovascular distribution in approximately 50% of patients (Fig. 12.11) [60, 61]. Foci of consolidation may be migratory on serial imaging. Common associated findings include ground-glass opacities in a random distribution (60%) (Fig. 12.12), air bronchograms (Fig. 12.13), and mild bronchial dilation. Lung volumes are typically preserved, and architectural distortion is generally absent.

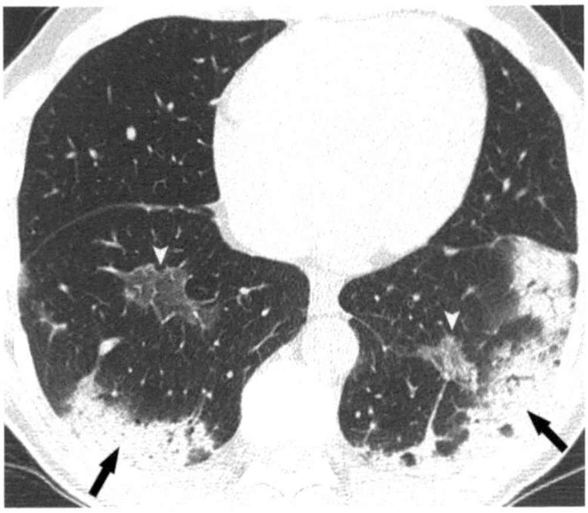

Fig. 12.11 Cryptogenic organizing pneumonia. HRCT image shows peripheral consolidation (*arrows*) in the lower lobes with a few foci of ground-glass opacity (*arrowheads*)

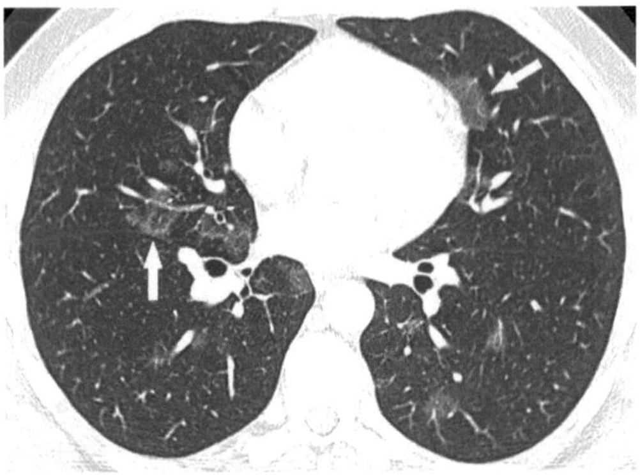

Fig. 12.12 Cryptogenic organizing pneumonia. HRCT image shows scattered foci of ground-glass opacity (*arrows*) in both lungs. Consolidation is more common than ground-glass opacity in COP

Small pleural effusions may occur in a small minority of patients. The reverse-halo sign (Fig. 12.14) was first described in the setting of OP as a relatively specific finding. This sign refers to a central region of ground-glass opacity surrounded by a > 2 mm crescent or ring of denser consolidation. Kim et al. reported the reverse-halo sign in 19% of biopsy proven cases of OP [62]. However, a reverse halo sign has since been reported in numerous separate entities [62]. Reticulation and honeycombing are uncommon to rare but when present are associated with an increased risk of progressive disease [63–65].

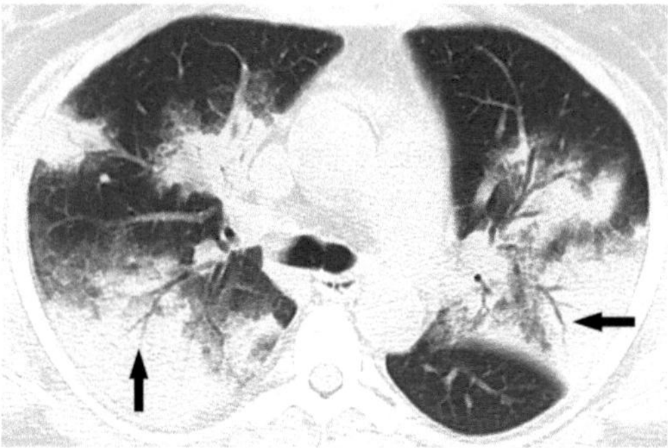

Fig. 12.13 Cryptogenic organizing pneumonia. HRCT image shows multiple foci of peripheral and peribronchial consolidation with air bronchograms (*arrows*)

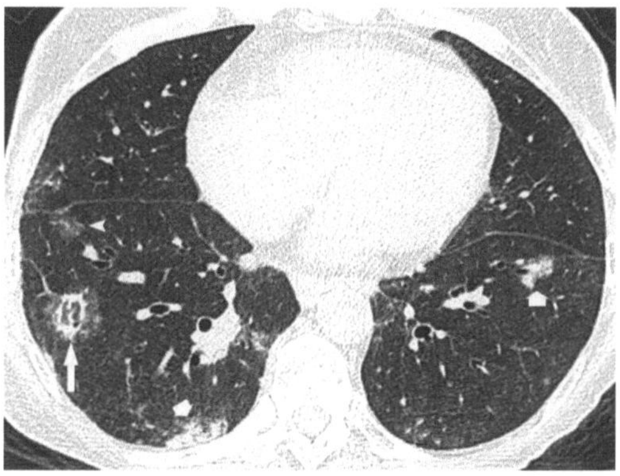

Fig. 12.14 Cryptogenic organizing pneumonia. HRCT image shows foci of consolidation (*wide arrows*) and ground-glass opacity (*arrowhead*) and a reverse halo sign (*thin arrow*), the latter characterized by central ground-glass opacity and a rim of consolidation

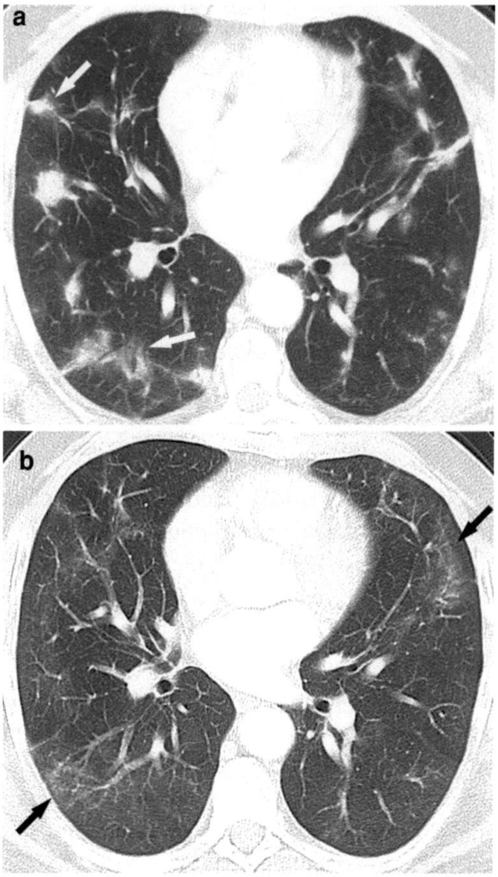

Fig. 12.15 Resolving cryptogenic organizing pneumonia. **a** HRCT image shows scattered of lung consolidation (*arrows*) in a peripheral and peribronchial distribution. **b** HRCT image obtained 2 weeks later shows patchy ground-glass opacity (*arrows*) where consolidation once was

With treatment, clinical and radiologic response is often striking. Symptomatic improvement may be expected within 1–2 days, while radiologic resolution occurs over several weeks (Fig. 12.15) [66]. Although relapse is not common, it does not worsen the long-term prognosis.

Respiratory Bronchiolitis, Respiratory Bronchiolitis–Interstitial Lung Disease, and Desquamative Interstitial Pneumonia

Respiratory bronchiolitis (RB), RB-associated interstitial lung disease (RB-ILD), and desquamative interstitial pneumonia (DIP) are included in the most recent IIP classification despite being almost invariably associated with cigarette smoking. RB, RB-ILD, and DIP represent a spectrum of smoking-related interstitial lung disease characterized by the accumulation of pigmented macrophages in the respiratory bronchioles and alveoli [67]. With RB, pigmented macrophages are limited primarily to the respiratory bronchioles whereas macrophage accumulation is more extensive with RB-ILD and diffuse in DIP. By definition, patients with RB are asymptomatic while those with RB-ILD and DIP may present with dyspnea, cough, and abnormal pulmonary function tests [68].

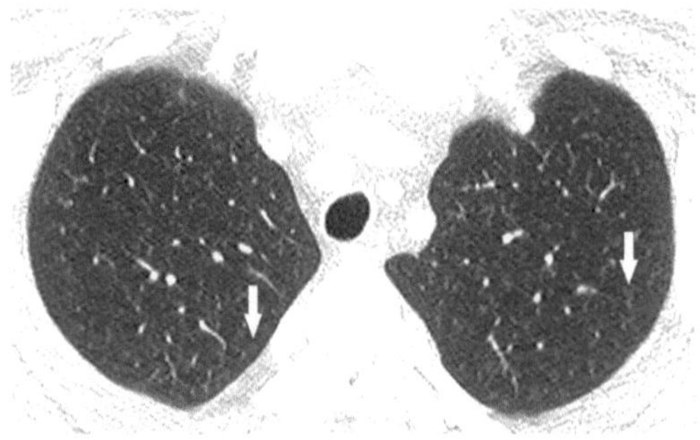

Fig. 12.16 Respiratory bronchiolitis. HRCT image shows scattered, poorly defined ground-glass attenuation nodules (*arrows*) in the upper lobes of this cigarette smoker

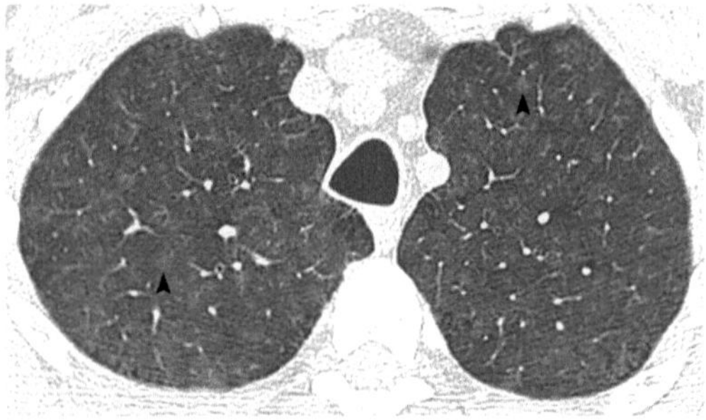

Fig. 12.17 RB-ILD. HRCT image shows diffuse, poorly defined centrilobular nodules (*arrowheads*) in the upper lobes of this heavy cigarette smoker who presented with dyspnea and cough

Characteristic HRCT findings of RB include mild, poorly defined centrilobular nodules in a mid and upper lung distribution (Fig. 12.16) with scattered, patchy ground-glass opacities [69]. Associated findings include occasional lobular air trapping and emphysema. With RB-ILD, the extent of poorly defined centrilobular nodules is greater (Fig. 12.17), and more extensive patchy ground-glass opacity may be present (Fig. 12.18) [70]. With smoking cessation, these parenchymal abnormalities are reversible to some degree [71].

DIP is rare and associated with more severe and diffuse parenchymal abnormality [72]. HRCT findings consist of diffuse ground-glass opacities with peripheral and lower lung predominance (Fig. 12.19) [12]. Reticular opacities are common but are often relatively mild and limited to a bibasilar distribution (Fig. 12.20). Small well-defined cysts may occur in areas of ground-glass opacity [73]. Centrilobular nodules are uncommon, while CT findings of respiratory bronchiolitis tend to be less severe than in RB-ILD [74]. DIP on CT may be indistinguishable from NSIP, acute or subacute hypersensitivity pneumonitis, and infections such as *Pneumocystis jiroveci* [67].

Acute Interstitial Pneumonia

Acute interstitial pneumonia (AIP) is diagnostically reserved for diffuse alveolar damage of unknown origin. Histologically, AIP is

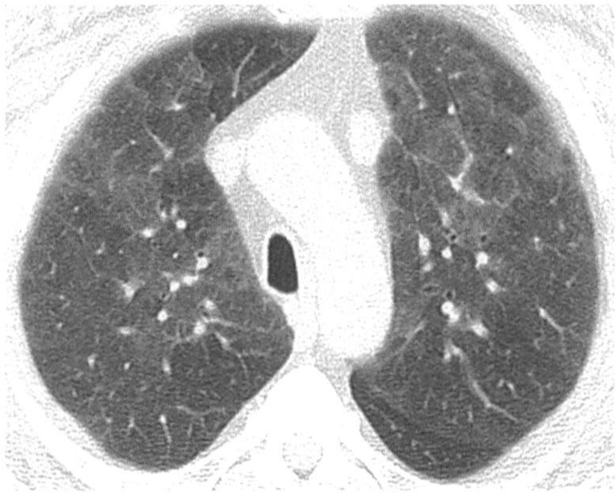

Fig. 12.18 RB-ILD. HRCT image shows patchy ground-glass opacities in the upper lobes of this heavy cigarette smoker who presented with dyspnea

indistinguishable from acute respiratory distress syndrome (ARDS) secondary to shock or sepsis. CT findings in the early exudative phase include dependent, subpleural consolidation and ground-glass opacities in a geographic, patchy, symmetric, and bilateral distribution (Fig. 12.21). Multiple foci of lobular sparing contribute to a geographic pattern. Greater than 50% of the lung parenchyma is typically involved [75].

In the subacute, organizing stage, traction bronchiectasis and architectural distortion progress with the duration of illness (Fig. 12.22). These findings are characteristically prominent relative to any degree of reticulation or honeycombing [76]. Pleural effusions are found in approximately 30%. While typically indistinguishable from ARDS, AIP is more commonly

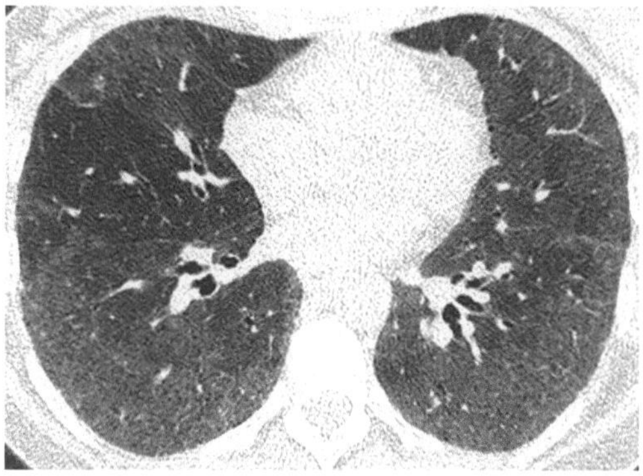

Fig. 12.19 Desquamative interstitial pneumonia in a heavy smoker. Low-dose HRCT shows extensive ground-glass opacity in the periphery of the lung bases. The HRCT findings of DIP can overlap those of NSIP

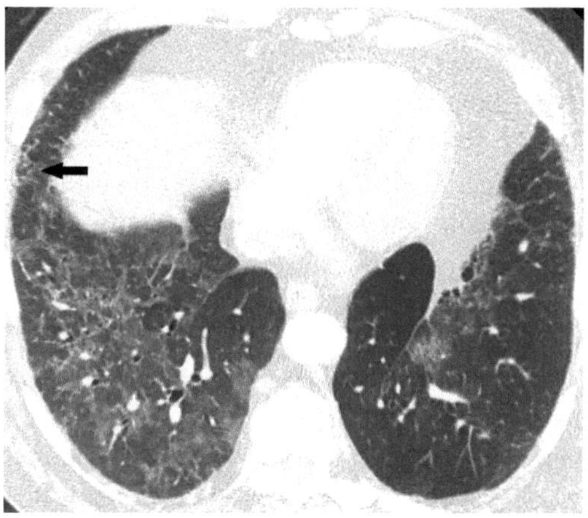

Fig. 12.20 Desquamative interstitial pneumonia in a heavy smoker. HRCT image shows patchy ground-glass opacity in the lower lobes. Mild subpleural reticulation (*arrow*) is present

lower lobe predominant in distribution with a greater prevalence of fibrotic changes [77, 78]. As with UIP and NSIP, the degree of fibrotic changes positively correlates with a worsened prognosis. ARDS, conversely, is more commonly associated with interlobular septal thickening. Differential considerations for an AIP/ARDS pattern include pulmonary edema, widespread infection, pulmonary hemorrhage, and acute eosinophilic pneumonia [67, 76, 79].

If a patient with AIP recovers, consolidation and ground-glass opacities typically clear in a progressive fashion, while residual areas of reticulation and hypoattenuation remain, particularly in the nondependent lung [76].

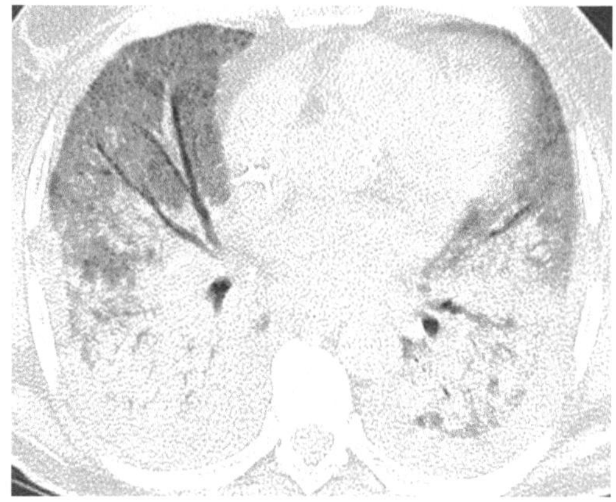

Fig. 12.21 Acute interstitial pneumonia. Low-dose HRCT image shows diffuse ground-glass opacity with superimposed septal thickening in the anterior lungs and consolidation in the dependent lungs

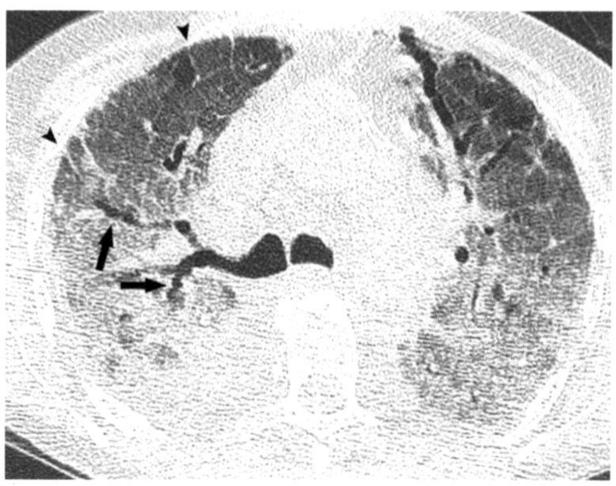

Fig. 12.22 Organizing phase of acute interstitial pneumonia. HRCT image shows ground-glass opacity and septal thickening (*arrowheads*) with dependent consolidation. Traction bronchiectasis (*arrows*) suggests developing fibrosis, although this is sometimes reversible

Lymphoid Interstitial Pneumonia

Lymphoid interstitial pneumonia (LIP) is a rare diagnosis most commonly seen in patients with Sjögren syndrome. Additional associations include other connective tissue and autoimmune diseases as well as AIDS, the latter particularly in children. Despite being a lymphoproliferative

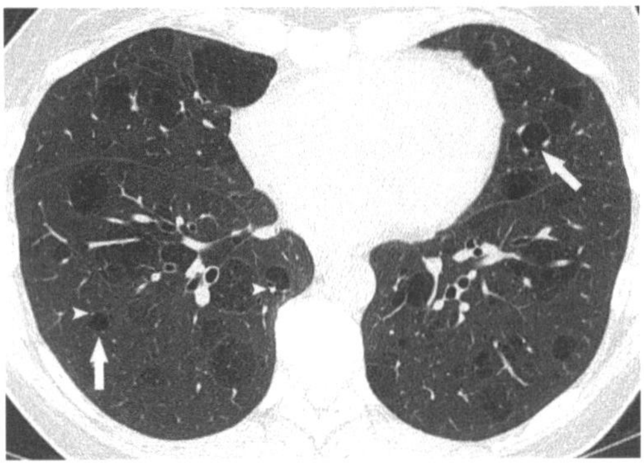

Fig. 12.23 Lymphoid interstitial pneumonia and Sjögren syndrome. HRCT image shows numerous thin-walled cysts (*arrows*) with adjacent vessels (*arrowheads*)

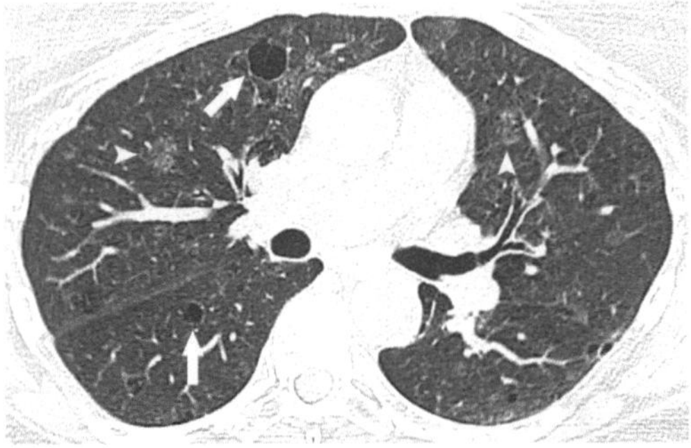

Fig. 12.24 Lymphoid interstitial pneumonia and Sjögren syndrome. HRCT image shows scattered thin-walled cysts (*arrows*) and scattered ground-glass attenuation opacities (*arrowheads*)

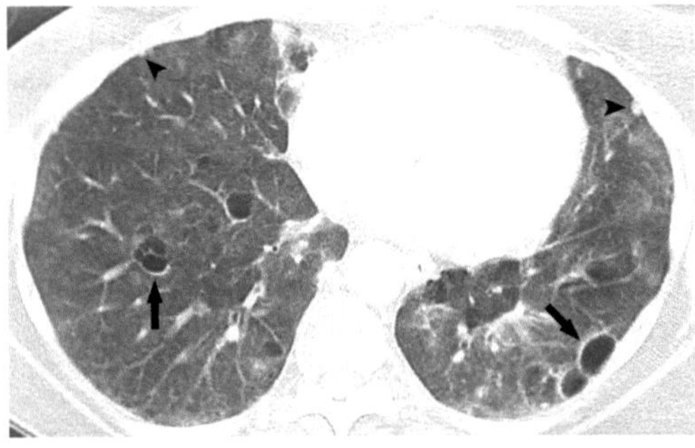

Fig. 12.25 Lymphoid interstitial pneumonia and Sjögren syndrome. HRCT image shows extensive ground-glass opacity, subpleural nodules (*arrowheads*), and scattered thin-walled cysts

disorder, LIP is included in the most recent classification system as an interstitial lung disease, given its inclusion in associated differential diagnoses of diffuse lung disease and its histologic pattern, which is characterized by a polyclonal lymphocytic and plasma cell infiltration of the alveolar septum [1].

The common HRCT findings of LIP include bilateral ground-glass opacity, thin-walled perivascular cysts located predominantly within the lower lobes, and poorly defined centrilobular nodules (Figs. 12.23, 12.24, 12.25). The cysts tend to range from 1 mm to 30 mm in diameter and are typically fewer in number compared with lymphangioleiomyomatosis. Less common findings include perilymphatic nodules and septal and bronchovascular thickening [67, 80–82]. Nodules or calcifications may develop in cysts, reflecting amyloid deposition.

Conclusion

In summary, HRCT is critical to evaluating patients with known or suspected diffuse lung disease. In patients with the appropriate clinical presentation, a highly confident diagnosis of UIP on HRCT is sufficient to establish a diagnosis of IPF. HRCT may also suggest the presence of other interstitial or diffuse lung diseases. Finally, consensus among the clinician, radiologist, and pathologist may be required to establish a diagnosis when the pieces of the diagnostic puzzle are not straightforward.

References

1. American Thoracic Society/European Respiratory Society International Multidisciplinary Consensus Classification of the Idiopathic Interstitial Pneumonias. Am J Respir Crit Care Med. 2002;165(2):277–304.
2. Liebow AA, Carington CB. The interstitial pneumonias. In: Simon M, Potchen EJ, LeMay M, editors. Frontiers in pulmonary radiology. New York: Grune and Stratton; 1969. p. 102–41.
3. Katzenstein AL. Katzenstein and askin's surgical pathology of non-neoplastic lung disease. Philadelphia: WB Saunders; 1997.
4. Müller NL, Colby TV. Idiopathic interstitial pneumonias: high-resolution CT and histologic findings. Radiographics. 1997;17:1016–22.

5. Raghu G, Collard HR, Egan JJ, et al. An official ATS/ERS/JRS/ALAT statement: idiopathic pulmonary fibrosis: evidence-based guidelines for diagnosis and management. Am J Respir Crit Care Med. 2011;183(6): 788–824.
6. Raghu G, Weycker D, Edelsberg J, et al. Incidence and prevalence of idiopathic pulmonary fibrosis. Am J Respir Crit Care Med. 2006;174:810–6.
7. Baumgartner KB, Samet JM, Coultas DB, et al. Occupational and environmental risk factors for idiopathic pulmonary fibrosis: a multicenter case-control study. Collaborating Centers. Am J Epidemiol. 2000;152:307–15.
8. Baumgartner KB, Samet JM, Stidley CA, et al. Cigarette smoking: a risk factor for idiopathic pulmonary fibrosis. Am J Respir Crit Care Med. 1994;150:670–5.
9. Kelly BG, Lok SS, Hasleton PS, et al. A rearranged form of Epstein-Barr virus DNA is associated with idiopathic pulmonary fibrosis. Am J Respir Crit Care Med. 2002;166:510–3.
10. Travis WD, Matsui K, Moss J, et al. Idiopathic nonspecific interstitial pneumonia: prognostic significance of cellular and fibrosing patterns: survival comparison with usual interstitial pneumonia and desquamative interstitial pneumonia. Am J Surg Pathol. 2000;24:19–33.
11. Nishimura K, Kitaichi M, Izumi T, et al. Usual interstitial pneumonia: histologic correlation with high-resolution CT. Radiology. 1992;182:337–42.
12. Johkoh T, Muller NL, Cartier Y, et al. Idiopathic interstitial pneumonias: diagnostic accuracy of thin-section CT in 129 patients. Radiology. 1999;211: 555–60.
13. American Thoracic Society; European Respiratory Society. Idiopathic pulmonary fibrosis: diagnosis and treatment: international consensus statement. Am J Respir Crit Care Med. 2000;161:646–64.
14. Iwai K, Mori T, Yamada N, et al. Idiopathic pulmonary fibrosis: epidemiologic approaches to occupational exposure. Am J Respir Crit Care Med. 1994;150:670–5.
15. Enomoto T, Usuki J, Azuma A, et al. Diabetes mellitus may increase risk for idiopathic pulmonary fibrosis. Chest. 2003;123:2007–11.
16. Steele MP, Speer MC, Loyd JE, et al. Clinical and pathologic features of familial interstitial pneumonia. Am J Respir Crit Care Med. 2005;172:1146–52.
17. Miyake Y, Sasaki S, Yokoyama T, et al. Occupational and environmental factors and idiopathic pulmonary fibrosis in Japan. Ann Occup Hyg. 2005;49:259–65.
18. Taskar VS, Coultas DB. Is idiopathic pulmonary fibrosis an environmental disease? Proc Am Thorac Soc. 2006;3:293–8.
19. Hwang JH, Misumi S, Sahin H, et al. Computed tomographic features of idiopathic fibrosing interstitial pneumonia: comparison with pulmonary fibrosis related to collagen vascular disease. J Comput Assist Tomogr. 2009;33:410–5.
20. Souza CA, Muller NL, Lee KS, et al. Idiopathic interstitial pneumonias: prevalence of mediastinal lymph node enlargement in 206 patients. AJR. 2006;186:995–9.
21. Maher TM. The diagnosis of idiopathic pulmonary fibrosis and its complications. Expert Opin Med Diagn. 2008;2:1317–31.
22. Mathieson JR, Mayo JR, Staples CA, et al. Chronic diffuse infiltrative lung disease: comparison of diagnostic accuracy of CT and chest radiography. Radiology. 1989;171:111–6.
23. Raghu G, Mageto YN, Lockhart D, et al. The accuracy of the clinical diagnosis of new-onset idiopathic pulmonary fibrosis and other interstitial lung disease: A prospective study. Chest. 1999;116: 1168–74.
24. Hunninghake GW, Zimmerman MB, Schwartz DA, et al. Utility of lung biopsy for the diagnosis of idiopathic pulmonary fibrosis. Am J Respir Crit Care Med. 2001;164:193–6.
25. Grenier P, Valeyre D, Cluzel P, et al. Chronic diffuse interstitial lung disease: diagnostic value of chest radiography and high-resolution CT. Radiology. 1991;179:123–32.
26. Lee KS, Primack SL, Staples CA, et al. Chronic infiltrative lung disease: comparison of diagnostic accuracies of radiography and low- and conventional-dose thin-section CT. Radiology. 1994;191:669–73.
27. Swensen SJ, Aughenbaugh GL, Myers JL. Diffuse lung disease: diagnostic accuracy of CT in patients undergoing surgical biopsy of the lung. Radiology. 1997;205:229–34.
28. Silva C, Muller NL, Lynch DA, et al. Chronic hypersensitivity pneumonitis: differentiation from idiopathic pulmonary fibrosis and nonspecific interstitial pneumonia by using thin-section CT. Radiology. 2008;246(1):288–97.
29. Mejia M, Carrillo G, Rojas-Serrano J, et al. Idiopathic pulmonary fibrosis and emphysema: decreased survival associated with severe pulmonary arterial hypertension. Chest. 2009;136: 10–5.
30. Nadrous HF, Pellikka PA, Krowka MJ, et al. The impact of pulmonary hypertension on survival in patients with idiopathic pulmonary fibrosis. Chest. 2005;128:616S–7S.
31. Lettieri CJ, Nathan SD, Barnett SD, et al. Prevalence and outcomes of pulmonary arterial hypertension in advanced idiopathic pulmonary fibrosis. Chest. 2006;129:746–52.
32. Martinez FJ, Safrin S, Weycker D, et al. The clinical course of patients with idiopathic pulmonary fibrosis. Ann Intern Med. 2005;142:963–7.
33. Panos RJ, Mortenson RL, Niccoli SA. Clinical deterioration in patients with idiopathic pulmonary fibrosis: causes and assessment. Am J Med. 1990; 88:396–404.
34. Papiris SA, Manali ED, Roussos C, et al. Clinical review: idiopathic pulmonary fibrosis acute

exacerbations–unravelling Ariadne's thread. Crit Care. 2010;14(6):246.
35. Collard HR, Moore BB, Flaherty KR, et al. Idiopathic Pulmonary Fibrosis Clinical Research Network Investigators, Acute exacerbations of idiopathic pulmonary fibrosis. Am J Respir Crit Care Med. 2007;176:636–43.
36. Kim DS, Park JH, Park BK, et al. Acute exacerbation of idiopathic pulmonary fibrosis: frequency and clinical features. Eur Respir J. 2006;27:143–50.
37. Parambil JG, Myers JL, Ryu JH. Histopathologic features and outcome of patients with acute exacerbation of idiopathic pulmonary fibrosis undergoing surgical lung biopsy. Chest. 2005;128: 3310–5.
38. Rice AJ, Wells AU, Bouros D, et al. Terminal diffuse alveolar damage in relation to interstitial pneumonias: an autopsy study. Am J Clin Pathol. 2003;119:709–14.
39. Churg A, Muller NL, Silva CIS, et al. Acute exacerbation (acute lung injury of unknown cause) in UIP and other forms of fibrotic interstitial pneumonias. Am J Surg Pathol. 2007;31:277–84.
40. Alhamed EH, Al-Boukai AA, Shaik SA, et al. Prediction of Pulmonary Hypertension in Patients with or without Interstitial Lung Disease: Reliability of CT Findings. Radiology May 2011; e-publication ahead of print.
41. Bouros D, Hatzakis K, Labrakis H, et al. Association of malignancy with diseases causing interstitial pulmonary changes. Chest. 2002;121:1278–89.
42. Travis WD, Hunninghake G, King TE Jr, et al. Idiopathic nonspecific interstitial pneumonia: report of an American Thoracic Society project. Am J Respir Crit Care Med. 2008;177:1338–47.
43. Cottin V, Donsbeck AV, Revel D, et al. Nonspecific interstitial pneumonia: individualization of a clinicopathologic entity in a series of 12 patients. Am J Respir Crit Care Med. 1998;158:1286–93.
44. Kim TS, Lee KS, Chung MP, et al. Nonspecific interstitial pneumonia with fibrosis: high-resolution CT and pathologic findings. AJR. 1998;171:1645–50.
45. Park CS, Jeon JW, Park SW, et al. Nonspecific interstitial pneumonia/fibrosis: clinical manifestations, histologic and radiologic features. Korean J Intern Med. 1996;11:122–32.
46. Park JS, Lee KS, Kim JS, et al. Nonspecific interstitial pneumonia with fibrosis: radiographic and CT findings in seven patients. Radiology. 1995;195:645–8.
47. Elliot TL, Lynch DA, Newell JD Jr, et al. High-resolution computed tomography features of nonspecific interstitial pneumonia and usual interstitial pneumonia. J Comput Assist Tomogr. 2005;29:339–45.
48. Jeong YJ, Lee KS, Muller NL, et al. Usual interstitial pneumonia and non-specific interstitial pneumonia: serial thin-section CT findings correlated with pulmonary function. Korean J Radiol. 2005; 6:143–52.
49. Flaherty KR, Travis WD, Colby TV, et al. Histopathologic variability in usual and nonspecific interstitial pneumonias. Am J Respir Crit Care Med. 2001;164:1722–7.
50. Tsubamoto M, Muller NL, Johkoh T, et al. Pathologic subgroups of nonspecific interstitial pneumonia: differential diagnosis from other idiopathic interstitial pneumonias on high-resolution computed tomography. J Comput Assist Tomogr. 2005;29:793–800.
51. Sumikawa H, Johkoh T, Ichikado K, et al. Usual interstitial pneumonia and chronic idiopathic interstitial pneumonia: analysis of CT appearance in 92 patients. Radiology. 2006;241:258–66.
52. Kligeman SF, Groshong S, Brown KK, et al. Nonspecific Interstitial Pneumonia: Radiologic, Clinical, and Pathologic Considerations. RadioGraphics. 2009;29: 73–87.
53. MacDonald SL, Rubens MB, Hansell DM, et al. Nonspecific interstitial pneumonia and usual interstitial pneumonia: comparative appearances at and diagnostic accuracy of thin-section CT. Radiology. 2001;221:600–5.
54. Flaherty KR, Toews GB, Travis WD, et al. Clinical significance of histological classification of idiopathic interstitial pneumonia. Eur Respir J. 2002;19:275–83.
55. Nicholson AG, Colby TV, du Bois RM, Hansell DM, Wells AU. The prognostic significance of the histologic pattern of interstitial pneumonia in patients presenting with the clinical entity of cryptogenic fibrosing alveolitis. Am J Respir Crit Care Med. 2000;162:2213–7.
56. Flaherty KR, Thwaite EL, Kazerooni EA, et al. Radiological versus histological diagnosis in UIP and NSIP: survival implications. Thorax. 2003;58:143–8.
57. Johkoh T, Muller NL, Colby TV, et al. Nonspecific interstitial pneumonia: correlation between thin-section CT findings and pathologic subgroups in 55 patients. Radiology. 2002;225:199–204.
58. Park IN, Kim DS, Shim TS, et al. Acute exacerbation of interstitial pneumonia other than idiopathic pulmonary fibrosis. Chest. 2007;132:214–20.
59. Nishiyama O, Kondoh Y, Taniguchi H, et al. Serial high resolution CT findings in nonspecific interstitial pneumonia/fibrosis. J Comput Assist Tomogr. 2000; 24:41–6.
60. Muller NL, Guerry-Force ML, Staples CA, et al. Differential diagnosis of bronchiolitis obliterans with organizing pneumonia and usual interstitial pneumonia: clinical, functional, and radiologic findings. Radiology. 1987;162:151–6.
61. Kim SJ, Lee KS, Ryu YH, et al. Reversed halo sign on high-resolution CT of cryptogenic organizing pneumonia: diagnostic implications. AJR. 2003;180: 1251–4.
62. Walker C, Tan-Lucien M, Chung JH. Reversed halo sign. J Thoracic Imaging. 2011;26:3.
63. Bouchardy LM, Kuhlman JE, Ball WC Jr, et al. CT findings in bronchiolitis obliterans organizing

pneumonia (BOOP) with radiographic, clinical, and histologic correlation. J Comput Assist Tomogr. 1993;17:352–7.
64. Cordier JF, Loire R, Brune J. Idiopathic bronchiolitis obliterans organizing pneumonia: definition of characteristic clinical profiles in a series of 16 patients. Chest. 1989;96:999–1004.
65. Lee J, Lynch D, Sharma S, et al. Organizing pneumonia: prognostic implication of high-resolution CT features. J Comput Assist Tomogr. 2003;27:260–5.
66. Lynch DA, Travis WD, King TE, et al. Idiopathic interstitial pneumonias: CT features. Radiology. 2005;236:10–21.
67. Myers JL, Veal CF Jr, et al. Respiratory bronchiolitis causing interstitial lung disease. A clinicopathologic study of six cases. Am Rev Respir Dis. 1987;135: 880–4.
68. Davies G, Wells AU, du Bois RM. Respiratory bronchiolitis associated with interstitial lung disease and desquamative interstitial pneumonia. Clin Chest Med. 2004;25:717–26. vi.
69. Remy-Jardin M, Remy J, Gosselin B, et al. Lung parenchymal changes secondary to cigarette smoking: pathologic-CT correlations. Radiology. 1993;186:643–51.
70. Holt R, Schmidt R, Godwin J, et al. High resolution CT in respiratory bronchiolitis-associated interstitial lung disease. J Comput Assist Tomogr. 1993;17:46–50.
71. Park JS, Brown KK, Tuder RM, et al. Respiratory bronchiolitis-associated interstitial lung disease: radiologic features with clinical and pathologic correlation. J Comput Assist Tomogr. 2002;26:13–20.
72. Ryu JH, Colby TV, Hartman TE, et al. Smoking-related interstitial lung diseases: a concise review. Eur Respir J. 2001;17:122–32.
73. Koyama M, Johkoh T, Honda O, et al. Chronic cystic lung disease: diagnostic accuracy of high-resolution CT in 92 patients. AJR. 2003;180:827–35.
74. Hartman TE, Primack SL, Swensen SJ, et al. Desquamative interstitial pneumonia: thin-section CT findings in 22 patients. Radiology. 1993;187:787–90.
75. Ichikado K, Johkoh T, Ikezoe J, et al. Acute interstitial pneumonia: high-resolution CT findings correlated with pathology. AJRl. 1997;168:333–8.
76. Johkoh T, Muller NL, Taniguchi H, et al. Acute interstitial pneumonia: thin-section CT findings in 36 patients. Radiology. 1999;211:859–63.
77. Tomiyama N, Muller NL, Johkoh T, et al. Acute respiratory distress syndrome and acute interstitial pneumonia: comparison of thin-section CT findings. J Comput Assist Tomogr. 2001;25:28–33.
78. Swigris JJ, et al. Acute interstitial pneumonia and acute exacerbations of idiopathic pulmonary fibrosis. Semin Respir Crit Care Med. 2006;27(6):659–67.
79. Thannickal VJ. Idiopathic interstitial pneumonia: a clinicopathological perspective. Semin Respir Crit Care Med. 2006;27(6):569–73.
80. Jonkoh T. Imaging of idiopathic interstitial pneumonias. Clin Chest Med. 2008;29.1:133–47.
81. Swigris JJ, Berry GJ, Raffin TA, et al. Lymphoid interstitial pneumonia: a narrative review. Chest. 2002;122(6):2150–64.
82. Das S, Miller RF. Lymphocytic interstitial pneumonitis in HIV infected adults. Sex Transm Infect. 2002; 79:88–93.

Occupational Lung Disease

13

Cris A. Meyer and James E. Lockey

Abstract

The term occupational lung disease encompasses the broad category of airway, lung parenchymal, and pleural disorders that occur due to the inhalation of natural occurring and manmade agents of various chemical and physical compositions. This chapter will describe the classic mineral dust exposures of asbestos, silica, and coal. In addition, examples of immune-mediated occupational lung disease will be reviewed including berylliosis, hard metal disease, and chronic hypersensitivity pneumonitis. In more recent years, airway diseases including occupational asthma have become the leading cause of work-related lung disorders in the industrialized world. While imaging is rarely necessary in occupational asthma, several entities associated with bronchiolitis obliterans will be discussed.

Keywords

Occupational lung disease • Pneumoconiosis • Asbestosis • Silicosis • Coal workers' pneumoconiosis • Berylliosis • Hypersensitivity pneumonitis • Bronchiolitis obliterans

Introduction

The term occupational lung disease encompasses a broad category of acute and chronic airway, lung parenchymal, and pleural disorders as related to the inhalation of natural occurring and manmade agents of various chemical and physical compositions. Historically, mineral dust induced pneumoconiosis from silica, coal, and asbestos exposures have been the most common occupational lung diseases. In more recent years, airway diseases including occupational asthma have become the leading cause of

C. A. Meyer (✉)
Department of Radiology
University of Wisconsin Hospital and Clinics,
600 Highland Avenue, Madison,
WI 53792-3252, USA
e-mail: cmeyer2@uwhealth.org

J. E. Lockey
Department of Environmental Health,
University of Cincinnati College of Medicine,
3223 Eden Ave., Kettering Lab, G16,
Cincinnati, OH 45267, USA
e-mail: james.lockey@uc.edu

J. P. Kanne (ed.), *Clinically Oriented Pulmonary Imaging*,
Respiratory Medicine, DOI: 10.1007/978-1-61779-542-8_13,

work-related lung disorders in the industrialized world [1–3]. The toxic effects of inhaled substances depend on physical characteristics such as size, shape, surface area, chemical composition, and dose to the target organ as indirectly reflected by the intensity and duration of exposure. Finally, an individual's immune system and genetics influence the type and extent of the pulmonary response to inhaled organic and inorganic substances [4].

The diagnosis of occupational lung disease depends on the combination of a thorough occupational exposure history, medical history and physical examination, and appropriate laboratory testing including pulmonary function and radiographic evaluation. In the setting of occupational lung disease, the radiologist plays an important role in the detection of radiographic patterns associated with specific occupational exposures, in monitoring disease progression, in the assessment for pulmonary impairment and in the diagnosis of potential infectious or neoplastic complications.

Pneumoconiosis refers to the reaction of the lung to inhaled mineral dust. The Work Related Lung Disease Surveillance Report 2002 produced by the Division of Respiratory Disease Studies at National Institute of Occupational Safety and Health (NIOSH) reported more than 31,000 deaths nationwide resulting from pneumoconiosis during the 10-year period from 1990 to 1999 [5]. While the death rates of coal workers' pneumoconiosis (CWP) and silicosis declined when comparing the periods of 1968–1981 to 1982–2000, the death rates from pulmonary asbestosis increased almost 400% [6]. Occupational lung disease remains a significant cause of morbidity and mortality among adults of working age and the annual estimated cost for occupational diseases including respiratory illness exceeds $26 billion [7].

This chapter will describe the classic mineral dust exposures: asbestos, silica, and coal. In addition, examples of immune-mediated occupational lung disease will be described including berylliosis, hard metal disease, and hypersensitivity pneumonitis (e.g. farmer's lung). Finally, several of the emerging entities recognized to cause occupational related airway disease will be described.

Non-Malignant Asbestos-Related Disease

It has been estimated that 40% of the US workforce or nearly 27 million individuals were exposed to asbestos between 1940 and 1979 [8]. Pulmonary asbestosis represented one-third of all pneumoconiosis deaths reported over the 10-year period between 1990 and 1999 [5]. Asbestos-related disease results in the death of 1 out of every 125 American males over 50 years of age [9].

Asbestos fibers are divided into two major groups: serpentine and amphibole [10]. Among the varieties of serpentine asbestos, chrysotile (white asbestos) accounted for 90% of asbestos used in the United States. Chrysotile fibers have a serpentine or curly configuration and are more easily fragmented and cleared from the lung in comparison to amphibole asbestos. The amphiboles, crocidolite (blue asbestos) and amosite (brown asbestos) were also used in various commercial applications. Amphibole fibers have a straight, rigid and needle-like configuration, are extremely durable in physiologic fluids and have a prolonged "residence" time in the lung parenchyma, which accounts for their increased fibrogenic and carcinogenic properties. Exposures have occurred in various industrial settings including asbestos mining and processing, construction and insulation, shipbuilding, and the manufacture and installation of asbestos textiles and other asbestos containing products [11]. Duration and time from initial asbestos exposure as well as job task characteristics are important factors when clinically evaluating a worker for potential asbestos-related pulmonary disorders.

Long, thin respirable-sized asbestos fibers can deposit in respiratory bronchioles and alveoli and translocate to the interstitial space and pleural surface. Parenchymal fibrosis is found around the respiratory bronchiole and in the subpleural interstitium. A small proportion of fibers is engulfed by macrophages and covered with an iron protein coating resulting in an asbestos body (also referred to as a ferruginous body). In a recent study, the presence of asbestos bodies in bronchial alveolar lavage (BAL) fluid of asbestos exposed individuals was associated with an increased prevalence of parenchymal disease (70% vs. 26%) [12]. Small airway dysfunction in asbestos-exposed individuals can result from peribronchial fibrosis and resultant airway narrowing and air trapping [13]. Recent studies suggest that individuals with lower levels of asbestos exposure may manifest a mild obstructive rather than restrictive pattern on pulmonary function tests, the latter of which has historically been associated with radiographic evidence of pulmonary asbestosis [13].

Pleural abnormalities are the most common finding in asbestos exposed individuals and manifest as pleural effusions, diffuse pleural thickening, and pleural plaques. Pleural effusions, while uncommon occuring in 3–7% of exposed workers, are typically the earliest manifestation of asbestos exposure, and classically occur within the first 5–10 years after exposure. The accompanying pleuritis involves the visceral and parietal pleura, and the fluid is exudative and often blood-tinged. The effusions usually resolve in 3–4 months leaving no residual findings except for potential residual blunting of the corresponding costophrenic angle [10]. Diagnosis requires a history of exposure and exclusion of other etiologies such as malignancy, infection, trauma or pulmonary infarction [14]. Asbestos-related pleural mesothelioma can present as a unilateral pleural effusion and should be considered in the differential diagnosis, particularly in older individuals with greater than 20- to 25-year latency from initial asbestos exposure.

Diffuse pleural thickening occurs in up to 13% of exposed individuals and appears to be the sequela of asbestos-related pleural effusion and the ensuing fibrosis and fusion of the visceral and parietal pleura [15]. Of all the pleural manifestations of asbestos exposure, diffuse pleural thickening has the most established relationship to a restrictive pattern on pulmonary function tests [16]. Several radiographic criteria have been proposed to define diffuse pleural thickening including uninterrupted pleural thickening of greater than 25% of the chest wall or absolute distance of pleural involvement in transaxial and craniocaudad dimensions. However, the best correlation with functional impairment remains that defined by the International Labour Organization (ILO) system—blunting of the costophrenic angle equal to or greater than that depicted on the ILO standard radiograph of t/t opacities, profusion 1/1 [17] (Fig. 13.1a). Diffuse pleural thickening rarely calcifies and generally has indistinct inner margins with the lung parenchyma in contrast to the sharp inner surface of hyalinized parietal pleural plaque. Thickening of the minor fissure is often an accompanying radiographic finding. CT reveals parietal and visceral pleural thickening in a continuous sheet extending over several rib interspaces sometimes with residual loculated pleural fluid and proliferation of the extrapleural fat.

Localized pleural thickening or pleural plaques are the most common manifestation of asbestos exposure occurring in up to 80% of exposed workers. Pleural plaques manifest radiographically 15–30 years after exposure and increase with intensity of exposure [18]. Data based on studies of workers exposed to amphibole fibers in Libby vermiculite support a dose–response relationship [19]. Chrysotile fiber fragments have been identified in up to 50% of plaques at electron microscopy [20]. Plaques are discrete bundles of acellular collagen arranged in a basket weave pattern and are located almost exclusively on the parietal pleura with a covering of mesothelial cells. Plaques are usually bilateral and typically located posterolaterally adjacent to ribs 6–9 and at the dome of the hemidiaphragms with sparing of the costophrenic angles; plaques will calcify over time in 15% of cases (Fig. 13.2). Previous chest radiography (CXR) studies report a predilection for left pleural plaques; however, a recent CT study fails to support this observation [21]. The detection rate for plaques on CXR is less sensitive at 13–53% compared to CT scans and is also less specific. Other processes including

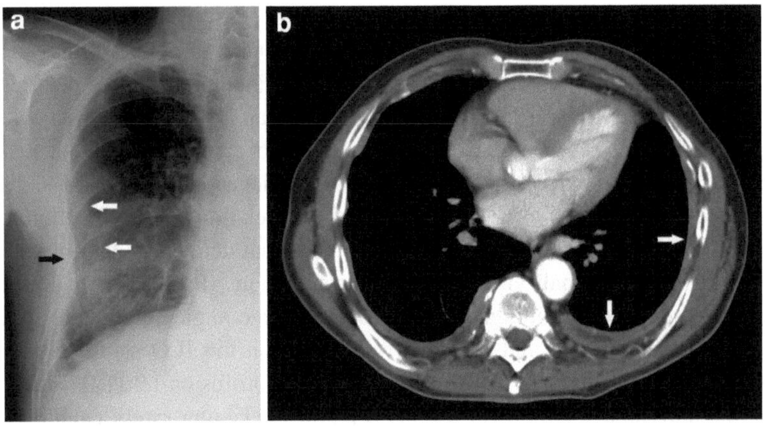

Fig. 13.1 **a** PA radiograph limited to the right lung reveals blunting of the right costophrenic angle and pleural thickening extending approximately half the distance up the lateral chest wall consistent with diffuse pleural thickening (*black arrow*). En face (*white arrows*) non-calcified pleural plaques are also present. **b** Contrast-enhanced chest CT in mediastinal windows with bilateral diffuse pleural thickening most pronounced on the left (*white arrows*) with small foci of calcification and proliferation of the extrapleural fat

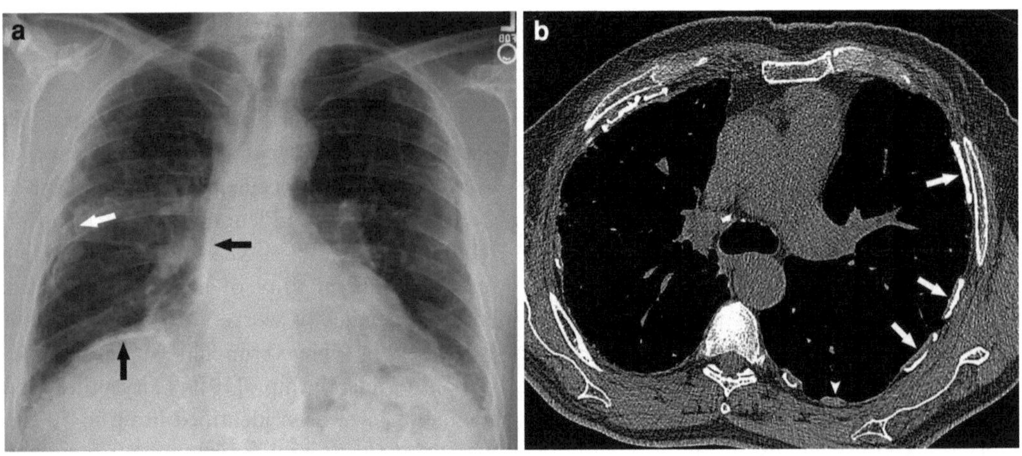

Fig. 13.2 **a** PA radiograph of calcified pleural plaque revealing the classic rolled edge appearance of plaque with a well-defined lateral margin and fading medial margin (*white arrow*). Calcified diaphragmatic and paraspinal pleural plaque is also present (*black arrows*). Coarse irregular linear interstitial markings in both costophrenic angles are due to asbestosis. **b** CT of calcified (*arrows*) and non-calcified parietal pleural plaque (*arrowheads*) with well-defined inner margins and a "mesa" configuration

extrapleural fat and pleural lipoma may simulate plaques on CXR (Fig. 13.3a). Distinguishing features of extrapleural fat include bilateral, symmetrical appearance that often extends into the major fissures and over the lung apices. Attenuation differences between fat and plaques are readily apparent on CT (Fig. 13.3b). The presence of pleural plaques documents a past history of asbestos exposure and, therefore, potential future risk for other asbestos-related diseases such as lung cancer and malignant mesothelioma. Pleural plaques alone are usually not associated with a clinically significant loss in lung function [16, 22].

Asbestosis is diffuse pulmonary fibrosis that usually develops 20 years or more after initial exposure and exhibits a definite dose–response relationship. Workers with interstitial fibrosis

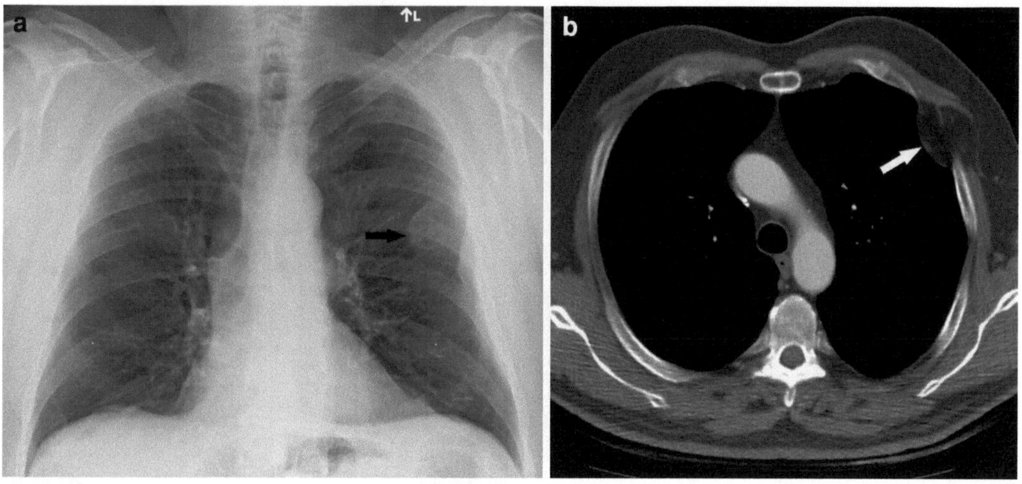

Fig. 13.3 **a** PA chest radiograph revealing an opacity in left mid lung zone with well-defined medial margin and fading lateral margin consistent with a pleural mass lesion of indeterminate etiology (*arrow*). **b** CT through this same region shows a fat attenuation lesion (*arrow*) consistent with an extrapleural lipoma and not a pleural plaque. Note that the low attenuation appearance of this lesion is identical to subcutaneous fat and contrast this with the dense non-calcified hyalinized plaque in Fig. 13.2b

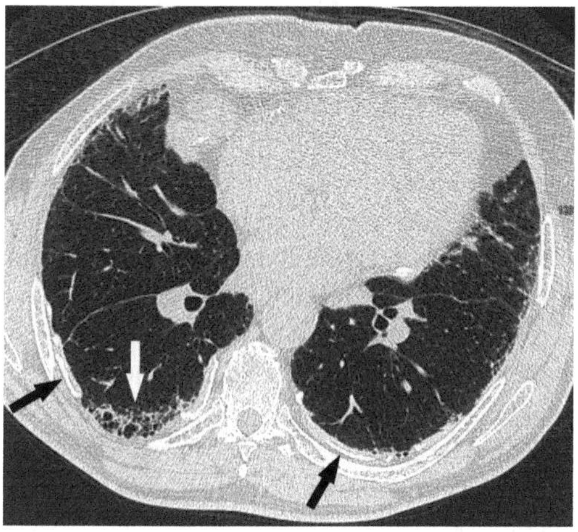

Fig. 13.4 Chest CT with subpleural linear irregular opacities and a region of honeycomb lung in the right lower lobe (*white arrow*) consistent with asbestosis. Calcified pleural plaques are also present (*black arrows*)

related to asbestos exposure also have pleural plaques in the majority of cases. CXR findings include low lung volumes, coarse irregular shadows, and a basilar and peripheral distribution of disease (Fig. 13.4a). HRCT findings include septal thickening, honeycomb lung, traction bronchiectasis, curvilinear subpleural lines, and parenchymal bands (Fig. 13.4b). Subpleural poorly defined centrilobular nodules have been described, likely reflecting the peribronchiolar fibrosis and, in combination with associated pleural findings, are useful in distinguishing asbestosis from other causes of pulmonary fibrosis [23]. It has been suggested that pleural tags and parenchymal bands are features more related to visceral pleural fibrosis and should be distinguished from the interstitial fibrosis characterizing asbestosis [24, 25]. Prone HRCT is useful for distinguishing mild fibrosis from dependent atelectasis. Remy-Jardin et al. demonstrated that low-dose CT examinations on a four-detector row helical CT system resulted in accurate depiction of asbestos-related pleuropulmonary disease compared with HRCT and may be a useful screening modality in the future [26]. Asbestos exposure puts an individual at higher risk for lung cancer, particularly those individuals with pulmonary asbestosis and a history of smoking. However, not all lung masses in patients with asbestosis are malignant. Lynch et al. characterized 43 unsuspected masses in 260 asbestos exposed individuals and reported round atelectasis as the most common cause in 11 patients, followed by 10 instances of fissural pleural plaques, 3 dense fibrotic bands, and 3 bronchogenic carcinomas;

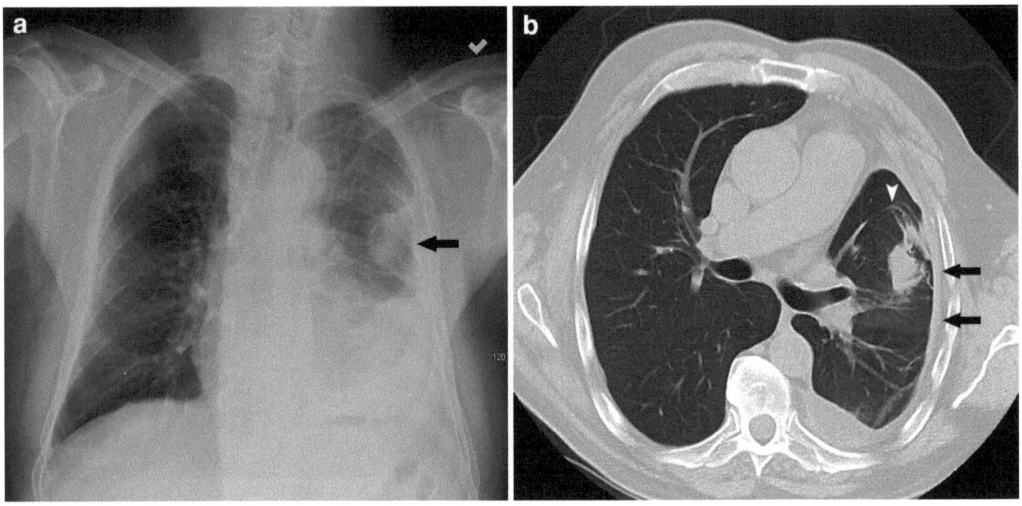

Fig. 13.5 **a** PA radiograph reveals diffuse left pleural thickening with volume loss and a focal mass-like opacity in the left mid zone (*arrow*). **b** CT of the chest through the mass confirms volume loss, pleural thickening (*arrows*), and swirling of vessels (*white arrowhead*) consistent with round atelectasis

the remaining 16 masses were stable on long-term follow-up and thus benign although not further characterized [27] (Fig. 13.5a). Round atelectasis is the most common benign mass associated with asbestos exposure. It is thought to be to the result of inflammatory reaction and fibrosis of the pleura that serves as a nidus for pleural buckling [28]. With progressive fibrosis, the buckled pleura serves as a lead point for subsequent atelectasis. Three radiographic signs must be present for the confident diagnosis of round atelectasis: pleural thickening, volume loss, and swirling of vessels ("comet tail" sign) (Fig. 13.5b). While typically benign, round atelectasis has been reported in association with mesothelioma [29]. FDG—PET may obviate the need for more invasive testing in patients with round atelectasis [30, 31]. Fissural pleural plaques and dense fibrotic bands can also appear as potential malignant lesions in asbestos exposed individuals [27].

Silicosis

Silicosis is caused by exposure to crystalline silica (silicon dioxide). Silica makes up nearly 25% of the earth's crust [32], and potential exposures occur in association with mining, quarrying, tunneling, stonecutting, polishing, sandblasting, foundry work, boiler scaling, and ceramics manufacturing. There are four manifestations of silica induced lung disease: acute silicoproteinosis, simple silicosis, complicated silicosis, and accelerated silicosis. Complications associated with silicosis include tuberculosis and a possible association with lung cancer [18]. Silica particles are ingested by macrophages that migrate to the lymphatics adjacent to the bronchioles. With macrophages death, inflammatory cytokines are released causing chronic fibrogenesis. The resulting nodular fibrotic foci contains layers of collagen and silica and are termed silicotic or hyalinized nodules, the unit lesions of silicosis. The ongoing release of crystalline silica results in a cascading fibrotic response, ultimately producing complicated silicosis with areas of conglomerate fibrosis. Deaths from silicosis have decreased from over 1000 per year in the 1960s to less than 200 per year in the 1990s [5].

Prior to the radiographic development of silicosis, exposures may lead to small airway dysfunction. This is characterized pathologically as fibrosis and pigmentation in the walls of the respiratory bronchioles [33]. A synergistic effect with cigarette smoking may lead to emphysema [34]. It has been postulated that symptomatic functional impairment in patients with mild silicosis is due to obstruction involving the small airways. Arakawa et al. [35] used paired inspiratory and expiratory HRCT and demonstrated a correlation between the presence of air trapping and spirometry in a small cohort of workers with silicosis.

Acute silicoproteinosis is a rare, rapidly progressive condition with death in 2–3 years due to extremely heavy exposures usually in an enclosed environment. Occasionally unusual occupations result in high intensity exposures that put workers at risk for acute silicoproteinosis. Most recently, an outbreak occurred in Turkey in the manufacturing of "distressed" denim using a sandblasting technique [36]. High intensity silica exposure results in proliferation of type II pneumocytes with copious surfactant production. Radiographically, the appearance is similar to pulmonary alveolar proteinosis with extensive bilateral airspace disease. A "crazy-paving" appearance of mosaic ground-glass with interlobular and intralobular septal thickening, multiple ill-defined centrilobular nodules, and lung consolidation is reported at HRCT [18, 37] (Fig. 13.6).

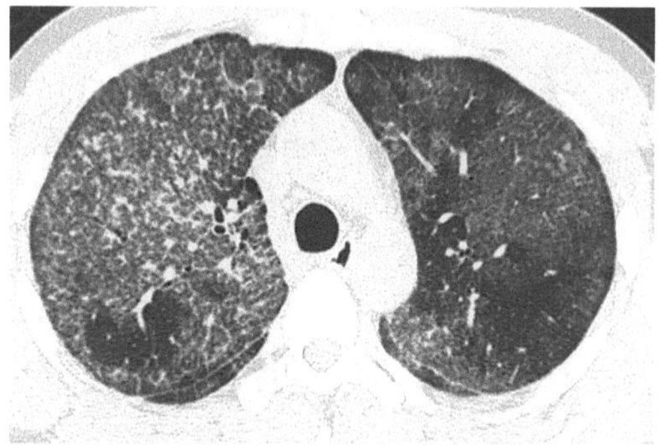

Fig. 13.6 HRCT of the chest in a stone mason's apprentice demonstrating patchy ground-glass opacity. There is superimposed interlobular and intralobular septal thickening in a "crazy-paving" pattern on the right consistent with acute silicoproteinosis

Simple silicosis usually manifests radiographically after a 10–20 year duration of exposure. The permissible exposure limits (PEL) established by Occupational Safety and Health (OSHA) for quartz is 0.1 mg/m^3 (time-weighted averages). At crystalline silica concentrations less than or equal to 0.5 mg/m^3, and with an exposure history of 2.0 mg/m^3-year, the cumulative risk of developing small opacities profusion category >1/0 is 1% [38]. The distribution of silicotic nodules largely depends on lymphatic drainage that in turn is dependent on pulmonary artery pressures, which are lower in the right lung. Chest wall excursion also contributes to "milking" of the lymphatics with the upper posterior chest wall having the least excursion. For these reasons, nodules are classically distributed with an upper lobe, posterior predominance, right-greater-than-left as noted on chest radiographs and CT [39] (Fig. 13.7). Multiple 2–5 mm nodules are characteristic, but occasionally larger opacities can occur and may calcify. Nodules are concentrated in a centrilobular distribution although may be perilymphatic at HRCT. In a perilymphatic distribution, nodules are seen along the bronchovascular bundles, the centrilobular core, and the subpleural interstitium. Irregular fibrosis around the respiratory bronchiole resulting in ill-defined or branching centrilobular opacities has been reported in the majority of patients in one HRCT review [40]. In keeping with the lymphatic clearance of particles, coalescent nodules in the subpleural interstitium may result in pseudoplaques; recent studies have reported a prevalence of localized pleural thickening from 32 to 58% resulting in the so-called "candle-wax" lesions [40–43] (Fig. 13.8). Hilar and mediastinal lymph node enlargement is often present and may precede parenchymal findings [44, 45]. In a study of silicotic patients 74% had hilar and/or mediastinal nodal enlargement and 66% had nodal calcification [40]. Eggshell (peripheral) calcification is the pattern most strongly associated with silicosis, although punctate nodal calcification was more commonly observed in one recent HRCT series [40] (Fig. 13.9).

Complicated silicosis is defined by the presence of large opacities (1 cm or greater in size) also termed conglomerate masses. These typically develop in the lung periphery and retract toward the hilum with resultant paracicatricial

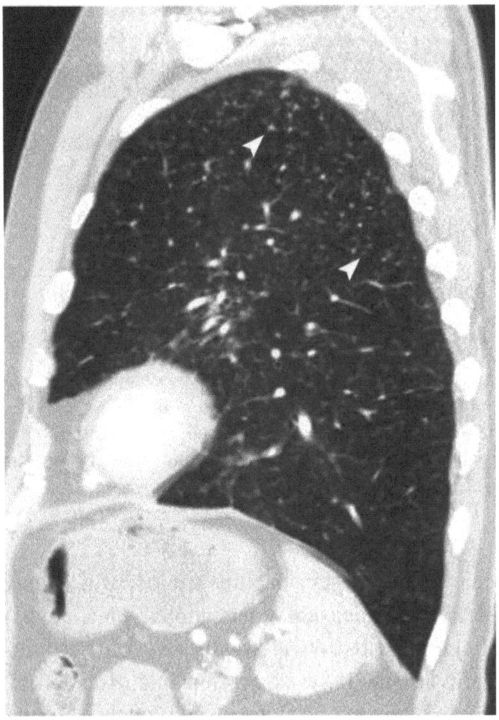

Fig. 13.7 Sagittal multiplanar reformat chest CT image in lung windows of a miner reveals a fine nodular pattern in the apicoposterior upper lobe and the superior segment of the lower lobe (*white arrowheads*). This distribution is typical of silicosis and coal workers' pneumoconiosis

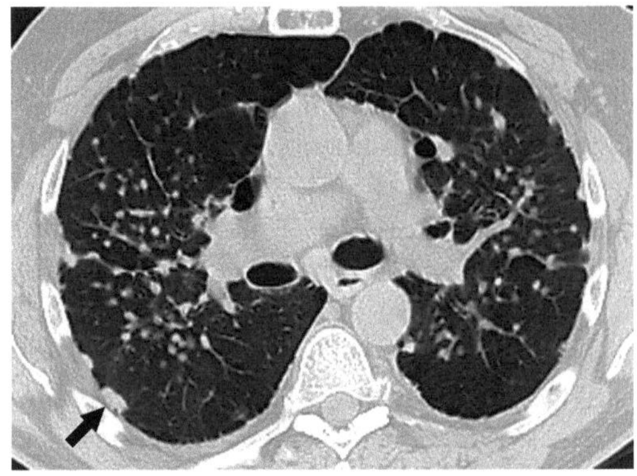

Fig. 13.8 Chest CT in lung windows revealing bilateral well-defined centrilobular nodules, greater on the right consistent with simple silicosis. Pseudoplaque formation (*arrow*) is the result of coalescence of subpleural nodules

emphysema. In one study of sandblasters, paracicatricial emphysema was associated with 72% of cases and all conglomerate masses occurred in the upper lobes with 92% posterior in location [45]. Conglomerate masses enlarge as progressive fibrosis incorporates the adjacent small nodules resulting in a decrease in the extent of background small opacities; calcification and air bronchograms have been reported in 64 and 70% of large opacities, respectively [46]. Calcification may reflect the incorporation of smaller calcified pneumoconiotic nodules (Fig. 13.9). Development of complicated pneumoconiosis is more common in silicosis than coal workers' pneumoconiosis because of the fibrogenic nature of free crystalline silica. Accelerated silicosis refers to the development of radiologic changes of complicated silicosis in individuals exposed to very high dust concentrations in as little as 4 years.

Due to the damaging effect of silica on the alveolar macrophages, there is an increased risk for developing tuberculosis, which has been reported in up to 25% of individuals with silicosis [47]. Conglomerate fibrosis may cavitate spontaneously or in association with tuberculosis and bronchogenic carcinoma (Fig. 13.10). Silica exposure has been linked to the development of chronic interstitial pneumonia (CIP), usual interstitial pneumonia, as well as systemic sclerosis and rheumatoid arthritis [48, 49]. In contrast to usual interstitial pneumonia, CIP demonstrates a more random distribution of fibrosis with homogeneous subpleural attenuation and less traction bronchiectasis [48].

Coal Workers' Pneumoconiosis

Coal miners exposed to increased dust burdens may develop simple or complicated (progressive massive fibrosis) coal workers' pneumoconiosis (CWP). CWP deaths accounted for nearly half of all pneumoconiosis related deaths in the 10-year period from 1990 to 1999 [5]. By the late 1990s, the prevalence of radiographically evident CWP was less than 2%, compared with over 10% in the early 1970s because of improved industrial hygiene [5]. Factors affecting the development

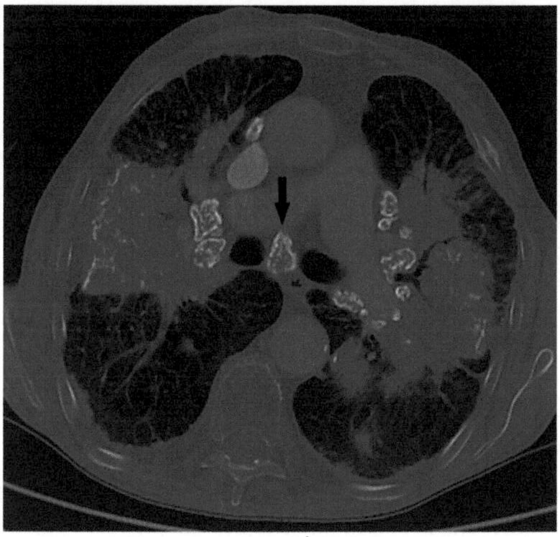

Fig. 13.9 Chest CT in bone windows shows large perihilar conglomerate fibrosis with extensive punctuate calcification due to incorporation of calcified silicotic nodules. Note the bilateral hilar and subcarinal lympadenopathy (*arrow*) with characteristic eggshell calcification

of CWP include concentration of coal dust exposure, mine size, work at the coalface, and hardness of coal or coal rank. Anthracite coal, for example, is harder than bituminous coal and, therefore, represents a higher risk for CWP [50]. Workers in smaller mines have an increased prevalence of CWP compared with mines with over 50 employees [51]. The mining methods, environmental control, and personal protective measures in addition to the proportion of other minerals such as mica, kaolin, and silica mixed with the coal dust impact the prevalence and severity of disease.

The deposition of 1–5 μm size particles occurs predominantly around the respiratory bronchiole. The unit lesion of CWP, the coal macule, is defined pathologically as a focal collection of coal dust containing macrophages at the division of the respiratory bronchiole, characteristically 1–4 mm in diameter with only occasional adjacent alveolar irregularities [52]. In contrast to the silicotic nodule, the coal macule does not contain hyalinization and laminated collagen. The visualization of an individual 3–5 mm lesion at chest radiography is unlikely, and their detection depends on density of lesions within the lung parenchyma and

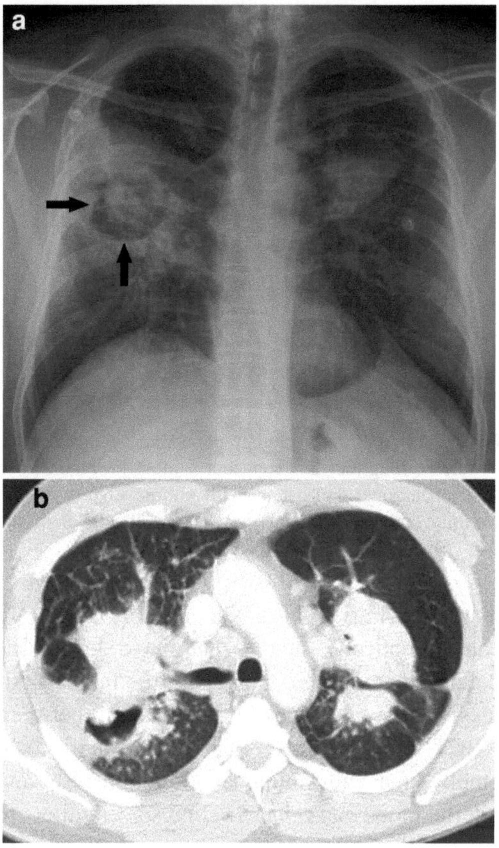

Fig. 13.10 **a** PA radiograph with bilateral perihilar large opacities and a background of fine nodularity consistent with complicated silicosis. Focal lucency in the right mid zone is due to a cavity (*arrows*). **b** CT confirms an irregular cavity in the posterior right lung that was stable over 5 years and the result of cavitation of a region of conglomerate fibrosis. In the acute setting in a patient with complicated silicosis, other considerations must include mycobacterial superinfection or cavitary neoplasm

the resultant summation shadows [53]. This explains the increased sensitivity of HRCT over CXR for subtle disease [54]. A threshold value of 8–10 g of dust accumulation in the lung has been associated with very mild forms of CWP (profusion 1/0), while total lung weight is roughly 40 g [55].

Simple CWP is defined clinically by the presence of small round opacities on CXR corresponding to the pathological coal macule and, similar to silicosis, manifests with an upper zone, posterior predominance, right-greater-

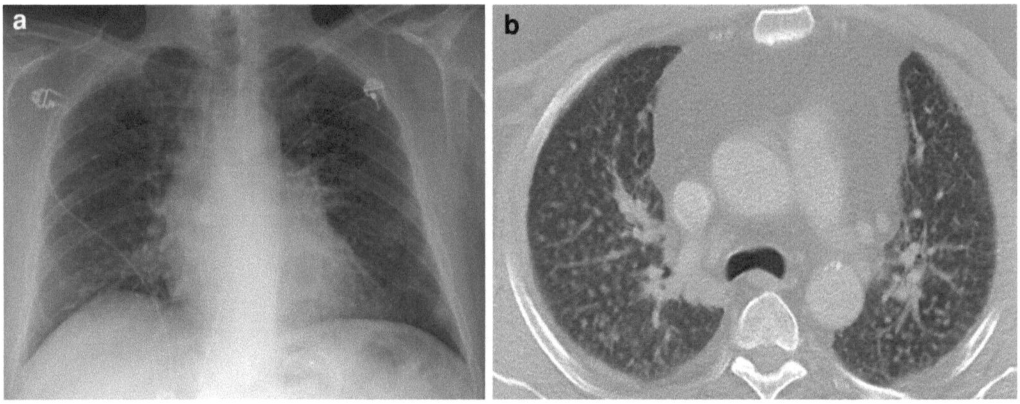

Fig. 13.11 **a** Frontal radiograph revealing diffuse fine nodules throughout all lung zones, most pronounced in the upper zones consistent with simple coal workers' pneumoconiosis. **b** CT of the chest at the level of the carina in the same patient shows diffuse ill-defined centrilobular nodules consistent with simple coal workers' pneumoconiosis

than-left (Fig. 13.11). Nodules in CWP are characteristically smaller and have less well-defined margins in comparison to silicotic nodules. There is a lack of correlation between HRCT findings of early CWP and focal emphysema with pulmonary function tests and arterial blood gas values leading some authors to suggest that subtle HRCT abnormalities should be classified as evidence of "exposure" rather than "disease" [56, 57]. The radiographic category of simple CWP, which for the most part is determined by the dust content of the lung, is not associated with respiratory symptoms or clinically significant loss in lung function. Patches of subpleural micronodules have been described resulting in "pseudoplaque" formation resulting from accumulation of particulate material in subpleural lymphatics [58].

Complicated CWP also termed progressive massive fibrosis (PMF) is defined by the presence of one or more opacities larger than 1 cm in greatest dimension. These large opacities are usually round or oval in shape and occur in the periphery of the lung with a lateral margin that parallels the pleural surface (Fig. 13.12a). The lesions may appear flat or lenticular on radiography or CT. Large opacities may cavitate and may contain calcifications. Distortion of the lung parenchyma with PMF and the incorporation of surrounding nodules results in an apparent regression of small opacities on the radiograph [59] (Fig. 13.12b). Large opacities are observed to retract toward the hila leaving paracicatricial emphysema in their wake and can be associated with clinically significant loss in lung function. Magnetic resonance imaging may be useful in distinguishing PMF from malignancy; PMF is reported to have low signal intensity relative to skeletal muscle while lung cancer is hyperintense on T2-weighted images [60].

Caplan syndrome (rheumatoid pneumoconiosis) is the association of CWP, serologic evidence of rheumatoid arthritis, and large (up to 5 cm) nodules at chest radiography. The Caplan nodule consists of a necrotic center surrounded by a cellular infiltrate of neutrophils, fibroblasts, giant cells, and dust-filled macrophages which form an annular ring pattern specific to Caplan nodules [61]. A broader definition of Caplan syndrome is currently described associated with other pneumoconiosis: asbestos, aluminum, dolomite, silica, and carbon [62].

Although not included in the radiologic definition of CWP, recent studies suggest that coal dust exposure, in the absence of CWP, can be associated with chronic obstructive pulmonary disease [63]. The extent of emphysema is reported to correlate better with dyspnea score

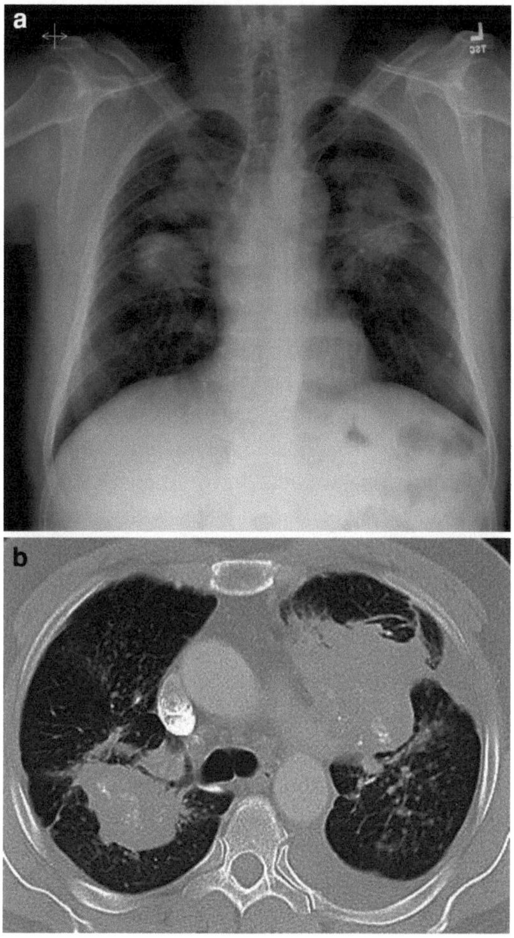

Fig. 13.12 **a** PA radiograph of a coal miner reveals large opacities in both upper zones, two on the right and one on the left, with hilar elevation. Large opacities are often lenticular in shape with an outer margin paralleling the shape of the chest wall as seen in this case. Note the paucity of background small nodules, a finding attributed to incorporation of these nodules into the regions of progressive massive fibrosis as they retract toward the hila. **b** Chest CT at the level of the carina in bone windows reveals bilateral large opacities with areas of punctuate calcification. There is a relative paucity of surrounding small centrilobular, ill-defined nodules consistent with coal workers' pneumoconiosis

and measures of pulmonary function (FEV_1 and D_{LCO}) than ILO classification [64]. A reticular pattern of irregular (linear) opacities has been reported in association with fine nodules and correlates better with the extent of emphysema [57, 65]; a significant association has been demonstrated between smoking and these irregular opacities in coal workers with one study of lung function abnormalities in working coal miners and irregular opacities only demonstrating findings in smokers [65, 66].

Immune Mediated Occupational Lung Disease

While the preceding disorders have concentrated on the effect of dust accumulation in the lung, the following entities primarily reflect immunologic reactions to occupational exposures within susceptible individuals. These include hard metal disease, berylliosis, and hypersensitivity pneumonitis.

Hard Metal Disease (Hard Metal Pneumoconiosis)

Hard metal alloys that contain cobalt in combination with tungsten carbide can cause interstitial lung disease called hard metal disease. These high strength alloys are used extensively in drilling, polishing, mining applications, and hard metal tipped tools. Cobalt is now recognized as the primary component of hard metal resulting in pulmonary toxicity. The clinical presentation can vary and can include features of hypersensitivity pneumonitis and asthma. Histologically, the presence of giant cell interstitial pneumonia (GIP) is virtually pathognomonic for hard metal disease. GIP is characterized by mononuclear infiltration of the interstitium and alveolar walls with giant cells in the air spaces. The presence of multinucleated giant cells on bronchoalveolar lavage in the appropriate clinical context obviates the need for biopsy [67]. A recent review of the HRCT findings reports bilateral ground-glass opacity or consolidation. Irregular linear opacities and traction bronchiectasis are also described; however, honeycombing is not typically present [68] (Fig. 13.13). UIP or DIP patterns have also been reported. In advanced disease, cystic spaces may occur and rarely, spontaneous pneumothorax [69]. With hypersensitivity

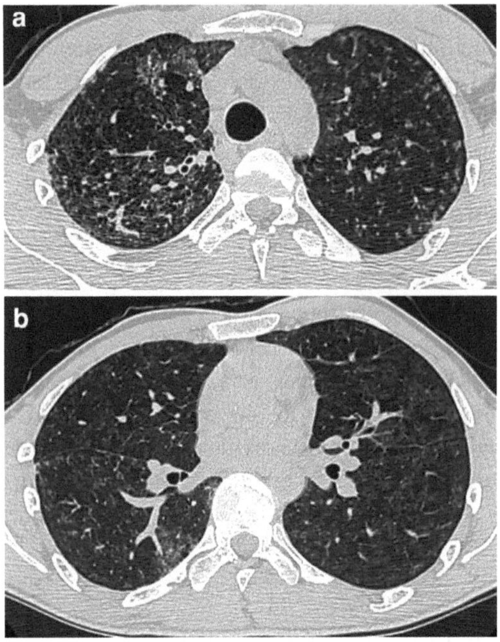

Fig. 13.13 Giant cell interstitial pneumonia in a 27-year-old man employed as a grinder. HRCT images through the upper and mid lung zones reveal mosaic ground-glass opacity and centrilobular nodules with right upper lobe reticulation. (Case courtesy of Dr. Keith Meyer, Department of Pulmonary Medicine, University of Wisconsin)

pneumonitis-like presentation the exposures are typically a shorter duration over 2–5 years and associated with flu-like symptoms and improvement with removal from exposure [70].

Berylliosis

Berylliosis is a granulomatous disorder resulting from exposure to beryllium from extraction from beryl ore and with processing of beryllium metal alloys and ceramics. Potential exposures can occur within aerospace, electronics, nuclear reactors, weapon production, manufacturing of bicycle frames and golf clubs, and the metal recycling industry. The total number of workers in the US with potential for exposure is estimated at 134,000 [71] and chronic beryllium disease (CBD) has been reported in up to 10% of exposed workers. The primary lung disease currently related to beryllium exposure, CBD, is an interstitial granulomatous process resulting from beryllium lymphocyte sensitization and proliferation. Sensitization may develop after as little as 3 months of exposure resulting in an antigen-specific lymphocyte mediated hypersensitivity response [72]. In workers with beryllium sensitization, progression to CBD can occur at a rate of 6–8% per year [73]. Sensitivity is detected with the beryllium lymphocyte proliferation test (BeLPT), which can be performed on blood or bronchoalveolar lavage fluid [74]. Epidemiologic studies have shown that on average, 50% of individuals with abnormal BeLPT will have chronic beryllium disease at clinical evaluation [75]. The resulting clinical syndrome and histology of noncaseating granulomas, mononuclear cell infiltrates, and interstitial fibrosis can be difficult to distinguish from sarcoidosis. Several studies have demonstrated that patients previously diagnosed with sarcoidosis were later found to have CBD [75]. CXR findings include upper zone predominant reticulonodular opacities and modest hilar lymphadenopathy (Fig. 13.14). HRCT findings similarly reflect granulomatous lung disease with fine nodules (57%), ground-glass opacity (32%), septal thickening (50%), and lymphadenopathy [76] (Fig. 13.15). Severe fibrosis and honeycombing may develop. Exposure to high concentrations of beryllium can cause acute berylliosis. This is manifested by inflammation of the airways and interstitium (chemical pneumonitis). Acute berylliosis is a rare disease when industrial environmental control measures are properly maintained.

Hypersensitivity Pneumonitis

Hypersensitivity pneumonitis (HP) is an immunologically mediated lung injury resulting from repeated inhalation of antigen in sensitized

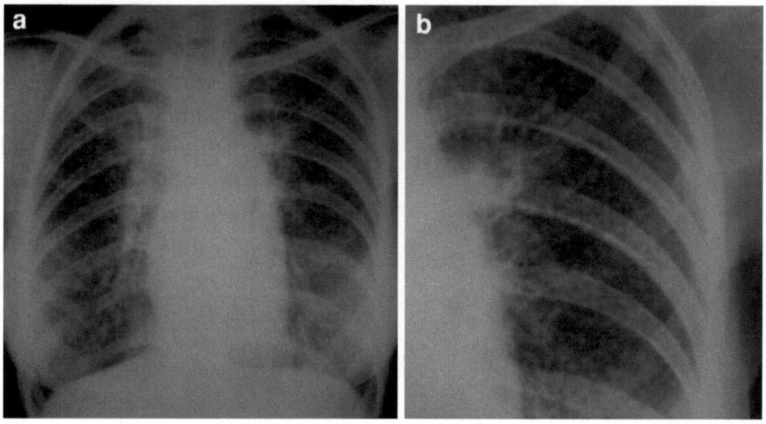

Fig. 13.14 **a** Berylliosis in a woman employed in an electronics factory. PA radiograph and magnified view of the left upper lung demonstrates diffuse fine nodules throughout the lungs with mediastinal and hilar lymphadenopathy. Note the radiographic similarity to sarcoidosis. **b** Berylliosis close-up

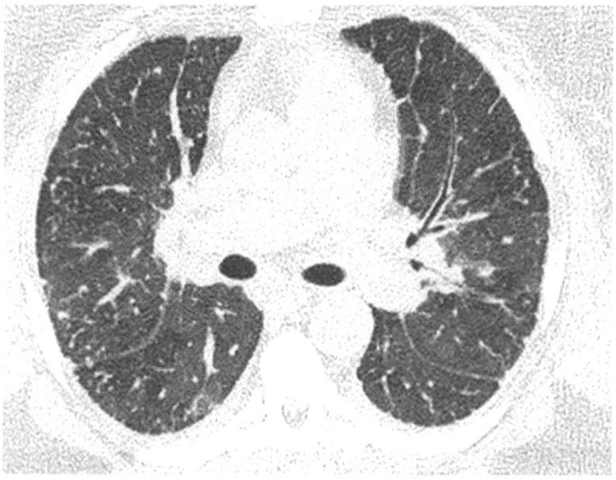

Fig. 13.15 HRCT of chronic berylliosis reveals perilymphatic small nodules and septal thickening. There is accompanying hilar and mediastinal lymphadenopathy manifesting as rounded contours to both hila and the subcarinal space

individuals. While a full exploration of this topic is beyond the scope of this chapter, common appellations of hypersensitivity pneumonitis include farmer's lung, mushroom worker's lung, humidifier lung, metal working fluid-associated hypersensitivity pneumonitis, and bird fancier's lung. The antigens associated with HP include various microbes that can contaminate organic produce, animal proteins, and small molecular weight chemical compounds such as isocyanates and trimetallic anhydrides. Recent case reports describe musicians with HP resulting from colonization of a saxophone with mold and a trombone with nontuberculous *Mycobacterium* and *Fusarium* species [77, 78].

Farmer's lung is a classic example of occupational HP caused by exposure to moldy livestock feed or compost most commonly contaminated with thermophilic actinomycetes. Organic as well as some inorganic antigens incite formation of IgG- and IgA-specific antibodies and a lymphocyte-mediated immune response resulting in an antigen-specific, lymphocytic alveolitis [79]. HP is a spectrum of disease classically grouped into acute, subacute, and chronic phases. Histologically, the subacute phase is characterized by interstitial lymphocyte infiltrates and loosely formed noncaseating small granulomas, cellular bronchiolitis, and nonspecific interstitial fibrosis; the severity of fibrosis may increase with chronic exposures. Patients characteristically present with flu-like symptoms 4–8 h after exposure. Acute HP such as with farmer's lung can clinically present like a viral pneumonia and the correct diagnosis missed or delayed in the absence of a complete occupational history. Pulmonary function tests are generally of a restrictive pattern with decreased lung volumes and diffusing capacity. Chest radiographic findings are nonspecific and may demonstrate ill-defined air space opacity in

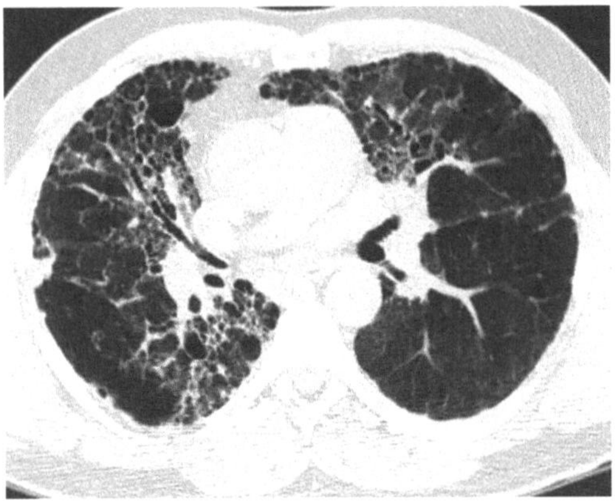

Fig. 13.16 Hypersensitivity pneumonitis in a 51-year-old farmer with hypersensitivity panel positive to *Micropolyspora faeni*. There is bilateral peribronchovascular fibrosis, bronchiectasis, and focal areas of hyperlucency consistent with chronic hypersensitivity pneumonitis

the acute setting and increased reticular markings with more chronic disease. In the subacute phase, HRCT characteristically demonstrates centrilobular micronodules, patchy ground-glass opacity, and lobular air trapping [80]. In chronic HP, findings include fibrosis accompanied by air trapping or emphysema with conflicting reports of zonal predominance [81] (Fig. 13.16). Diagnosis is based on the appropriate exposure history and compatible clinical and radiographic evaluation.

Airway Centric Occupational Lung Disease

Occupational Asthma

The definition of asthma is based on a combination of symptoms and significant variability in airflow as measured by pulmonary function. Occupational asthma is asthma that has been caused by exposures within the workplace [2] and is the most common form of occupational lung disease. It is estimated to cause 1 in 10 cases of adult-onset asthma and globally to cause 38,000 deaths per year [82, 83]. A recent American College of Chest Physicians (ACCP) consensus statement emphasizes the importance of a thorough medical and occupational history, exposure assessment, and targeted diagnostic tests in establishing this diagnosis. These tests may include spirometry before and after administration of bronchodilators, serial peak expiratory flow measurements, nonspecific bronchoprovocation testing (methacholine challenge), and dermatologic and serologic immunological testing; radiographic evaluation is not generally necessary [84, 85].

Nylon Flock Worker's Lung

When nylon is cut into short pieces to coat a material, ultrafine respirable fibers of synthetic material are created. These small fibers may result in a "non-specific interstitial pneumonia (NSIP)-like" pattern at HRCT described as patchy ground-glass, diffuse micronodular disease, or peripheral honeycombing [83]. Pathologically, the lung manifestations include a lymphocytic bronchiolitis and peribronchiolitis with lymphoid hyperplasia. Acute alveolar injury might also be present including diffuse alveolar damage and organizing pneumonia [86].

Bronchiolitis Obliterans Related to Flavoring Agents

Various occupational exposures have been linked to clinical findings consistent with bronchiolitis obliterans, an obstructive airway disease involving the respiratory bronchioles [87]. Recently food flavoring exposures have been linked to BO in occupational settings, particularly butter flavorings such as diacetly previously used in microwave popcorn production [88, 89]. Workers involving with mixing butter flavorings demonstrated decrements in forced expiratory volume in one second (FEV1) and airway obstruction on pulmonary function tests [90]. HRCT is superior to conventional thick section CT in the evaluation of small airways disease, and thin section CT images are easily reconstructed from the volumetric data sets

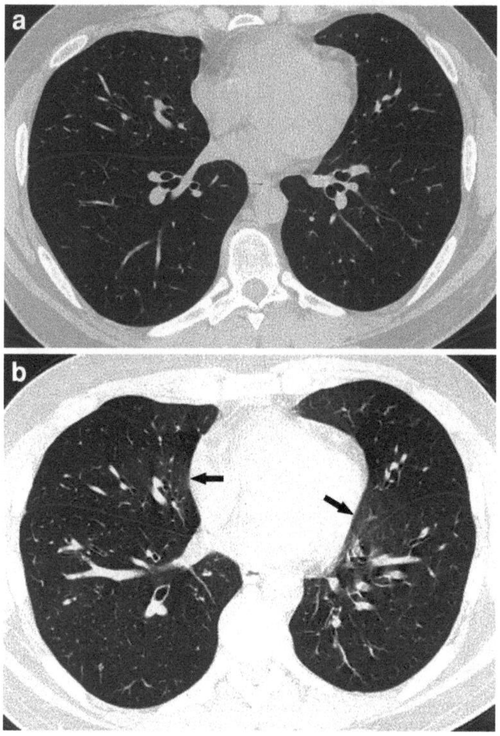

Fig. 13.17 Bronchiolitis obliterans in a flavor worker at a microwave popcorn factory. Inspiratory HRCT (**a**) reveals mild fusiform bronchiectasis while the diffuse air trapping is better appreciated on the expiratory HRCT (**b**) as extensive areas of persistent hyperlucent lung. Normal expiratory lung attenuation is seen in only a few central regions of the middle lobe and lingula (*arrows*)

obtained on current generation multidetector CT scanners without additional radiation exposure. Expiratory imaging may be a useful adjunct to standard inspiratory CT imaging in subtle cases by accentuating regional air trapping. End expiratory HRCT imaging has been reported to alter the initial HRCT interpretation in up to 15% of cases [91]. At end-expiration, normal lung parenchyma is expected to increase in attenuation while regions of air trapping remain lucent. HRCT findings of flavoring agent related to BO include mosaic attenuation at inspiratory images, which is shown to represent air trapping on end-expiratory HRCT images, as well as patchy areas of fibrosis [89] (Fig. 13.17). As in other causes of BO, bronchiectasis may accompany these findings.

Thesaurosis

Hair dressers are exposed to a wide variety of chemicals both absorbed and inhaled that can result in bronchial inflammation. The greatest extent of airway symptoms is associated with exposure to bleaching powder and hair spray; reduction in PFT values of FEV_1, maximum mid-expiratory flow, and peak expiratory flow suggest changes of obstructive pulmonary disease [92]. Histologic evaluation reveals a mononuclear cell infiltration with foreign body granuloma, numerous intra-alveolar and interstitial vacuolated macrophages, and foreign body-type multinucleated giant cells [93]. HRCT findings reported in a single case described homogeneous ground-glass opacity [94] (Fig. 13.18).

World Trade Center Lung

The collapse of the World Trade Center (WTC) towers on Sept 11, 2001 produced large amounts of medium (2.5–10 μm) and large size (>10 μm) alkaline particulate material representing a mixture of fiberglass, asbestos, aluminum and calcium silicates, and polycyclic hydrocarbons; in the subsequent 3 months, fine particulate material from multiple fires was also produced [95]. The majority of clinical respiratory symptoms are related to damage to the respiratory tract mucosa resulting in cough and dyspnea. Several cases of pulmonary fibrosis have been reported subsequent to the incident including granulomatous pneumonitis and accelerated pulmonary fibrosis [82]. Exposure to WTC dust has also been linked to bronchial hyper-reactivity, asthma, and bronchiolitis obliterans [96]. Finally, symptomatic WTC recovery workers have demonstrated air trapping as a manifestation of

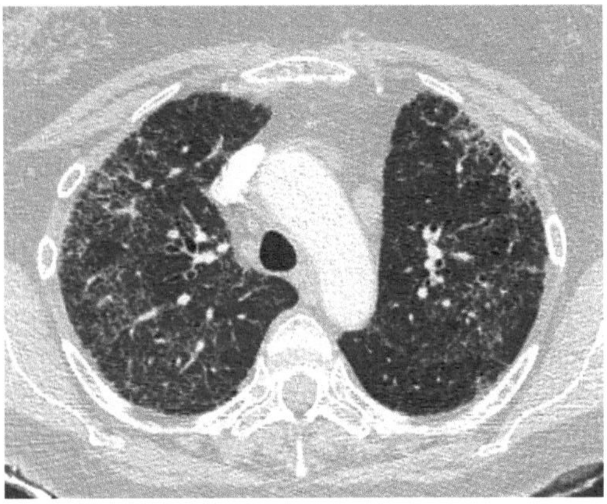

Fig. 13.18 Thesaurosis in a woman with no other risk factors who worked as a hairdresser for 43 years. There is bilateral reticular and ground-glass opacities with focal areas of air trapping in a pattern suggestive of chronic hypersensitivity pneumonitis. Lung biopsy confirmed bronchiolocentric predominant interstitial fibrosis. (Case courtesy of Dr. Keith Meyer, Department of Pulmonary Medicine, University of Wisconsin)

small airways disease at HRCT that correlated to duration of exposure [97].

Conclusion

The true economic and health impact of occupational lung disease remains inadequately defined. While our knowledge of the health effects of exposures associated with asbestos, silica, and coal are well-defined, new industrial exposures resulting in immune mediated reactions and airway disease such as asthma and bronchiolitis obliterans continue to evolve. Knowledge of radiologic manifestations of occupational lung disease in combination with an appropriate occupational history remains fundamental to the understanding, diagnosis, and prevention of this diffuse group of lung disorders.

References

1. Balmes J, Becklake M, Blanc P, et al. American thoracic society statement: occupational contribution to the burden of airway disease. Am J Respir Crit Care Med. 2003;167:787–97.
2. Mapp CE, Boschetto P, Maestrelli P, Fabbri LM. Occupational asthma. State of the Art. Am J Respir Crit Care Med. 2005;172:280–305.
3. Meyer JD, Holt DL, Chen Y, et al. SWORD'99: Surveillance of work-related respiratory disease in the UK. Occup Med. 2001;51:204–8.
4. Yucesoy B, Luster MI. Genetic susceptibility in pneumoconiosis. Toxicol Lett. 2007;168:249–54.
5. Work-Related Lung Disease Surveillance Report 2002. Division of Respiratory Disease Studies. National Institute of Occupational Safety and Health. U.S. Department of Health and Human Services. Public Health Service Centers for Disease Control and Prevention. Publication Dissemination, EID May 2003.
6. Attfield MD, Wood JM, Antao VC, Pinheiro GA. Changing patterns of pneumoconiosis mortality, United States, 1968–2000. MMWR Weekly. 2004;53: 627–32.
7. Leigh JP, Markowitz SB, Fahs M, Shin C, Landrigan P. Occupational injury and illness in the United States: estimates of costs, morbidity, and mortality. Arch Int Med. 1997;157:1557–68.
8. Ohar J, Sterling DA, Bleecker E, Donahue J. Changing patterns in asbestos-induced lung disease. Chest. 2004;125:744–53.
9. Kazan-Allen L. Asbestos and mesothelioma: worldwide trends. Lung Cancer. 2005;49S(1):S3–8.
10. Peacock C, Copley SJ, Hansell DM. Asbesto-related benign pleural disease. Clin Rad. 2000;55:422–32.
11. Niklinski J, Niklinska W, Chyczewska E, Laudanski J, Naumnik W, Chyczewski L, Pluygers E. The epidemiology of asbestos-related diseases. Lung Cancer. 2004;45S:S7–15.
12. Vathesatogkit P, Harkin TJ, Addrizzo-Harris DJ, et al. Clinical correlation of asbestos bodies in BAL fluid. Chest. 2004;126:966–71.
13. Churg A, Wright JL, Wiggs B, et al. Small airways disease and mineral dust exposure: prevalence, structure, and function. Am Rev Respir Dis. 1985;131: 139–43.
14. Martensson G, Hagberg S, Pettersson K, et al. Asbestos pleural effusion: a clinical entity. Thorax. 1987;42:646–51.
15. Solomon A. Radiological features of asbestos-related visceral pleural changes. Am J Ind Med. 1991;19: 339–55.
16. Copley SJ, Wells AU, Rubens MB, Chabat F, Sheehan RE, Musk AW, Hansell DM. Functional consequences of pleural disease evaluated with chest radiography and CT. Radiology. 2001;220:237–43.
17. Ameille J, Matrat M, Paris C, Joly N, Raffaelli C, Brochard P, Iwatsubo Y, Pairon JC, Letourneux M. Asbestos-related pleural diseases: dimensional criteria are not appropriate to differentiate diffuse pleural thickening from pleural plaques. Am J of Ind Med. 2004;45:289–96.
18. Kim JS, Lynch DA. Imaging of nonmalignant occupational lung disease. J Thorac Imaging. 2002; 17:238–60.

19. Rohs AM, Lockey JE, Dunning KK, Shukla R, Fan H, Hilbert T, Borton E, Wiot J, Meyer C, Shipley RT, LeMasters GK, Kapil V. Low-level fiber-induced radiographic changes caused by Libby vermiculite. Am J Resp Crit Care Med. 2008;177:630–7.
20. Sebastien P, Janson X, Gaudichet A, Hirsch A, Bignon J. Asbestos retention in human respiratory tissues: comparative measurements in lung parenchyma and in parietal pleura. IARC Sci Publ. 1980;30:237–46.
21. Gallego JC. Absence of left-sided predominance in asbestos-related pleural plaques. Chest. 1998;113: 1034–6.
22. Schwartz DA, Galvin JR, Yagla SJ, Speakman SB, Merchant JA, Hunninghake GW. Restrictive lung function and asbestos-induced pleural fibrosis: a quantitative approach. J Clin Invest. 1993;91:2685–92.
23. Akira M, Yamamoto S, Inoue Y, et al. High-resolution CT of asbestosis and idiopathic pulmonary fibrosis. Am J Roentgenol. 2003;181:163–9.
24. Gevenois PA, de Maertelaer V, Madani A, et al. Asbestosis, pleural plaques and diffuse pleural thickening: three distinct benign responses to asbestos exposure. Eur Respir J. 1998;11:1021–7.
25. Bergin CJ, Castellino RA, Blank N, et al. Specificty of high-resolution CT findings in pulmonary asbestosis: do patients scanned for other indications have similar findings? AJR. 1994;163:551–5.
26. Remy-Jardin M, Sobaszek A, Duhamel A, et al. Asbestos-related pleuropulmonary diseases: evaluation with low-dose four-detector row spiral CT. Radiology. 2004;233:182–90.
27. Lynch DA, Gamsu G, Ray CS, et al. Asbestos-related focal lung masses: manifestations on conventional and high-resolution CT scans. Radiology. 1988;169: 603–7.
28. Menzies R, Fraser R. Round atelectasis. Pathologic and pathogenetic features. Am J Surg Pathol. 1987;11: 674–81.
29. Munden RF, Libshitz HI. Round atelectasis and mesothelioma. AJR Am J Roentgenol. 1998;170: 1519–22.
30. McAdams HP, Erasmus JJ, Patz EF, et al. Evaluation of patients with round atelelctasis using 2-[18F]-fluoro-2-deoxy-D-glucose PET. JCAT. 1998;22: 601–4.
31. Gilkeson RC, Adler LP. Rounded atelectasis. Evaluation with (18)PET Scan. Clin Positron Imaging. 1998;1:229–32.
32. Silvestri S. Commentary: change in the world of occupational health: silica control then and now. J Public Health Policy. 2005;26:203–5.
33. Churg A, Wright JL. Small airways disease and mineral dust exposure. Pathol Annu. 1983;18:233–51.
34. Cowie RL, Mabena SK. Silicosis, chronic airflow limitation and chronic bronchitis in South African gold miners. Am Rev Respir Dis. 1991;143:80–4.
35. Arakawa H, Gevenois PA, Saito Y, et al. Silicosis: expiratory thin-section CT assessment of airway obstruction. Radiology. 2005;236:1059–66.
36. Alper F, Akgun M, Onbas O, Araz O. CT findings in silicosis due to sandblasting. Eur Radiol. 2008;18: 2739–44.
37. Marchiori E, Souza CA, Barbassa TG, Escuissato DL, Gasparetto EL, Souza SA. Silicoproteinosis: high-resolution CT findings in 13 patients. AJR. 2007;189:1402–6.
38. Hughes JM, Weill H, Checkoway H, et al. Radiographic evidence of silicosis risk in the diatomaceous earth industry. Am J Respir Crit Care Med. 1998;158:807–14.
39. Remy-Jardin M, Remy J, Farre I, Marquette CH. Computed tomographic evaluation of silicosis and coal worker's pneumoconiosis. Radiol Clin North Am. 1992;30:1155–76.
40. Antao VCS, Pinheiro GA, Terra-Filho M, Kavakama J, Muller NL. High resolution CT in silicosis. Correlation with radiographic findings and functional impairment. JCAT. 2005;29:350–6.
41. Zeren EH, Colby TV, Roggli VL. Silica-induced pleural disease. Chest. 1997;112:1436–8.
42. Craighead JE, Kleinerman J, Abraham JL, Gibbs AR, Green FH, Harley RA, Ruettner JR, Vallyathan NV, Juliano EB. Diseases associated with exposure to silica and nonfibrous silicate minerals. Arch Pathol Lab Med. 1988;112:673–720.
43. Lopes AJ, Mogami R, Capone D, Tessarollo B, De Melo PL, Jansen JM. High-resolution computed tomography in silicosis: correlation with chest radiography and pulmonary function tests. J Bras Pneumol. 2008;34:264–72.
44. Cox-Ganser JM, Burchfiel CM, Fekedulegn D, Andrew ME, Ducatman BS. Silicosis in lymph nodes: the canary in the miner? J Occup Environ Med. 2009;51:164–9.
45. Marchiori E, Ferreira A, Saez F, et al. Conglomerated masses of silicosis in sandblasters: High-resolution CT findings. Eur J of Rad. 2006;59: 56–9.
46. Ferreira AS, Moreira VB, Ricardo HMV, Coutinho R, Gabetto JM, Marchiori E. Progressive massive fibrosis in silica-exposed workers. High-resolution computed tomography findings. J Bras Pneumol. 2006;32:523–8.
47. Chong S, Lee KS, Chung MJ, et al. Pneumoconiosis: comparison of imaging and pathologic findings. Radiographics. 2006;26:59–77.
48. Arakawa H, Johkoh T, Honma K, Saito Y, Fukushima Y, Shida H, Suganuma N. Chronic interstitial pneumonia in silicosis and mix-dust pneumoconiosis. Chest. 2007;131:1870–6.
49. Sirajuddin A, Kanne JP. Occupational lung disease. J Thorac Imaging. 2009;24:310–20.
50. Antao VCS, Petsonk EL, Sokolow LZ, et al. Rapidly progressive coal worker's pneumoconiosis in the United States: geographic clustering and other factors. Occup Environ Med. 2005;62:670–4.
51. Laney AS, Attfield MD. Coal workers' pneumoconiosis and progressive massive fibrosis are increasingly more prevalent among workers in

small underground coal mines in the United States. Occup Environ Med. 2010;67:428–31.
52. Kleinerman J, Green F, Harley RA, Lapp L, Laqueur W, Naeye RL, Pratt P, Taylor G, Wiot J, Wyatt J. Pathology standards for coal worker's pneumoconiosis. Arch Pathol Lab Med. 1979;103:375–85.
53. Carstairs LS. The interpretation of shadows in the restricted area of a lung field on the chest radiograph. Proc R Soc Med. 1961;54:978–80.
54. Remy-Jardin M, Degreef JM, Beauscart R, et al. Coal worker's pneumoconiosis: CT assessment in exposed workers and correlation with radiographic findings. Radiology. 1990;177:363–71.
55. Rossiter CE. Relation between content and composition of coal workers' lungs and radiological appearances. Br J Ind Med. 1972;29:31–4.
56. Collins LC, Willing S, Bretz R, Harty M, Lane E, Anderson WH. High-resolution CT in simple coal workers' pneumoconiosis. Lack of correlation with pulmonary function tests and arterial blood gas values. Chest. 1993;104:1156–62.
57. Gevenois PA, Pichot E, Dargent F, Dedeire S, Vande Weyer R, De Vuyst P. Low grade coal worker's pneumoconiosis. Comparison of CT and chest radiography. Acta Radiolgica. 1994;35:351–6.
58. Remy-Jardin M, Beuscart R, Sault MC, et al. Subpleural micronodules in diffuse infiltrative lung diseases: evaluation with thin-section CT scans. Radiology. 1990;177:133–9.
59. Vallyathan V, Brower PS, Green FHY, et al. Radiographic and pathologic correlation of coal worker's pneumoconiosis. Am J Respir Crit Care Med. 1996;154:741–8.
60. Matsumoto S, Miyake H, Oga M, et al. Diagnosis of lung cancer in a patient with pneumoconiosis and progressive massive fibrosis using MRI. Eur Radiol. 1998;8:615–7.
61. Gough J, Rivers D, Seal RME. Pathological studies of modified pneumoconiosis in coal-miners with rheumatoid arthritis (Caplan's syndrome). Thorax. 1955;10:9–18.
62. Wilson AG, Hansell DM. Immunologic Diseases of the Lungs in Imaging of Diseases of the Chest. In: Armstrong P, Wilson AG, Dee P, Hansell DM, editors. Philadelphia: Mosby; 2000, p. 565.
63. Yildiz OA, Gulbay BE, Saryal S, Karabiyiikoglu G. Evaluation of the relationship between radiological abnormalities and both pulmonary function and pulmonary hypertension in coal workers' pneumoconiosis. Respirology. 2007;12:420–6.
64. Bauer TT, Heyer CM, Duchna HW, Andreas K, Weber A, Schmidt EW, Ammenwerth W, Schultze-Wernignhaus G. Radiological findings, pulmonary function and dyspena in underground coal miners. Respiration. 2007;74:80–7.
65. Lyons JP, Ryder RC, Campbell H, et al. Significance of irregular opacities in the radiology of coal worker's pneumoconiosis. Br J Ind Med. 1974;31: 36–44.
66. Amandus HE, Lapp NL, Jacobsen G, Reger RB. Significance of irregular opacities in the radiographs of coalminers in the USA. Br J Ind med. 1976;33:13–7.
67. Nemery B, Verbeken EK, Demedts M. Giant cell interstitial pneumonia (hard metal lung disease, cobalt lung). Semin Resp Crit Care Med. 2001;22:435–47.
68. Choi JW, Lee KS, Chung MP, et al. Giant cell interstitial pneumonia: high-resolution CT and pathologic findings in four adult patients. AJR. 2005;184:268–72.
69. Gotway MB, Golden JA, Warnock M, Koth LL, Webb R, Reddy GP, Balmes JR. Hard metal lung disease: high-resolution computed tomography appearance. J of Thorac Imag. 2002;17:314–8.
70. Okuno K, Kobayashi K, Kotani Y, Ohnishi H, Ohbayashi C, Nishimura Y. A case of hard metal lung disease resembling a hypersensitive pneumonia in radiological images. Int Med. 2010;49:1185–89.
71. Henneberger PK, Goe SK, Miller WE, Doney B, Groce DW. Industries in the United States with airborne beryllium exposure and estimates of the number of current workers potentially exposed. J Occup Environ Hyg. 2004;1:648–59.
72. Maier LA. Clinical approach to chronic beryllium disease and other nonpneumoconiotic interstitial lung diseases. J Thorac Imaging. 2002;17:273–84.
73. Newman LS, Mroz MM, Balkissoon R, Maier LA. Beryllium sensitization progresses to chronic beryllium disease: a longitudinal study of disease risk. Am J Respir Crit Care Med. 2005;171:54–60.
74. Tomas LHS. Beryllium hypersensitivity and chronic beryllium lung disease. Curr Opin Pulm Med. 2009;15:165–9.
75. Newman LS, Mroz MM, Balkissoon R, Maier LA. Screening for Chronic Beryllium Disease. From the authors. Am J Respir Crit Care Med. 2005;172:1230.
76. Sharma N, Patel J, Mohammed TLH. Chronic beryllium disease: computed tomographic findings. J Comput Assist Tomogr. 2010;34:945–8.
77. Metersky ML, Bean SB, Meyer JD, Mutambudzi M, Brown-Elliott BA, Wechsler ME, Wallace RJ. Trombone player's lung: a probable new cause of hypersensitivity pneumonitis. Chest. 2010;138:754–6.
78. Metzger F, Haccuria A, Reboux G, Nolard N, Dalphin JC, DeVuyst P. Hypersensitivity pneumonitis due to molds in a saxophone player. Chest. 2010;138:724–6.
79. Spurzem JR, Romberger DJ, Von Essen SG. Agricultural lung disease. Clin Chest Med. 2002;23:795–810.
80. Cormier Y, Brown M, Worthy S, Racine G, Muller NL. High-resolution computed tomographic characterstics in acute farmer's lung and in its follow-up. Eur Respir J. 2000;16:56–60.
81. Malinen AP, Erkinjuntti-Pekkanen RA, Partanen PLK, Rytkonen HT, Vanninen RL. Long-term sequelae of Farmer's lung disease in HRCT: a 14 year follow-up of 88 patients and 83 matched control farmers. Eur Radiol. 2003;13:2212–21.

82. Lombardo LJ, Balmes JR. Occupational asthma: a review. Environ Health Perspect. 2000;108:697–704.
83. Goldyn SR, Condos R, Rom WN. The burden of exposure-related diffuse lung disease. Semin Respir Crit Care Med. 2008;29:591–602.
84. Tarlo SM, Liss GM, Blanc PD. How to diagnose and treat work-related asthma. Pol Arch Med Wewn. 2009;119:660–5.
85. Stenton SC. Review series: occupational and environmental lung disease: occupational asthma. Chronic Respir Dis. 2010;7:35–46.
86. Boag AH, Colby TV, Fraire AE, et al. The pathology of interstitial lung disease in nylon flock workers. Am J Surg Pathol. 1999;23:1539–45.
87. Schachter EN. Popcorn worker's lung. N Engl J Med. 2002;347:360–1.
88. Lockey J, McKay R, Bareth E, Dahlsten J, Baughman JR. Bronchiolitis obliterans in the food flavoring manufacturing industry. Am J Respir Crit Care Med. 2002;165:A461.
89. Kreiss K, Gomaa A, Kullman G, Fedan K, Simoes E, Enright PL. Clinical bronchiolitis obliterans in workers at a microwave-popcorn plan. N Engl J Med. 2002;5:330–8.
90. Lockey JE, Hilbert TJ, Levin LP, Ryan PH, White KL, Borton EK, Rice CH, McKay RT, LeMasters GK. Airway obstruction related to diacetyl exposure at microwave popcorn production facilities. Eur Respir J. 2009;34:63–71.
91. Arakawa H, Webb WR, McCowin M, Katsou G, Lee KN, Seitz RF. Inhomogeneous lung attenuation at thin-section CT: diagnostic value of expiratory CT scans. Radiology. 1998;206:89–94.
92. Hahemis N, Boskabady MH, Nazari A. Occupational exposures and obstructive lung disease: a case-control study in hairdressers. Respir Care. 2010;55: 895–900.
93. Gebbers JO, Burkhardt A, Tetzner C, Rudiger HW, Wichert PV. Hairspray Lung. Schweiz Med Wschr. 1980;110:610.
94. Nagata N, Kawajiri T, Hayashi T, Nakanishi K, Nikaido Y, Kido M. Interstitial pneumonitis and fibrosis associated with the inhalation of hair spray. Respiration. 1997;64:310–2.
95. Lioy PJ, Weisel CP, Millette JR, et al. Characterization of the dust/smoke aerosol that settled east of the World Trade Center (WTC) in lower Manhattan after the collapse of the WTC 11 September 2001. Environ Health Perspect. 2002;110:703–14.
96. Mann JM, Sha KK, Kline G, Breuer FU, Miller A. World trade center dyspnea: bronchiolitis obliterans with functional improvement: a case report. Am J Ind Med. 2005;48:225–9.
97. Mendelson DS, Roggeveen M, Levin SM, Herbert R, de la Hoz RE. Air trapping detected on end-expiratory high-resolution computed tomography in symptomatic world trade center rescue and recovery workers. J Occup Environ Med. 2007;49:840–5.

Hemoptysis

14

Kristie M. Guite, Trina J. Hollatz, and Jeffrey P. Kanne

Abstract

Hemoptysis can range from mild blood-tinged sputum to massive, life-threatening expectoration of blood. The causes of hemoptysis are myriad, ranging from neoplasm to infection to vasculitis. Imaging, particularly CT, plays a central role in identifying the cause of hemoptysis and localizing the site of bleeding, helping to guide intervention. This chapter reviews the etiologies of hemoptysis and illustrates their respective imaging findings.

Keywords

Hemoptysis · Neoplasm · Computerized tomography · Infection · Vasculitis · Pulmonary thromboembolism

Introduction

Hemoptysis, expectoration or coughing up blood originating from the lower respiratory tract, has numerous etiologies. Non-pulmonary bleeding from the gastrointestinal tract or upper airway bleeding can have a similar presentation and can be confused with true hemoptysis. Presentation may vary, ranging from a single episode of blood-streaked mucus to acutely life-threatening massive hemoptysis. Thirty percent of patients with hemoptysis have an identifiable cause with the remaining classified as idiopathic, in which subtle airway or parenchymal disease is presumed to be responsible [1]. In the US, the three most common causes of non-massive hemoptysis in order of decreasing frequency are bronchiectasis and acute and chronic bronchitis. Worldwide,

K. M. Guite (✉)
Department of Radiology, University of Wisconsin School of Medicine and Public Health, E3/366 Clinical Science Center, 600 Highland Ave, Madison, WI 53562, USA
e-mail: kguite@uwhealth.org

T. J. Hollatz
Department of Pulmonary Medicine, Division of Pulmonary & Critical Care, University of Wisconsin School of Medicine and Public Health, 600 Highland Ave, MMC #9988, Madison, WI 53792, USA

J. P. Kanne
Department of Radiology, University of Wisconsin School of Medicine and Public Health, 600 Highland Ave, MC 3252, Madison, WI 53792-3252, USA
e-mail: jkanne@uwhealth.org

J. P. Kanne (ed.), *Clinically Oriented Pulmonary Imaging*, Respiratory Medicine, DOI: 10.1007/978-1-61779-542-8_14,

however, tuberculosis remains the most common cause of non-massive hemoptysis [2].

Massive hemoptysis is an uncommon but life-threatening manifestation of hemoptysis, accounting for only 1.5–5% of patients. Mortality rates from massive hemoptysis range from 9 to 38% [3]. No uniform consensus exists for the definition of massive hemoptysis. Reported volumes range from 100 to 600 mL of expectorated blood over a 24-hour period [4, 5]. It is estimated that approximately 400 mL of blood within the alveolar space causes significant impairment of gas exchange. However, volumes less than 400 mL can also be life threatening because of asphyxiation. The volume of blood loss is most useful in management and less helpful in diagnosis.

The most common causes of massive hemoptysis include bronchogenic carcinoma, necrotizing pneumonia, mycetoma, polyangiitis, vasculitis, and coagulopathies [6–8]. Tuberculosis remains the leading cause of massive hemoptysis in locations where tuberculosis is endemic such as parts of Africa and East Asia. Several studies have attempted to elucidate prognosticating factors for poor outcome in patients with massive hemoptysis. Bleeding rates equal to or greater than 1,000 mL within a 24 h period, aspiration of blood into the contralateral lung, massive bleeding requiring single lung ventilation, and bronchogenic carcinoma as the underlying cause have been associated with higher mortality [5, 9].

In order to better understand hemoptysis, it is first important to understand the blood supply to the lungs. The lungs have a dual source blood supply. Ninety-five percent of the blood supply is delivered in the low-pressure pulmonary arteries and is responsible for gas exchange. Only 5% of the lung blood supply arises from the high-pressure systemic bronchial arteries, which typically arise from the aorta and rarely from the intercostal arteries.

While hemoptysis can result from hemorrhage anywhere in the lower respiratory tract, bronchial arterial hemorrhage accounts for approximately 90% of cases of hemoptysis. Chronic inflammation or infectious processes can result in pathologic alterations in the bronchial vascular anatomy including friable walls and pseudoaneurysm formation. In addition, the bronchial arteries can become enlarged and tortuous with increased arterial blood flow and formation of new collateral pathways as the normal capillary beds become engorged [10].

Etiologies and Diagnosis

The workup of hemoptysis is guided by history and physical examination; however, there is no consensus on the exact appropriate diagnostic workup. Clinical evaluation usually includes laboratory analysis in combination with radiologic imaging, bronchoscopy, or both. The initial step in evaluating a patient with reported hemoptysis is to attempt to determine whether the hemorrhage is arising from the lower respiratory tract or elsewhere such as the gastrointestinal tract or upper aerodigestive tract. Patients with gastrointestinal hemorrhage presenting as hemoptysis may report a history of abdominal pain, nausea, vomiting, or "coffee-ground" colored expectorant. Clinical clues to upper airway and nasopharyngeal bleeding include post-nasal drip and blood in the oropharynx.

Etiologies of hemoptysis can be grouped into four different categories based on the location from where the bleeding arises: tracheobronchial (Table 14.1), local and diffuse pulmonary parenchymal (Table 14.2), primary vascular (Table 14.3), and miscellaneous or rare (Table 14.4). Clinical history such as exposures, travel, and other signs and symptoms in addition to physical findings may help point to the cause of hemoptysis.

Laboratory findings that can be helpful include a complete blood count to determine the extent of blood loss, platelet count, coagulation labs including prothrombin time and INR, or D-dimer in patients considered low risk for pulmonary embolus to exclude that diagnosis. If there are

Table 14.1 Tracheobronchial etiologies of hemoptysis

Tracheobronchial Etiology		Clinical Presentation
Neoplasm	Adenocarcinoma Small cell carcinoma Squamous cell carcinoma Endobronchial metastasis Kaposi sarcoma → HIV infection Bronchial carcinoid	Fatigue, weight loss Smoking history Carcinoid symptoms
Inflammation	Bronchitis (acute or chronic) Bronchiectasis	Acute onset Infectious symptoms
Broncholithiasis		lithoptysis (rare)
Airway trauma		Airway trauma Foreign body

Table 14.2 Pulmonary parenchymal etiologies of hemoptysis

Pulmonary Parenchymal Etiology		Clinical Presentation
Focal	Abscess	Cough with copious or purulent sputum
	Tuberculosis	Immunosuppression, travel
	Mycetoma (fungus ball)	
	Lung contusion	Trauma
Diffuse	Goodpasture syndrome	Renal failure, proteinuria, hematuria Antiglomerular basement membrane antibody
	Idiopathic pulmonary hemosiderosis	Iron deficiency anemia
	Wegener granulomatosis	Saddle nose with rhinitis and septal perforation Renal insufficiency
	Lupus	Fever, cough, dyspnea Butterfly and malar rash
	Behçet disease	Mucocutaneous ulcers
	Other connective tissue diseases (systemic sclerosis, etc.)	

Table 14.3 Primary vascular etiologies of hemoptysis

Primary Vascular Etiology	Clinical Presentation
Arteriovenous malformation	Mucocutaneous telangiectasia or peripheral cyanosis
Pulmonary embolism	Pleuritic chest pain, tachycardia, calf or leg swelling/pain Risk factors
Elevated pulmonary venous pressure (esp. mitral stenosis, left ventricular failure)	Clinical findings of heart failure: dyspnea on exertion, orthopnea, fatigue, paroxysmal nocturnal dyspnea, frothy pink sputum, lower extremity edema

findings concerning for a pulmonary-renal syndrome, urinalysis can be used to evaluate for hematuria or proteinuria, and antibody blood tests could include c-ANCA, p-ANCA, and anti-GBM antibodies. When infectious symptoms are present, sputum cultures and bronchoalveolar lavage

Table 14.4 Miscellaneous etiologies of hemoptysis

Miscellaneous Etiology	Clinical Presentation
Pulmonary endometriosis	Menstruating female, cyclic symptoms
Systemic coagulopathy or use of anticoagulants or thrombolytic agents	
von Willebrand disease, hemophilia, thrombocytopenia	History of abnormal bleeding
Lymphangioleiomyomatosis	Progressive cystic lung disease that occurs almost exclusively in women
Radiation	
Drug reactions	
Iatrogenic	

may help direct therapy. If the etiology of hemoptysis is suspected to be a gastrointestinal source, an acidic pH and a dark red or coffee-ground color of expectorated blood products are confirmatory. In contrast, true hemoptysis from a respiratory source tends to be bright red or pink and frothy in appearance with an alkaline pH.

Following a thorough history, physical examination and pertinent labs, chest imaging is usually warranted. Chest radiographs have been reported to be able to identify the etiology of massive hemoptysis in approximately 35% of patients, usually identifying findings of tuberculosis, neoplasm, and extensive bronchiectasis. Chest radiographs are rarely normal in massive hemoptysis, and normal radiographs make malignancy as a source of hemoptysis very unlikely [11].

Computed tomography, particularly with volumetric high-resolution technique, is superior to radiography in determining the etiology of hemoptysis and may help to localize the source of bleeding. CT can accurately determine the etiology of hemoptysis in 60–77% of patients, in contrast to bronchoscopy, which can determine the etiology in only 2.5–8% of patients [6, 11, 12]. Furthermore, CT has been shown to be more effective in correct localization of bleeding in patients with massive hemoptysis in 70–89% of patients [9, 13].

There are a number of signs and symptoms that are considered red flags and warrant concern and evaluation for life-threatening bleeding or malignancy. Pulmonary malignancies often carry a poor prognosis and rarely present with life-threatening hemoptysis. Clinical clues to underlying malignancy consist of constitutional symptoms including malaise, weight loss, and fatigue. Patients with dyspnea at rest or decreased/absent breath sounds are concerning for massive/life-threatening bleeding. Lastly, patients with pulmonary artery catheters with hemoptysis should also be aggressively evaluated and treated.

Tracheobronchial

Table 14.1 shows the tracheobronchial etiologies of hemoptysis.

Neoplasm

Neoplasm should be strongly considered for any patient with a significant smoking history and hemoptysis. Approximately 20% of patients with pulmonary neoplasms will develop hemoptysis with approximately 3% of patients developing massive hemoptysis [14]. A variety of pulmonary neoplasms can cause hemoptysis including primary endobronchial tumors and primary intraparenchymal tumors that directly extend into the airways, although endobronchial lesions most commonly result in hemoptysis. Non-small cell and small cell lung carcinoma (Fig. 14.1), endobronchial metastatic tumors,

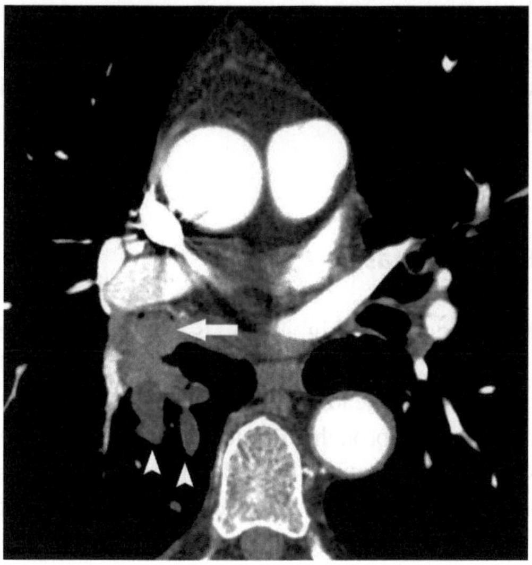

Fig. 14.1 Squamous cell carcinoma of the lung. Contrast-enhanced CT image shows a soft tissue nodule (*arrow*) in the bronchus intermedius resulting in mucoid impaction in right lower lobe superior segmental bronchi (*arrowheads*)

Kaposi sarcoma, and bronchial carcinoid can all produce hemoptysis.

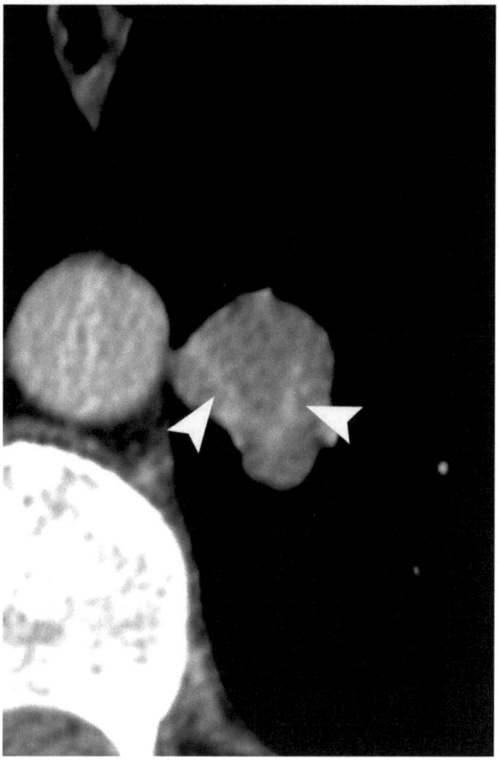

Fig. 14.2 Typical carcinoid. Contrast-enhanced CT image shows a heterogeneous soft tissue nodule in the left lower lobe. Note the hypervascular foci (*arrowheads*) within the tumor

Carcinoid

Bronchial carcinoids (Fig. 14.2) are neuroendocrine tumors arising from bronchial and bronchiolar epithelium and may derive from existing Kulchitsky cells, neuroepithelial bodies, or pluripotential bronchial epithelial stem cells. They range from low-grade (typical carcinoids) to very aggressive (atypical carcinoids) tumors. Bronchial carcinoids are uncommon and constitute 1–2% of all pulmonary malignancies [15]. Approximately 50% of patients present with hemoptysis. Other signs and symptoms include cough, fever, wheezing, and chest pain [16, 17].

Approximately 80% of bronchial carcinoids are endobronchial and occur within the central airways including the main, lobar, or segmental bronchi. They may also extend into the pulmonary parenchyma. On CT, carcinoid tumors tend to be round, oval, or lobulated and well defined. Carcinoid is a highly vascular tumor, which intensely enhances following intravenous contrast administration. Eccentric calcification is seen in about 30% of histologic specimens; calcification is rarely seen on chest radiography but is easily identified on CT [18, 19]. If a carcinoid is more peripheral in location, a solitary pulmonary nodule is more likely to be seen. When a carcinoid is large enough to result in obstruction, associated peripheral atelectasis, air trapping, or mucoid impaction can be seen on chest imaging.

Inflammatory

Inflammatory etiologies of tracheobronchial sources of hemoptysis include acute or chronic bronchitis and bronchiectasis.

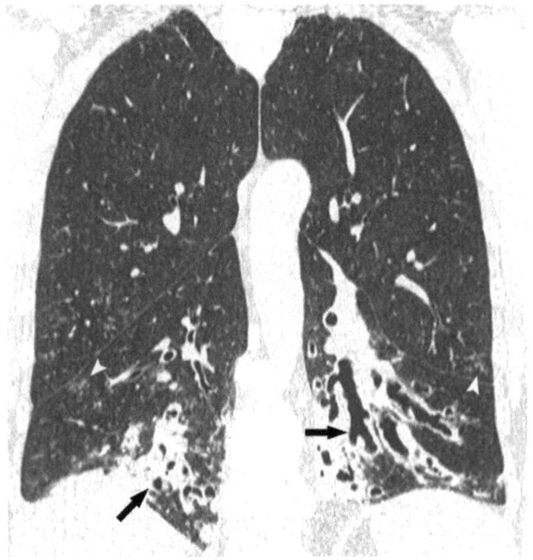

Fig. 14.3 Bronchiectasis. Coronal reformatted volumetric HRCT image shows bilateral lower lobe bronchiectasis (*arrows*). Bronchiectasis is the most common cause of hemoptysis

Acute and Chronic Bronchitis

Patients with acute bronchitis present with an acute history of cough and other respiratory tract signs and symptoms. Acute bronchitis is a respiratory tract infection that results in inflammation of the airways and development of friable mucosa as well as rupture of small superficial vessels leading to hemoptysis. It is self-limiting and may present with sputum production with or without hemoptysis. Bronchitis has been reported to cause approximately 26% of cases of hemoptysis [20]. In acute bronchitis, radiographs are often normal but may show bronchial wall thickening.

Chronic bronchitis is typically seen in adult patients and is considered a form of chronic obstructive pulmonary disease. Chronic bronchitis is a clinical diagnosis and is defined as sputum production that lasts for at least 3 months over at least two consecutive years. Chronic bronchitis has not only similar radiographic findings to acute bronchitis but also can have findings of pulmonary hypertension or cor pulmonale such as an enlarged right ventricle, enlarged central pulmonary arteries, and peripheral artery tapering. On HRCT, bronchial wall thickening and mucus within the bronchi can be seen.

Bronchiectasis

Bronchiectasis (Fig. 14.3) is an irreversible process characterized by chronic bronchial inflammation leading to abnormal dilation of one or more bronchi. Bronchiectasis has a wide variety of causes. Clinically, bronchiectasis is similar to chronic bronchitis with recurrent infections, sputum production, dyspnea, weight loss, and hemoptysis, the latter of which is seen in approximately 27% of patients [21]. Like carcinoid, hemoptysis may be the only clinical finding in bronchiectasis. Hemoptysis is secondary to bronchial artery hypertrophy and abnormal bronchial arterial walls.

Chest radiographs are abnormal in 80–90% of patients with bronchiectasis; however, the findings are nonspecific and include the tram track lines and dilated bronchi. On high resolution CT, bronchiectasis is defined as dilated bronchi with a bronchoarterial ratio >1:1.0–1.5 (bronchi are equal to or larger in size than the adjacent pulmonary artery), or bronchi seen touching or within 1 cm of the pleural or mediastinum. There is a spectrum of CT findings of bronchiectasis which has been traditionally classified into cylindrical, varicose, and cystic bronchiectasis, in order of increasing severity.

Broncholithiasis

Broncholithiasis (Fig. 14.4) is defined as calcified material protruding into the lumen of a bronchus and is usually the sequela of remote granulomatous infection such as tuberculosis or histoplasmosis. Broncholithiasis usually develops from erosion of an adjacent calcified lymph node into the affected bronchial lumen. A cough with or without hemoptysis is the most common

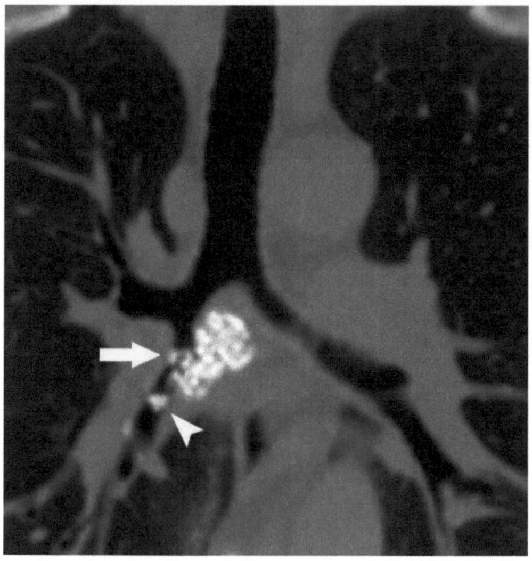

Fig. 14.4 Broncholithiasis. Coronal oblique reformatted volumetric HRCT image shows a large calcified subcarinal lymph node extending into the bronchus intermedius (*arrow*). Note the small calcific fragment (*arrowhead*) located distally. Histoplasmosis is the most common cause of broncholiths in the United States

presenting clinical symptom. Rarely, patients will expectorate calcified debris, termed lithoptysis [22].

Radiographic findings of broncholithiasis include airway obstruction such as atelectasis, mucoid impaction, bronchiectasis, and expiratory air trapping. However, unless large, the broncholith may be occult on the chest radiograph. CT, especially volumetric HRCT with multiplanar reformations, is superior to radiography for detecting broncholiths [23, 24]. Other findings of bronchial obstruction such as atelectasis, obstructive pneumonitis, or bronchiectasis are also readily apparent on CT.

Aspiration of Foreign Bodies

Accidental foreign body aspiration (Fig. 14.5) occurs most commonly in children whereas foreign body aspiration in adults more commonly is the result of trauma (e.g. teeth) or iatrogenic. The history often indicates aspiration of foreign bodies as the etiology of hemoptysis. Aspirated foreign bodies are evident on the chest radiograph only in 10–15% of patients [25]. Indirect findings such as atelectasis may be apparent.

Pulmonary Parenchymal

Table 14.2 shows the pulmonary parenchymal etiologies of hemoptysis.

Focal Infection

Focal sources of pulmonary hemorrhage include a wide variety of infections. Bacterial pneumonia findings on radiographs and CT range from nodules to consolidation that may be focal or diffuse. History of cough, fever, or infectious symptoms in conjunction with radiographic findings is essential in confirming this diagnosis.

Pulmonary Abscess

Hemoptysis is an atypical presentation in patients with a pulmonary abscess (Fig. 14.6). Up to 40% of patients with pulmonary abscesses can develop hemoptysis, although less than 10% have massive hemoptysis [26]. Patients with lung abscesses tend to present with symptoms of cough, fever, and rigors for greater than 2 weeks. Lung abscesses typically form after approximately 7–14 days following the appearance of consolidation on imaging. They tend to be solitary, more commonly seen in the lower lobes, and most commonly associated with anaerobic organisms, although *Staphylococcus aureus* and gram-negative rod infections can also result in abscess formation. Abscesses are typically treated with long-term antibiotics with fewer than 15% of patients requiring surgical intervention. Surgical intervention is reserved for patients not responding to antibiotic therapy, patients with underlying malignancy, severe hemoptysis, or patients with complicated infection such as empyema or bronchopleural fistula.

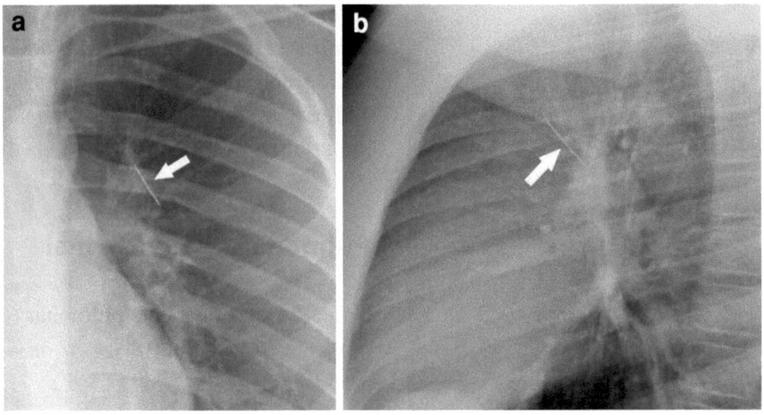

Fig. 14.5 Aspirated sewing needle. Coned-down PA (**a**) and lateral (**b**) radiographs show a linear metallic foreign body (*arrows*) in the left upper lobe

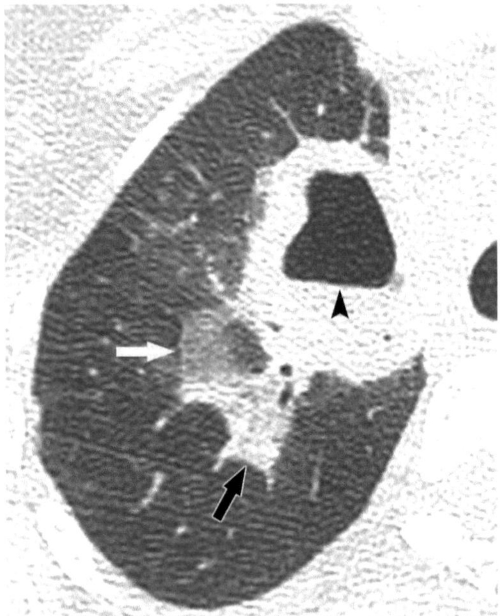

Fig. 14.6 Anaerobic pulmonary abscess. HRCT image shows a thick-walled cavity in the right upper lobe containing an air-fluid level (*arrowhead*). Surrounding ground-glass opacity (*white arrow*) and consolidation (*black arrow*) presumably represent hemorrhage in this patient who presented with hemoptysis

Radiographic findings suggestive of abscess include air-fluid levels and thick walled cavities. On CT, the wall is irregular and usually >4 mm. Intra-abscess air-fluid levels or gas bubbles may be present, and peripheral rim enhancement following administration of intravenous contrast can be seen.

Tuberculosis

Tuberculosis (TB) is the most common cause of hemoptysis worldwide. Risk factors for TB include immunosuppression, travel to or emigration from endemic areas, and living in close quarters (homeless shelters, prisons, nursing homes) and may be the initial clue in this diagnostic consideration. At least one quarter to one-third of patients with TB develop hemoptysis [27].

Primary TB is less common than reactivation TB and tends to be a self-limiting and non-destructive process in patients with a normal immune system. Primary TB is also thought of as a disease of childhood. However, the incidence of primary TB is increasing in the adult population primarily because of the AIDS epidemic and the rising number of transplant recipients. Findings of pneumonia are seen on radiographs including lung consolidation, ipsilateral hilar lymphadenopathy, atelectasis, and pleural effusion. Cavities are uncommon in primary TB. In approximately two-thirds of patients, consolidation resolves. In the remaining one-third of patients, residual scar develops and can, an entity known as a Ghon complex.

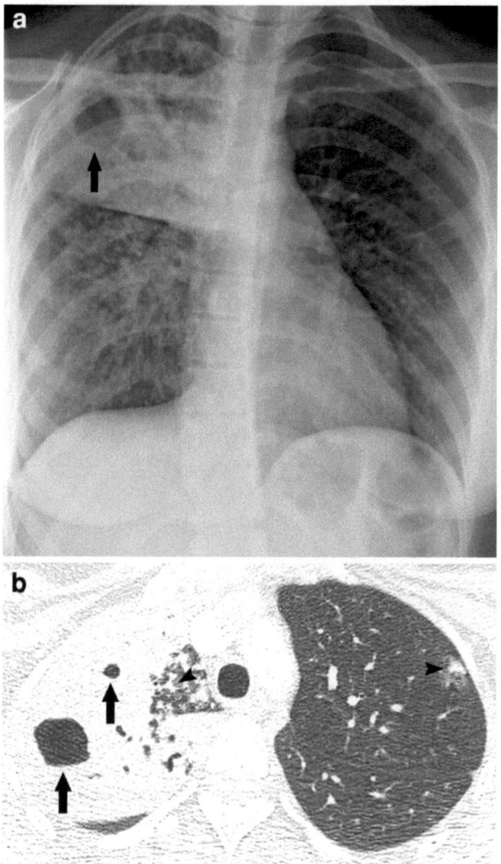

Fig. 14.7 Reactivation tuberculosis. **a** PA radiograph shows dense right upper lobe consolidation containing an air-filled cavity (*arrow*). Scattered poorly defined nodules reflect endobronchial spread of inflammatory debris and blood products. **b** HRCT image shows cavities (*arrows*) surrounding by dense consolidation in the right upper lobe. Smaller nodules are in both lungs (*arrowheads*)

Post-primary or reactivation TB (Fig. 14.7) is a destructive infection that usually results in cavity formation. Besides cavity formation, reactivation TB can have a variety of appearances including round discrete nodules and patchy or confluent lung consolidation. Cavities tend to have thick and irregular walls and are most often located in the upper lobes. Lymphadenopathy is notably absent in reactivation TB. Cavities that develop adjacent to a small or medium pulmonary artery branch can result in a pseudoaneurysm formation, otherwise known as a Rasmussen aneurysm. A Rasmussen aneurysm may rupture, resulting in hemoptysis that may be severe and possibly result in death.

Fungal Infections

The incidence of fungal pulmonary infections is increasing as the immunocompromised patient population increases. Aspergillosis is one of the more common pulmonary fungal infections and has several different infection patterns including mycetoma (aspergilloma), chronic necrotizing, angioinvasive, and allergic bronchopulmonary aspergillosis. Allergic bronchopulmonary aspergillosis is not typically associated with hemoptysis and will not be discussed here.

Mycetomas or fungus balls (Fig. 14.8) are saprophytic fungal growths, usually within a pre-existing cavity, without tissue invasion. While many patients are asymptomatic, 50–85% of patients will initially present with hemoptysis [28, 29]. On radiographs, the earliest sign may be pleural thickening, which can appear before the cavity is apparent. The fungus ball is a solid round or oval mobile mass in a lung cavity and can be seen on radiographs and CT. The mass is often separated from the cavity wall by a focus of air resulting in an "air crescent sign." Additionally, gravitational shift of the intracavitary mass may be identifiable with changes in patient position.

Chronic necrotizing aspergillosis occurs in patients with low-grade immunocompromise such as COPD, alcoholism, corticosteroid use, diabetes, or TB. This is a disease similar in histopathology to tuberculosis; however, tissue necrosis and granuloma formation are not present. Patients with chronic necrotizing aspergillosis less frequently present with hemoptysis, which occurs in about 15% [30]. Radiographs typically mimic the appearance of TB and show a progressive but slowly growing unilateral or bilateral foci consolidation or pulmonary nodules with or without cavitation and adjacent pleural thickening. In addition to these findings, CT may show an endobronchial or hilar mass.

Invasive aspergillosis (Fig. 14.9) occurs almost exclusively in patients with neutropenia. Hemoptysis is an uncommon presentation in

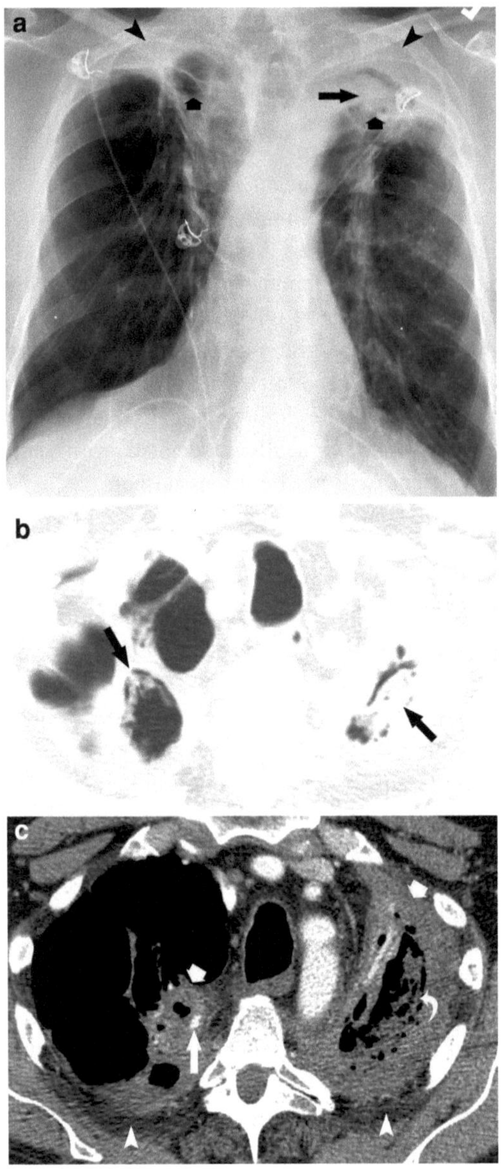

Fig. 14.8 Aspergilloma. **a**. PA radiograph shows extensive upper lobe fibrosis with bilateral cavities (*wide arrows*). A soft tissue mass (*thin arrow*) fills the left upper lobe cavity. Note thickening of the pleural and extrapleural tissues (*arrowheads*), indicating the chronic inflammatory nature of this process. **b**. Contrast-enhanced CT image (lung window settings) shows heterogeneous soft tissue masses (*arrows*) typical of aspergillomas filling the cavities. **c**. Contrast-enhanced CT image depicts the thick cavity walls (*wide arrows*) and hypertrophy of the extrapleural fat (*arrowheads*). Aspergillomas (*curved arrow*) typically contain pockets of air. A pulmonary artery pseudoaneurysm (*thin arrow*) has formed in the right upper lobe cavity wall

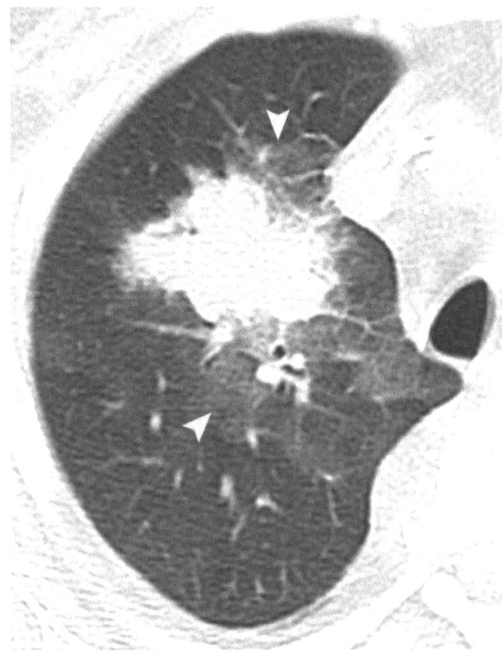

Fig. 14.9 Invasive pulmonary aspergillosis in a patient with neutropenia and acute myelogenous leukemia. HRCT image shows a consolidative right upper lobe mass with a halo of ground-glass opacity (*arrowheads*). While not pathognomonic, the CT halo sign is highly suggestive of invasive aspergillosis in the correct clinical setting

invasive aspergillosis. On radiographs, nonspecific rapidly progressing pulmonary nodules or areas of consolidation with or without a cavity can be seen. Nodules or subpleural, wedge-shaped areas of consolidation can be seen on CT. The characteristic ground-glass halo surrounding pulmonary nodules representing hemorrhage from angioinvasion can also be seen but is not specific for aspergillosis, as it is also seen with *Candida*, herpes simplex virus, cytomegalovirus, and Wegener granulomatosis. Direct extension of invasive aspergillosis into bronchial and pulmonary arteries can lead to development of mycotic pseudoaneurysms. *Aspergillus* infection is not limited to the anatomic barriers of the lung and can extend into the mediastinum where mycotic pseudoaneurysms of the aorta and aortic branches may form. Like TB, these aneurysms can rupture, result in hemoptysis that may be massive in nature, and possibly result in death.

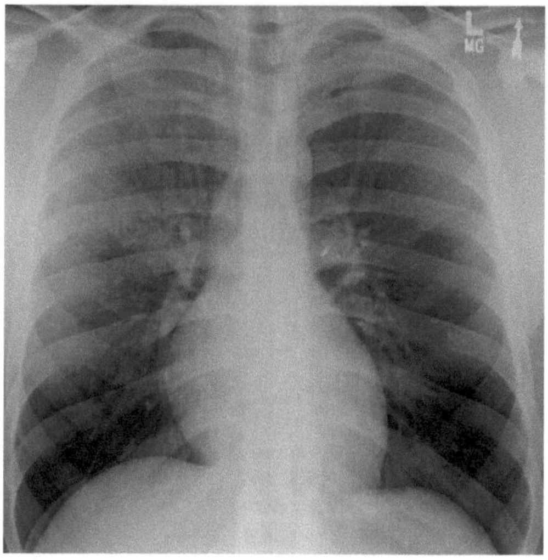

Fig. 14.10 Pulmonary contusion in a football player. PA radiograph shows ill-defined hazy opacity in the right upper lung. Contusion should begin clearing within 48–72 h after injury

Trauma

Pulmonary Contusion

Pulmonary contusion (Fig. 14.10) is the most common lung injury resulting from blunt chest trauma, found especially in unrestrained drivers in motor vehicle collisions after deceleration injuries. Pulmonary contusions are most commonly seen at the site of trauma; however *contrecoup* injury (on the opposite side) can occur. Following injury, capillary disruption and hemorrhage fill the alveolar spaces resulting in parenchymal contusion. Hemoptysis is the most common clinical sign, seen in 50% of patients. Contusions are commonly associated with other injuries to the chest or mediastinum, including pneumothorax or pneumomediastinum. Underlying pulmonary laceration may be obscured until contusion clears.

Contusion is usually evident on the chest radiograph at the time of presentation or develops shortly thereafter. Radiographic findings of contusion are often nonspecific ranging from irregular confluent or discrete nodular opacities to dense consolidation. A non-segmental and non-gravitationally dependent distribution should suggest pulmonary contusion in the acute trauma setting. CT is more specific than chest radiography for not only depicting the extent of contusion but also for detecting associated injuries such as pulmonary laceration, pneumothorax, hemothorax, mediastinal injury, and chest wall injury. Contusion typically begins to clear within 48–72 h, resolving by 10–14 days [31]. Developing lung opacities 24 h after trauma or failure to resolve within 10–14 days should suggest an alternative underlying process such as aspiration pneumonia.

Diffuse Alveolar Hemorrhage

Diffuse alveolar hemorrhage (DAH) is recognized as a clinical syndrome comprising hemoptysis, anemia, diffuse alveolar airspace opacities, and hypoxemia. Only about two-thirds of patients with DAH present with hemoptysis. The most common causes of DAH include Wegner granulomatosis (32%), Goodpasture syndrome (13%), idiopathic pulmonary hemosiderosis (IPH) (13%), collagen vascular diseases (13%), and microscopic polyangiitis (MPA) (9%) [32].

Goodpasture Syndrome (Anti-Glomerular Basement Membrane Antibody Disease)

Acute Goodpasture syndrome (Fig. 14.11) is an idiopathic autoimmune syndrome consisting of a triad of renal failure, alveolar hemorrhage, and antiglomerular basement membrane antibodies. Up to 10% of patients present with DAH without renal involvement; however, 90% of patients with both pulmonary and renal involvement have hemoptysis and anemia. Radiographs may be normal early in the disease process. With increased alveolar hemorrhage, extensive bilateral ground-glass opacity, often in a perihilar distribution, develops and can progress to patchy consolidation with relative sparing of the lung periphery. Fibrosis can develop with recurrent

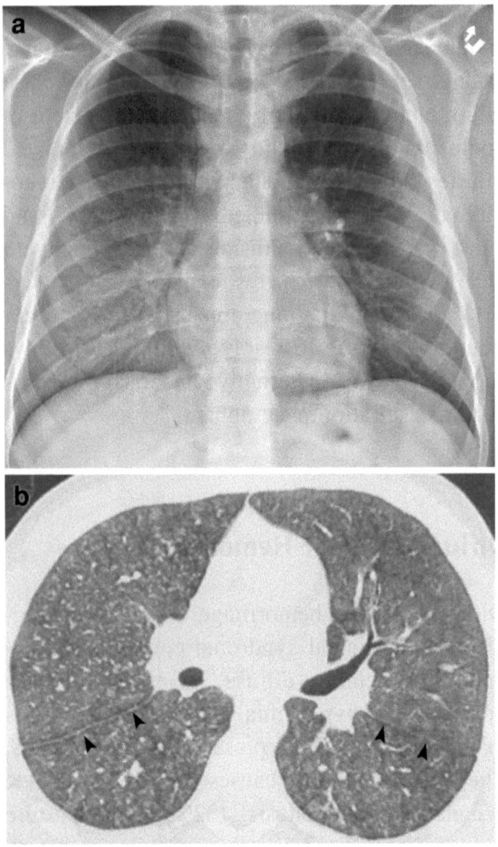

Fig. 14.11 Goodpasture syndrome with diffuse alveolar hemorrhage. **a** PA radiograph of a patient presenting with acute hemoptysis and hypoxia shows patchy hazy opacities in both lungs, more so on the right. **b** HRCT image shows extensive nodular ground-glass opacities with sparing of the subpleural lung including along the major fissures (*arrowheads*)

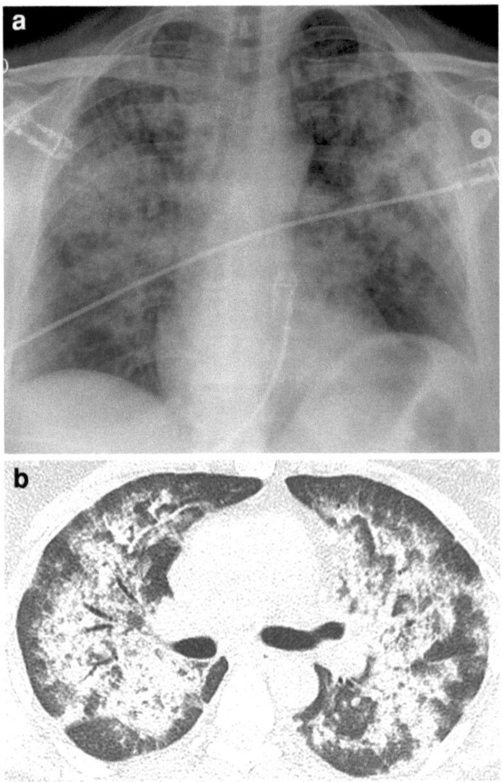

Fig. 14.12 Wegener granulomatosis with diffuse alveolar hemorrhage. **a** Portable AP radiograph shows bilateral patchy perihilar consolidation with relative sparing of the periphery. **b** HRCT image shows extensive bilateral lung consolidation with relative sparing of the subpleural lung. Diffuse alveolar hemorrhage may be the presenting manifestation of Wegener granulomatosis

hemorrhage and is characterized on CT primarily by reticulation with or without traction bronchiectasis.

Wegner Granulomatosis

Wegner granulomatosis is a systemic autoimmune small vessel vasculitis. Clinical findings of rhinitis and sinusitis with mucosal hemorrhage, saddle nose deformity, and septal perforation can be helpful in the diagnosis.

Wegner granulomatosis has a variety of appearances; however, this section will focus primarily on diffuse alveolar hemorrhage (Fig. 14.12). Approximately 10% of patients with Wegner granulomatosis develop diffuse alveolar hemorrhage [33]. On radiographs, findings are nonspecific and can include patchy or diffuse airspace opacities that may be ground-glass or areas of focal consolidation. These findings can be widespread; however, they tend to be more prominent in the perihilar region in the mid and lower lungs. On CT, findings are nonspecific with diffuse ground-glass opacities. The diagnosis can be suggested by the other CT findings such as cavitary nodules or masses, ground-glass opacities, or consolidation with our without pleural effusions.

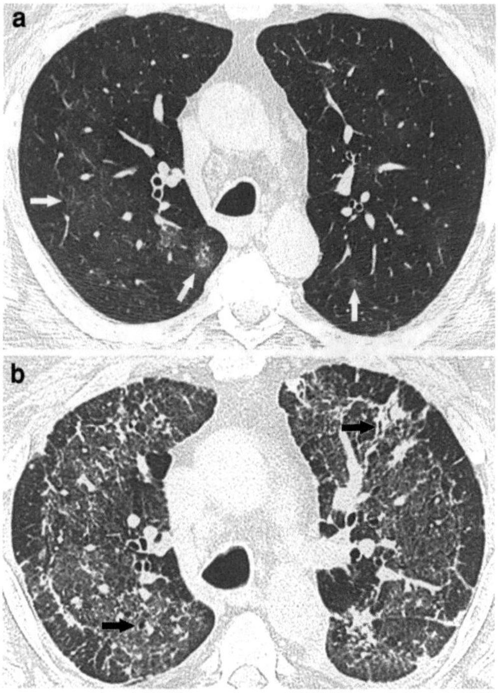

Fig. 14.13 Idiopathic pulmonary hemosiderosis. **a** HRCT shows patchy ground-glass opacity (*arrows*) reflecting alveolar hemorrhage. **b** HRCT image 4 years later shows ground-glass opacity from acute hemorrhage superimposed on fibrosis characterized by new reticular opacities and traction bronchiectasis (*arrows*)

Idiopathic Pulmonary Hemosiderosis

Idiopathic pulmonary hemosiderosis (IPH) is a rare syndrome characterized by chronic anemia secondary to repeated episodes of pulmonary hemorrhage (Fig. 14.13). It most commonly occurs in patients under the age of 30, and the etiology is unknown but believed to be autoimmune. Nearly all adults will develop hemoptysis [34]. On radiographs, IPH can manifest as diffuse alveolar opacities and acutely may even have appearance as symmetric perihilar distribution. These findings typically resolve in 2 weeks. Late findings include fibrosis that results from the inflammatory response to blood products. On HRCT, ground-glass opacities representing alveolar hemorrhage are usually bilateral and located predominantly in the mid and lower lungs. Pulmonary fibrosis can ensue with recurrent hemorrhage.

Sarcoidosis

Sarcoidosis is a granulomatous disorder with >90% of patients having respiratory tract involvement. Sarcoidosis may be clinically silent and detected incidentally or cause cough and progressive dyspnea. Patients can present with mild or massive hemoptysis, but diffuse alveolar hemorrhage is rare in sarcoidosis. Hemoptysis related to sarcoidosis occurs in patients with advanced disease and is more often related to cavitary formation and bronchiectasis. Radiographs typically show bilateral hilar enlargement and right paratracheal lymphadenopathy with or without pulmonary opacities. When present, the parenchymal findings are reticulonodular opacities predominantly in the mid and upper lungs in a peribronchovascular and subpleural distribution. On HRCT, a perilymphatic distribution of micronodules is characteristic (Fig. 14.14). Late findings on CT include honeycombing, traction bronchiectasis, and reticulation.

Systemic Lupus Erythematosis

Approximately 4% of patients with SLE will develop DAH (Fig. 14.15) [35], and hemoptysis is the presenting feature of SLE in approximately 11% of patients [36]. When imaging findings of DAH are seen in conjunction with pleural and pericardial effusion, SLE should be considered, especially in young women.

Behçet Disease

Behçet disease is a vasculitis that involves both small and large arteries, and most common in 25–30 year old patients of Mediterranean and far Eastern descent. Pulmonary involvement occurs in less than 15% of patients; however, hemoptysis is the leading cause of death in these patients primarily from rupture of a large intrathoracic aneurysm [37, 38]. Although the diagnosis is more commonly based on clinical

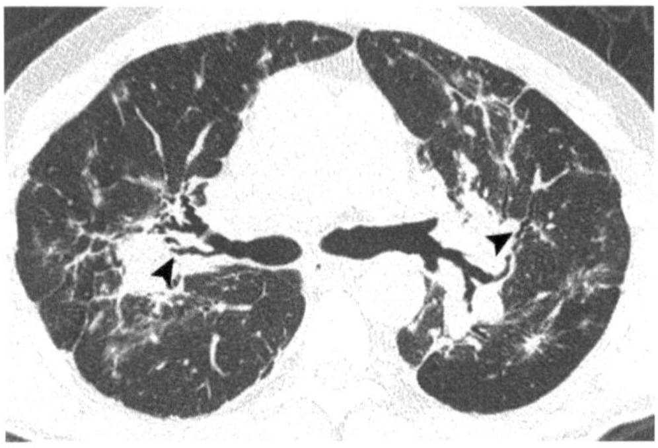

Fig. 14.14 Sarcoidosis. HRCT image shows bilateral and symmetric perilymphatic nodules and thickening of the bronchovascular bundles. Traction bronchiectasis (*arrowheads*) has developed as a consequence of fibrosis

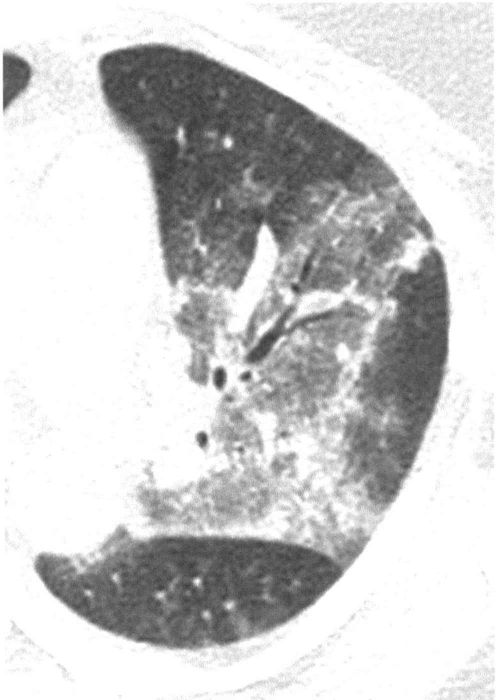

Fig. 14.15 Systemic lupus erythematosis. HRCT image shows extensive ground-glass opacity with patchy consolidation in the left upper lobe in this patient who presented with dyspnea and hemoptysis

findings including mucocutaneous ulceration, there are characteristic radiologic findings of the disease. On radiographs, focal and diffuse airspace opacities and mediastinal or hilar

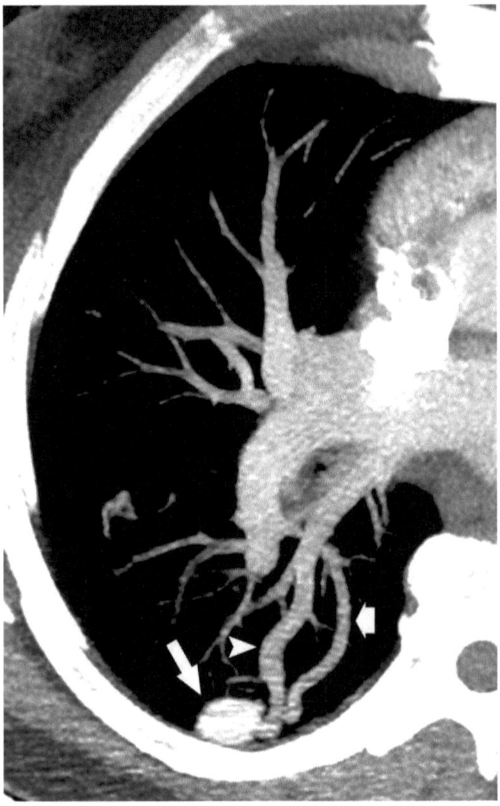

Fig. 14.16 Pulmonary arteriovenous malformation. Maximum intensity projection (MIP) from a contrast-enhanced CT scan shows contrast filling the nidus of the arteriovenous malformation (*thin arrow*). A single feeding pulmonary artery (*wide arrow*) and draining pulmonary vein (*arrowhead*) are present

enlargement from pulmonary arterial aneurysms are the main findings. Subpleural and wedge-shaped or ill-defined rounded areas of lung consolidation representing focal vasculitis with hemorrhage, infarction, and inflammation can also be seen [39].

Primary Vascular

Table 14.3 shows the primary vascular etiologies of hemoptysis.

Pulmonary Arteriovenous Malformations

Pulmonary arteriovenous malformations (PAVM) (Fig. 14.16) are abnormal connections between arteries and veins in the lungs and are a rare

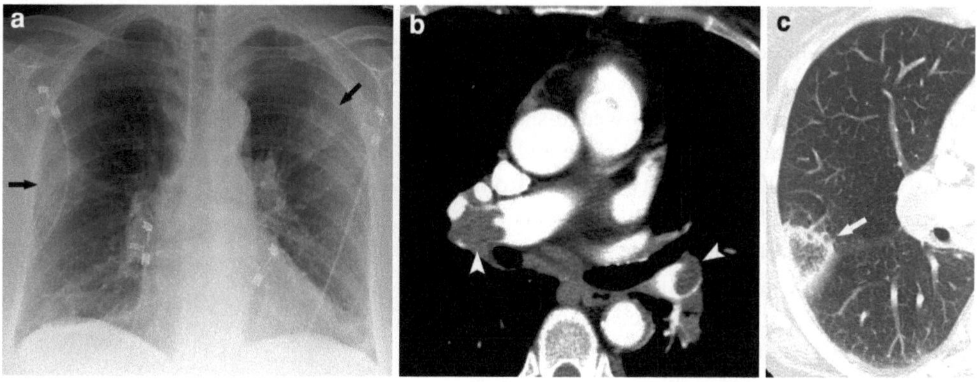

Fig. 14.17 Acute pulmonary thromboembolism with infarction. **a** Portable AP radiograph shows poorly defined wedge-shaped opacities (*arrows*) in the periphery of the lungs. **b** Contrast-enhanced CT image shows bilateral acute pulmonary thromboemboli (*arrowheads*). **c** Contrast-enhanced CT image (lung window settings) shows the characteristic wedge-shaped appearance of an infarct in the right lung with peripheral consolidation (*arrow*) and central ground-glass opacity

cause of hemoptysis. Hemoptysis is the third most common symptom in PAVMs; the hemoptysis may be massive, is more common during the later half of pregnancy, and is rarely fatal. Most PAVMs are congenital, and approximately 70% of patients have Osler-Weber-Rendu syndrome, also known as hereditary hemorrhagic telangiectasia (HHT). Most patients do not present until adulthood [40]. Patients with HHT are at risk for septic emboli, which can result in stroke or cerebral abscesses.

Nearly all patients with HHT have some radiographic abnormality. Sharply defined single or multiple oval or lobulated opacities are the most common radiographic finding [41]. HRCT is much more useful in characterizing a PAVM by characterizing its size, location, and arterial supply and venous drainage. Common CT findings are single or multiple pulmonary nodules with enlarged feeding vessels, draining vessels, or both [42]. Arteriovenous malformations with feeding arteries >3 mm in diameter are typically treated by endovascular embolization. If coil embolization is not feasible or unsafe, resection can be considered. CTA is useful for following patients with treated PAVMs as it can assess whether or not a treated PAVM remains occluded.

Pulmonary Embolus

Patients with pulmonary emboli may be asymptomatic or present with a wide range of signs and symptoms including pleuritic chest pain, shortness of breath, hemoptysis, fever, and tachycardia. Approximately 10% of patients present with hemoptysis, and hemoptysis is typically an indicator of pulmonary infarction [43]. CT angiography is the imaging study of choice in patients with suspected pulmonary embolism. Pulmonary hemorrhage in the setting of acute pulmonary embolism typically manifests as peripheral, often wedge-shaped focal ground-glass opacity or consolidation in the distribution of a visible pulmonary artery filling defect.

Pulmonary Infarction

Pulmonary infarction (Fig. 14.17) is usually the result of acute pulmonary thromboembolism, although only 10% of thromboemboli result in infarction [44]. Pulmonary infarction typically presents on the chest radiograph as peripheral, wedge-shaped focus of lung consolidation with a truncated apex that is directed toward the ipsilateral hilum, eponymously known as "Hampton's hump". Infarcts >4 cm can undergo central cavitation. Infarcts may be multiple depending on the extent of thromboembolic disease, and pleural effusions may develop. CT findings of infarction include a wedge-shaped opacity that contacts the pleural surface and has convex borders. A linear opacity directed from the apex toward the hilum, which represents the feeding vessel. Additionally, there may be areas more centrally of low attenuation or surrounding halo due to adjacent hemorrhage. Air bronchograms are conspicuously absent. Infarction may take weeks to months to resolve and may leave a linear focus of scar. Infarcts classically resolve from the periphery to the center, similar to the "melting of an ice cube" [45].

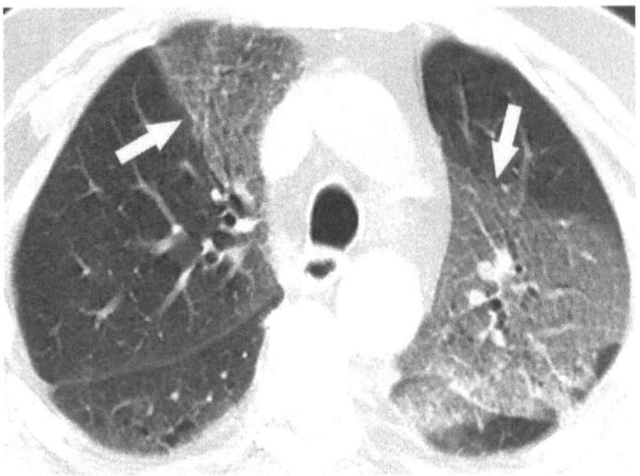

Fig. 14.18 Radiation pneumonitis in a patient with lung carcinoma. HRCT image shows confluent ground-glass opacity in both lungs. Note the sharp margins (*arrows*) between the ground-glass opacity and normal lung reflecting the confines of the radiation field

Miscellaneous

Table 14.4 shows the miscellaneous etiologies of hemoptysis.

Coagulopathy

A relatively common cause for pulmonary hemorrhage is systemic coagulopathy from the use of anticoagulants or thrombolytic agents. Rare bleeding disorders such as hemophilia or coagulopathy secondary to thrombocytopenia are considered when more common etiologies are excluded. For example, pulmonary endometriosis is extremely rare with few case reports in the literature. This diagnosis is suggested with patient history of cyclic hemoptysis that correlates with menstrual cycles [46].

Radiation-Induced Lung Injury

Radiation therapy can result in inflammation or irritation and inflammation of the bronchial mucosa. Many factors affect the potential for bronchial mucosal injury: the method of irradiation, the volume of irradiated lung, the total dosage and frequency of irradiation, and associated chemotherapy. Acute radiation pneumonitis (Fig. 14.18) occurs approximately 4–12 weeks following radiation therapy and infrequently presents with hemoptysis. After 6–12 months of radiation, pulmonary fibrosis can develop.

Radiation pneumonitis appears as perivascular haziness that often progresses to patchy alveolar opacities in the region of radiation exposure. Effusions and rib fractures may also be present. Fibrosis often appears as coarse reticular opacities with bronchiectasis. On CT, initially there are ground-glass opacities in the radiated pulmonary parenchyma that progress to areas of consolidation with sharp edges that are related to the region of radiation and not anatomic boundaries. These opacities resolve, and linear scarring with possible parenchymal loss can be seen.

Drug Reaction

Many medications have been reported to cause hemoptysis. Chemotherapeutic agents are most commonly implicated. For example, a known side effect in patients taking bevacizumab with non-small cell lung cancer is severe and massive hemoptysis. Chemotherapeutic agents in conjunction with chest radiation also increase the risk for hemoptysis. Drug-induced vasculitis is relatively rare reported with drugs such as sulfasalazine or hydralazine, which result in a lupus-like vasculitis.

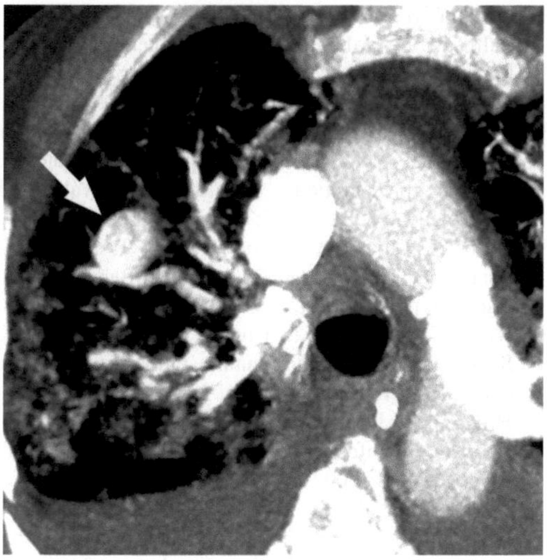

Fig. 14.19 Pseudoaneurysm from malpositioned pulmonary artery catheter. MIP from contrast-enhanced CT scan shows a large pseudoaneurysm (*arrow*) in the right upper lobe. Pulmonary artery pseudoaneurysm rupture can cause massive hemoptysis and is frequently fatal

Iatrogenic

Iatrogenic causes of hemoptysis are not common but are important to recognize. Balloon-tip pulmonary artery catheter placement or manipulation can result in pulmonary artery rupture or pseudoaneurysm formation (Fig. 14.19) and subsequently can lead to hemoptysis [47]. Major complications with balloon-tip pulmonary artery catheter placement occur in approximately 17% of patients, with only 0.2% being related to pulmonary artery rupture. However, the mortality rate when pulmonary artery rupture occurs is nearly 50% [48]. Transbronchial or percutaneous biopsies are an additional iatrogenic cause of hemoptysis.

References

1. Savale L, Parrot A, Khalil A, et al. Cryptogenic hemoptysis: from a benign to a life-threatening pathologic vascular condition. Am J Respir Crit Care Med. 2007;175(11):1181.
2. Knott-Craig CJ, Oostuizen JD, Rossouw G, et al. Management and prognosis of massive hemoptysis. J Thorac Cardio vasc Surg. 1993;105:394–7.
3. Hirshberg B, Biran I, Glazer M, Kramer MR. Hemoptysis: etiology, evaluation, and outcome in a tertiary referral hospital. Chest. 1997;112:440–4.
4. Colice GL. Hemoptysis. Three questions that can direct management. Postgrad Med. 1996;100:227–36.
5. Corey R, Hla KM. Major and massive hemoptysis: reassessment of conservative management. Am J Med Sci. 1987;294:301–9.
6. McGuinness G, Beacher JR, Harkin TJ, et al. Hemoptysis: prospective high-resolution CT/bronchoscopic correlation. Chest. 1994;105:1155–62.
7. Shigemura N, Wan IY, Yu SCH. Multidisciplinary management of life-threatening massive hemoptysis: a 10-year experience. Ann Thorac Surg. 2009; 87:849–53.
8. Fartoukh M, Khalil A, Louis L, et al. An integrated approach to diagnosis and management of severe haemoptysis in patients admitted to the intensive care unit: a case series from a referral centre. Respir Res. 2007;8:11–20.
9. Dweik R, Stoller JK. Role of bronchoscopy in massive hemoptysis. Clin Chest Med. 1999; 20: 89–105.
10. Deffebach ME, Charan NB, Lakshminarayan S, Butler J. The bronchial circulation: small, but a vital attribute to the lung. Am Rev Respir Dis. 1987;135:463–81.
11. Khalil A, Soussan M, Mangiapan G, Fartoukh M, Parrot A, Carette MF. Utility of high-resolution chest CT scan in the emergency management of hemoptysis in the intensive care unit: severity, localization and aetiology. BJR. 2007;80:21–5.
12. Millar AB, Boothroyd AE, Edwards D, Hetzel MR. The role of computed tomography (CT) in the investigation of unexplained haemoptysis. Respir Med. 1992;86:39–44.
13. Revel MP, Fournier LS, Hennebicque AS, et al. Can CT replace bronchoscopy in the detection of the site and cause of bleeding in patients with large or massive hemoptysis? AJR Am J Roentgenol. 2002; 179:1217–24.
14. Kvale PA, Selecky PA, Prakash UB. American College of Chest Physicians. Palliative care in lung cancer: ACCP evidence-based clinical practice guidelines (2nd edition). Chest. 2007;132(suppl):368S–403S.
15. Modlin IM, Lye KD, Kidd M. A 5-decade analysis of 13, 715 carcinoid tumors. Cancer. 2003;97:934–59.
16. Fraser RG, Paré JAP, Paré PD, Fraser RS, Genereux GP. Neoplasms of pulmonary neuroendocrine cells. Philadelphia: Saunders; 1991. p. 1476–97.
17. Rosado de Christenson ML, Abbott GF, Kirejczyk WM, Galvin JR, Travis WD. Thoracic carcinoids: radiologic-pathologic correlation. RadioGraphics. 1999;19: 707–36.
18. Magid D, Siegelman SS, Eggleston JC, Fishman EK, Zerhouni EA. Pulmonary carcinoid tumors: CT assessment. J Comput Assist Tomogr. 1989;13:244–7.
19. Zwiebel BR, Austin JHM, Grimes MM. Bronchial carcinoid tumors: assessment with CT of location

and intratumoral calcification in 31 patients. Radiology. 1991;179:483–6.
20. Reisz G, Stevens D, Boutwell C, Nair V. The causes of hemoptysis revisited. Review of the etiologies of hemoptysis between 1986 and 1995. Mo Med. 1997;94:6335.
21. King PT, Holdsworth SR, Freezer NJ, Villanueva E, Holmes PW. Characterization of the onset and presenting clinical features of adult bronchiectasis. Respir Med. 2006;100(12):2183.
22. Antao VCS, Pinheiro GA, Jansen JM. Broncholithiasis and Lithoptysis Associated with Silicosis. Eur Respir J. 2002;20(4):1057–9.
23. Conces DJ Jr, Tarver RD, Vix VA. Broncholithiasis: CT features in 15 patients. AJR Am J Roentgenol. 1991;157:249–53.
24. Adler O, Peleg H. Computed tomography in diagnosis of broncholithiasis. Eur J Radiol. 1987;7:211–2.
25. Armstrong P, Wilson AG, Dee P, Hansell DM. Imaging of diseases of the chest. 2nd ed. ed. St. Louis, O: Mosby; 1995. p. 453–7.
26. Estrera SE, Platt MR, Lawrence JM, Shaw RR. Primary lung abscess. J Thorac Cardiovasc Surg. 1980;79:275–82.
27. El-Khushman H, Momani JA, Sharara AM, et al. The pattern of active pulmonary tuberculosis in adults at King Hussein Medical Center, Jordan. Saudi Med J. 2006;27(5):633–6.
28. Glimp RA, Bayer AS. Pulmonary aspergilloma. Diagnostic and therapeutic considerations. Arch Intern Med. 1983;143(2):303.
29. Shapiro MJ, Albelda SM, Mayock RL, McLean GK. Severe hemoptysis associated with pulmonary aspergilloma. Percutaneous intracavitary treatment. Chest. 1988;94(6):1225.
30. Franquet T, Müller NL, Giménez A, Domingo P, Plaza V, Bordes R. Semiinvasive pulmonary aspergillosis in chronic obstructive pulmonary disease: radiologic and pathologic findings in nine patients. Am J Roentgenol. 2000;174:51–6.
31. Rivas LA, Fishman JE, Munera F, et al. Multislice CT in thoracic trauma. Radiol Clin North Am. 2003;41:599–616.
32. Lara AR, Schwarz MI. Diffuse alveolar hemorrhage. Chest. 2010;137:1164–71.
33. Frank TJ, Koss MN. Pulmonary capillaritis. Curr Opin Pulm Med. 2000;6:403–35.
34. Milman N, Pedersen FM. Idiopathic pulmonary haemosiderosis. Epidemiology, pathogenic aspects and diagnosis. Respir Med. 1998;92(7):902.
35. Zamora MR, Warner ML, Tuder R, Schwarz MI. Diffuse alveolar hemorrhage and systemic lupus erythematosus. Clinical presentation, histology, survival, and outcome. Med Baltimore. 1997;76(3):192–202.
36. Collard HR, Schwarz MI. Diffuse alveolar hemorrhage and systemic lupus erythematosus. Clinical presentation, histology, survival, and outcome. Medicine. 1997;76(3):192–202.
37. Hiller N, Liberman S, Chajek-Shaul T, Bar-Ziv J, Shaham D. Thoracic manifestations of Behcet on CT. RadioGraphics. 2004;24:801–8.
38. Hiller N, Lieberman S, Chajek-Shaul T, Bar-Ziv J, Shaham D. Thoracic manifestations of Behçet disease at CT. Radiographics. 2004;24:801–8.
39. Hillar N, Lieberman S, Chajek-Shaul T, et al. Thoracic manifestations of Behcet disease at CT. Radiographics. 2004;24(3):801–8.
40. Hodgson CH, Burchell HB, Good CA, Claggett OT. Hereditary hemorrhagic telangiectasis and pulmonary arteriovenous fistula. Circulation. 2006;114: 48–9.
41. Jaskolka J, Wu L, Chan RP, Faughnan ME. Imaging of hereditary hemorrhagic telangiectasia. Am J Roentgenol. 2004;183(2):307.
42. Remy J, Remy-Jardin M, Giraud F, Wattinne L. Angioarchitecture of pulmonary arteriovenous malformations: clinical utility of three-dimensional helical CT. Radiology. 1994;191:657–64.
43. Miniati M, Prediletto R, Formichi B, et al. Accuracy of Clinical Assessment in the Diagnosis of Pulmonary Embolism. Am J Respir Crit Care Med. 1999;159(3):864–71.
44. Greaves MS, Hart EM. Brown, K, et. al. Pulmonary Thromboembolism: Spectrum of CT Findings. AJR. 1995;165:1359–63.
45. Woesner M, Sanders I, White G. The melting ice sign in Resolving Transient Pulmonary Infarction. AJR. 1971;3(4):782–90.
46. Guidry GG, George RB, Payne DK. Catamenial hemoptysis: a case report and review of the literature. J La State Med Soc. 1990;142(11):27–30.
47. Abreu AR, Campos MA, Krieger BP. Pulmonary artery rupture induced by a pulmonary artery catheter: a case report and review of the literature. J Intensive Care Med. 2004;19(5):291–6.
48. Poplausky MR, Rozenblit G, Rundback JH, Crea G, Maddineni S, Leonardo R. Swan-Ganz catheter-induced pulmonary artery pseudoaneurysm formation: three case reports and a review of the literature. Chest. 2001;120:2105–11.

Non-AIDS Immunologic Diseases

15

Stephen A. Quinet and Jeffrey P. Kanne

Abstract

The broad category of noninfectious inflammatory pulmonary diseases encompasses a wide variety of pathologic entities with myriad clinical presentations. This chapter seeks to guide the informed, judicious use of imaging in the initial work-up and subsequent follow-up of patients with these often widely disparate conditions. The topics to be covered in this chapter include sarcoidosis, common variable immunodeficiency, primary immunodeficiencies (X-linked agammaglobulinemia, X-linked immunoproliferative syndrome), low-grade lymphoproliferative disorders (follicular bronchiolitis, lymphoid interstitial pneumonia, Castleman disease, lymphomatoid granulomatosis), and allergic bronchopulmonary aspergillosis.

Keywords

Non-infectious inflammatory • Sarcoidosis • Primary immunodeficiencies • Low-grade lymphoproliferative disorders • Allergic bronchopulmonary aspergillosis

Introduction

The broad category of noninfectious inflammatory pulmonary diseases encompasses a wide variety of pathologic entities with myriad clinical presentations. The topics to be covered in this chapter include sarcoidosis, common variable immunodeficiency (CVID), primary immunodeficiencies (X-linked agammaglobulinemia, X-linked immunoproliferative syndrome), low-grade lymphoproliferative disorders (follicular bronchiolitis, lymphoid interstitial pneumonia, Castleman disease, lymphomatoid granulomatosis), and allergic bronchopulmonary aspergillosis (ABPA).

Sarcoidosis

Clinical Presentation

Sarcoidosis is a granulomatous inflammatory disease of unknown etiology that can affect any organ in the body, with pulmonary, dermatologic,

S. A. Quinet (✉) · J. P. Kanne
Department of Radiology,
University of Wisconsin School of Medicine and Public Health, 600 Highland Ave, Madison, WI 53792-3252, USA
e-mail: squinet@uwhealth.org

J. P. Kanne (ed.), *Clinically Oriented Pulmonary Imaging*,
Respiratory Medicine, DOI: 10.1007/978-1-61779-542-8_15,

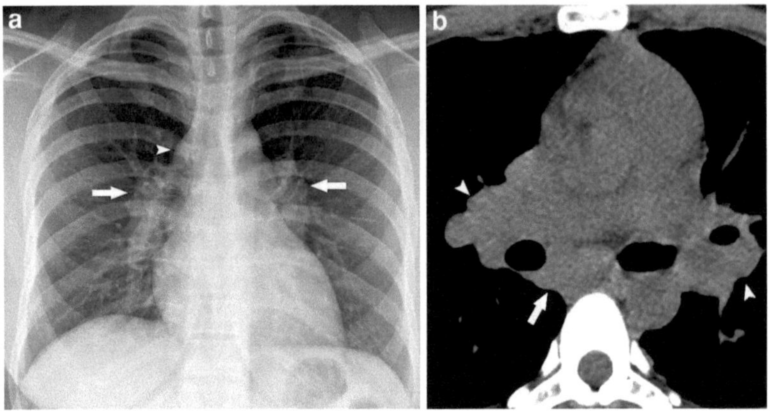

Fig. 15.1 *Stage* 1 sarcoidosis. **a** PA radiograph shows bilateral hilar (*arrows*) and right paratracheal (*arrowhead*) lymphadenopathy with no appreciable lung abnormalities. **b** Unenhanced CT image shows bilateral hilar (*arrowheads*) and subcarinal (*arrow*) lymphadenopathy

and ocular findings most common. In genetically susceptible people, an autoimmune response to a dynamic interplay of infectious, organic agents, and inorganic particles leading to the characteristic pathologic finding of noncaseating granulomas has been proposed as a potential etiology of sarcoidosis [1, 2]. The emphasis of this section will be on the pulmonary manifestations of the disease. Pulmonary involvement is present in over 90% of patients with sarcoidosis, manifesting as a variety of nonspecific signs and symptoms, including nonproductive cough, dyspnea, and wheezing [1]. Constitutional symptoms such as fatigue, weight loss, and fever are common. Sarcoidosis is an important consideration in the evaluation of fever of unknown origin (FUO) [3]. Up to 50% of patients are asymptomatic at initial presentation with incidentally detected radiographic abnormalities [1, 2]. Physical examination often reveals no findings suggestive of pulmonary involvement, despite radiographic abnormalities. Crackles, particularly auscultated anteriorly, may be present and are more common in advanced disease. Sarcoidosis usually manifests clinically prior to the fourth decade of life, with a second peak in women over age 50. Sarcoidosis disproportionately affects African–Americans and Northern Europeans [4].

Utility of Imaging in Diagnosis and Management

The chest radiograph is frequently obtained early in the work-up of patients presenting with pulmonary or systemic symptoms and is often the first diagnostic modality to suggest the diagnosis of sarcoidosis. An established staging system based on radiographic findings exists, though these patterns do not necessarily correlate with chronology of disease [2]. There are five radiographic stages: stage 0 (normal chest radiograph), stage 1 (hilar or mediastinal lymphadenopathy without visible parenchymal involvement) (Fig. 15.1), stage 2 (hilar or mediastinal lymphadenopathy with visible parenchymal involvement) (Fig. 15.2), stage 3 (parenchymal involvement without lymphadenopathy) (Fig. 15.3), and stage 4 (Fig. 15.4) (irreversible/end-stage fibrosis). When lung abnormalities are present radiographically, they often manifest as bilateral, symmetric, upper-lobe predominant linear, nodular, or reticulonodular opacities.

While the majority of patients with sarcoidosis have abnormalities on chest radiograph at the time of diagnosis, up to 10% may have no radiographic findings [5]. It has been suggested that in the correct clinical setting, further evaluation with CT imaging is unnecessary unless

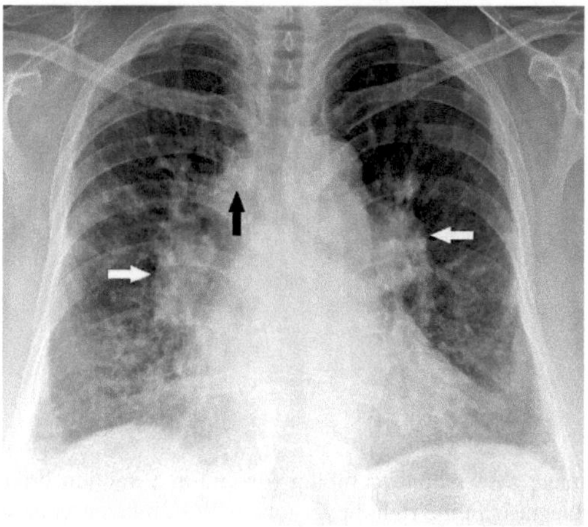

Fig. 15.2 *Stage* 2 sarcoidosis. PA radiograph shows bilateral hilar (*white arrows*) and right paratracheal (*black arrow*) lymphadenopathy and diffuse nodular and linear opacities in the lungs

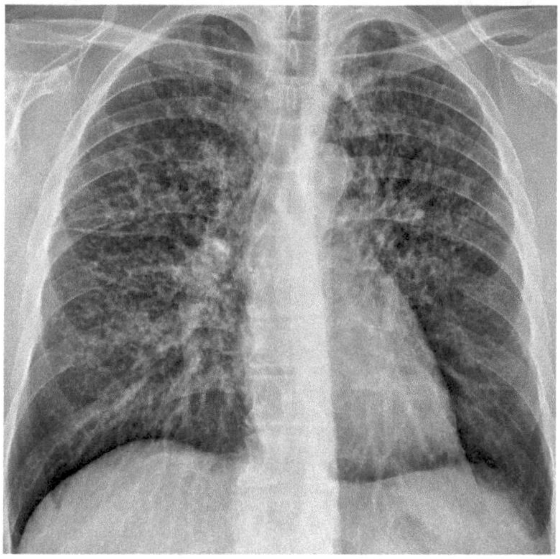

Fig. 15.3 *Stage* 3 sarcoidosis. PA radiograph shows diffuse linear and nodular opacities in both lungs without apparent lymphadenopathy

the radiographic appearance is unusual for sarcoidosis or if the patient presents with hemoptysis [2]. Additionally, chest CT may be useful with a normal chest radiograph but high clinical suspicion for sarcoidosis [5]. It has been estimated that 80–90% of patients with stage I disease radiographically have lung lesions visible on CT or present pm transbronchial biopsy [6]. CT is also of utility in detecting specific complications of sarcoidosis, such as superimposed infection, aspergilloma, bronchiectasis, pulmonary fibrosis, or malignancy [3, 5]. However, CT of the chest has also been described in the literature as a "standard investigation" to further assess extent of pulmonary involvement, increase diagnostic confidence, and identify potential sites for biopsy [1]. Nevertheless, because treatment of pulmonary sarcoidosis is most often guided by results of pulmonary function tests, in the absence of a specific clinical question, further evaluation of the chest with CT provides limited additional clinical utility and exposes the patient to unnecessary ionizing radiation.

Sarcoidosis has myriad potential presentations within the lungs and mediastinum on chest CT. As on radiographs, hilar and mediastinal lymph node enlargement is common. Although the classic radiographic appearance of sarcoidosis includes bilateral hilar lymphadenopathy, right paratracheal and aortopulmonary window lymph node enlargement are more frequently seen on CT. Lymph nodes may calcify in up to 50% of patients. Early in the disease process, faint central calcification may be present, manifesting as increased attenuation centrally within the lymph nodes (Fig. 15.5). With more chronic disease, coarse peripheral, so-called eggshell pattern, calcification may be present (Fig. 15.6).

In active sarcoidosis, granulomas can present as small, irregular nodules in a perilymphatic distribution on CT and are found in close association with the bronchovascular bundles, subpleural interstitial space, and interlobar fissures (Fig. 15.7). A centrilobular distribution in a patchy, upper-lobe predominant pattern is common. Granulomas may coalesce to form massive, ill-defined conglomerate airspace consolidation, sometimes with air-bronchograms (Fig. 15.8). The CT finding of smaller nodules at the periphery of a larger coalescent mass has been termed the "galaxy" sign (Fig. 15.9) and can be seen in sarcoidosis, but can occur in the setting of other granulomatous inflammatory processes or neoplasms. Patchy areas of ground-glass opacity may also be evident, likely reflecting tiny granuloma.

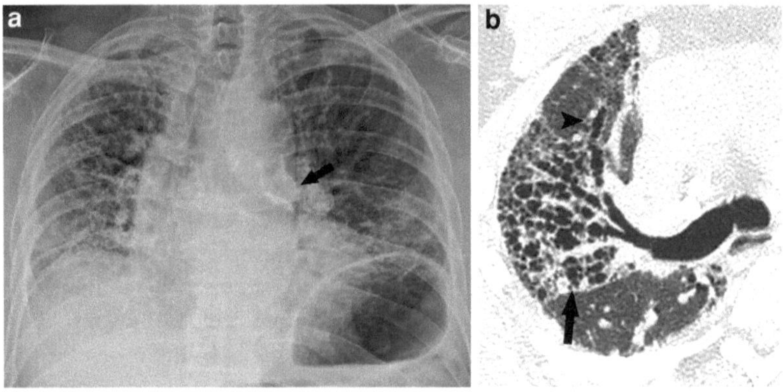

Fig. 15.4 *Stage* 4 sarcoidosis. **a** PA radiograph shows pulmonary fibrosis characterized by architectural distortion and reticulation. A peripheral calcified enlarged left mediastinal lymph node (*arrow*) is present. **b** HRCT image shows honeycombing (*arrow*) and traction bronchiectasis in the right upper lobe with significant volume loss

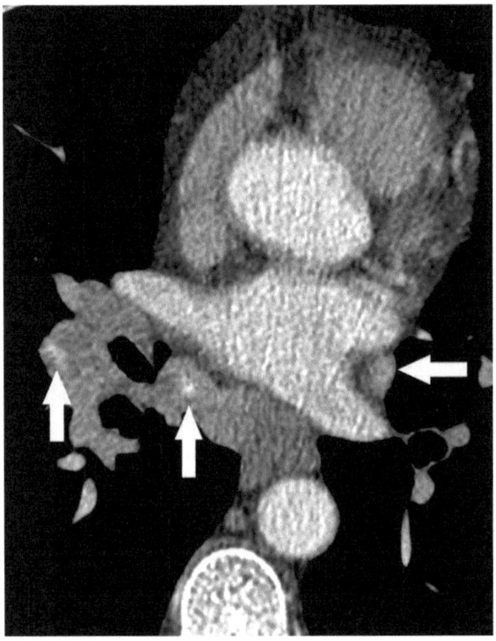

Fig. 15.5 Sarcoidosis and lymphadenopathy. Contrast-enhanced CT image shows bilateral hilar and subcarinal lymphadenopathy with faint central calcification (*arrows*). This appearance is highly suggestive of sarcoidosis but can be seen with other granulomatous processes such as fungal infection

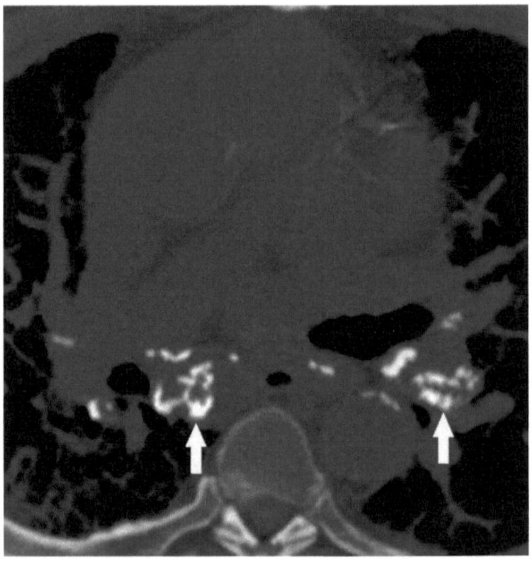

Fig. 15.6 Sarcoidosis and lymphadenopathy. Unenhanced CT image shows lymphadenopathy with coarse peripheral calcification (*arrows*), referred to as "egg shell" calcification. Lymph node calcification in silicosis and coal workers' pneumoconiosis can have a similar appearance

Chronic sarcoidosis may progress to fibrosis, which initially manifests as reticular opacities in a patchy, upper lobe predominant distribution. Peribronchial fibrosis is seen as perihilar masses with upward displacement of the hila and posterior displacement of the upper lobe and main bronchi. The findings of conglomerate fibrosis are similar in appearance to progressive massive fibrosis associated with silicosis, coal workers' pneumoconiosis, and talcosis. Associated architectural distortion is often present. Emphysema, bullae, peribronchovascular bundle thickening, and traction bronchiectasis may also be seen.

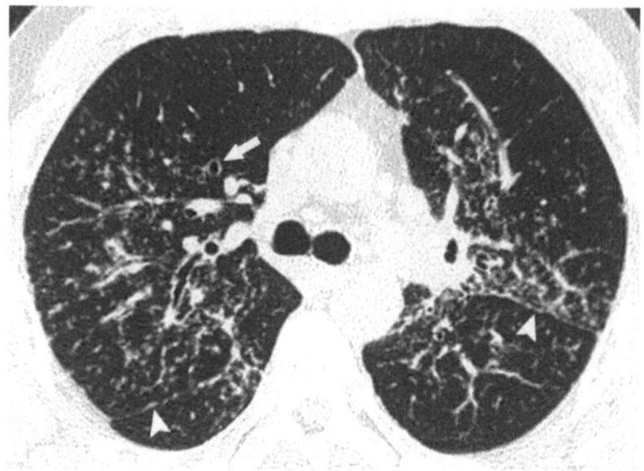

Fig. 15.7 Sarcoidosis. HRCT image shows numerous tiny irregular nodules in a perilymphatic distribution, which includes peribronchovascular, subpleural, and centrilobular regions. Perilymphatic nodules often can be best appreciated along the pulmonary fissures (*arrowheads*). This distribution of nodules is highly suggestive of sarcoidosis

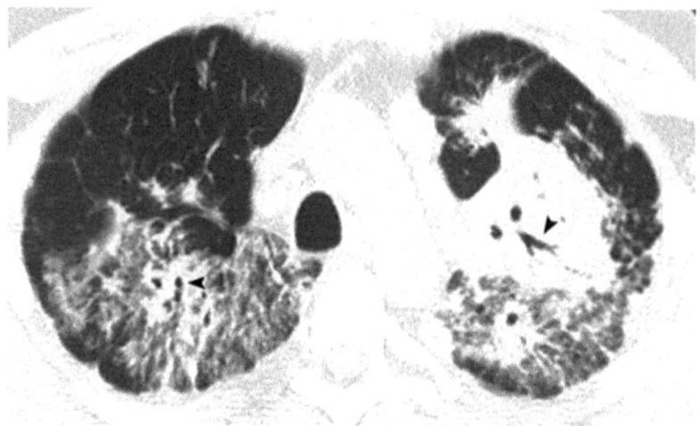

Fig. 15.8 Sarcoidosis with conglomerate fibrosis. HRCT image shows bilateral upper lobe peribronchial consolidation with air bronchograms (*arrowheads*) with associated architectural distortion. Conglomerate fibrosis in sarcoidosis can have a similar appearance to progressive massive fibrosis associated with silicosis, coal workers' pneumoconiosis, and talcosis

Honeycombing is an unusual imaging finding and tends to have mid- and upper-lung zone predominance and may involve the central, peribronchovascular lung. Development of an intracavitary aspergilloma (Fig. 15.10) is not uncommon in end-stage disease.

Sarcoidosis may involve the airways (Fig. 15.11), demonstrated on CT by bronchial or bronchiolar nodular wall thickening or stenosis or both. Endobronchial nodules may be present. Pleural involvement manifests as pleural effusions and pleural thickening. CT of the chest may also reveal cardiomegaly, which may suggest cardiomyopathy or other cardiac involvement. Likewise, enlargement of the central pulmonary arteries, most often in the setting of fibrosis, can reflect pulmonary hypertension, but is not specific. Echocardiography and right heart catheterization are more sensitive than CT for the detection of pulmonary hypertension.

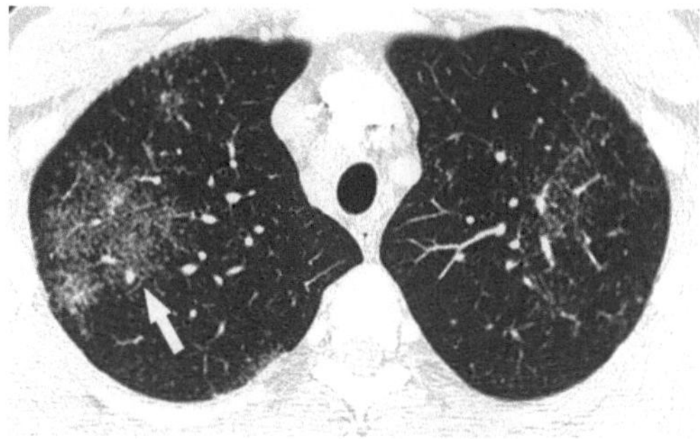

Fig. 15.9 Sarcoidosis with the galaxy sign. HRCT image shows bilateral tiny nodules around the bronchovascular bundles and subpleural lung. Nodules have coalesced (*arrow*) in the right upper lobe, a finding referred to as the "galaxy sign."

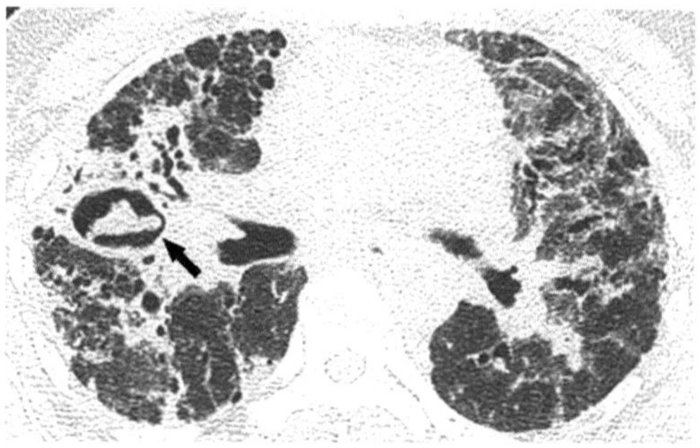

Fig. 15.10 End-stage sarcoidosis with aspergilloma. HRCT image shows extensive peribronchial fibrosis in the upper lobes associated with bronchovascular bundle thickening and traction bronchiectasis. The soft tissue mass (*arrow*) in the right upper lobe cavity is typical of an aspergilloma

Nuclear medicine imaging, particularly with gallium, can be used to detect nonspecific sites of inflammation throughout the body. The "lambda sign" (positive uptake in bilateral hilar and right paratracheal lymph nodes) and the "panda sign" (positive uptake in the bilateral salivary glands) are suggestive of sarcoidosis [3]. FDG-PET may

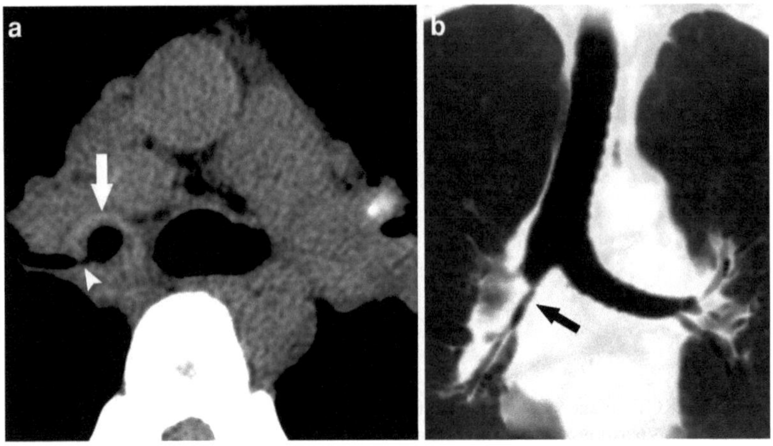

Fig. 15.11 Sarcoidosis with airway involvement. **a** Unehanced CT image shows circumferential thickening (*arrow*) of the right main bronchus with luminal stenosis. The orifice of the right upper lobe bronchus (*arrowhead*) is quite stenotic. **b** Coronal minimum intensity projection shows high-grade stenosis of the bronchus intermedius (*arrow*). Courtesy of Arlene Sirajuddin, M.D. (Chicago, IL)

be useful for determining extent of organ involvement and determining potential radiographically occult biopsy sites, if diagnosis is uncertain based on clinical findings and prior imaging [2, 3]. MRI is useful for determining presence and extent of cardiac or central nervous system involvement.

Common Variable Immunodeficiency

Clinical Presentation

Primary immunodeficiencies are diseases defined by genetic defects that primarily affect the immune system. CVID is characterized by hypogammaglobulinemia and is the most common primary immunodeficiency encountered in clinical practice [7]. Levels of IgA, IgG, or IgM are at least two standard deviations below mean for age and are associated with defective antibody response to protein and polysaccharide antigens [8]. Patients with CVID are prone to developing autoimmune diseases, including idiopathic thrombocytopenia purpura, vasculitis, seronegative spondyloarthropathies, pernicious anemia, systemic lupus erythematosus, and anti-IgA IgG antibodies [9]. Antibody-related defects in CVID predispose patients to infection, and it is recurrent sinopulmonary infections that most commonly suggest the diagnosis [7]. The infectious agents most frequently associated with both upper and lower respiratory tract infections include encapsulated organisms (e.g., *H. influenzae, S. pneumoniae)*, atypical bacteria (e.g., *Mycoplasma* spp.), and *Pseudomonas* [7, 9]. Systemic infection (e.g., viral hepatitis, herpes zoster) and gastrointestinal complications (e.g., giardiasis) are also common. Chronic pulmonary complications have been described as the primary cause of morbidity in patients with CVID [7]. Specifically, morbidity in patients with CVID is most often due to acute-on-chronic respiratory infections resulting in respiratory failure [10]. In addition to complications of recurrent pneumonia, many patients with CVID develop obstructive lung disease, such as chronic bronchitis and asthma. Restrictive lung disease evidenced by pulmonary function testing has been found to correlate with evidence of fibrosis on chest CT in CVID patients [9].

CVID can also manifest as systemic granulomatous disease characterized histologically by noncaseating granulomas, resembling sarcoidosis. Granulomatous disease may occasionally be the initial presentation of CVID, which may delay its diagnosis [7]. Recent evidence suggests that

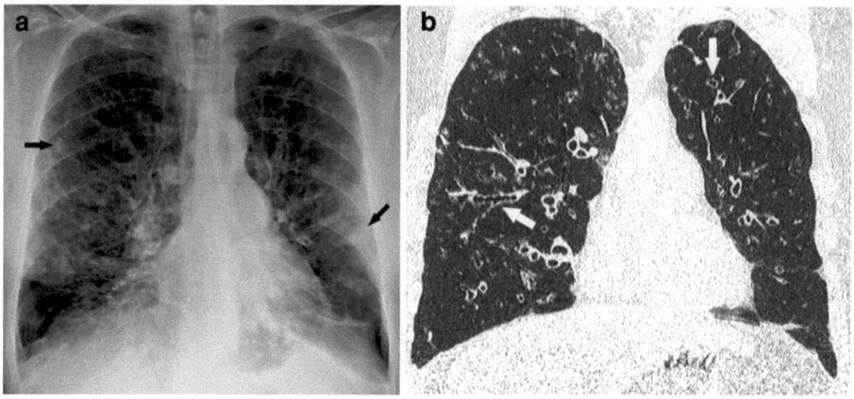

Fig. 15.12 Common variable immunodeficiency. **a** PA radiograph shows pulmonary hyperinflation with bronchial wall thickening and scattered linear and nodular (*arrows*) opacities. **b** Coronal reformation from HRCT shows diffuse bronchial wall thickening and bronchiectasis (*arrows*), accounting for the linear opacities on the chest radiograph. Small nodules are scattered throughout both lungs

human herpesvirus-8 (HHV-8) may be a cause of systemic granulomatous disease and lymphoproliferative disorders in some patients with CVID [7]. Patients with CVID are also at risk of both hematological and solid-organ malignancies, especially non-Hodgkin lymphoma and gastric cancer [7]. Development of mucosa-associated lymphoid tissue (MALT) lymphoma has also been described in CVID patients [9].

Because of the heterogeneity in clinical presentation of CVID, an average diagnostic delay of 5.5 years from time of initial symptoms has been reported in adults and 2.5 years in children [10]. There is a bimodal distribution of age of presentation of CVID, with an initial peak in mid-childhood and a second, larger peak in early to mid-adulthood, when most patients present.

Utility of Imaging in Diagnosis and Management

Chest radiograph findings are nonspecific and most commonly include bronchial wall thickening, bronchiectasis, linear opacities, and reticulation with a middle and lower lung zone predominance (Fig. 15.12). Small nodules can also be seen without a zonal predominance [11]. Historically, CT findings in CVID have included bronchiectasis and features of lymphoid hyperplasia, lymphoid interstitial pneumonia (LIP), granulomatous disease, and organizing pneumonia. Though CT findings of pulmonary disease in CVID are varied, Tanaka et al. identified three predominant CT patterns in a review of cases: airway disease, nodules, and parenchymal opacification. The predominant findings in the airways disease group most commonly seen were bronchiectasis and centrilobular nodules, the latter indicative of small airways disease. This pattern is thought to be a consequence of repeated infections. Bronchiectasis is best demonstrated by CT, and some groups have advocated HRCT for all CVID patients at the time of diagnosis to establish baseline lung disease, with repeat CT every 12–24 months, depending on pulmonary symptoms to assess disease progression [9]. It has been shown that bronchiectasis most commonly occurs in the middle and lower lobes and lingula, presumably reflecting gravity-facilitated mucociliary clearance in the upper lobes [8].

Patchy ground-glass opacities without zonal predominance are also described (Fig. 15.13). In the group with the CT pattern of nodules (Fig. 15.14), nodules were found to be peribronchial or random. Histologically, one case of each of these patterns correlated with non-caseating granulomas and mixed organizing pneumonia and lymphoid interstitial pneumonia (LIP), respectively. Thus, a primarily nodular

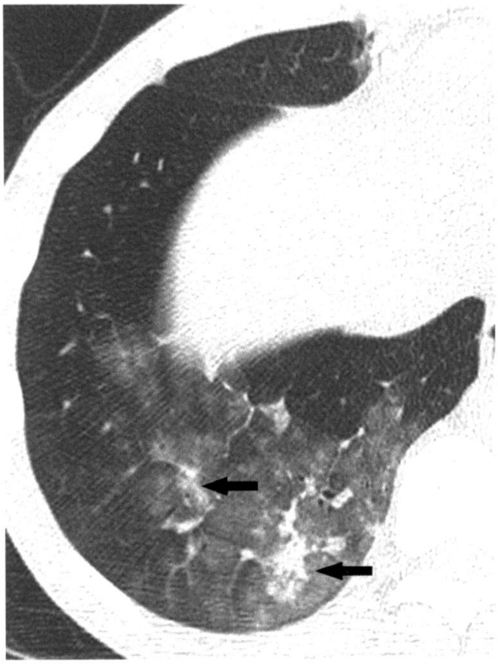

Fig. 15.13 Common variable immunodeficiency. HRCT image of the right lung shows patchy ground-glass opacity with a few foci of consolidation (*arrows*) in the right lower lobe

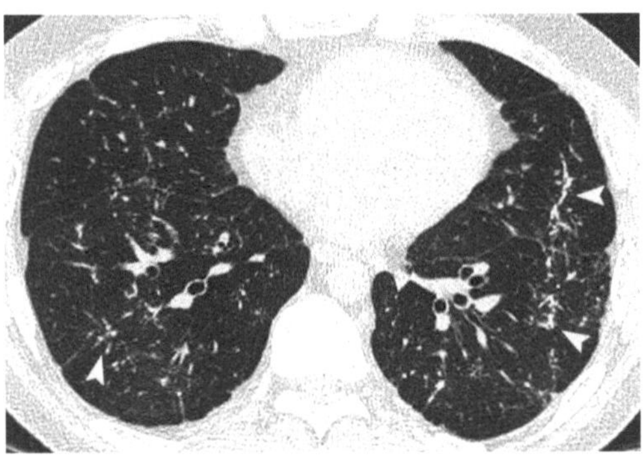

Fig. 15.14 Common variable immunodeficiency. HRCT image shows multiple calcified and noncalcified nodules (*arrowheads*) clustered in both lungs, presumably reflecting noncaseating granulomata

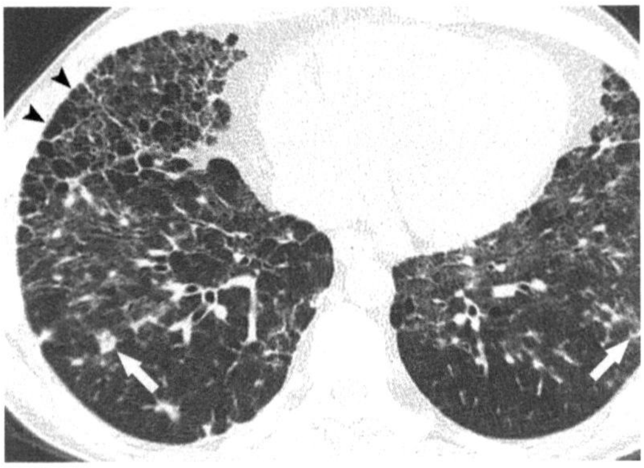

Fig. 15.15 Common variable immunodeficiency. HRCT image shows bilateral irregular nodules (*arrows*), mild bronchial wall thickening, and peripheral honeycombing (*arrowheads*). End-stage fibrosis is typically the result of recurrent pulmonary infections and chronic inflammation

pattern may be consistent with granulomatous disease, lymphoproliferative disease, or both. In the parenchymal opacification group (Fig. 15.15), predominant findings included middle and lower lung zone ground-glass opacities, reticulation, and centrilobular nodules. Histological samples from this group showed organizing pneumonia, LIP, and non-necrotizing granulomas. Recurrent pulmonary infections and chronic inflammation can lead to end-stage fibrosis, often manifesting as peripheral honeycombing.

An entity known as granulomatous-lymphocytic interstitial lung disease (GLILD) is characterized by a combination of granulomatous and lymphoproliferative processes (LIP, follicular bronchiolitis, and lymphoid hyperplasia) has been described in association with CVID [9, 12]. GLILD is defined histopathologically and characterized by a spectrum of findings that include follicular hyperplasia, reactive lymphoid hyperplasia, LIP, and granulomatous inflammation [12]. It has been reported that CVID patients with GLILD have worse prognosis and decreased median survival, likely related to increased prevalence of lymphoproliferative disorders and autoimmune disease [12]. As is the case with lymphoproliferative disorders in general with CVID, HHV-8 has been found in the majority of patients with CVID and GLILD [12]. HRCT has been shown to be useful in monitoring progression of pulmonary disease in CVID patients receiving intravenous immunoglobulin (IVIg) in the absence of clinical symptoms or changes in pulmonary function testing [9].

X-Linked Agammaglobulinemia

Clinical Presentation

As described above, primary immunodeficiencies are a clinically and genetically heterogeneous group of over 150 disorders characterized by abnormalities affecting the innate and adaptive immune systems [13]. These diseases often manifest clinically as recurrent pulmonary infections, with the offending organism predicated on the deficient arm of the immune system. X-linked agammaglobulinemia (XLA) is characterized by deficiency in all immunoglobulin subclasses and circulating B cells. This defect predisposes XLA patients to recurrent infections with encapsulated bacteria as well as *Mycoplasma* [8]. Sinopulmonary infections often begin to develop after 6 months of age, after titers of circulating maternal IgG wane. As is the case with patients with CVID, there is often a considerable delay between onset of symptoms and establishment of a diagnosis of XLA.

Utility of Imaging in Diagnosis and Management

As would be expected with any other patient initially presenting with nonspecific pulmonary symptoms, the chest radiograph is often the first imaging examination obtained in patients with pulmonary manifestations of XLA. The most common chest radiographic findings of recurrent pulmonary infection include interstitial fibrosis, bronchiectasis, and pleural thickening [14]. Patients with milder disease evident only on HRCT may have normal chest radiographs. On CT, bronchiectasis has been shown to be widespread or lower lobe predominant [14]. Bronchiectasis is less common compared to patients with CVID, likely related to early age of onset of symptoms and earlier diagnosis in patients with XLA as well as the autoimmunity and immune dysregulation occurring in CVID [15]. Additionally, parenchymal scarring is not an uncommon finding on chest CT of patients with XLA. Other less reproducible findings on CT include nonspecific ground-glass opacities, pleural thickening, emphysema, bullae, atelectasis, and small parenchymal nodules [14]. Findings on CT have not consistently been shown to correlate with PFTs. Kailunainen et al. advocate for routine CT scanning of patients with primary agammaglobulinemia given CT's superior sensitivity over radiography in determining the presence and extent of pulmonary disease. Additionally, CT is useful in monitoring effects of treatment for patients with primary immunodeficiencies, especially given the well-documented phenomenon of clinically silent progression of pulmonary disease in this patient population receiving IVIg.

X-Linked Lymphoproliferative Syndrome

Clinical Presentation

X-linked lymphoproliferative disease (XLP) is an inherited immunodeficiency characterized by the clinical triad of susceptibility to Epstein–Barr virus (EBV) infection manifesting as fulminant infectious mononucleosis, dysgammaglobulinemia, and lymphoma [16]. XLP disproportionately affects males, and patients typically present at ages 2–5 years old after infection with EBV, after which T- and B-cell lymphoproliferation and hemophagocytic lymphohistiocytosis (HLH) develop. Less common clinical features include aplastic anemia, lymphoid vasculitis, lymphomatoid granulomatosis, and autoimmune manifestations including psoriasis and colitis [16]. However, it should be noted that XLP can manifest in the absence of prior EBV exposure [17].

Abnormal humoral immune response is characteristic of XLP and is more common in patients with prior EBV exposure. As such, recurrent sinopulmonary infections are common

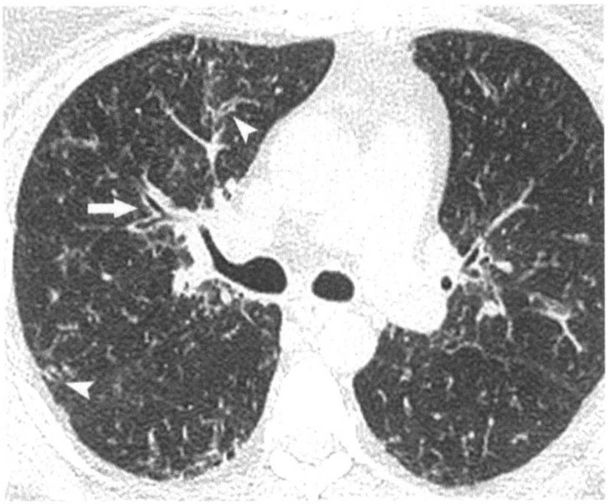

Fig. 15.16 Follicular bronchiolitis associated with rheumatoid arthritis. HRCT image shows scattered tiny irregular nodules in both lungs. The central bronchial walls are mildly thickened (*arrow*), and there is mild bronchiectasis (*arrowheads*)

initial presentations of this entity. Gastrointestinal, cutaneous, and systemic manifestations are also possible, but less common initial presentations. Approximately one-third of patients with XLP will initially present with lymphoma [16]. In XLP, lymphoma often arises as a result of malignant transformation of EBV-infected B cells. Half of these cases are Burkitt lymphoma. The remainder is most often a diverse histological spectrum of B-cell origin.

XLP should be suspected clinically with any male patient presenting with severe EBV infection, a male child with HLH in childhood or adolescence, or a male patient with hypogammaglobulinemia. Clinical suspicion is increased with a family history of maternally related males with similar clinical history.

Utility of Imaging in Diagnosis and Management

XLP is generally diagnosed with molecular diagnostics and genetic analysis. The role of imaging in the diagnosis of XLP has not been extensively studied. Radiographs and CT would be expected to identify sequela of recurrent pulmonary infections, including bronchiectasis. Additionally, CT is sensitive to the detection of lymphoma in the chest as well as pulmonary lymphomatoid granulomatosis.

Low Grade Lymphoproliferative Disorders

Follicular Bronchiolitis

Clinical Presentation

Follicular bronchiolitis is lymphoid hyperplasia of bronchus-associated lymphoid tissue [18]. It is characterized histologically by lymphoid follicles with reactive germinal centers in a peribronchial and peribronchiolar distribution [19]. Lymphoid hyperplasia may be found in isolation or may be found in association with bronchiectasis, chronic bronchitis, asthma, or other conditions. Follicular bronchiolitis occurs in three clinical settings: collagen vascular disease (especially rheumatoid arthritis and Sjögren syndrome), congenital or acquired immunodeficiency (e.g., CVID or AIDS), or is idiopathic. The idiopathic variant of follicular bronchiolitis tends to occur in middle-aged or older patients. Follicular bronchiolitis may be associated with hypersensitivity reactions to an unspecified, yet to be determined, antigen [18].

Follicular bronchiolitis may manifest clinically with pulmonary symptoms including cough, dyspnea, and recurrent pneumonia or with constitutional symptoms, including fever, fatigue, and weight loss. Results of PFTs are nonspecific and may be normal or show restrictive, obstructive, or mixed patterns. Serum rheumatoid factor may be positive in patients with collagen vascular disease. Hypo- or hypergammaglobulinemia may be present in patients with immunodeficiencies.

Utility of Imaging in Diagnosis and Management

Radiographs of patients with follicular bronchiolitis may show a nonspecific reticular or reticulonodular pattern [6]. Lymphoid hyperplasia

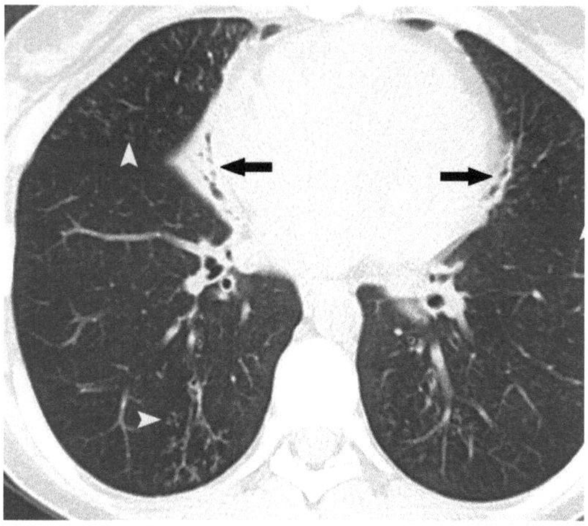

Fig. 15.17 Follicular bronchiolitis associated with rheumatoid arthritis. CT image shows tree-in-bud opacities (*arrowheads*) and right middle lobe and lingular bronchiectasis (*arrows*). This appearance can also be seen as infectious bronchiolitis

and enlarged lymphoid follicles manifest on CT as bilateral centrilobular nodules, often less than 3 mm, but can measure up to 12 mm, with or without tree-in-bud pattern [19] (Fig. 15.16). There is variable association of small peribronchial nodules and areas of ground-glass opacity. Less common CT manifestations of follicular bronchiolitis include bronchial wall thickening, bronchiectasis (Fig. 15.17), interlobular septal thickening, and peribronchovascular consolidation [18].

Lymphoid Interstitial Pneumonia

Clinical Presentation

Lymphoid interstitial pneumonia (LIP) is a benign lymphoproliferative disorder defined by proliferation of polyclonal lymphocytes and plasma cells within the pulmonary interstitium. Histologically, LIP is characterized by polymorphous inflammatory interstitial infiltrate that diffusely expands alveolar septa [19]. The inflammatory infiltrate consists of lymphocytes, histiocytes, and plasma cells. Together with follicular bronchiolitis, LIP is considered part of the histological spectrum of pulmonary lymphoid hyperplasia, and the two entities may be difficult to distinguish histologically. Additionally, there is considerable overlap in the histologic appearance of LIP and cellular nonspecific interstitial pneumonia (NSIP). This distinction is made based on the more extensive infiltrate with distortion and expansion of the alveolar framework seen with LIP [19].

LIP is often associated with underlying collagen vascular (most commonly Sjögren syndrome, rheumatoid arthritis, or systemic lupus erythematosus) or immunodeficiency disease (most commonly AIDS or CVID). Importantly, LIP is an AIDS-defining illness if found in a child less than 13 years old with underlying HIV infection [19]. LIP is also associated with allogeneic bone marrow transplantation and drug reaction [19]. The clinical manifestation of LIP in these patients is usually related to the underlying disease process. An idiopathic LIP syndrome exists, most often presenting in middle age (40–50 years). Cough and dyspnea are common symptoms, which may be progressive, particularly if left untreated.

Utility of Imaging in Diagnosis and Management

The radiographic appearance of LIP is variable and nonspecific, most commonly including lower lung-zone predominant reticular or reticulonodular opacities. A nodular pattern or lung consolidation is a less common appearance [6]. HRCT findings of LIP include bilateral ground-glass opacities (Fig. 15.18), poorly defined centrilobular nodules, thickening of bronchovascular bundles, and interlobular septal thickening [18]. Ground-glass opacities and consolidation are more common in patients with immunodeficiency and reflect alveolar infiltration [6]. Poorly defined centrilobular nodules (Fig. 15.19) are more common in the presence of collagen vascular disease and AIDS and are reflective of lymphocytic infiltration involving

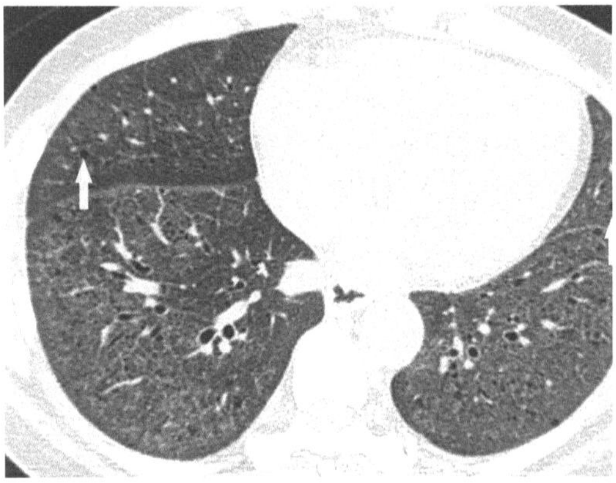

Fig. 15.18 Lymphoid interstitial pneumonia associated with undefined connective tissue disease. HRCT image shows diffuse ground-glass opacity with scattered reticular opacities and thin-walled cysts (*arrows*)

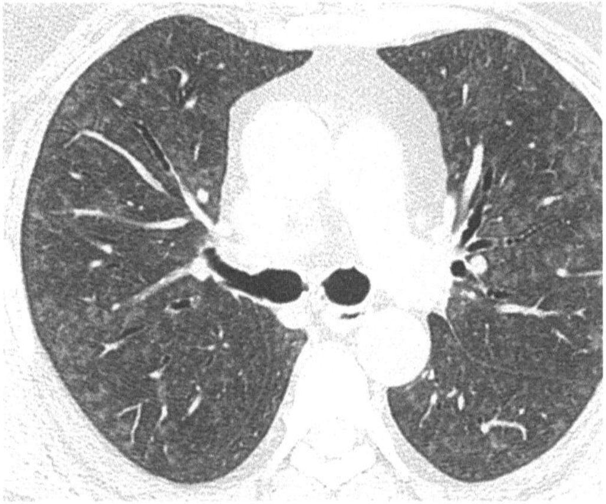

Fig. 15.19 Lymphoid interstitial pneumonia associated with Sjögren syndrome. HRCT image shows diffuse ground-glass attenuation nodules located primarily in a centrilobular distribution. Courtesy of Arlene Sirajuddin, M.D. (Chicago, IL)

bronchioles [6]. Small, well-defined perilymphatic nodules with or without septal thickening reflect interstitial infiltration, most commonly seen with underlying AIDS. Few, scattered or diffuse thin-walled cysts (Fig. 15.20) are also commonly seen, particularly with Sjögren syndrome and collagen vascular disease. These are thought to arise secondary to over-distended airspaces distal to bronchioles from partial obstruction by lymphocytic infiltrate [18]. Progressive fibrosis is associated with increased mortality. Development of low-grade B-cell lymphoma has been described as a rare complication.

LIP is often associated with restrictive pattern on PFTs and reduced DLCO. Serum dysproteinemia consisting of polyclonal hypergammaglobulinemia is present in 75–80% of patients with LIP [6, 19].

Castleman Disease

Clinical Findings

Castleman disease (CD) was originally described in 1956 in a case series of several patients presenting with localized mediastinal lymph node hyperplasia [20]. CD has also been called angiofollicular mediastinal lymph node hyperplasia, angiomatous lymphoid hamartoma, and giant mediastinal lymph node hyperplasia. Two histologic variants exist: hyaline-vascular type and plasma-cell type. CD is also described clinically as localized or multicentric.

Hyaline-vascular type CD is usually localized, affecting a single lymph node or localized group of nodes [20]. This type accounts for up to 70% of cases of CD without sex predilection [21]. The hyaline-vascular type often manifests as an isolated mediastinal mass in asymptomatic young adults. Chains of lymph nodes may also be involved and other possible sites of involvement include cervical, axillary, and abdominal lymph nodes [21]. Histologically, hyaline-vascular CD is characterized by follicular hyperplasia, lymphocytes forming concentric rings around hypervascular, atrophic germinal centers. Vascular proliferation between follicles and penetrating through germinal centers with perivascular hyalinization is common [20, 22]. The pathogenesis is unknown, but follicular dendritic cell abnormalities and vascular endothelial growth factor (VEGF) have been suggested as contributing factors. Complete cure after surgical resection is typical.

Plasma-cell type is most often multicentric, but may represent up to almost 25% of localized

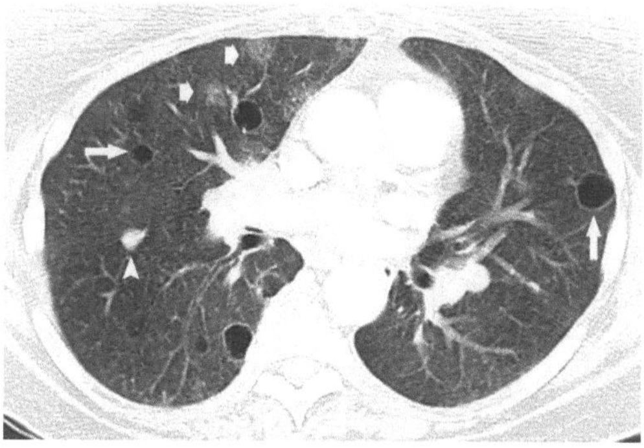

Fig. 15.20 Lymphoid interstitial pneumonia associated with Sjögren syndrome. CT image shows diffuse ground-glass opacity with bilateral thin-walled cysts (*thin arrows*) and ground-glass attenuation nodules in the right lung (*wide arrows*). The perifissural nodule (*arrowhead*) in the right lower lobe is most likely an enlarged intrapulmonary lymph node

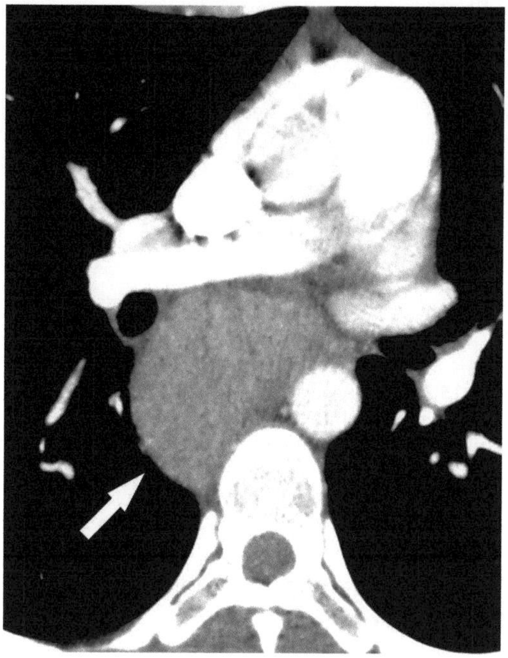

Fig. 15.21 Localized hyaline-vascular Castleman disease. Contrast-enhanced CT image shows a large, homogeneous mediastinal mass (*arrow*) with relatively high attenuation. Courtesy of Tan-Lucien Mohammed, M.D. (Cleveland, OH)

CD [20]. The localized type affects a similar demographic as hyaline-vascular type, while the multicentric form affects an older population, typically in the fifth or sixth decade. Both variants of plasma-cell type CD are commonly associated with fevers, night sweats, and malaise. Physical examination may reveal splenomegaly and generalized lymphadenopathy. Laboratory abnormalities include hypergammaglobulinemia, anemia, thrombocytopenia, elevated transaminases, hypoalbuminuria, and elevated erythrocyte sedimentation rate. Additionally, patients may present with marked edema, pleural effusions, and ascites [21]. Histologically, plasma-cell type is nonspecific and is characterized by sheets of plasma cells surrounding reactive germinal centers [22]. Both localized and multicentric plasma-cell type CD are associated with increased levels of interleukin-6 (IL-6). The localized form behaves similar to hyaline-vascular type, in that surgical excision is curative, while the multicentric form generally requires systemic therapy [20]. Both forms of plasma-cell type are associated with POEMS syndrome (polyneuropathy, organomegaly, endocrinopathy, monoclonal gammopathy, and skin changes).

A distinct variant of CD associated with HHV-8 infection has been described and typically affects immunosuppressed individuals, particularly those infected with HIV. This entity has been variably referred to as HHV-8-associated or plasmablastic multicentric CD. Patients with this type of CD experience similar constitutional symptoms, physical exam findings, and laboratory derangements as do patients with plasma-cell type. This entity can progress to HHV-8 associated plasmablastic lymphoma, a form of large B-cell lymphoma [20]. Additionally, this patient population is at risk for development of microlymphomas, KSHV-associated germinotropic lymphoproliferative disorder, and Kaposi sarcoma.

Finally, another category of exclusion known as multicentric CD, not otherwise specified exists. This entity presents most commonly in the sixth decade, but is otherwise similar in clinical presentation to plasma-cell type CD. However, multicentric CD not otherwise specified patients are at increased risk for development of non-Hodgkin lymphoma.

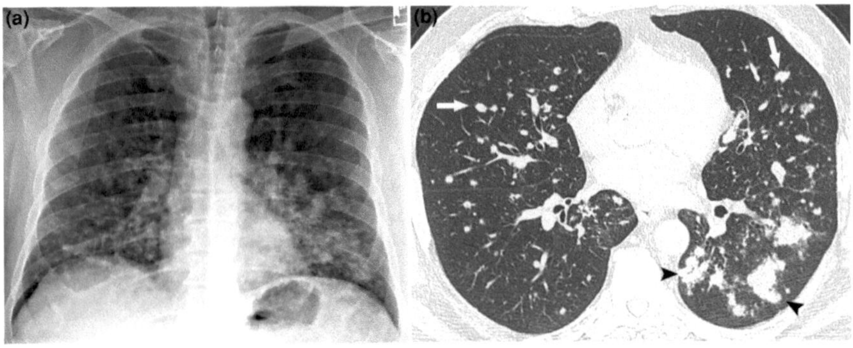

Fig. 15.22 Lymphomatoid granulomatosis. **a** PA chest radiograph shows bilateral mid and lower lung predominant irregular nodules. **b** HRCT image shows diffuse irregular nodules (*arrows*) of varying sizes with more focal mass-like peribronchial consolidation (*arrowheads*) in the left lower lobe

Utility of Imaging in Diagnosis and Management

CD may present as an incidentally detected, solitary mediastinal mass on chest radiography, especially in patients with hyaline-vascular type CD. Multicentric CD may also present as multifocal lymphadenopathy on chest radiograph. Contrast-enhanced CT typically shows early, dense enhancement of the mediastinal mass (Fig. 15.21) or involved lymph nodes. Lymph nodes may calcify. Multicentric CD may rarely involve the pulmonary parenchyma and manifests as poorly defined centrilobular nodules, thin-walled cysts, thickening of the peribronchovascular bundles, and interlobular septal thickening. These findings may be reflective of LIP [18].

Lymphomatoid Granulomatosis

Clinical Findings

Lymphomatoid granulomatosis (LYG) was first described in a case series by Liebow in 1972 as an entity with overlapping features of Wegener granulomatosis and lymphoma [23]. LYG has also been called angiocentric lymphoma and angiocentric immunoproliferative reaction [18]. LYG tends to occur in middle-aged adults, with 2:1 male to female predominance. Fever and cough are the most common presenting symptoms. Extrapulmonary findings most commonly occur in the skin and central nervous system, but the heart and kidneys may also be involved. Mortality is high, with most deaths occurring within the first 2 years.

Histologically, LYG is characterized by nodular mixed mononuclear cell infiltrate with prominent vascular invasion and areas of necrosis replacing lung parenchyma [23]. Epstein–Barr virus (EBV) infection is present in the majority of cases. Three histologic grades exist, depending on degree of cellular atypia and proportion of large B cells in the infiltrate [23]. Progression to histologically overt lymphoma in both lymph nodes and other lymphoreticular sites has been well-documented. It has been proposed that grades 2 and 3 LYG be classified as a large B-cell lymphoma. Grade 1 is rare and thought to likely represent poorly sampled or early lymphoma (grade 2 or 3 LYG) [23]. Immunophenotyping is required to distinguish LYG lymphoma from other types of lymphoma. Additionally, LYG should not be diagnosed in patients with history of solid organ transplantation or methotrexate use because of the considerable overlap histologically with post-transplant lymphoproliferative disease (PTLD) and iatrogenic immunodeficiency-associated lymphoproliferative disease [23].

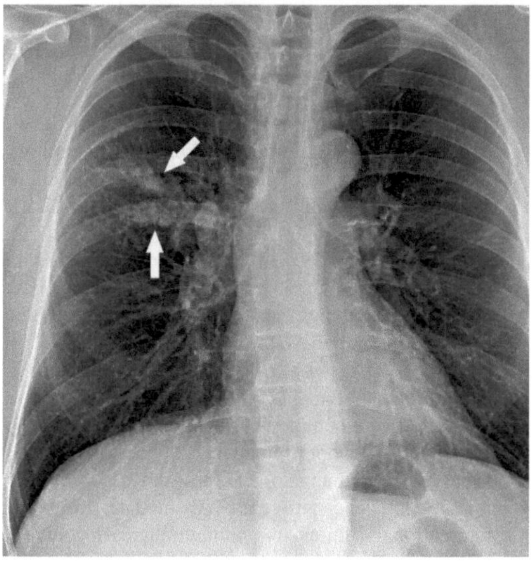

Fig. 15.23 Allergic bronchopulmonary aspergillosis. PA radiograph shows a branching tubular opacity (*arrows*) in the right upper lobe giving the "finger-in-glove" appearance. Courtesy of Jonathan Chung, M.D. (Denver, CO)

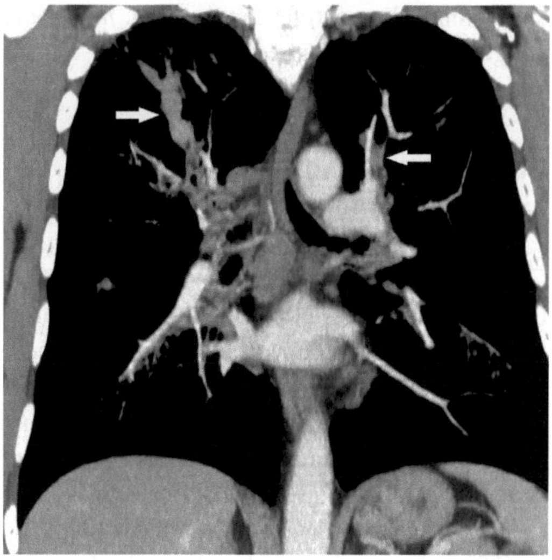

Fig. 15.24 Allergic bronchopulmonary aspergillosis. Coronal maximum intensity projection from contrast-enhanced CT shows high attenuation secretions (*arrows*) filling dilated upper lobe bronchi. This appearance is highly specific for ABPA

Utility of Imaging in Diagnosis and Management

Bilateral nodules or foci of consolidation (Fig. 15.22) are typically present on the chest radiograph at the time of presentation [23]. CT shows mid- and basal-predominant, poorly defined nodules in a peribronchovascular distribution that may progress rapidly and cavitate, simulating Wegener granulomatosis. Nodules may coalesce to form mass-like consolidation, which may contain air bronchograms [18]. Coarse irregular opacities, small thin-walled cysts, and pleural effusions have been described [18, 23].

Allergic Bronchopulmonary Aspergillosis

Clinical Presentation

Allergic bronchopulmonary aspergillosis (ABPA) is an allergic pulmonary disorder caused by hypersensitivity reaction to *Aspergillus fumigatus*. ABPA often presents in young adults with history of asthma or atopy and in up to 10% of patients with cystic fibrosis [6]. ABPA is an under-diagnosed condition associated with up to 10 years latency between onset of symptoms and diagnosis [24]. There is no sex predilection, and most patients present in the third or fourth decade of life. Common presenting signs and symptoms include cough, wheezing, fever, bronchial hyper-reactivity, and hemoptysis. Expectoration of black–brown mucous plugs is common.

The pathogenesis of ABPA is incompletely understood but is thought to occur from exposure to large concentrations of *A. fumigatus* spores in genetically susceptible individuals. Spores develop into hyphae, leading to impaired mucociliary clearance, compromise of the mucoepithelial barrier, and subsequent activation of the innate immunity of the lung. A cytokine and chemokine-mediated inflammatory cascade activates mast cells and eosinophils with resultant increased levels of circulating IgE and eosinophil-mediated damage of lung parenchyma and subsequent airway remodeling [24].

Supportive laboratory findings include serum antibodies specific to *A. fumigatus*, elevated circulating IgE, reactive skin test to *A. fumigatus* antigen, and peripheral eosinophilia.

Utility of Imaging in Diagnosis and Management

Characteristic radiographic findings of ABPA include patchy areas of consolidation and central bronchiectasis with upper lobe predominance. "Toothpaste and finger-in-glove" (Fig. 15.23) opacities resulting from mucoid secretions impacted within dilated airways are characteristic [24]. Lobar or segmental atelectasis may reflect bronchial obstruction by mucus plugs.

CT is more sensitive to detection of pulmonary complications of ABPA than radiography. Upper lobe predominant central bronchiectasis, mucous plugging, and bronchial wall thickening are common. Other common CT findings include centrilobular nodules with tree-in-bud opacities reflecting mucoid impaction of bronchioles, atelectasis, and areas of mosaic attenuation with air trapping on expiration [24]. The presence of high attenuation secretions in dilated bronchi (Fig. 15.24), a reflection of calcium oxalate deposition, is an appearance highly specific for ABPA [6].

References

1. Dempsey OJ, Paterson EW, Kerr KM, et al. Sarcoidosis. Brit Med J. 2009;339:620–5.
2. Iannuzzi MC, Rybicki BA, Teirstein AS. Sarcoidosis. N Engl J Med. 2007;357:2153–65.
3. Costabel U, Ohshimo S, Guzman J. Diagnosis of sarcoidosis. Curr Opin Pulm Med. 2008;14:455–61.
4. Judson MA. The diagnosis of sarcoidosis. Clin Chest Med. 2008;29:415–27.
5. Mihailovic-Vucinic V, Jovanovic D. Pulmonary sarcoidosis. Clin Chest Med. 2008;29:459–73.
6. Webb WR, Higgins CB. Thoracic imaging: pulmonary and cardiovascular radiology. 2nd ed. Lippincott: North American Edition; 2010.
7. Park MA, Li JT, Hagan JB, et al. Common variable immunodeficiency: a new look at an old disease. Lancet. 2008;372:489–509.
8. Notarangelo LD, Plebani A, Mazzolari E. Genetic causes of bronchiectasis: primary immune deficiencies and the lung. Respiration. 2007;74:264–75.
9. Busse PJ, Farzan S, Cunningham-Rundles C. Pulmonary complications of common variable immunodeficiency. Ann Allergy Asthma Immunol. 2007;98:1–9.
10. Thickett KM, Kumararantne DS, Banerjee AK, et al. Common variable immune deficiency: respiratory manifestations, pulmonary function and high-resolution CT scan findings. Q J Med. 2002;95: 655–62.
11. Tanaka N, Kim JS, Bates CA. Lung diseases in patients with common variable immunodeficiency: chest radiographic and computed tomographic findings. J Comput Assist Tomogr. 2006;30:28–838.
12. Torigian DA, LaRosa DF, Levinson AI. Granulomatous-lymphocytic interstitial lung disease associated with common variable immunodeficiency: CT findings. J Thorac Imaging. 2008;23:162–9.
13. Geha RS, Notarangelo LD, Casanova J. Primary immunodeficiency diseases. An update from the international union of immunological societies primary immunodeficiency diseases classification committee. J Allergy Clin Immunol. 2007;120: 776–94.
14. Kainulainen L, Varpula M, Liippo K. Pulmonary abnormalities in patients with primary hypogammaglobulinemia. J Allergy Clin Immunol. 1999;104:1031–6.
15. Aghamohammadi A, Allahverdi A, Abolhassani H, et al. Comparison of pulmonary diseases in common variable immunodeficiency and X-linked agammaglobulinaemia. Respirology. 2010;15:289–95.
16. Rezaei N, Mahmoudi E, Aghamohammadi A. X-linked lymphoproliferative syndrome: a genetic condition typified by the triad of infection, immunodeficiency and lymphoma. Brit J Haemotology. 2010;152:13–30.
17. Gilmour KC, Gaspar HB. Pathogenesis and diagnosis of X-linked lymphoproliferative disease. Expert Rev Mol Diagn. 2003;3(5):549–61.
18. Do KH, Lee JS, Seo JB, et al. Pulmonary parenchymal involvement of low-grade lympholiferative disorders. J Comput Assist Tomogr. 2005;29:825–30.
19. Guinnee DG Jr. Update on nonneoplastic pulmonary lymphoproliferative disorders and related entities. Arch Pathol Lab Med. 2010;134:691–701.
20. Cronin DMP, Warnke RA. Castleman Disease: an update on classification and the spectrum of associated lesions. Adv Anat Pathol. 2009;16: 236–46.
21. Dham A, Peterson BA. Castleman disease. Curr Opin Hematol. 2007;14:354–9.
22. Bragg DG, Chor PJ, Murray KA. Lymphoproliferative disorders of the lung: histopathology, clinical manifestations, and imaging features. Am J Radiol. 1994;163:273–81.
23. Katzenstein AA, Doxtader E, Narendra S. Lymphomatoid granulomatosis: insights gained over 4 decades. Am J Surg Pathol. 2010;34:e35–48.
24. Agarwal R. Allergic bronchopulmonary aspergillosis. Chest. 2009;135:805–26.

The Critically Ill Patient

16

Jie C. Nguyen and Jeffrey P. Kanne

Abstract

Various imaging examinations are used to monitor critically ill patients, including radiography, bedside ultrasound, and computed tomography. However, portable chest radiography is the most common imaging examination performed in the intensive care unit. The extracted imaging findings can improve or significantly alter clinical management. An understanding of the imaging appearances of various cardiopulmonary disease processes and the typical appearances and locations of life support devices is essential for early diagnosis and correction of iatrogenic complications.

Keywords

Critically ill · Intensive care · Radiography · Tubes · Lines · Balloon pump · Mediastinum · Cardiomegaly · Opacities · Pleural effusion · Septic emboli · Atelectasis

Imaging Modalities

Imaging plays a vital role in the care and management of the critically ill patient. Although the most commonly used imaging examination in the intensive care unit (ICU) is the portal chest radiograph, computed tomography (CT) and bedside ultrasound (US) are being used more frequently in order to confirm a suspected diagnosis or limit the differential diagnosis. Specifically, US can confirm and characterize the complexity of a fluid collection as well as assist in therapeutic interventions. The anatomic detail of CT is superior to that of radiography, allowing for better characterization of pleural and pulmonary disease.

Portable Radiography

The use of daily routine portable chest radiographs in the ICU has been favored because of

J. C. Nguyen (✉) · J. P. Kanne
Department of Radiology, University of Wisconsin School of Medicine and Public Health, 600 Highland Ave, MC 3252, Madison, WI 53792-3252, USA
e-mail: jnguyen@uwhealth.org

J. P. Kanne
e-mail: jkanne@uwhealth.org

J. P. Kanne (ed.), *Clinically Oriented Pulmonary Imaging*,
Respiratory Medicine, DOI: 10.1007/978-1-61779-542-8_16,

its relatively low cost and minimal risk to the patient and possibility of detecting a clinically unexpected abnormality [1–4]. However, this "overuse" mode of practice has been under increasing scrutiny after recent publication of prospective, larger scale studies failing to establish the efficacy of routine radiographs [5–11]. Specifically, these studies showed that "routine" chest radiographs did not significantly alter patient care or outcome when compared to radiographs obtained "on-demand" when a patient's clinical status worsened or did not improve as expected. Furthermore, on-demand radiographs are more likely to show an important abnormality. Hejblum et al. [10] analyzed results from ICUs at 21 different centers and showed no difference in the length of stay, duration of mechanical ventilation, need for diagnostic, therapeutic interventions, or mortality when comparing "routine" to "on-demand" chest radiographs. A meta-analysis of over 7,000 ICU patients also showed no statistically significant in the length of stay, ventilator days, or mortality [11]. In the current era of increased medical cost awareness, these authors argued that although daily routine radiographs are of relatively low cost, their overwhelming number still leads to significant unnecessary expenditure of health care dollars [7, 9].

Although portable radiographs have low specificity for cardiopulmonary diseases, they are an efficient mean for early detection of malpositioned support devices and procedural complications. Portable chest radiographs have a number of limitations resulting from both patient and technical factors. The inability to better position the patient or to control respiration can obscure a small pneumothorax or underestimate the size of a pleural effusion. Evaluation of the posterior costophrenic sulcus is nearly impossible on a single anteroposterior (AP) view, often because of relatively high positioning of the diaphragm and respiratory motion [12]. Additionally, radiographs provide limited information about subtle mediastinal and chest wall disease. Routine bedside AP radiographs magnify the cardiac silhouette as a result of its relative anterior location and thus further location from the cassette or detector plate. Wires of monitoring devices located outside of the patient can obscure the courses and locations of internal support devices. Although many of these limitations cannot be corrected, awareness of the specific clinical question can help the technologist better optimize the imaging environment and the radiologist better address the clinical question of interest. For example, sensitivity for detection of small pneumothoraces or mobile effusion can be improved with semi-upright or lateral decubitus views, respectively.

Computed Tomography

CT is often obtained in the setting of clinical deterioration or failure to respond to empirical treatment, as a method of problem solving [13–15]. Miller et al. [13] compared over 100 CT scans with recent bedside radiographs and showed that CT found new and clinically important findings in 30% of patients and resulted in management change in 22% of patients. With superior spatial resolution, CT is now considered the reference standard for diagnosis of pneumothorax, pleural effusion, lung consolidation, atelectasis, and other lung abnormalities [16]. For example, CT has near 100% sensitivity for detection of small pneumothoraces, especially those that are located anteriorly in a supine patient [17, 18]. Wall et al. [18] found 10 of 35 traumatic pneumothoraces to be clinically and radiographically occult, and, of these, 7 required chest tube drainage. Additionally, CT can detect small and medium pleural effusions and distinguish them from lung opacities. Kitazono et al. [19], in reviewing 100 surgical ICU patients, found small and medium pleural effusions were radiographically occult in 55% of patients and were misdiagnosed in 45% of patients, and pulmonary opacities were occult on 34% of radiographs. CT can also accurately characterize the distribution of lung abnormalities, narrowing the differential diagnosis. Finally, CT is superior to radiography for evaluating the mediastinum for cardiovascular pathology, mediastinitis, or lymphadenopathy.

Chest CT, in contrast to abdominal CT, usually does not require intravenous contrast, because of the intrinsic contrast between thoracic structures. Contrast is only required to evaluate the internal components of cardiovascular structures such as evaluation for pulmonary embolism or subtle aortic dissection.

Ultrasound

Although ICU imaging mainly relies on bedside chest radiography and CT, the use of portable US is increasing. Not only can US provide for quick, ionizing radiation-free diagnosis of pericardial and pleural effusions, but also it can guide therapeutic interventions. Whereas radiographs are often insensitive in distinguishing between small pleural effusion and lung consolidation, ultrasound is extremely sensitive in detecting pleural effusions and estimating their volumes [20]. In the case of pleural effusion of uncertain etiology and duration, US allows assessment for internal loculations and debris, which favor an exudative effusion, predict lower success rates for small-bore catheter drainage, and suggest better outcome from early surgical debridement [21]. Additionally, sonographically detectable hyperemia surrounding an air-fluid cavity on color Doppler ultrasound favors lung abscess over empyema [22]. Recent studies have shown an expanded role of bedside ultrasound for detecting peripheral lung consolidation, assessing for improved aeration, and, in the setting of trauma, detecting lung contusion and diaphragmatic perforation [23–27]. More challenging and newer applications include detection of pneumothorax and assistance in placement of a double-lumen endotracheal tube [28]. The use of ultrasound for cardiac assessment is well established and is beyond the scope of this chapter.

The main disadvantage of ultrasound is its operator dependency. Additionally, ultrasound of the chest is often limited to the superficial tissues, such as chest wall, pleura, and peripheral lung tissue, because sound waves are attenuated by normally aerated lung. The closely spaced ribs also limit the size of the acoustic window.

Magnet Resonance Imaging

The use of magnet resonance imaging (MRI) in the critical care setting is mostly limited to evaluation of neurological pathology, which is beyond the scope of this chapter. The need for various support and monitoring devices and the longer duration of MRI examinations make this technique more cumbersome and less desirable for the critically ill patient.

Monitoring and Support Devices

Endotracheal Tubes

The optimum endotracheal tube (ETT) position (Fig. 16.1) is subject to debate. Nevertheless, radiographic assessment is based on the tube's tip location relative to the carina and clavicles. Conrardy et al. [29] found that the ETT position is highly dependent on the patient's head position. Using these results, Goodman et al. [30] recommended the following guidelines for the assessment of ETT: if the neck is in neutral position, with the mandible projecting over C5–C6, the ETT tip should be 5 ± 2 cm from the carina; if the neck is flexed, with the mandible projecting over T1 or below, the ETT tip should be 3 ± 2 cm from the carina; if the neck is extended, with the mandible projecting over C3–C4, the ETT tip should be 7 ± 2 cm from the carina.

Malpositioning of the ETT can be clinically occult, especially when intubation occurs emergently [31–34]. For example, Gary et al. [32] reviewed 112 ICU intubations and found 22 clinically occult malpositioned tubes, all of which were discovered only on post-intubation chest radiograph. These studies proved that the "standard" clinical assessment, which includes auscultation for equal breath sounds, ballottement of the balloon in the suprasternal notch, and identification of 21 cm and 23 cm marking for average sized women and men, respectively, at the teeth or gum, can be inadequate [34]. To date,

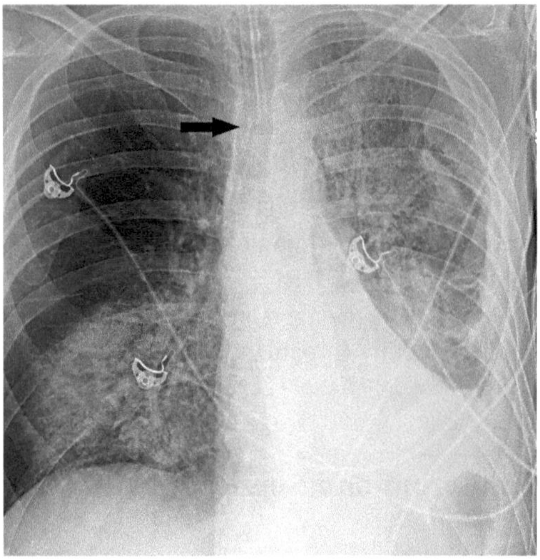

Fig. 16.1 Endotracheal tube. AP radiograph shows endotracheal tube tip (*arrow*) at the level of the thoracic inlet. The patient's head is in neutral position. Multifocal lung consolidation is from pneumonia, and there is a small, partially loculated left pleural effusion

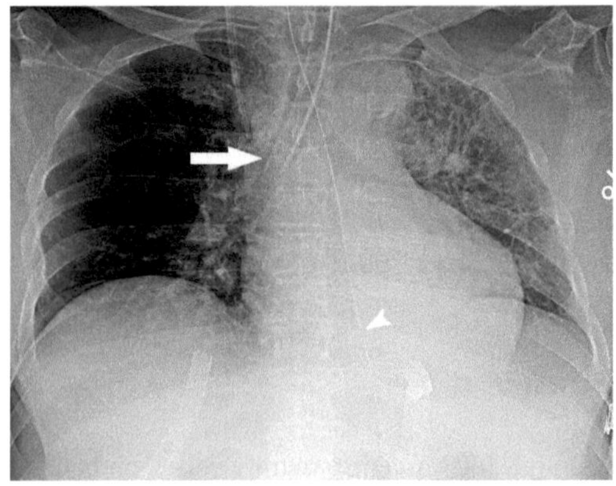

Fig. 16.2 Malpositioned endotracheal tube immediately following liver transplant. AP radiograph shows the tip (*arrow*) of the endotracheal tube in the right main bronchus. The nasogastric tube side port (*arrowhead*) is in the lower esophagus, and optimally should be advanced

chest radiography is recommended following intubation to confirm appropriate positioning. While in most institutions these studies are obtained urgently, Lotano et al. [35], in reviewing over 100 ICU intubations performed by experienced operators, argue that confirmatory radiographs do not need to be urgently obtained.

ETT placement that is too low is more common than placement that is too high and typically results in more immediate complications, particularly main bronchial intubation (Fig. 16.2). Main bronchial intubation occurs more frequently on the right because of the straighter and more vertically oriented course of the right main bronchus. ETTs placed too high can lead to inadvertent extubation or vocal cord injury.

Tracheostomy Tubes

Tracheostomy tube placement is becoming more common in the ICU setting and is used mainly for patients with respiratory failure requiring long-term airway maintenance. Routine post-tracheostomy chest radiography is not recommended because of low yield reported in several studies [36–40]. Postoperative atelectasis is the most common complication. Pneumothorax is rare, occurring in 0–3% of patients, and correlates with a difficult operative course and clinical deterioration [38].

Although early complications with tracheostomy tube placement are uncommon, awareness of the radiographic findings suggesting a complication is critical for prompt detection and therapy. The tracheostomy tube should project and parallel the tracheal air column with its tip within the superior or mid intrathoracic trachea (Fig. 16.3). Unlike ETTs, tracheostomy tubes should not move relative to the patient's head position. Tracheostomy tubes typically occupy two-thirds of the diameter of the tracheal air column. A newly placed or replaced tracheostomy tube may be surrounded by subcutaneous and superior mediastinum air (Fig. 16.4). However, pneumothorax, increased mediastinal density, or abnormal convex mediastinal contours reflecting hematoma can be emergent postoperative complications.

Venous Access Catheters

Venous access catheters are commonly used in the ICU setting. These devices include

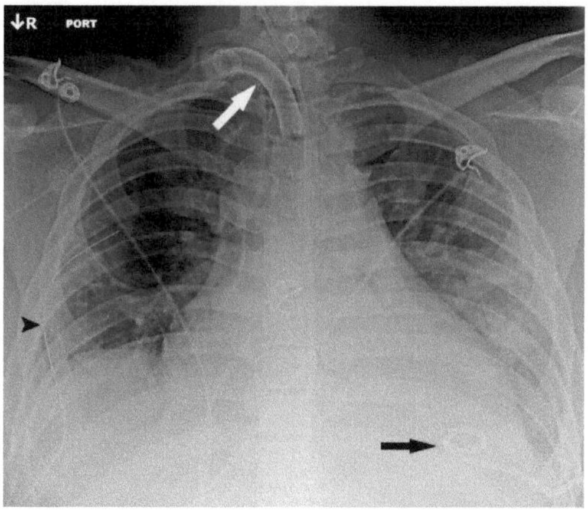

Fig. 16.3 Tracheostomy. AP radiograph shows a tracheostomy cannula (*white arrow*) in expected position with the tip projecting over the upper tracheal air column. A left pleural pigtail catheter (*black arrow*) is also present. Note that the side port (*arrowhead*) of the large bore right pleural drain is medial to the inner margin of the ribs

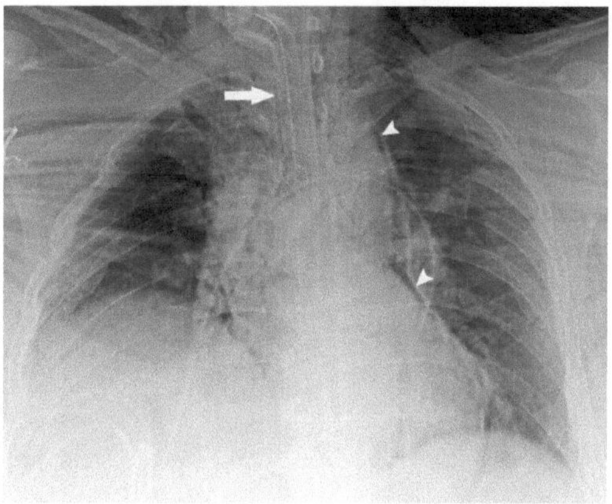

Fig. 16.4 Pneumomediastinum following tracheostomy. AP radiograph shows tracheostomy cannula (*arrow*) projecting over the tracheal air column. Pneumomediastinum has developed, characterized by air (*arrowheads*) outlining the mediastinal contours. Subcutaneous gas, as depicted here, is frequently a consequence of pneumomediastinum

temporary central lines, entering via internal jugular (IJ), subclavian, or femoral routes. Long-term venous access can be obtained with tunneled central lines, peripherally inserted central catheters (PICC), or subcutaneous ports. The tip of these catheters should be within the superior vena cava (SVC) (Fig. 16.5). The origin of the SVC usually lies to the right of midline at the level of the first intercostal space. The tip of the catheter should be vertical, paralleling the spine, away from the vessel wall. If the tip of the catheter is located within the superior SVC, just above the right main bronchus, and has a curved distal tip, azygos vein cannulation should be suspected (Fig. 16.6). Oblique or lateral radiographs are usually confirmatory.

Routine post-procedural chest radiography is not required following image-guided central venous line placement [41, 42] or catheter exchange over a wire [43]. A few studies have challenged the need for routine radiographic assessment following uncomplicated bedside line placement [44–46]. However, post-procedural imaging confirmation remains the current recommended standard [47, 48].

Post-procedural radiography can determine the catheter tip position and identify any immediate complications such as pneumothorax, vessel perforation (Fig. 16.7), catheter kinking, or discontinuity. Evaluation of a nonfunctioning catheter often begins with a radiograph to determine catheter position and to assess for kinking or fragmentation. Further evaluation with fluoroscopy, ultrasound, or CT may be required to assess for fibrin sheath formation or associated venous thrombosis (Fig. 16.8).

Pulmonary Artery Catheters

Since its introduction in 1970s, the balloon-tipped pulmonary artery catheter has been used with varying degrees of popularity in the ICU to monitor the hemodynamic status in the critically ill patient or patients in the immediate postoperative period. The catheter is often inserted via the IJ approach, with subclavian and femoral vein insertions much less commonly used. The catheter courses through the right atrium, into the right ventricle, and finally through the right ventricular outflow tract into the pulmonary arterial system. During pressure recording, the balloon-tipped catheter is wedged within a peripheral pulmonary artery. However, when the catheter is not in use, the balloon is deflated with

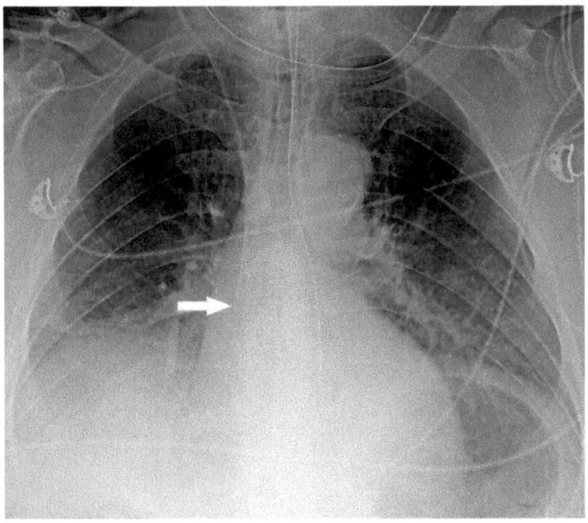

Fig. 16.5 Central venous catheter. AP radiograph shows the tip of the right internal jugular central venous catheter (*arrow*) at or near the cavoatrial junction. Endotracheal and gastric tubes are in expected positions, as well

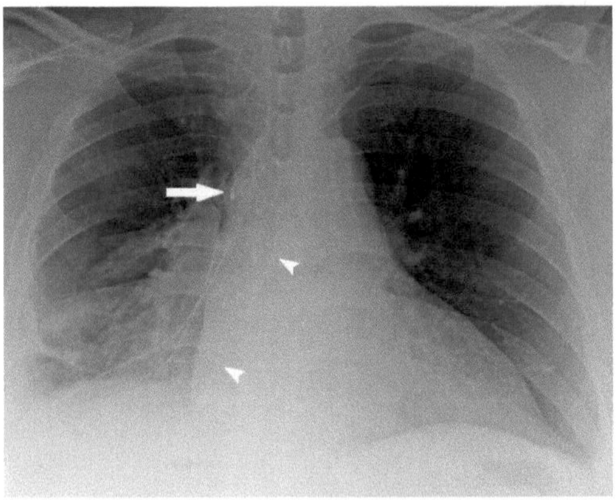

Fig. 16.6 Malpositioned PICC. AP radiograph shows foreshortening and abnormal angulation of the tip of the PICC (*arrow*), suggesting cannulation of the azygos vein. A metallic stent (*arrowheads*) has been placed in the gastric conduit

the catheter tip withdrawn into the main pulmonary artery (Fig. 16.9). The precise optimal location of the pulmonary artery catheter has not been defined. Suggested locations include 2 cm from the pulmonary hilum, [49] cardiac border, or 3–5 cm from the midline [50].

Serious complication rates from pulmonary artery catheter usage are estimated to be 4% and predominately include pulmonary hemorrhage, septicemia, and ventricular tachycardia [51]. The most serious complication, pulmonary artery rupture, which has a reported 50% morality rate, is rare with an incidence of 0.031% [52]. Other complications include formation of a pulmonary artery pseudoaneurysm (Fig. 16.10), intracardiac knotting, cardiac perforation, and thromboembolism [53, 54]. Postprocedural radiography remains the standard of care to ensure proper catheter placement; however, Houghton and colleagues challenged this practice [53]. In their study of 390 catheters, they found that clinical assessment can exclude 99% of malpositioned catheters, and, thus, they argued that if the catheter is not manipulated and remains secure, additional imaging should be obtained only if there is clinical suspicion of migration [53].

Chest radiography can adequately assess catheter tip location and detect distal catheter looping. New mediastinal fullness or density should raise the question of hematoma. A new round or ovoid opacity in the lung should be viewed with suspicion for a pseudoaneurysm if it persists or enlarges. Contrast-enhanced CT pulmonary angiography can be performed in hemodynamically stable patients with suspected pulmonary artery pseudoaneurysm for assessment and surgical planning [54].

Intra-Aortic Conterpulsation Balloon

Since its introduction in 1962, intra-aortic counterpulsation balloons (IACB) have been increasingly used in the setting of cardiogenic shock to improve left ventricular function. The device is 26 cm long and is typically inserted through a femoral approach. The inflation-deflation timing is electrically linked to the electrocardiogram to allow inflation to occur during diastole and deflation to occur during systole, better augmenting coronary artery perfusion and decreasing afterload, respectively [55].

The long length of this device increases risk of complications from proximal and distal vessel occlusion, making radiographic confirmation of its position critical. Ideally, the proximal tip of the IACB should be within the proximal descending aorta, just distal to the origin of the left subclavian artery (Fig. 16.11). Proximal

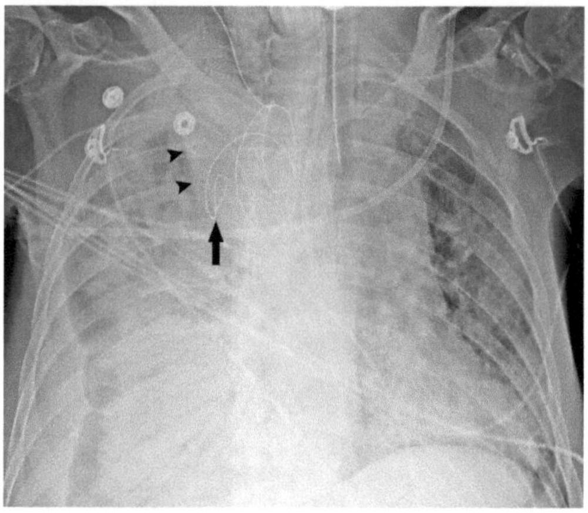

Fig. 16.7 Mediastinal hematoma following attempted central line placement. AP radiograph shows retained guidewire (*arrow*) coiled in the right upper mediastinum. Increased attenuation and lateral convexity (*arrowheads*) in the right upper mediastinum reflects the subsequent hematoma

positioning toward the aortic root risks cerebral vessel thromboembolism from great vessel occlusion. Distal positioning into the abdominal aorta risks bowel ischemia from abdominal artery occlusion [55, 56]. In addition to immediate radiography following IACB placement, periodic routine radiographs are also recommended to detect clinically occult device migration (Fig. 16.12) [55]. Because the device can change in position by 1–4.5 cm between recumbent and sitting positions, follow-up radiographs are best obtained with similar patient positioning [57].

Other major complications, which can be radiographically subtle, include aortic dissection and balloon rupture with intravascular gas. Subtle loss of aortic definition, in the context of clinical deterioration, warrants further evaluation with a contrast-enhanced CT angiogram to exclude aortic injury. Dunkman et al. [58] found aortic dissections are associated with severe atherosclerotic disease and difficult device placement.

Chest Tubes

Chest tubes are standard management for pneumothorax, hemothorax, empyema, chylothorax, and bronchopleural fistula. The ideal position of the tube depends on the intrathoracic

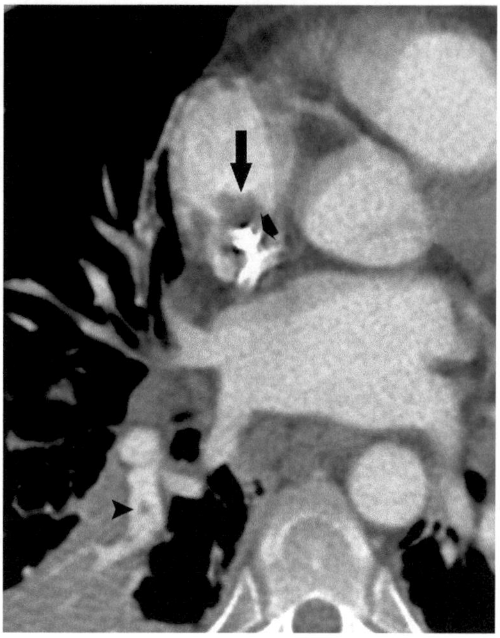

Fig. 16.8 Septic venous thrombosis in this patient presenting with staphylococcal sepsis and pneumonia. Contrast-enhanced CT image shows a filling defect (*long arrow*) adherent to the tip of the central venous catheter (*short arrow*). Note the embolized thrombus (*arrowhead*) in a right lower lobe segmental pulmonary artery

content being evacuated. Specifically, optimal tube position for fluid drainage is in a dependent location at the posterior base in contrast to a non-dependent position at the anterior apex for air [59, 60]. There are two classes of chest tubes. The larger diameter, straight catheter is often placed surgically or emergently at the bedside (Fig. 16.13). These larger catheters contain an end hole and a side port. The side port disrupts the radiopaque catheter line. The smaller diameter, pigtail drainage catheters (Fig. 16.14) are often placed by interventional radiology. These catheters contain an end hole and multiple side ports along the inner margin of the looped portion of the distal catheter.

Traditionally, frontal chest radiographs have been used to confirm appropriate positioning, monitor progress, and assess lung re-expansion. However, multiple studies comparing radiography with subsequent CT evaluation have shown the insensitivity of single frontal radiographs for detection of possible complications [59, 61–65].

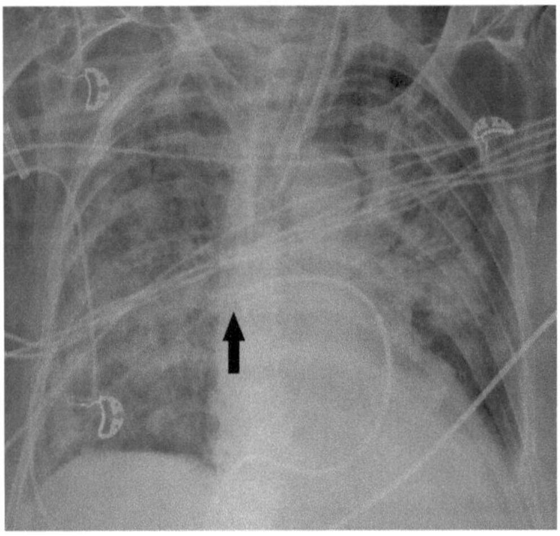

Fig. 16.9 Properly positioned pulmonary artery catheter. AP radiograph shows pulmonary artery catheter tip at the right mediastinal border. Extension into the lung periphery may result in pulmonary artery pseudoaneurysm or rupture

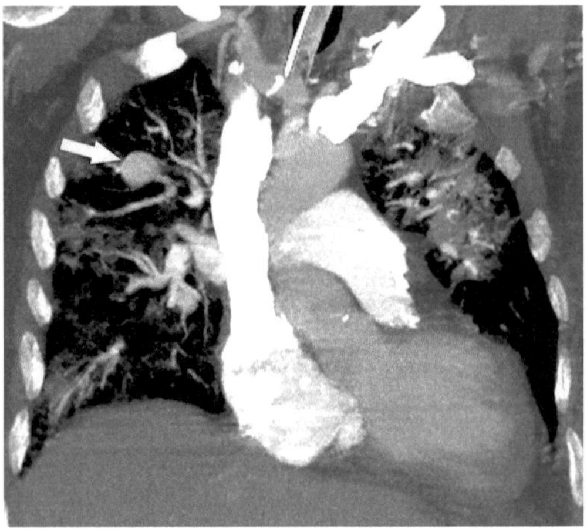

Fig. 16.10 Pulmonary artery pseudoaneurysm resulting from malpositioned pulmonary artery catheter. Coronal maximum intensity projection (MIP) from CT pulmonary angiogram shows a right upper lobe pulmonary artery pseudoaneurysm (*arrow*). Pulmonary artery rupture is associated with a nearly 50% mortality rate

Although adding a lateral view improves sensitivity, this is often not feasible because of multiple support devices and possible other injuries preventing proper positioning [61]. Additionally, with published complications rates of up to 37% for emergent chest tube placement, CT may be useful to assess positioning when patients fail to respond as expected to tube placement [62, 63].

Nevertheless, bedside chest radiographs are more accessible and are often the first imaging test of choice. Familiarity with possible radiographically detectable complications is important. The tip and side ports of the tube should be located medial to the inner margin of the ribs and peripheral to the visceral pleura.

Transdiaphragmatic chest tube placement occurs when the tube enters too low, below the lateral insertion of the diaphragm, with possible associated new pneumoperitoneum, liver, or splenic injury. Although transdiaphragmatic placement can be apparent on radiographs, CT is more sensitive [59]. Intrapulmonary tube placement is often difficult to diagnose on radiographs; however, parenchymal injury should be suspected with new or increasing lung consolidation surrounding the tube, abrupt increase in pulmonary or pleural opacity, increasing pneumothorax, or new chest wall gas [64]. Similarly, mediastinal placement (Fig. 16.15) is also difficult to assess on radiographs. Unless the tube crosses into the contralateral hemithorax, determining the lateral convex margin of the mediastinum on a two-dimensional image can be difficult. The significance of intrafissural tube placement remains controversial. Webb and Maurer found an intrafissural location to be

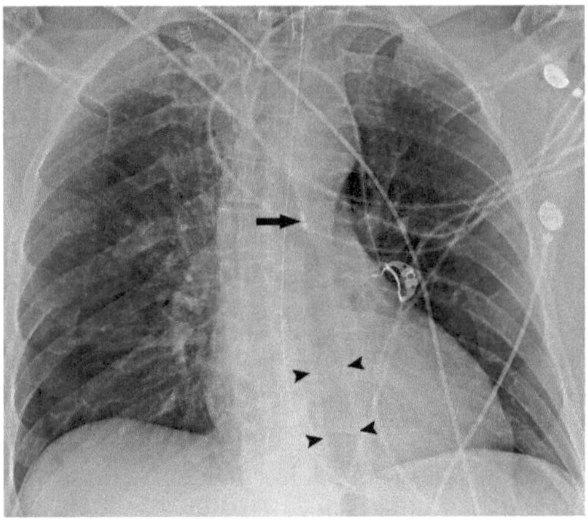

Fig. 16.11 Intra-aortic counterpulsation balloon. AP radiograph shows the tip (*arrow*) of the IACB in the proximal descending thoracic aorta. The balloon (*arrowheads*) may be visible during diastole

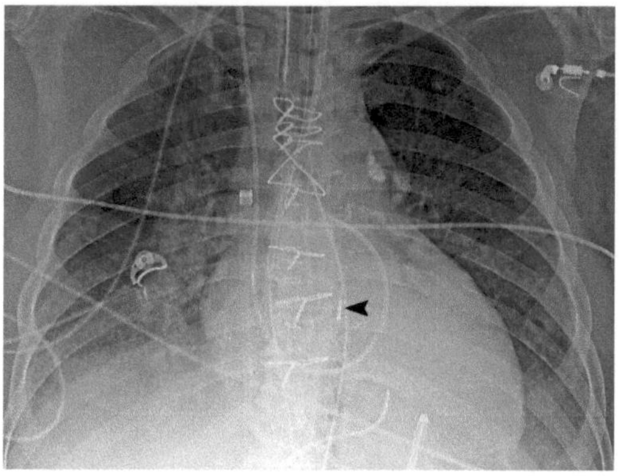

Fig. 16.12 Malpositioned IACB. AP radiograph shows the tip of the IACB (*arrowhead*) in the distal descending thoracic aorta. Mild lung edema is present

associated with tube dysfunction; however, Curtin found no significant tube dysfunction [66–68]. Subcutaneous tube placement results in either the entire or a portion of the tube, with its side port(s) peripheral to the ribs or skin margin. Subcutaneous gas is often present. Pneumothoraces may enlarge or fail to resolve.

Unenhanced CT scans allow for precise tube localization in the setting of inadequate tube drainage, clinical deterioration, or an inconclusive radiograph [59]. Additionally, CT can help assess undrained, loculated pleural fluid collections, and unsuspected lung disease.

Mediastinal Drains

Mediastinal drains are often placed after cardiac or esophageal surgery [69]. Although postoperative radiographs are routinely obtained at most institutions, increasing evidence indicates that in the setting of uncomplicated surgery and no other clinical indication, chest radiography rarely shows a significant abnormality requiring intervention [70, 71].

Mediastinal drains are similar to the large bore pleural drains and are often oriented vertically, projecting over the heart. Apparent changes in heart size or mediastinal contours may suggest drain dysfunction or reflect early postoperative complications such as hematoma or abscess. Technical differences between examinations should be taken into consideration as variable degree of inspiration and recumbent positioning can affect the mediastinal size and shape. CT can

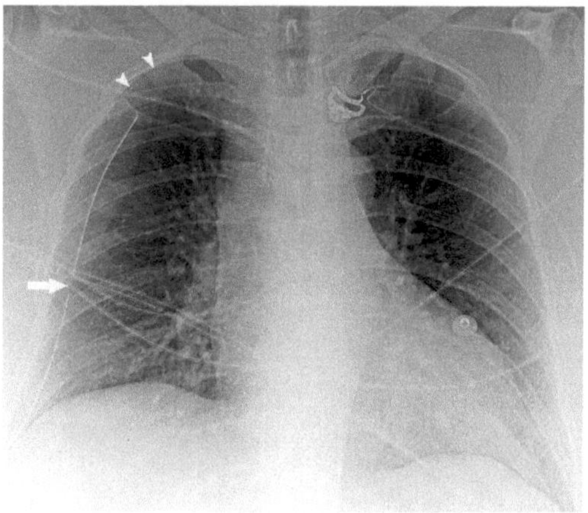

Fig. 16.13 Pneumothorax and large bore pleural drain. AP radiograph shows a large bore right pleural drain with side port (*arrow*) medial to the inner rib margin. A small pneumothorax (*arrowheads*) remains

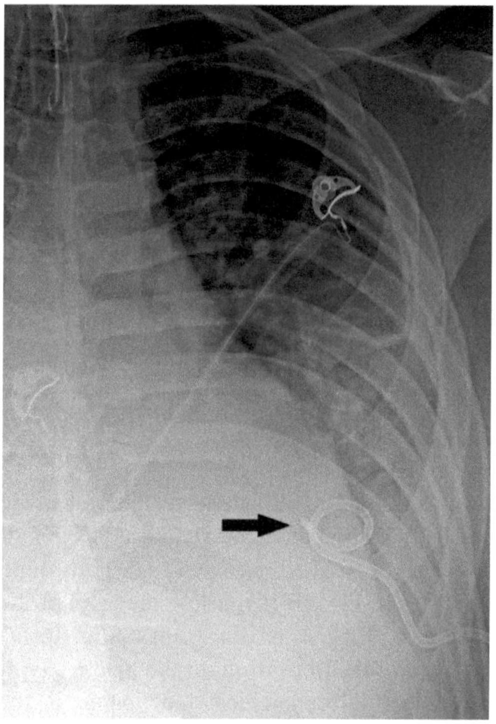

Fig. 16.14 Pigtail pleural drain. Coned-down view of AP radiograph shows a pigtail catheter (*arrow*) in the left pleural space with associated pleural effusion and atelectasis

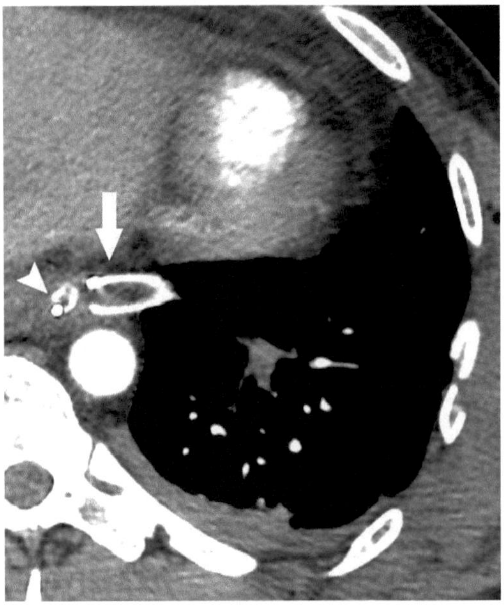

Fig. 16.15 Malpositioned emergently placed pleural drain in trauma patient. Contrast-enhanced CT image shows tip of left pleural drain (*arrow*) in the mediastinum, abutting the wall of the esophagus. Note the drain's close proximity to the nasogastric tube (*arrowhead*)

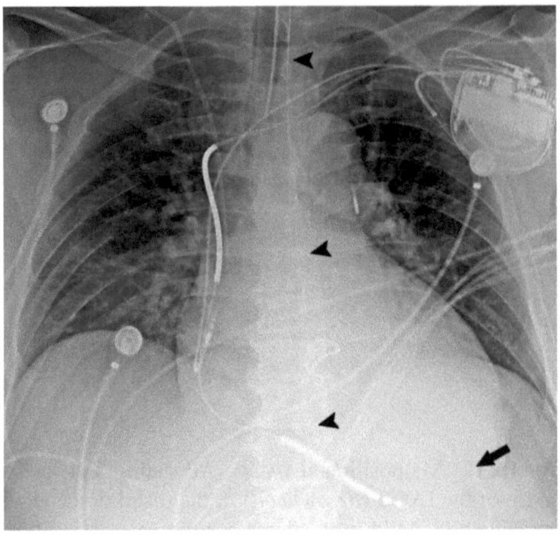

Fig. 16.16 Nastogatric tube. AP radiograph shows the nasogastric tube (*arrowheads*) coursing below the diaphragm into the stomach. The side port (*arrow*) should be located below the gastroesophageal junction

be used to evaluate for vascular injury, mediastinal hematoma, mediastinitis, and undrained fluid collections.

Enteric Tubes

Nasogastric (NG) and enteric feeding tubes are frequently used in the ICU. The ideal position of the NG tube includes both tip and side port within the stomach (Fig. 16.16), below the level of the diaphragm. Enteric feeding tubes (Fig. 16.17) ideally have their tips distal to the pylorus, typically at the duodenojejunal junction or in the proximal jejunum, in order to minimize gastroesophageal reflux and subsequent aspiration. The duodenojejunal junction is the superior most small bowel fixation point, located within the left superior abdomen, held in place by the ligament of Treitz.

The most serious complication of these tubes is airway insertion (Fig. 16.18) with resultant pneumothorax, pleural effusion, pneumonia, or abscess. Clinical signs and symptoms of airway insertion may be lacking secondary to depressed sensorium, impaired gag reflex, or recent intubation [72]. Malpositioned smaller bore enteric feeding tubes are more likely to be clinically occult than the larger NG tubes [73, 74]. The most common location of the malpositioned tube is within the right low lobe bronchi [75]. Chest radiographic findings indicating airway insertion of gastric tubes include the tube projecting over the airway lateral to the expected location of the esophagus and above the diaphragm.

Other complications include coiled tube within the oropharynx and esophageal perforation with possible mediastinitis [76, 77]. Although coiled tube can be easily detected with radiography, early esophageal perforation or mediastinitis may be radiographically occult. Clinical deterioration with new mediastinal fullness, pneumomediastinum, or left pleural effusion, should prompt further evaluation with CT. The overall rate of tube malposition resulting in

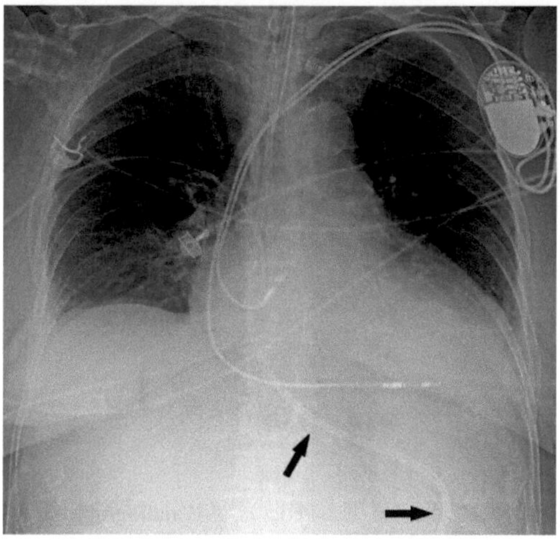

Fig. 16.17 Enteric feeding tube. AP radiograph shows an enteric feeding tube (*arrows*) coursing below the diaphragm into the stomach and then beyond the field of view

complications ranges from 0.3% to 7.6% in various ICU settings [76–78]. Post-procedural radiographs are recommended before initiation of tube feeds.

Approach to ICU Chest Imaging

Various approaches to examining a chest radiograph exist, all of which include a systematic method. In the following section, various mediastinal and lung disease processes will be discussed.

Mediastinum

Cardiac Abnormalities

Cardiomegaly is a common finding on ICU portal chest radiographs and may simply be an artifact resulting from low lung volume, patient position, or technical factors such as the AP projection. Additionally, respiratory motion can give the suggestion of vascular engorgement and an ill-defined diaphragm, mimicking pulmonary edema. Therefore, correlation with the patient's clinical status can help distinguish artifact from disease. In ambiguous situations, repeat radiographs with technique optimization and upright AP positioning (when possible) may suffice. CT is typically reserved for problem solving.

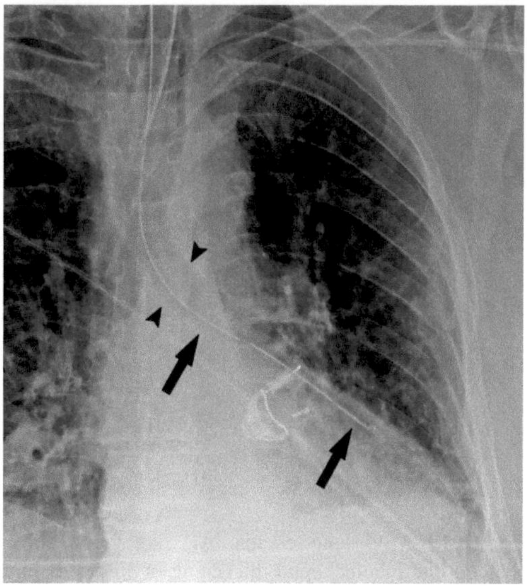

Fig. 16.18 Malpositioned nasogastric tube. Coned-down view of AP radiograph shows a nasogastric tube (*arrow*) extending into the left lower lobe. Note how the tube parallels the course of the left main bronchus (*arrowheads*)

In the setting of acute cardiac enlargement and depressed cardiac output, bedside radiographs are often not specific for distinguishing between cardiomegaly and pericardial effusion. Although CT can clearly distinguish pericardial effusion from cardiomegaly, bedside ultrasound is often the preferred diagnostic examination and allows for simultaneous drainage of pericardial fluid.

Cardiomegaly can be diffuse or focal. Diffuse cardiomegaly is often the common endpoint of a variety of cardiac diseases and is often irreversible. Conversely, focal cardiomegaly can suggest a specific pathology, which may be amenable to treatment. For example, left ventricular hypertrophy and ultimately dilation can occur with systemic hypertension, aortic valve stenosis, and mitral valve regurgitation. Left ventricular hypertrophy results in elevation of the cardiac apex while dilation results in

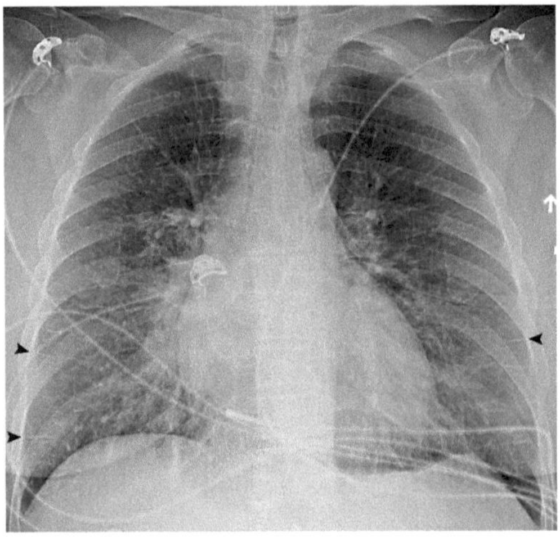

Fig. 16.19 Mild lung edema. AP radiograph shows bilateral interlobular septal thickening or Kerley B lines (*arrowheads*) and slight indistinctness of the pulmonary vessels. Kerley B lines are generally 1–2 cm in length, run perpendicular to the pleura, and tend to be more pronounced in the lower lungs

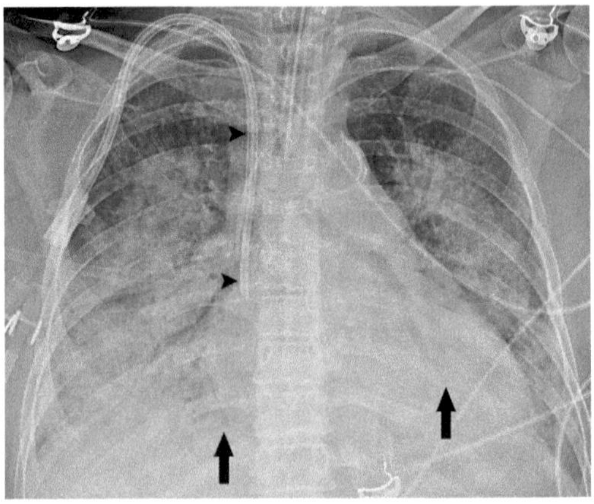

Fig. 16.20 Severe lung edema. AP radiograph shows bilateral dense lung consolidation with relative peripheral sparing in this patient with renal failure. Note bilateral air bronchograms (*arrows*). A large bore dual lumen hemodialysis catheter (*arrowhead*) has been placed via a right internal jugular venous approach

lateralization of the left cardiac boarder. Similar pathological processes can affect the right ventricle with pulmonary valve stenosis, pulmonary hypertension, and tricuspid valve regurgitation. However, subtle changes in right ventricular size may not be apparent on a portable AP radiograph.

Lung

Diffuse Lung Opacities

Pulmonary Edema

There are many causes of pulmonary edema [79] with cardiogenic and permeability edema being the two most commonly encountered in the ICU. Cardiogenic pulmonary edema can be roughly divided into predominately interstitial edema (Fig. 16.19) or alveolar flooding (Fig. 16.20) and is often seen in the setting of left heart or renal failure. A positive relationship exists between pulmonary capillary wedge pressures (PCWP) and the radiographic severity of the pulmonary edema, progressing from interstitial edema into alveolar flooding. Specifically, 12–17 mmHg PCWP corresponds to loss of subsegmental and segmental vessel definition with vascular cuffing; 17–20 mmHg PCWP corresponds to lymphatic congestion with better appreciation of the peripheral interlobular septal lines, better known as Kerley B lines, and small pleural effusions. Progressive elevation of the PCWP to or above 25 mmHg leads to alveolar flooding. In contrast to other alveolar filling processes, hydrostatic alveolar edema typically develops and clears rapidly [79–81].

Acute respiratory distress syndrome (ARDS) (Fig. 16.21) is the most common cause of noncardiogenic pulmonary edema in the ICU and results from underlying increased capillary basement membrane permeability in the setting of normal PCWP. The increased permeability is secondary to diffuse alveolar damage, which can be the result of chemical or infectious exposure, in combination with secondary autoimmune mediated response. Temporal progression of ARDS has been commonly divided into three stages: exudative, proliferative, and fibrotic. During the exudative stage, interstitial edema develops with rapid progression to alveolar edema, consolidation, and air bronchograms, often more peripheral and basal in distribution, mimicking hydrostatic pulmonary edema. However, Kerley B lines and

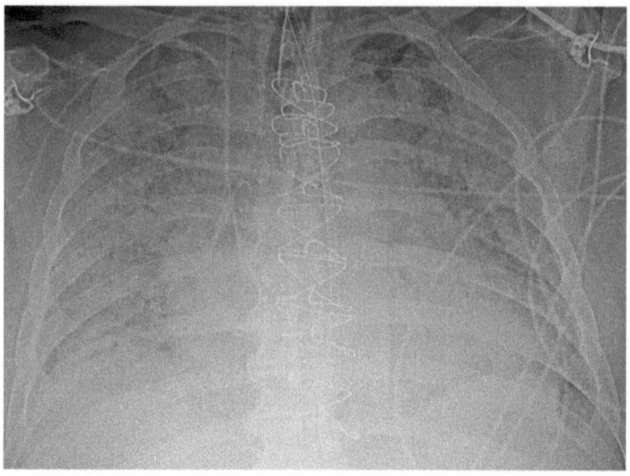

Fig. 16.21 Acute respiratory distress syndrome (ARDS). AP radiograph shows diffuse lung consolidation without apparent pleural effusions. Distinguishing ARDS from diffuse lung edema may be difficult on chest radiography; however, whereas edema may rapidly decrease, ARDS evolves more slowly

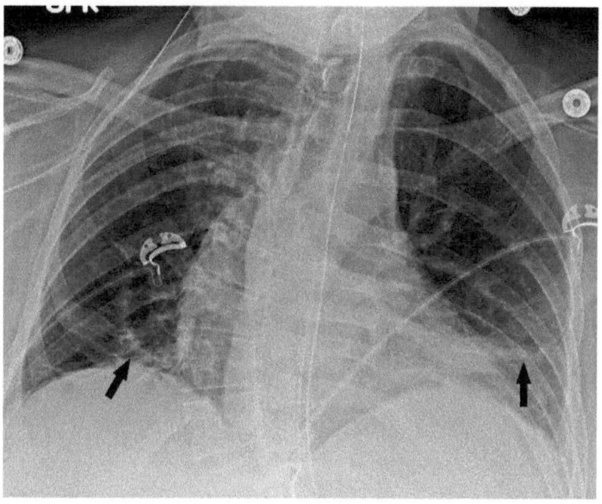

Fig. 16.22 Linear atelectasis. AP radiograph shows low lung volumes with linear consolidation (*arrows*) in both lung bases that is characteristic of linear or plate-like atelectasis

cardiomegaly are uncommon. During the proliferative phase (days 5–10), the exudative fluid with high protein content is organized with regeneration of the alveolar lining, resulting in increased pulmonary opacity and consolidation. Some patients progress to the fibrotic stage with subpleural and intrapulmonary cyst and scar formation [79, 82, 83].

Focal Lung Opacities

Focal lung opacities include non-homogeneous distribution of airspace opacities, which can range from a solitary focus to bilateral abnormalities. These can coalesce to form diffuse lung opacity. The most common causes of focal lung opacities in the critically ill patient include atelectasis, aspiration, and infection.

Atelectasis

In an intubated, bed-bound patient with low inspiratory volume, atelectasis is extremely common. On the portable chest radiograph, atelectasis may range from a linear or plate-like appearance (Fig. 16.22) to diffuse lobar consolidation (Fig. 16.23). Displacement of the normal pulmonary fissure is a direct sign of atelectasis. Indirect signs of atelectasis include hypoinflation, increased attenuation of the atelectatic segment, ipsilateral mediastinal shift, and elevation of the ipsilateral hemidiaphragm.

Aspiration

In a supine patient, aspiration favors the posterior upper lobes and lower lobe superior segments. The right lung may be more extensively involved given the relatively straight course of the right main bronchus. The clinical severity and radiographic appearance of aspiration depend on both the amount and composition of the aspirated fluid (Fig. 16.24). Aspiration of acidic gastric contents can cause a reactive pneumonitis with resulting lung consolidation. Aspiration of particulates can cause bronchial obstruction and subsequent atelectasis. Patients with an altered level of consciousness, impaired gag reflex, esophageal dysmotility, or distal intestinal obstruction are at high risk for aspiration. The inflation balloon of endotracheal tubes does not produce a complete seal within the proximal trachea and, therefore, does not prevent aspiration.

Pneumonia

Pneumonia can be focal or diffuse (Fig. 16.25). In the critically ill patient, bilateral, multifocal bronchopneumonia is most commonly seen.

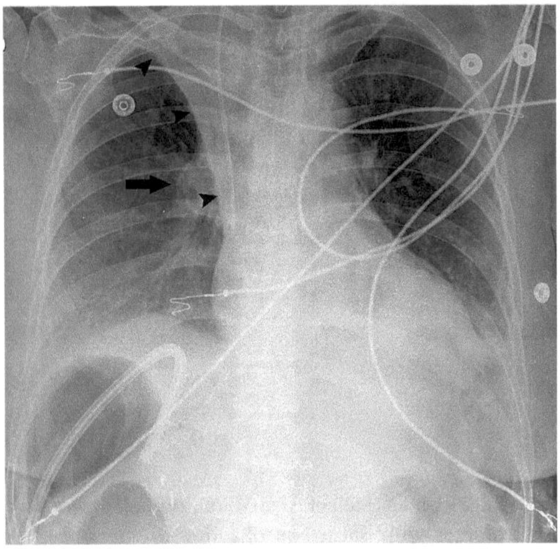

Fig. 16.23 Lobar atelectasis. AP radiograph shows collapse of the right upper lobe. Note upward and medial rotation of the pulmonary fissure (*arrowheads*) and upward displacement of the right hilum (*arrow*)

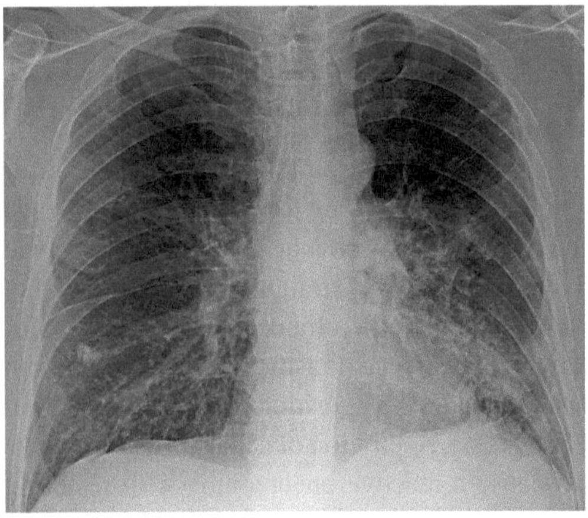

Fig. 16.24 Aspiration. AP radiograph shows coarse bilateral lower lobe and perihilar consolidation, greater on the left. The gravitationally dependent distribution and coarse appearance are typical of aspiration, the latter reflecting filling of large and small airways with aspirated material

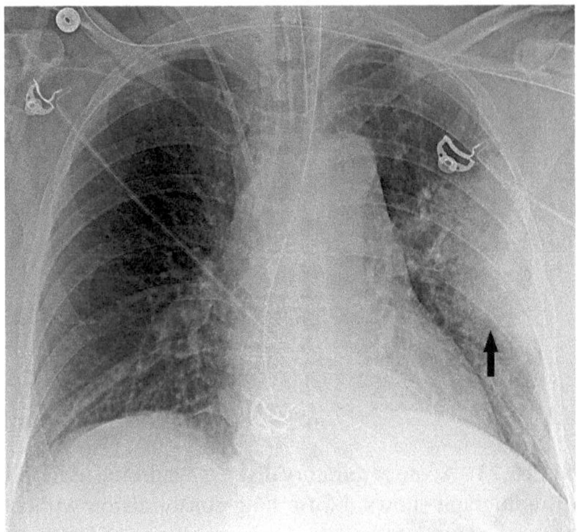

Fig. 16.25 Hospital acquired pneumonia. AP radiograph shows peripheral consolidation (*arrow*) in the mid right lung. The unilateral and non-gravitationally dependent distribution along with lack of significant volume loss favors pneumonia over atelectasis or aspiration

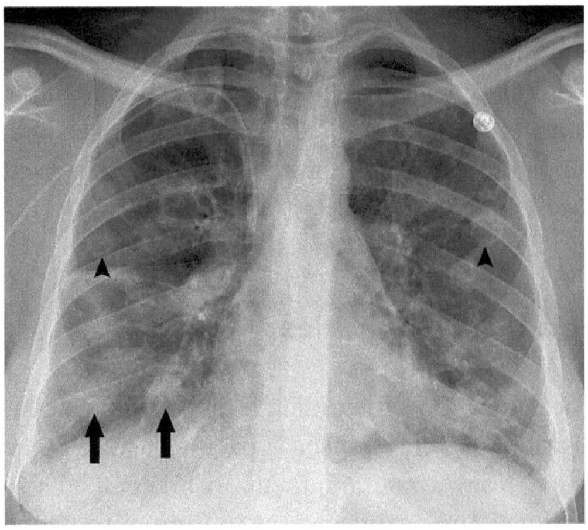

Fig. 16.26 Septic emboli. Frontal radiograph shows bilateral lung nodules (*arrows*) with a basal and peripheral predominance. Some of the nodules are cavitary (*arrowheads*)

Distinguishing pneumonia from aspiration or atelectasis can be difficult on a single radiograph. However, change over time may favor one process over the other. For example, atelectasis may wax and wane over serial radiographs whereas pneumonia typically develops more slowly and gradually clears with treatment. For patients with delayed clinical improvement or clinical deterioration, chest CT may be indicated to assess for developing complications such as parenchymal necrosis, abscess formation, parapneumonic effusion, or empyema.

Pleural Effusion

Supine radiographs are only moderately sensitive and specific for evaluation of pleural effusion; specifically, 175–525 mL of pleural fluid can accumulate on a supine radiograph before lateral costophrenic sulcus blunting becomes apparent [84, 85]. Lateral and PA chest radiographs perform minimally better, with sensitivities of 85.7% and 82.1% and specificities 87.5% and 81.3%, respectively, compared to 78.4% and 76.4% for AP chest radiographs [86]. Therefore, diagnostic and possible therapeutic ultrasound or CT is often used [87]. Bedside ultrasound can help better characterize the fluid collection and distinguishing simple from complex fluid collections, the latter of which are more likely to contain fibrous bands and dependent debris. However, only fluid analysis can definitively distinguish sterile from infected fluid.

Septic Pulmonary Emboli

Septic pulmonary emboli (Fig. 16.26) result from hematogenous dissemination of infection lodged within the peripheral pulmonary arteries, with sudden appearance and often rapid development of multiple peripheral round or triangular ill-defined, patchy lung opacities. Imaging findings can mimic sterile pulmonary embolism, pulmonary metastases, tuberculosis, and other cavitary diseases of the lung. However, the rapid development and evolution of pulmonary septic emboli along with clinical signs of bacteremia help to distinguish it from other relatively indolent disease processes [88]. Chest CT shows peripheral nodules with or without surrounding ground-glass opacity, the latter suggestive of hemorrhage. The lesions may have varying degrees of central low attenuation suggestive of necrosis or developing cavitation. Common sources of septic pulmonary emboli include infected cardiac valves, infected intravenous catheters, and thrombophlebitis. Delay in treatment can lead to development of lung abscess, empyema, bronchopleural fistula, shock, and death [89, 90].

Conclusion

Chest imaging is an important diagnostic component in the evaluation of critically ill patients. The chest radiograph continues to be the most commonly performed diagnostic imaging procedure in the ICU. Optimizing technical and patient factors can greatly improve the diagnostic quality of the exam, allowing for prompt detection of potentially life-threatening conditions. However, severe limitations exist, and bedside ultrasound and chest CT can be used to better address clinical questions and improve medical decision making.

References

1. Gray P, Sullivan G, Ostryzniuk P, et al. Value of postprocedural chest radiographs in the adult intensive care unit. Crit Care Med. 1992;20(11): 1513–8.
2. Hall JB, White SR, Karrison T. Efficacy of daily routine chest radiographs in intubated, mechanically ventilated patients. Crit Care Med. 1991;19(5): 69–93.
3. Janower ML, Jennas-Nocera Z, Mukai J. Utility and efficacy of portable chest radiographs. AJR. 1984; 142(2):265–7.
4. Bekemeyer WB, Crapo RO, Calhoon S, et al. Efficacy of chest radiography in the respiratory intensive care unit: a prospective study. Chest. 1984;88(5):691–5.
5. Graat ME, Choi G, Wolthuis EK, et al. The clinical value of daily routine chest radiographs in a mixed medical-surgical intensive care unit is low. Critical Care. 2006;10(1):R11.
6. Graat ME, Kroner A, Spronk PE, et al. Elimination of daily routine chest radiographs in a mixed medical-surgical intensive care unit. Intensive Care Med. 2007;33(4):639–44.
7. Hendrikse KA, Gratama JW, Hove W, et al. Low value of routine chest radiographs in a mixed medical-surgical ICU. Chest. 2007;132(3):823–8.
8. Krivopal M, Shlobin OA, Schwartzstein RM. Utility of daily routine portable chest radiographs in mechanically ventilated patients in the medical ICU. Chest. 2003;123(5):1607–14.
9. Graham RJ, Meziane MA, Rice TW, et al. Postoperative portable chest radiographs: optimum use in thoracic surgery. J Thorac Cardiovasc Surg. 1998;115(1):45–50.
10. Hejblum G, Chalumeau-Lemoine L, Ioos V, et al. Comparison of routine and on-demand prescription of chest radiographs in mechanically ventilated adults: a multicentre, cluster-randomized, two-period crossover study. Lancet. 2009;374(9702):1687–93.
11. Oba Y, Zaza T. Abandoning daily routine chest radiography in the intensive care unit: meta-analysis. Radiology. 2010;255(2):386–95.
12. Wandtke JC. Bedside chest radiography. Radiology. 1994;190(1):1–10.

13. Miller WT Jr, Tino G, Friedburg JS. Thoracic CT in the intensive care unit: assessment of clinical usefulness. Radiology. 1998;209(2):491–8.
14. Snow N, Bergin KT, Horrigan TP. Thoracic CT scanning in the critically ill patients: information obtained frequently alters management. Chest. 1990; 97(6):1467–70.
15. Mirvis SE, Tobin KD, Kostrubiak I, et al. Thoracic CT in detecting occult disease in critically ill patients. AJR. 1987;148(4):685–9.
16. Bouhemad B, Zhang M, Lu Q, et al. Clinical review: bedside lung ultrasound in critical care practice. Crit Care. 2007;11(1):205–14.
17. Esposito RA, Boyd A, Spencer FC. The value of computed tomography in postoperative pneumothorax following open heart surgery. Ann Thor Surg. 1986;42(6):699–701.
18. Wall SD, Federle MP, Jeffrey RB, et al. CT diagnosis of unsuspected pneumothorax after blunt abdominal trauma. AJR. 1983;141(5):919–21.
19. Kitazono MT, Lau CT, Parada AN, et al. Differentiation of pleural effusions from parenchymal opacities: accuracy of bedside chest radiography. AJR. 2010;194(2):407–12.
20. Peris A, Tutino L, Zagli G, et al. The use of point-of-care bedside lung ultrasound significantly reduces the number of radiographs and computed tomography scans in critically ill patients. Anesth Analg. 2010;111(3):667–92.
21. Chen CH, Chen W, Chen HJ, et al. Transthoracic ultrasonography in predicting the outcome of small-bore catheter drainage in empyemas or complicated parapneumonic effusions. Ultrasound Med Biol. 2009;35(9):1468–74.
22. Chen HJ, Yu YH, Tu CY, et al. Ultrasound in peripheral pulmonary air-fluid lesions. Color Doppler imaging as an aid in differentiating empyema and abscess. Chest. 2009;135(6):1426–32.
23. Bouhemad B, Zhang M, Lu Q, et al. Clinical reviews: bedside lung ultrasound in critical care practice. Crit Care. 2007;11(1):205.
24. Alptekin B, Tran DT, Lisbon A, et al. Bedside ultrasonography in the differential diagnosis of pulmonary pathologies in the intensive care unit. J Clin Anesth. 2006;18(7):534–6.
25. Arbelot C, Ferrari F, Bouhemad B, et al. Lung ultrasound in acute respiratory distress syndrome and acute lung injury. Curr Opin Crit Care. 2008; 14(1):70–4.
26. Rocco M, Carbone I, Morelli A, et al. Diagnostic accuracy of bedside ultrasonography in the ICU: feasibility of detecting pulmonary effusion and lung contusion in patients on respiratory support after severe blunt thoracic trauma. Acta Anaesthesiol Scand. 2008;52(6):776–84.
27. Lichtenstein DA, Meziere GA, Lagoueyte JF, et al. A-lines and B-lines: lung ultrasound as a bedside tool for predicting pulmonary artery occlusion pressure in the critically ill. Chest. 2009;136(4):1014–20.
28. Sustic A, Protic A, Cicvaric T, et al. The addition of a brief ultrasound examination to clinical assessment increases the ability to confirm placement of double-lumen endotracheal tubes. J Clin Anesth. 2010;22(4): 246–9.
29. Conrardy PA, Goodman LR, Lainge F, et al. Alteration of endotracheal tube position. Flexion and extension of the neck. Crit Care Med. 1976; 4(1):7–12.
30. Goodman LR, Conrardy PA, Laing F, et al. Radiographic evaluation of the endotracheal tube position. AJR. 1976;127(3):433–4.
31. Brunel W, Coleman DL, Schwartz DE, et al. Assessment of routine chest roentgenograms and the physical examination to confirm endotracheal tube position. Chest. 1989;96(5):1043–5.
32. Gray P, Sullivan G, Ostryzniuk P, et al. Value of postprocedural chest radiographs in the adult intensive care unit. Crit Care Med. 1992;20(11): 1513–8.
33. Schwartz DE, Lieberman JA, Cohen NH. Women are at greater risk than men for malpositioning of the endotracheal tube after emergent intubation. Crit Care Med. 1994;22(7):1127–31.
34. Owen RL, Cheney FW. Endobronchial intubation: a preventable complication. Anesthesiology. 1987; 67(2):255–7.
35. Lotano R, Gerber D, Aseron C, et al. Utility of postintubation chest radiographs in the intensive care unit. Crit Care. 2000;4(1):50–3.
36. Hoehne F, Ozaeta M, Chung R. Routine chest X-ray after percutaneous tracheostomy is unnecessary. Am Surg. 2005;71(1):51–3.
37. Haddad SH, Aldawood AS, Arabi YM. The diagnostic yield and clinical impact of a chest X-ray after percutaneous dilatational tracheostomy: a prospective cohort study. Anaesth Intensive Care. 2007;35(3):393–7.
38. Datta D, Onyirimba F, McNamee MJ. The utility of chest radiographs following percutaneous dilatational tracheostomy. Chest. 2003;123(5):1603–6.
39. Kumar VM, Grant CA, Hughes MW, et al. Role of routine chest radiograph after percutaneous dilatational tracheostomy. Br J Anaesth. 2008; 100(5):663–6.
40. Tarnoff M, Moncure M, Jones F, et al. The value of routine posttracheostomy chest radiograph. Chest. 1998;113(6):1647–9.
41. Lucey B, Varghese JC, Haslam P, et al. Routine chest radiographs after central line insertion: mandatory postprocedural evaluation or unnecessary waste of resources? Cardiovasc Intervent Radiol. 1999;22(5): 381–4.
42. Caridi JG, West JH, Stavropoulos SW, et al. Internal jugular and upper extremity central venous access in interventional radiology: is a postprocedure chest radiograph necessary? AJR. 2000;174(2):363–6.
43. Palesty JA, Amshel CE, Dudrick SJ. Routine chest radiographs following central venous

recatheterization over a wire are not justified. Am J Surg. 1998;176(6):618–21.
44. Lessnau KD. Is chest radiography necessary after uncomplicated insertion of a triple-lumen catheter in the right internal jugular vein, using the anterior approach? Chest. 2005;127(1):220–3.
45. Gray P, Sullivan G, Ostryzniuk P, et al. Value of postprocedural chest radiographs in the adult intensive care unit. Crit Care Med. 1992;20(11):1513–8.
46. Farrell J, Walshe J, Gellens M, et al. Complications associated with insertion of jugular venous catheters for hemodialysis: the value of postprocedural radiograph. Am J Kidney Dis. 1997;30(5):690–2.
47. Maffessanti M, Bortolotto P, Kette F. Malpositions and complications following central venous catheterization in relation to the access site. Radio Med. 1988;75(6):609–12.
48. Gladwin MT, Slonim A, Landucci DL, et al. Cannulation of the internal jugular vein: Is postprocedural chest radiographs always necessary? Crit Care Med. 1999;27(9):1819–23.
49. Zarshenas Z, Sparschu RA. Catheter placement and misplacement. Crit Care Clin. 1994;10(2):417–36.
50. Miller JA, Singireddy S, Maldjian R, et al. A reevaluation of the radiographically detectable complications of percutaneous venous access lines inserted by four subcutaneous approaches. Am Surg. 1999;65(2):125–30.
51. Boyd KD, Thomas SJ, Gold J, et al. A prospective study of complications of pulmonary artery catheterization in 500 consecutive patients. Chest. 1983;84(3):245–9.
52. Kaerney TJ, Shabot MM. Pulmonary artery rupture associated with Swan-Ganz catheter. Chest. 1995;108(5):1349–52.
53. Houghton D, Cohn S, Schell V, et al. Routine daily chest radiography in patients with pulmonary artery catheters. Am J Crit Care. 2002;11(3):261–5.
54. Poplausky MR, Rozenblit G, Rundback JH, et al. Swan-Ganz catheter-induced pulmonary artery pseudoaneurysm formation: three case reports and a review of the literature. Chest. 2001;120(6):2105–11.
55. Hyson EA, Ravin CE, Kelley MJ, et al. Intraaortic counterpulsation balloon: radiographic considerations. AJR. 1977;128(6):915–8.
56. Chiles C, Vail CM, Coblentz CL, et al. Intra-aortic balloon pumps: an update on radiographic recognition. Can Assoc Radiol J. 1991;42(4):257–60.
57. O'Rourke MF, Shepherd KM. Protection of the aortic arch and subclavian artery during intraaortic balloon pumping. J Thorac Cardiovasc Surg. 1973;65(4):543–6.
58. Dunkman WB, Leinbach RC, Buckley MJ, et al. Clinical and hemodynamic results of intraaortic balloon pumping and surgery for cardiogenic shock. Circulation. 1972;46(3):465–77.
59. Gayer G, Rozenman J, Hoffmann C, et al. CT diagnosis of malpositioned chest tubes. Br J Radiol. 2000;73(871):786–90.
60. Miller KS, Sahn SA. Chest tubes. Indications, technique, management and complications. Chest. 1987;91(2):258–64.
61. Stark DD, Federle MP, Goodman PC. CT and radiographic assessment of tube thoracostomy. AJR. 1983;141(2):253–8.
62. Lim KE, Tai SC, Chan CY, et al. Diagnosis of malpositioned chest tubes after emergency tube thoracostomy: is computed tomography more accurate than chest radiograph? Clin Imaging. 2005;29(6):401–5.
63. Baldt MM, Bankier AA, Germann PS, et al. Complications after emergency tube thoracostomy: assessment with CT. Radiology. 1995;195(2):539–43.
64. Landay M, Oliver Q, Estrera A, et al. Lung penetration by thoracostomy tubes: imaging findings on CT. J Thorac Imaging. 2006;21(3):197–204.
65. Heim P, Maas R, Tesch C. Pleural drainage in acute thoracic trauma. Comparison of the radiologic image and computer tomography. Aktuelle Radiol. 1998; 8(4):163–8.
66. Webb WR, LaBerge JM. Radiographic recognition of chest tube malposition in the major fissure. Chest. 1984;85(1):81–3.
67. Maurer JR, Friedman PJ, Wing VW. Thoracostomy tube in an interlobar fissure: Radiologic recognition of a potential problem. AJR. 1982;139(6):1155–61.
68. Curtin JJ, Goodman LR, Quebbeman EJ, et al. Thoracostomy tubes after acute chest injury: relationship between location in a pleural fissure and function. AJR. 1994;163(6):1339–42.
69. Bjessmo S, Hylander S, Vedin J, et al. Comparison of three different chest drainages after coronary artery bypass surgery: a randomized trial of 150 patients. Eur J Cardiothorac Surg. 2007;31(3):372–5.
70. Khan T, Chawla G, Daniel R, et al. Is routine chest X-ray following mediastinal drain removal after cardiac surgery useful? Eur J Cardiothorac Surg. 2008;34(3):542–4.
71. Rao PS, Abid Q, Khan KJ, et al. Evaluation of routine postoperative chest x-ray in the management of the cardiac surgical patient. Eur J Cardiothorac Surg. 1996;12(5):724–9.
72. Miller KS, Tomlinson JR, Sahn SA. Pleuropulmonary complications of enteral tube feedings. Chest. 1985;88(2):230–3.
73. Biggart M, McQuillan PJ, Choudhry AK, et al. Dangers of placement of narrow bore nasogastric feeding tubes. Ann R Coll Surg Engl. 1987;69(3):119–21.
74. Hand RW, Kempster M, Levy JH, et al. Inadvertent transbronchial insertion of narrow-bore feeding tubes into the pleural space. JAMA. 1984;251(18):2396–7.
75. Bankier AA, Wiesmayr MN, Henk C, et al. Radiographic detection of intrabronchial malpositions of nasogastric tubes and subsequent complications in intensive care unit patients. Intensive Care Med. 1997;23(4):406–10.
76. McWey RE, Curry NS, Schabel SI, et al. Complications of nasoenteric feeding tubes. Am J Surg. 1988;155(2):253–7.

77. Ghahremani GG, Gould RJ. Nasoenteric feeding tubes. Radiographic detection of complications. Dig Dis Sci. 1986;31(6):574–85.
78. Valentine RJ, Turner WW Jr. Pleural complications of nasoenteric feeding tubes. JPEN. 1985;9(5): 605–7.
79. Gluecker T, Capasso P, Schnyder P, et al. Clinical and radiologic features of pulmonary edema. Radiographics. 1999;19(6):1507–31.
80. Milne EN, Pistolesi M, Miniati M, et al. The radiologic distinction of cardiogenic and noncardiogenic edema. AJR. 1985;144(5):879–84.
81. Meszaros WT. Lung changes in left heart failure. Circulation. 1973;47(4):859–71.
82. Greene R. Adult respiratory distress syndrome: acute alveolar damage. Radiology. 1987;163(1):57–66.
83. Holter JF, Weiland JE, Pacht ER, et al. Protein permeability in the adult respiratory distress syndrome. J Clin Invest. 1986;78(6):1513–22.
84. Woodring JH. Recognition of pleural effusion on supine radiographs: how much fluid is required? AJR. 1984;142(1):59–64.
85. Ruskin JA, Gurney JW, Thorsen MK, et al. Detection of pleural effusions on supine chest radiographs. AJR. 1987;148(4):681–3.
86. Brixey AG, Luo Y, Skouras V, et al. The efficacy of chest radiographs in detecting parapneumonic effusions. Respirology. 2011;16(6):1000–4.
87. Halvorsen RA Jr, Thompson WM. Ascites or pleural effusion? CT and ultrasound differentiation. Crit Rev Diagn Imaging. 1986;26(3):201–40.
88. Fred HL, Harle TS. Septic pulmonary embolism. Dis Chest. 1969;55(6):483–6.
89. Griffith GL, Maull KI, Schatello CR. Septic pulmonary embolization. Surg Gynecol Obstet. 1977;144(1):105–8.
90. Jaffe RB, Koschmann EB. Septic pulmonary emboli. Radiology. 1970;96(3):527–32.

Image Guided Thoracic Interventions 17

Daniel Barnes, Kayvan Amjadi, and Jean M. Seely

Abstract

This chapter describes the major types of thoracic interventional procedures, including radiofrequency ablation, transthoracic needle biopsy of lung, mediastinal and pleural disease, thoracentesis, and pleural chest tube drainage. The clinical indications for these procedures, risks and complications of each procedure, and where appropriate, a description of how they are performed are covered. This chapter should be relevant to the chest clinician to better understand risks and benefits of interventional chest procedures, hopefully leading to a better understanding of the appropriate use of each procedure and to help explain them to their patients.

Keywords

Radiofrequency ablation (RFA) · Transthoracic lung biopsy · Percutaneous thoracic biopsy · Pleural biopsy · Mediastinal biopsy · Thoracentesis · Pleural chest tube drainage

The role of the interventional thoracic radiologist has significantly increased in the last decade. Its scope now encompasses both diagnostics and therapeutics with significant overlap between the two. This chapter will describe the different types of thoracic interventional procedures, the clinical indications for them, and where appropriate, a description of how they are performed. The interventional procedures that will be covered include radiofrequency (RF) ablation of lung lesions; transthoracic needle biopsy of lung, mediastinal, and pleural disease; thoracentesis; and chest tube drainage.

For all interventional procedures, patients should be adequately consented, including discussion of benefits and possible complications of the procedure. Many of these complications are

D. Barnes
Central Manchester University Hospitals NHS Foundation Trust, Oxford Road, Manchester, M13 9WL, UK
e-mail: daniel_barnes_50@msn.com

K. Amjadi
Department of Medicine,
The Ottawa Hospital, 1053 Carling Avenue, Ottawa, ON K1Y 4E9, Canada

K. Amjadi
Interventional Pulmonology, Civic Hospital, 1053 Carling Avenue, Ottawa, ON K1Y 4E9, Canada

J. M. Seely (✉)
Department of Medical Imaging, The Ottawa Hospital, University of Ottawa, 501 Smyth Rd., Ottawa, ON K1H 8L6, Canada
e-mail: jeseely@ottawahospital.on.ca

J. P. Kanne (ed.), *Clinically Oriented Pulmonary Imaging*,
Respiratory Medicine, DOI: 10.1007/978-1-61779-542-8_17,

Table 17.1 Indications for Radiofrequency Ablation (RFA)

Patients with lung tumors <3 cm who cannot undergo surgery, chemotherapy, and/or radiotherapy
Patients with lung tumors <3 cm who have failed prior treatment
Patients with metastatic lung disease and ≤5 lesions
Patients with intractable chest wall pain or hypertrophic osteoarthropathy

generic such as pain, bleeding, and infection. However, complications specific to an individual procedure will be discussed in the relevant sections. Likewise, any abnormality in a patient's clotting profile must be addressed. Generally a patient's International Normalized Ratio (INR) should be below 1.3; however, thoracentesis can be performed at INR up to 1.5 without any increased risks [1]. Most institutions have helpful local policies and resources guiding physicians regarding anticoagulation of patients on a case-by-case basis perioperatively.

Radiofrequency Ablation of Lung Tumors

Image-guided RF thermal ablation has been used as an effective treatment for malignant lesions, both primary and secondary, since it was first used to treat hepatic lesions in the 1990s [2]. Since then, RF ablation has grown to encompass the treatment of renal, splenic, prostatic, brain, and breast masses [3, 4]. RF ablation of lung malignancies in humans was first reported in 2000 [5], and the technique has grown steadily and is now recognized as a safe and effective treatment for patients with both primary and metastatic thoracic malignancies (see Table 17.1).

This minimally invasive therapy works on the basis of thermal injury to the tumor with eventual coagulative necrosis and death of the affected tissue [4]. The equipment varies between manufacturers, but the basic design is the same, consisting of a RF generator to supply the current, a needle electrode that is inserted

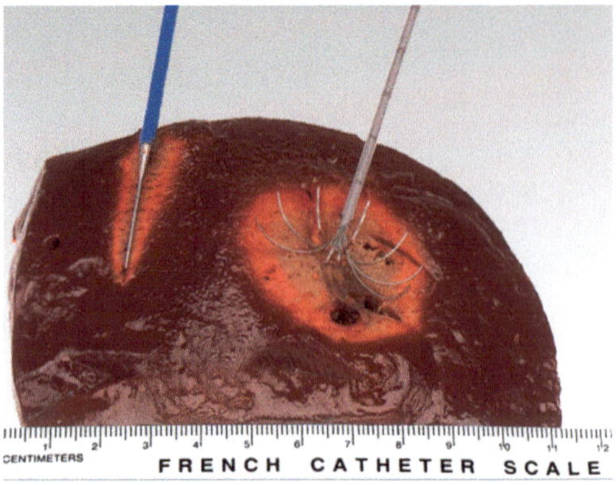

Fig. 17.1 Picture depicting the differing areas of thermal injury achieved by the linear versus the array probes (LeVeen RF electrode) on a piece of liver. (Obtained with permission from Boston Scientific)

into the patient, and a grounding pad to insulate the patient from thermal injury. The patient forms part of the 'electrical circuit', and when the AC current is applied, the exposed tip of the probe generates frictional heat, which in turn causes heating of the adjacent tissue mass and, when above 60°C, results in cell death [6]. The lung is well suited to this type of treatment as the surrounding air causes an insulating effect around the mass allowing the required temperature to be achieved with increased efficiency and thus reducing the treatment time. There are two principle probe designs, either a simple linear probe, like a biopsy needle, or a probe with multiple deployable 'tines' at the end that form an 'array' and an 'umbrella' appearance as shown in Fig. 17.1 [6]. The deployable version allows a larger area to be treated with a single probe, as compared to the linear probes.

Although the procedure can theoretically be performed under a variety of imaging modalities (ultrasound or fluoroscopy), practically most RF ablations of lung lesions are carried out under CT guidance to provide the most accurate positioning of the probe and evidence of treatment progression. The patient is positioned as required, taking into account patient comfort (a single treatment can take upwards of 15 min) and the safest and usually shortest route to the lesion. Using appropriate local anesthetic, the probe is inserted under CT guidance into the

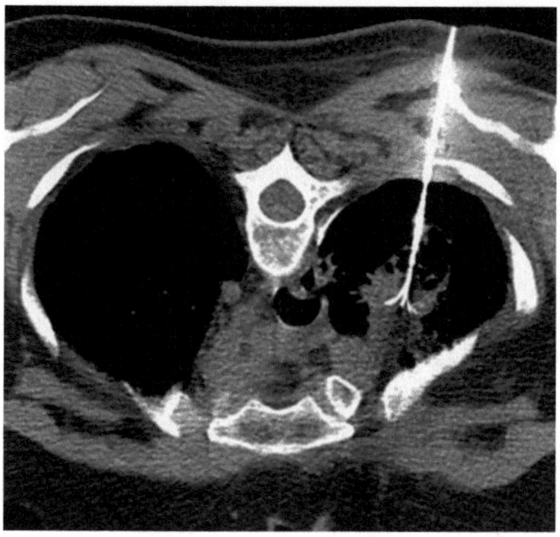

Fig. 17.2 Axial CT scan showing the array type probe with its tines deployed in the center of the tumor

center of lesion, and the tines are deployed as shown in Fig. 17.2. The length of the tines is chosen to correspond to the size of the tumor being treated. Then, using an appropriate treatment protocol, which varies with the apparatus, the RF ablation is performed. Depending on the size of the lesion, multiple treatments may be required for a single lesion for complete ablation, and this is judged by interval CT scans throughout the procedure [6].

An important part of the procedure is giving appropriate sedation and analgesia. In our experience, this is particularly important towards the end of a treatment when patient's pain and agitation are most pronounced. Although some earlier studies report using general anesthesia [4, 7] many centers now perform the procedure using conscious sedation with no significant problems [3, 8, 9]. After the procedure, the patient should be carefully monitored and appropriate analgesia given. In our center, the patient is always admitted for overnight observation regardless of the presence or absence of complications.

The main complications of RF ablation include pneumothorax, pain, and pleural effusions (see Table 17.3). A review of the current literature relating to this topic reports the pneumothorax rate at 28% with 14% requiring chest tube insertion [8]. Interestingly, several studies have found no correlation between the probe size and rate of pneumothorax, which may relate to the fact that the probe in effect heat-seals its own path when withdrawn. Other rarer complications have been reported including acute respiratory distress syndrome, massive hemoptysis [3], third degree burns due to suboptimal grounding of the patient, vocal cord palsy [7], tumor destruction syndrome (myalgia and fever), and brachial plexus nerve injury [4, 10] (see Table 17.2).

Appropriate patient selection is vital and should be carried out in a multidisciplinary setting, as it is often the last treatment option available. Although surgery and radiation

Table 17.2 Complications of RFA

Pneumothorax 15–29% (14% requiring chest tube insertion) [11]
Hemoptysis 0–12% [11]
Pneumonia 0–22% [11]
Pulmonary abscess 0–6% [11, 12]
Hemothorax 0–2% [11]
Bronchopleural fistula 1% [11] Exacerbation of COPD 0–6% [11]
Acute respiratory distress syndrome 0–3% [11]
Inflammation-related aseptic pleuritis and interstitial pneumonia 1.2% [12]
Third degree burns due to inadequate grounding of the patient 1% [11]
Vocal cord palsy 1% [11]
Tumor destruction syndrome (myalgia and fever) 1%
Neural injury such as phrenic, brachial plexus, or recurrent laryngeal nerve injury <1%
Continuous chest wall pain <1%
Tumor tract seeding 1% [11]
Death 0.6% [12]

Table 17.3 Limitations of RFA

Less effective if tumor >3 cm
Larger probes, saline injections necessary to increase heat production-tumor necrosis in larger tumors
Unable to achieve tumor necrosis when adjacent to large vascular structures

therapy are still the best primary treatment options for primary lung cancers and metastases, these may not be possible due to the stage of the tumor and comorbidities. With regard to pulmonary metastases, many patients are not eligible for surgery due to unfavorable histology (particularly with colorectal carcinoma), extent of disease elsewhere in the body, high risk of recurrence, and other comorbidities [9].

These patients, along with those with locally recurrent tumors who have exhausted other treatment options including chemotherapy and radiotherapy, are potential candidates for RF treatment. The conventional primary aim of RF ablation of lung tumors is cure, or at least local control. However, RF ablation can be used for symptomatic relief in certain situations, one of which is hypertrophic osteoarthropathy (HOA). This disabling condition is a secondary complication of some primary lung tumors and is characterized by digital clubbing, arthralgia and arthritis, and periostitis [13]. The pain associated with HOA can be crippling and often resistant to conventional analgesics [13]. RF ablation of the primary lung cancer in these patients has shown to provide symptomatic relief, particularly reducing arthralgia and swelling [13, 14]. Some patients also choose to undergo RFA as their primary treatment. Patients who have already undergone ablation of a lung tumor may be candidates for repeat ablations, as there is no limit to the total number of ablations that can be performed in the lung.

Over the last decade, a number of studies and case series looking at outcome data on RF treatment of pulmonary lesions have been published. Although there are no randomized trials comparing RF ablation against other treatment modalities, published data indicate that RF ablation is effective [15]. The largest multicenter intention to treat trial involving both primary and metastatic lung cancer reported cancer-specific survival of 92% (78–98%) at 1 year and 73% (54–86%) at 2 years in patients with stages 1–4 NSCLC, 91% (78–96%) at 1 year and 68% (54–80%) at 2 years in patients with colorectal metastases, and 93% (67–99%) at 1 year and 67% (48–84%) at 2 years in patients with other metastases [9]. This compares favorably with the 2-year survival of only 36% for external beam radiotherapy for primary lung cancer [16]. These data also compare favorably with the 2-year survival data from the international registry for metastases following surgical resection, which is approximately 60% [8]. With regard to metastatic disease, only one lung should be treated at a time and only up to three lesions within one lung during a treatment.

The only real tumor variable that appears to affect outcome is size (see Table 17.3). Several series have shown that the efficacy of treatment diminishes with increasing size of the tumor [15]. One such study reported 100% necrosis if the tumor was <3 cm but only 23% if >3 cm [3]. In our center, only lesions 3 cm or smaller are generally treated (see Fig. 17.3).

The contraindications to RF ablation of lung tumors include the patient being too unwell to undergo the procedure; the inability to stop anticoagulation; and technical factors such as tumor invading vital mediastinal structures, tumor abutting the heart, and implanted pacemakers and defibrillators. Patients with pacemakers and defibrillators may be treated with special precautions taken to inactivate the devices during the procedure ('safe mode').

Appropriate and timely follow-up imaging is vital. This can be performed with CT, MRI, or PET-CT. However, at present the mainstay is contrast-enhanced CT. Most reports advocate close follow-up, particularly early after treatment. Follow-up interval is variable, but many centers advocate follow-up at 6 weeks, then regularly every 3–6 months. The large RAPTURE study imaged subjects immediately after the procedure, at 1 month, then at 3 month intervals for 2 years [9].

Imaging findings following RF ablation are well described [3, 4, 7]. Immediately after therapy there is a characteristic increase in the size of the lesion and a decrease in its attenuation (density). A halo of ground-glass opacity is typically apparent (Fig. 17.3b) with the aim of having at least 5 mm halo surrounding the lesion immediately after treatment, as this finding is associated with complete necrosis of the mass

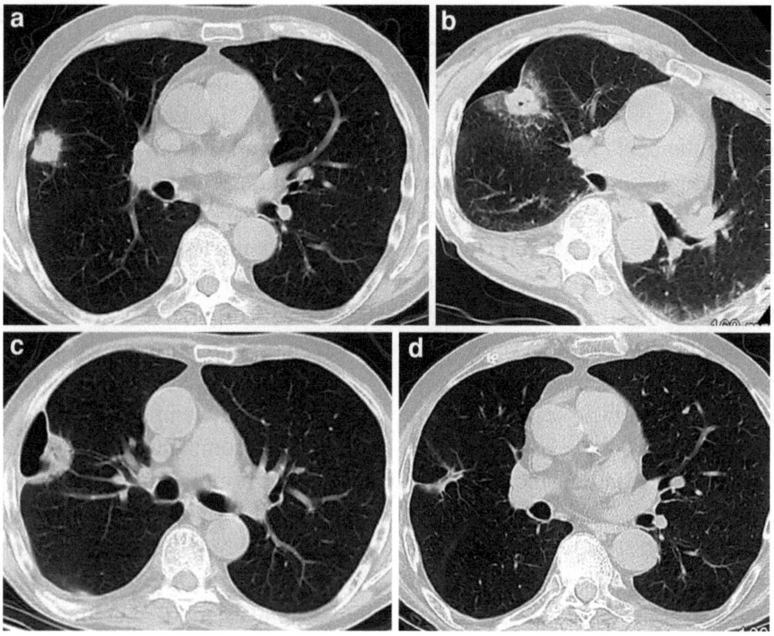

Fig. 17.3 **a** Axial CT scan depicting a peripheral nodule immediately prior to treatment. Due to peripheral location and size <3 cm, it is an optimal lesion for RF ablation therapy. **b** Axial CT scan taken immediately after the RF ablation. Note the ground-glass halo around the lesion consistent with successful treatment. There is a small post-procedure pneumothorax lateral to the tumor. **c** Axial CT scan 6 weeks following treatment showing a more solid lesion with resolution of the ground-glass halo. The pneumothorax has become loculated. **d** Axial CT scan 1 year following treatment. The tumor remnant has shrunken to become a linear scar. The pneumothorax has resolved

[3]. The appearance in the next 48–72 h is sometimes called the 'cockade phenomenon' due to its appearance of multiple concentric rings surrounding the lesion [4]. These changes are thought to be as a result of tumor necrosis, damaged normal lung, and the associated inflammatory response that ensues. At 1 month after treatment, the size of the tumor often appears larger as the whole treated area, and the surrounding halo becomes denser, corresponding to the area of necrosis, which includes the ablated tumor and surrounding lung (Fig. 17.3c). From 3 months onwards, the mass should decrease in size and often becomes wedge or linear shaped (Fig. 17.3d). Cavitation may occur in up to 20% of patients and often resolves [6]. Incomplete tumor ablation and tumor reoccurrence can be detected by contrast enhancement. As a rule, non-viable tumor will not enhance. The only caveat to this is a recognized thin rim of peripheral enhancement that can occur and generally resolves over the first 3 months and is thought to be as a result of peripheral hyperemia [3]. New enhancement of the mass is indicative of new tumor growth. PET-CT can be used to assess residual or new tumor growth when CT is inconclusive [8].

Overall, RFA provides an effective alternative to conventional therapy for pulmonary metastases, previously treated lung carcinoma, as well as primary treatment in patients in whom conventional therapy is not indicated. Careful patient selection and appropriate imaging following the procedure are vital. Within the first 4–6 weeks, physicians can expect an increase in tumor size. However, any growth beyond this time should be viewed with suspicion for disease progression.

Image Guided Percutaneous Thoracic Biopsies

The detection of thoracic lesions, including pleural and mediastinal, but particularly parenchymal, is occurring with increasing frequency and at an earlier stage. The reasons for this include cancer screening programs and the increased reliance on imaging for day-to-day clinical management. Image-guided transthoracic needle biopsy (TTNB) is now a vital tool in the assessment of many thoracic lesions because it is cost effective and minimally invasive when compared to open thoracotomy or thoracoscopy. TTNB facilitates appropriate clinical decisions including therapeutic strategies if malignant, appropriate treatment if infective, or no further course of action if benign.

Specific indications for TTNB include irregular suspicious lesions, encompassing those that are semi-solid, solid, or have incomplete calcification; lesions in patients with a history of malignancy; and patients with mediastinal or pleural masses or pleural thickening. The parenchymal and mediastinal lesions will be discussed together while the pleural disease will be considered separately.

The most commonly used modalities for image-guided percutaneous thoracic biopsies are fluoroscopy and CT. However, there has been a trend towards predominantly CT-guided thoracic biopsies, particularly of mediastinal and pleural lesions [17]. Although ultrasound (US) guidance can be used [18], particularly for very peripheral and mediastinal lesions, there are inherent limitations in this technique resulting from the lack of penetration of US waves through air and lung tissue. It is not a particularly widely used technique, typically reserved for pleural or subpleural lesions.

Biopsies can be performed by either fine needle aspiration (FNA), which provides a sample for cytological analysis, or by cutting (core) needle biopsy (CNB), which provides a specimen for histological analysis. Examples of the needles are shown in Fig. 17.4. Early reports found cytology to be inferior to histology for cell typing malignant lesions [19]. However, the presence of a cytopathologist at the time of biopsy has shown to increase the diagnostic accuracy of the FNA [20]. Overall diagnostic accuracy varies from 65 to 95% depending on the technique, nodule size, and modality used [21].

The accuracies of FNA and CNB are comparable, with sensitivities of 0.86–0.98 vs. 0.92–0.98, respectively [19, 22]. In a study where individual lesions were biopsied by both FNA and CNB techniques, diagnostic accuracy for malignancy and cell typing of epithelioid tumors was comparable [23]. However, for non-epithelioid tumors such as lymphoma and other mediastinal lesions like thymoma, CNB was superior to FNA [23]. This is likely due to the fact the tissue architecture plays a major part in the diagnosis and that the diagnosis often requires multiple ancillary studies such as immunohistochemistry [23]. Bocking et al. recommended that all mediastinal masses should be biopsied using CNB technique to increase diagnostic accuracy [22].

Size does matter when considering the biopsy of a nodule. At our institution, biopsies are being requested on smaller and smaller lesions. There are significant limitations with this as the diagnostic accuracy of the biopsy falls as the lesion becomes smaller. One study found that for nodules <15 mm, the diagnostic accuracy for malignancy was 70% vs. 81% for larger lesions [21]. Another study showed that results for 47 lesions measuring 0.8–1.0 cm were considerably better (sensitivity, 88%; accuracy, 92%) than those for 10 lesions measuring 0.5–0.7 cm (sensitivity, 50%; accuracy, 70%) [24]. In our institution, we have extensive experience biopsying lesions as small as 7–8 mm. Nevertheless, anecdotally in lesions of this size in the lower lobes and in challenging patients, the accuracy is probably around 50%. If a biopsy result is 'non-diagnostic', the radiologist and referring physician should discuss whether to repeat the biopsy, follow the lesion with sequential imaging, or obtain a surgical biopsy.

CNB has a significantly higher accuracy than FNA for the diagnosis of benign lesions, commonly granulomas [23, 24]. This was demonstrated in a study where the sensitivity of FNA for the diagnosis of necrotizing granulomas was only 2.2% compared to 91% for CNB [25]. If the pre-test probability of malignancy is low and if FNA yields no malignant cells, CNB is performed whenever possible. It is essential in these cases to have a cytotechnologist present to review the slides at the time of the biopsy to determine if the sample is non-diagnostic, in which case the radiologist can then proceed with CNB. At our institution, a cytotechnologist is present for all percutaneous thoracic biopsies, providing rapid assessment of the material before the procedure is completed.

Often the aim of the biopsy is to confirm or refute the presence of malignancy. However, when a patient is immunocompromised or has a hematological malignancy, the differential diagnosis may be broad and include inflammation, infection, and hemorrhage. The role of the percutaneous biopsy in these patients has been found to be very beneficial, altering management in 61% [25].

Technique

Under image guidance, local anesthetic is infiltrated into the subcutaneous tissues down to the pleura. Depending on the biopsy technique being used, either an introducer or FNA needle is inserted into the lesion under image guidance. If an introducer is used, then either a CNB or FNA needle is inserted through the introducer needle and the samples are taken. Examples of the biopsy needles and introducers are shown in Fig. 17.4.

A CT scan is required for planning purposes in every patient before undergoing the biopsy. Generally, the shortest path to the lesion is taken. Although crossing fissures should be avoided if possible, if the shortest distance includes crossing a fissure, this may be the preferred route. A transfissural approach has not been shown to increase the pneumothorax rate [26]. Care is taken to avoid adjacent bulla or vessels. An example of a lesion seen on chest radiography and the subsequent successfully biopsied under fluoroscopic guidance is shown in Fig. 17.5. CT guidance is almost always used for more difficult lesions and those that cannot be adequately identified such as the ground-glass attenuation lesion shown in Fig. 17.6.

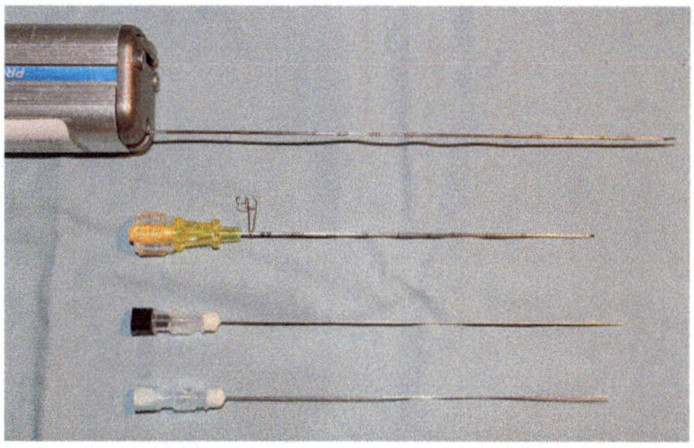

Fig. 17.4 Picture showing the apparati used for percutaneous lung biopsies. At the top is a 20G cutting needle biopsy gun with a 19G introducer below it. The lower two needles are a 22G FNA needle (*black hub*) and a 25G FNA needle (*blue hub*)

In order to reduce the rate of complications, needle manipulation should only occur during suspended respiration. When explaining the biopsy to a patient, it is prudent to 'coach' the patient on breathing instructions as this can often make the difference between a difficult and an easy biopsy, particularly with a smaller lesion. Once the procedure is complete, it is important to monitor the patient closely. Chest radiography is routinely used to detect any post-procedural pneumothorax. While many institutions observe patients for 2–4 h following TTNB, one study showed that patients without pneumothorax can be discharged safely 30 min after TTNB [27]. At our institution, we obtain a chest radiograph 30 min following the biopsy, repeating in 30–60 min if a pneumothorax is present. Patients are discharged if they are asymptomatic and if chest radiography shows no pneumothorax or a small, stable pneumothorax. Discharge instructions include returning to the hospital in case of worsening chest pain, hemoptysis, or shortness of breath. If there is an enlarging or clinically significant pneumothorax, a pleural drain is inserted, and, whenever possible, the patient is discharged home with a Heimlich

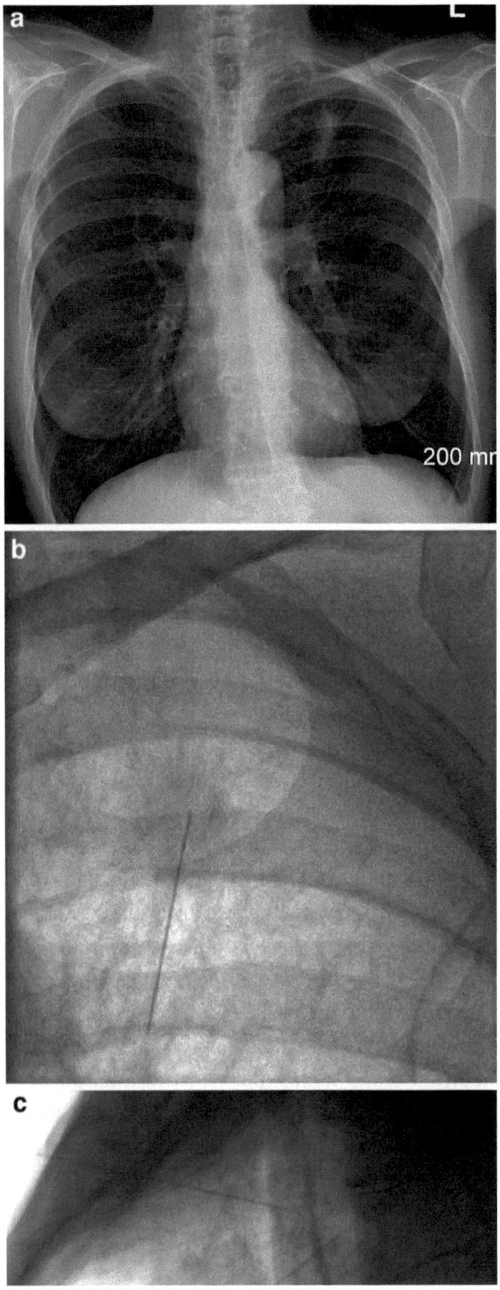

Fig. 17.5 **a** Chest radiograph shows a poorly-defined lesion in the left upper lobe. **b**, **c** Fontal and lateral images from the fluoroscopically guided biopsy of the lesion in Fig. 17.5a. The two images show how the radiologist can be confident of a good sample as the tip of the FNA needle can be seen within the lesion on both AP and lateral views

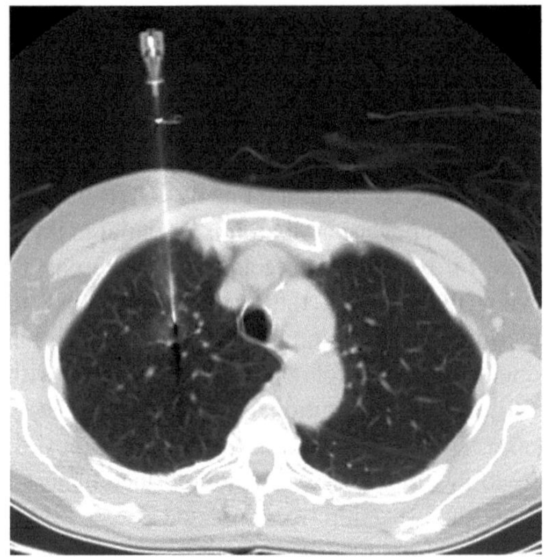

Fig. 17.6 Axial CT showing a CT guided biopsy of a small central ground-glass attenuation lesion that was occult on fluoroscopy

valve attached. They are instructed to return to the department 24–48 h later to be re-evaluated and to have the drain removed.

The most common complications of TTNB are hemorrhage and pneumothorax. In a large study by Yeow et al. looking at 660 CT-guided lung biopsies, the pneumothorax rate was 23% with 1% of patients requiring pleural drain insertion. There were no mortalities. Pneumothorax rate increased with lesions less than 2 cm and with lesions in a subpleural location. The risk of hemorrhage was also associated with a lesion size less than 2 cm and a distance of more than 2.1 cm from the pleural surface. Interestingly, larger needle size was not a predictor of pneumothorax or bleeding. Use of a 25 gauge needle has been shown to be accurate and effective with a lower pneumothorax rate, particularly in patients with underlying emphysema [28, 29]. The small caliber and increased flexibility of the needle (Fig. 17.7) presumably account for the improved safety profile.

Major complications are rare and include tension pneumothorax, massive hemoptysis, cardiac tamponade, and air embolus. The major

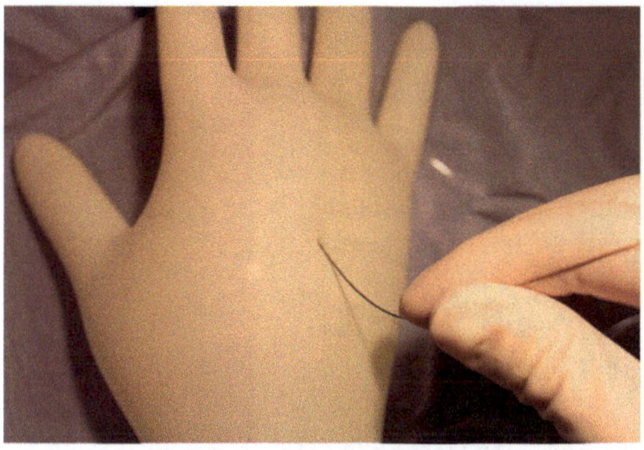

Fig. 17.7 Image showing the flexibility of a 25 gauge FNA needle, thought to minimize pneumothorax rate during biopsy

complications typically occur during or immediately after the procedure and require prompt action. Air embolus should be strongly considered if the patient develops acute neurologic signs or symptoms. Immediate CT scanning of the head and chest should be performed. If available, hyperbaric chamber treatment may be indicated for air embolus [30].

Overall, TTNB plays a vital role in the management of patients with both mediastinal and parenchymal lesions. The imaging modality chosen depends on operator preference and availability, although most biopsies are performed under CT guidance. The accuracy for diagnosing malignancy is high for both FNA and CNB. However, when the pre-test probability of malignancy is low or intermediate, CNB may be preferred given its higher accuracy for benign lesions.

Pleural Biopsies

Pleural biopsies play an important role in the investigation of both undiagnosed exudative pleural effusions and pleural thickening (both generalized and focal). There are many causes of pleural thickening including asbestos related pleural disease, infection, and trauma. However, the aim of a biopsy is to distinguish malignancy, particularly mesothelioma, from benign causes (Fig. 17.8).

Although surgical biopsies remain the gold standard for pleural thickening, patient and economic factors limit the practicality of this technique. Thoracoscopy, although very accurate with a sensitivity for malignancy of 93% [31], is often not readily available and requires the presence of pleural fluid to safely enter the pleural space. It is also an invasive procedure with reported major complication rates of 1.9–15% [32]. In 2001, image guided pleural CNB was shown by Adams and Gleeson to be a minimally invasive and safe means of obtaining adequate tissue for a histologic diagnosis of the cause of pleural thickening, with an overall accuracy of 91% [32]. This technique should be considered as a first line test for investigating suspected malignant pleural thickening (see Table 17.4).

Table 17.4 Indications for pleural biopsy

Nodular, mediastinal, or circumferential pleural thickening >4–5 mm

Historically, pleural biopsies have been performed blindly using an Abrams or Cope needle. The blind technique has a sensitivity of 79% for TB, in which the pleural thickening is usually generalized. However in cases of malignancy where thickening is patchy, basal, or midline, the sensitivity is much lower at 47% [33].

Image-guided pleural biopsies can be performed using either US or CT guidance, although CT is the predominant modality used. One important study by Maskell et al. reported a sensitivity of 87% for malignancy using CT-guided technique compared to a sensitivity of 47% using a blind approach [33]. Subsequently, this had led to a decline in the number of blind pleural biopsies being performed [34].

Pleural biopsies can be performed with either FNA or CNB technique. However, in contrast to percutaneous lung biopsy, these techniques are not equally effective in the diagnosis of malignancy. CNB is more sensitive than FNA with values of 88% and 78%, respectively [32]. Furthermore, the CNB is significantly superior to FNA for diagnosing mesothelioma with sensitivities of 93% and 50%, respectively [32].

Although less frequently used, US-guided pleural biopsies are effective because the

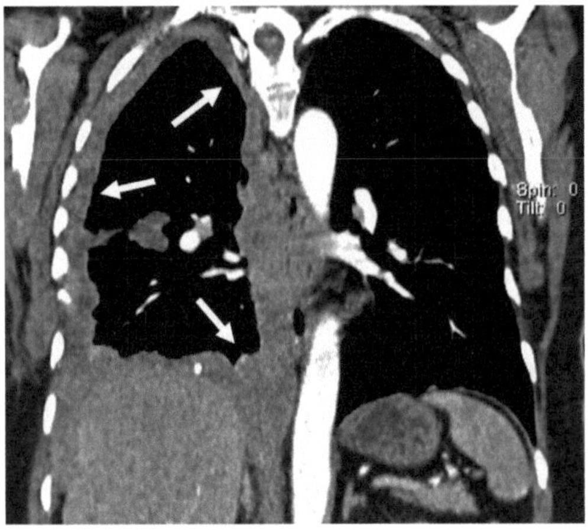

Fig. 17.8 Coronal CT of the thorax, showing diffusely thickened pleura encasing the right hemithorax and extending into the minor fissure. Arrows denote the pleural thickening. This was diagnosed as a mesothelioma with CNB

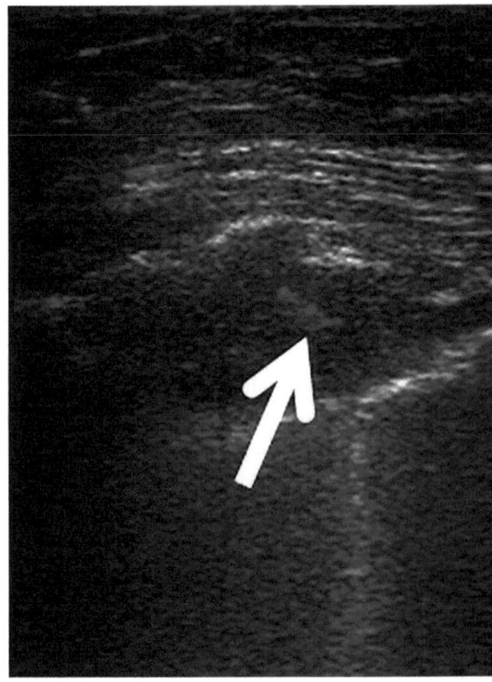

Fig. 17.9 Axial image of a pleural mass being biopsied under ultrasound guidance. The arrow points to the tip of the biopsy needle within the lesion

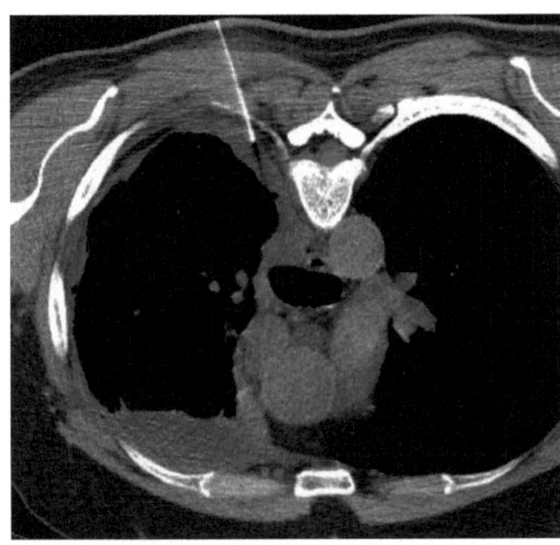

Fig. 17.10 Prone image of an axial chest CT shows the 'parallel' approach of the biopsy needle into the pleural thickening, thereby maximizing the tissue sample yield

peripheral location of the pleura is ideal for US. Furthermore, no ionizing radiation is used. Heilo et al. reported a sensitivity of 77% for US-guided pleural biopsies for the diagnosis of mesothelioma, similar to that of CT-guided biopsy and significantly higher than blind biopsy [35]. An example of an US-guided pleural biopsy is shown in Fig. 17.9.

The most important principle of pleural biopsy is to use image guidance to maximize sampling of as much viable tissue as possible, and obtaining the biopsy parallel to the plane of the pleural thickening ensures that the maximal amount of tissue is sampled (Fig. 17.10). This approach can result in an adequate sample even when pleural thickness is less than 5 mm [36]. Out our institution, TTNB is only performed with pleural thickening of 5 mm or more. When mesothelioma is suspected, CNB should be used.

Complications of percutaneous pleural biopsies are low, occurring in less than 1% of patients [37], and include pneumothorax, hemothorax, and laceration of the underlying abdominal viscera. Although not a direct complication of a percutaneous pleural biopsy, tumor seeding along the biopsy tract can occur in patients with mesothelioma with reported rates ranging from 4 [38] to 20% [39]. Post-procedural radiotherapy has been shown to reduce this risk [40], although it is not universally employed. One advantage of image-guided pleural biopsy over thoracoscopy and surgical biopsy is the lower rate of tumor seeding. In one recent study, the incidence of needle track seeding was 4% for image-guided CNB and 22% for surgical biopsy [38]. Overall, image-guided percutaneous pleural biopsy is safe and effective. It has comparable sensitivities to surgical biopsies and thoracoscopy and is safer, less invasive, and less costly and requires less time.

Thoracentesis

Pleural effusions are extremely common with a myriad of causes including both pulmonary and non-pulmonary causes. The commonest etiologies are thoracic malignancy, infections, and cardiac dysfunction. Many pleural effusions do not require sampling, and the patient's history and non-invasive investigations can often provide the most likely diagnosis. A common example of this is bilateral pleural effusions in the presence of cardiac dysfunction; the fluid should only be sampled if either the patient is not responding to treatment or if there are atypical features. Clinical features which should prompt fluid sampling include a suspected exudate, particularly TB and malignancy, or if the effusion fails to respond to therapy.

Many clinicians are extremely competent at sampling pleural effusions, particularly if they are large. However, one of the commonest indications for an image-guided thoracentesis is an unsuccessful blind 'dry tap'. Other indications for an image-guided aspiration include a small or loculated effusion [41]. Pleural aspiration is also performed for pneumothoraces, although image guidance is not usually required.

There are no specific contraindications to thoracentesis other than those that typically prohibit any invasive procedure. US is almost always used for image guidance. Rarely, a loculated pneumothorax will require fluoroscopy or CT guidance for drainage.

The important role of US-guided pleural aspiration has been well documented in several studies. Following failed blind aspiration, US-guided aspiration is successful in up to 88% of patients [42–44]. The procedure itself is relatively simple. The general convention is to use image guidance to mark the site for aspiration rather than follow the needle into the fluid in real-time. After anesthetizing the skin and subcutaneous tissues, the fluid can be aspirated. It is important that enough fluid be obtained for adequate analysis, usually at least 50 mL (45). Generally a thoracic radiologist will send the sample analysis for protein, lactose dehydrogenase, glucose, cell count and differential, pH, Gram stain, cytology, and microbiological culture. However, if more specific tests are required, these should be specified in advance.

The primary complication from a thoracentesis is pneumothorax, the incidence of which is greatly decreased when using image guidance. One study demonstrated that US-guided needle placement resulted in no pneumothoraces as compared to a rate of 29% when performed without image guidance, regardless of effusion size [45]. Another study showed similar results of 3% pneumothorax rate with image guidance in contrast to 18% without image guidance. Furthermore, the number of patients requiring drainage of pneumothorax was also lower in the image-guided cohort [46].

A less common but potentially serious complication is visceral puncture, particularly to the spleen and liver. One interesting study compared clinical and US guidance for the potential site for aspiration of pleural fluid on the same patients and showed that using US not only increased the yield and accuracy but also would have prevented organ puncture in 10% of patients [41].

A rare but potentially catastrophic complication is lung re-expansion pulmonary edema (RPE), which has a mortality rate of up to 20% [47]. The rate of RPE has been quoted as high as 14%, but a more recent investigation puts the figure at less than 1% [48]. Limiting the initial amount of fluid drainage to less than 1.5 L has been suggested to minimize the risk of RPE. However, there appears to be no safe volume, and volumes of up 6.5 L have been removed with no consequence [48]. Animal studies suggest a correlation between the drop in intrapleural pressure during thoracentesis and the development of RPE. Risk for RPE is minimal if pleural pressure is kept above −20 mmHg and quite high if pleural pressure is below −40 mmHg [49, 50]. Thus, using intrapleural manometry has been suggested while removing large volumes of pleural fluid to minimize the risk of RPE. Development of chest pain during thoracentesis has been shown to be associated with significant drop in pleural pressures. In the absence of manometry, ceasing drainage when patients report chest pain has been suggested [51]. Furthermore, the fact that pneumothorax rate increases with volume of fluid aspirated should be considered when deciding how much fluid to drain [52].

Many non-radiologists are now performing US-guided aspirations, particularly those involved with critical and respiratory care, with good results. A study by Mayo et al. reported a pneumothorax rate of only 1.3% in 232 aspirations in patients on ventilators [53]. A more recent study of over 900 US examinations performed by respiratory physicians found a 99.6% accuracy in detecting pleural fluid [54]. Of the 558 patients in this study who underwent a procedure, only 0.5% had a major complication, similar to results reported in other studies [54].

Chest Tube Insertion

The insertion of a chest tube into the pleural space is a common procedure. The indications for insertion include complicated pleural collections and pneumothoraces. Complicated pleural collections are those that fail to resolve without drainage and can include loculated or non-loculated parapneumonic effusion, empyema, malignant effusion, and hemothorax (infected or sterile). Drainage is required to control infection, allow lung re-expansion, and prevent long-term complications such as pleural fibrosis (fibrothorax) and trapped lung [55]. Drainage of malignant pleural effusion is required for effective pleurodesis. The choice of a percutaneous versus a surgical approach in patients with established collections remains controversial. If the collection has been present for more than 6 weeks, surgical approach may be the best option, since patients often develop a thick, fibrotic visceral pleural peel that limits lung re-expansion despite drainage of the effusion.

Many chest drains can be safely inserted without image guidance in the mid axillary line just above the level of the 6th rib. However, for cases of smaller or loculated collections or for those that are posteriorly located, image guidance is generally required. Imaging modality used is operator specific, but as with thoracentesis, US is generally preferred. CT guidance is typically reserved for complex loculated collections or those obscured by bone. As expected, several studies have shown efficacy of US guidance for chest tube insertion, with success rate approaching 100% [56]. Another study showed image-guided chest tube insertion was successful in 77% of cases where a clinically inserted tube had failed [57]. One particular advantage of image guidance is that drains can be inserted into particular locules within a complex collection with good effect [58–60]. For difficult collections or for those that are not adequately seen on US, CT guidance should be used [57].

Catheters for pleural drainage vary in size from larger bore drains (22–34 French) favored by surgeons to the smaller ones preferred by radiologists (8–14 French). The small tubes used have multiple drainage holes allowing for rapid drainage and form a pigtail, maximizing patient comfort and safety (see Fig. 17.11). The ‘pig tail’ will form in any space, correctly within the pleural space (as shown in Fig. 17.12), but generally do not form the shape of a ‘pig tail’ if they are present in a solid organ (see Fig. 17.13).

The catheter can be inserted either directly using a trocar method or a modified Seldinger technique. Traditionally, the latter technique is preferred because of perceived lower complication rates and reduced patient discomfort. Although it is generally accepted that the Seldinger technique using smaller drains is less painful for the patient, there is some debate as to whether it is in fact safer with continued reports of adverse outcomes [61]. In our institution, we primarily use the trocar technique with excellent results. Problems are likely to occur with either

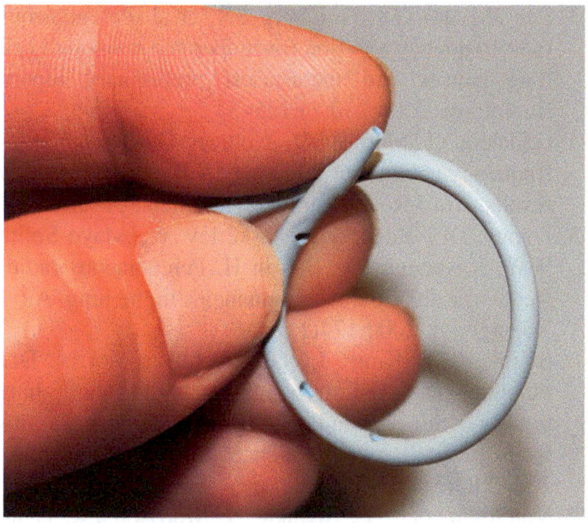

Fig. 17.11 Picture shows the end of a pigtail catheter with the 'pigtail' formed. The multiple drainage holes are easy to see

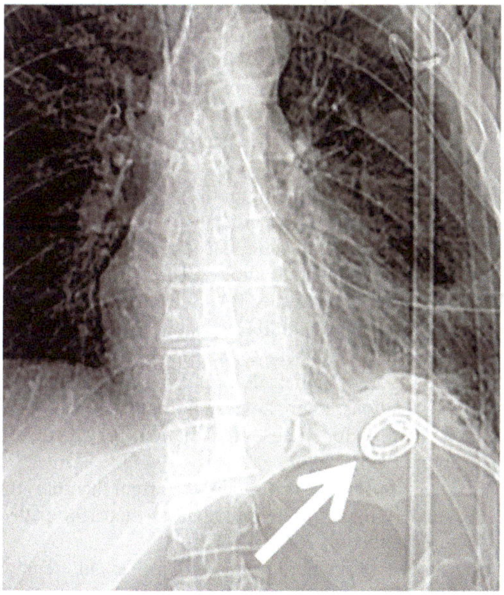

Fig. 17.12 Scout of a chest CT demonstrates good position of the left pigtail catheter (*arrow*) in the posterior left costophrenic recess

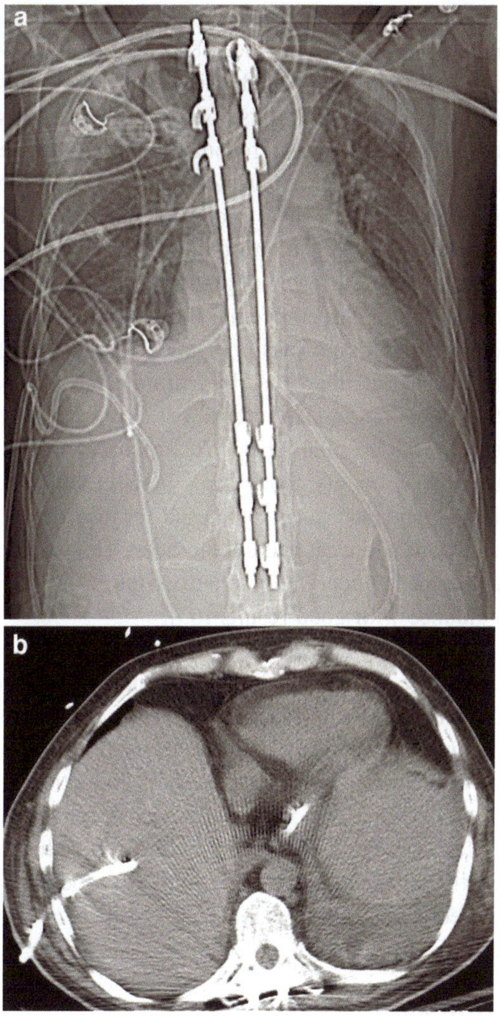

Fig. 17.13 **a** Scout view of a CT shows poor position of a right pigtail pleural catheter, as evidenced by the lack of formation of the pigtail, which was confirmed on abdominal CT (Fig. 17.13b) to be within the liver. The patient later expired from complications of tube removal. **b** Axial CT shows the catheter within the liver

technique when less experienced operators are not trained or supervised adequately.

Although many believe that larger bore drains are required for some collections, particularly empyemas, published studies do not support this stance. A very recent study by Rahman et al. reviewing the insertion of over 400 chest tubes for infection found that the size of the chest tube (ranging from <10F to >20F) was not associated with any significant difference in the number of patients who required surgery or died. However, patients who received smaller drains reported less pain [62]. Smaller drains should be inserted wherever possible.

Complications associated with chest tube insertion include pain, infection, drain dislodgement, and drain blockage. The commonest of these appears to be drain blockage with an incidence of approximately 8% [48]. Post-procedural drain care and flushing can reduce this complication. Routine use of fibrinolytic agents for empyemas is not recommended after one large randomized controlled trial showed no significant reduction in mortality, frequency of surgery, or length of hospital stay [63]. However, new recent data suggest has shown that in the setting of an empyema, the combination of intrapleural tissue plasminogen activator (tPA) and DNAase improves fluid drainage, reduces the rate of surgical referral, and reduces the length of hospital stay. Treatment with the individual agents alone was ineffective [64]. Image guidance can also be used for insertion of chest tubes to treat pneumothoraces. This can be performed under both fluoroscopic and CT guidance with good results [65].

Overall image-guided thoracentesis and chest tube insertion play a very important role in the management of patients with suspicious pleural effusions and collections from a variety of etiologies. The main benefit is reduction in complications and increased success rate after failed unguided attempts at the procedures, particularly in cases of small or loculated collections.

Summary

This chapter describes the major image-guided thoracic interventional procedures, including RF ablation; TTNB of lung, mediastinal, and pleural disease; thoracentesis, and pleural chest tube drainage. Clinical indications, risks, complications, and practical description are described.

References

1. McVay PA, Toy PT. Lack of increased bleeding after paracentesis and thoracentesis in patients with mild coagulation abnormalities. Transfusion. 1991;31(2): 164–71.
2. Goldberg SN, Gazelle GS, Solbiati L, et al. Ablation of liver tumors using percutaneous RF therapy. Am J Roentgenol. 1998;170(4):1023–8.
3. Lee JM, Jin GY, Goldberg SN, et al. Percutaneous radiofrequency ablation for inoperable non-small cell lung cancer and metastases: preliminary report. Radiology. 2004;230(1):125–34.
4. Gadaleta C, Mattioli V, Colucci G, et al. Radiofrequency ablation of 40 lung neoplasms: preliminary results. Am J Roentgenol. 2004;183(2):361–8.
5. Dupuy DE, Zagoria RJ, Akerley W, Mayo-Smith WW, Kavanagh PV, Safran H. Percutaneous radiofrequency ablation of malignancies in the lung. Am J Roentgenol. 2000;174(1):57–9.
6. Steinke K, King J, Glenn DW, Morris DL. Percutaneous radiofrequency ablation of lung tumors with expandable needle electrodes: tips from preliminary experience. Am J Roentgenol. 2004;183(3):605–11.
7. VanSonnenberg E, Shankar S, Morrison PR, et al. Radiofrequency ablation of thoracic lesions: part 2, initial clinical experience–technical and multidisciplinary considerations in 30 patients. Am J Roentgenol. 2005;184(2):381–90.
8. Chan VO, McDermott S, Malone DE, Dodd JD. Percutaneous radiofrequency ablation of lung tumors: evaluation of the literature using evidence-based techniques. J Thorac Imaging. 2011;26(1):18–26.
9. Lencioni R, Crocetti L, Cioni R, et al. Response to radiofrequency ablation of pulmonary tumours: a prospective, intention-to-treat, multicentre clinical trial (the RAPTURE study). Lancet Oncol. 2008;9(7):621–8.
10. Hiraki T, Gobara H, Mimura H, et al. Brachial nerve injury caused by percutaneous radiofrequency ablation of apical lung cancer: a report of four cases. J Vasc Interv Radiol. 2010;21(7):1129–33.
11. Rose SC, Thistlethwaite PA, Sewell PE, Vance RB. Lung cancer and radiofrequency ablation. J Vasc Interv Radiol. 2006;17(6):927–51. quiz 951.
12. Nomura M, Yamakado K, Nomoto Y, et al. Complications after lung radiofrequency ablation: risk factors for lung inflammation. Br J Radiol. 2008;81(963):244–9.
13. Nguyen S, Hojjati M. Review of current therapies for secondary hypertrophic pulmonary osteoarthropathy. Clin Rheumatol. 2010;30(1):7–13.
14. Kishi K, Nakamura H, Sudo A, et al. Tumor debulking by radiofrequency ablation in hypertrophic pulmonary osteoarthropathy associated with pulmonary carcinoma. Lung Cancer. 2002; 38(3):317–20.
15. de Baere T, Palussiere J, Auperin A, et al. Midterm local efficacy and survival after radiofrequency ablation of lung tumors with minimum follow-up of 1 year: prospective evaluation. Radiology. 2006; 240(2):587–96.
16. Talton BM, Constable WC, Kersh CR. Curative radiotherapy in non-small cell carcinoma of the lung. Int J Radiat Oncol Biol Phys. 1990;19(1):15–21.
17. Gohari A, Haramati LB. Complications of CT scan-guided lung biopsy: lesion size and depth matter. Chest. 2004;126(3):666–8.

18. Savage C, Zwischenberger JB. Image-guided fine needle aspirate strategies for staging of lung cancer. Clin Lung Cancer. 2000;2(2):101–10. discussion 111–102.
19. Klein JS, Salomon G, Stewart EA. Transthoracic needle biopsy with a coaxially placed 20-gauge automated cutting needle: results in 122 patients. Radiology. 1996;198(3):715–20.
20. Austin JH, Cohen MB. Value of having a cytopathologist present during percutaneous fine-needle aspiration biopsy of lung: report of 55 cancer patients and metaanalysis of the literature. Am J Roentgenol. 1993;160(1):175–7.
21. Kothary N, Lock L, Sze DY, Hofmann LV. Computed tomography-guided percutaneous needle biopsy of pulmonary nodules: impact of nodule size on diagnostic accuracy. Clin Lung Cancer. 2009;10(5):360–3.
22. Bocking A, Klose KC, Kyll HJ, Hauptmann S. Cytologic versus histologic evaluation of needle biopsy of the lung, hilum and mediastinum. Sensitivity, specificity and typing accuracy. Acta Cytol. 1995;39(3):463–71.
23. Gong Y, Sneige N, Guo M, Hicks ME, Moran CA. Transthoracic fine-needle aspiration vs concurrent core needle biopsy in diagnosis of intrathoracic lesions: a retrospective comparison of diagnostic accuracy. Am J Clin Pathol. 2006;125(3):438–44.
24. Wallace MJ, Krishnamurthy S, Broemeling LD, et al. CT-guided percutaneous fine-needle aspiration biopsy of small (< or =1-cm) pulmonary lesions. Radiology. 2002;225(3):823–8.
25. Thiessen R, Seely JM, Matzinger FR, et al. Necrotizing granuloma of the lung: imaging characteristics and imaging-guided diagnosis. Am J Roentgenol. 2007;189(6):1397–401.
26. Ayyappan AP, Souza CA, Seely J, Peterson R, Dennie C, Matzinger F. Ultrathin fine-needle aspiration biopsy of the lung with transfissural approach: does it increase the risk of pneumothorax? Am J Roentgenol. 2008;191(6):1725–9.
27. Dennie CJ, Matzinger FR, Marriner JR, Maziak DE. Transthoracic needle biopsy of the lung: results of early discharge in 506 outpatients. Radiology. 2001;219(1):247–51.
28. Oikonomou A, Matzinger FR, Seely JM, Dennie CJ, Macleod PJ. Ultrathin needle (25 G) aspiration lung biopsy: diagnostic accuracy and complication rates. Eur Radiol. 2004;14(3):375–82.
29. VanSonnenberg E, Goodacre BW, Wittich GR, Logrono R, Kennedy PT, Zwischenberger JB. Image-guided 25-gauge needle biopsy for thoracic lesions: diagnostic feasibility and safety. Radiology. 2003;227(2):414–8.
30. Hare S, Gupta A, Souza CA, Matzinger F, Seely J. Systemic arterial air embolism after percutaneous lung biopsy. Clin Radiol. 2011;66(7):589–96.
31. Blanc FX, Atassi K, Bignon J, Housset B. Diagnostic value of medical thoracoscopy in pleural disease: a 6-year retrospective study. Chest. 2002;121(5): 1677–83.
32. Adams RF, Gleeson FV. Percutaneous image-guided cutting-needle biopsy of the pleura in the presence of a suspected malignant effusion. Radiology. 2001; 219(2):510–4.
33. Maskell NA, Gleeson FV, Davies RJ. Standard pleural biopsy versus CT-guided cutting-needle biopsy for diagnosis of malignant disease in pleural effusions: a randomised controlled trial. Lancet. 2003;361(9366):1326–30.
34. Gopal M, Romero AB, Baillargeon J, Sharma G. Trends in pleural biopsies between 1996 and 2006 at a tertiary medical center. Am J Med Sci. 2010; 339(4):345–9.
35. Heilo A, Stenwig AE, Solheim OP. Malignant pleural mesothelioma: US-guided histologic core-needle biopsy. Radiology. 1999;211(3):657–9.
36. Adams RF, Gray W, Davies RJ, Gleeson FV. Percutaneous image-guided cutting needle biopsy of the pleura in the diagnosis of malignant mesothelioma. Chest. 2001;120(6):1798–802.
37. Qureshi NR, Gleeson FV. Imaging of pleural disease. Clin Chest Med. 2006;27(2):193–213.
38. Agarwal PP, Seely JM, Matzinger FR, et al. Pleural mesothelioma: sensitivity and incidence of needle track seeding after image-guided biopsy versus surgical biopsy. Radiology. 2006;241(2):589–94.
39. Screaton NJ, Flower CD. Percutaneous needle biopsy of the pleura. Radiol Clin North Am. 2000; 38(2):293–301.
40. Boutin C, Rey F, Viallat JR. Prevention of malignant seeding after invasive diagnostic procedures in patients with pleural mesothelioma. A randomized trial of local radiotherapy. Chest. 1995;108(3):754–8.
41. Diacon AH, Brutsche MH, Soler M. Accuracy of pleural puncture sites: a prospective comparison of clinical examination with ultrasound. Chest. 2003; 123(2):436–41.
42. Hirsch JH, Rogers JV, Mack LA. Real-time sonography of pleural opacities. Am J Roentgenol. 1981;136(2):297–301.
43. Kohan JM, Poe RH, Israel RH, et al. Value of chest ultrasonography versus decubitus roentgenography for thoracentesis. Am Rev Respir Dis. 1986; 133(6):1124–6.
44. O'Moore PV, Mueller PR, Simeone JF, et al. Sonographic guidance in diagnostic and therapeutic interventions in the pleural space. Am J Roentgenol. 1987;149(1):1–5.
45. Grogan DR, Irwin RS, Channick R, et al. Complications associated with thoracentesis. A prospective, randomized study comparing three different methods. Arch Intern Med. 1990;150(4): 873–7.
46. Raptopoulos V, Davis LM, Lee G, Umali C, Lew R, Irwin RS. Factors affecting the development of pneumothorax associated with thoracentesis. Am J Roentgenol. 1991;156(5):917–20.

47. Mahfood S, Hix WR, Aaron BL, Blaes P, Watson DC. Reexpansion pulmonary edema. Ann Thorac Surg. 1988;45(3):340–5.
48. Havelock T, Teoh R, Laws D, Gleeson F. Pleural procedures and thoracic ultrasound: British thoracic society pleural disease Guideline 2010. Thorax. 2010;65(Suppl 2):ii61–76.
49. Pavlin J, Cheney FW Jr. Unilateral pulmonary edema in rabbits after reexpansion of collapsed lung. J Appl Physiol. 1979;46(1):31–5.
50. Miller WC, Toon R, Palat H, Lacroix J. Experimental pulmonary edema following re-expansion of pneumothorax. Am Rev Respir Dis. 1973;108(3): 654–6.
51. Feller-Kopman D, Walkey A, Berkowitz D, Ernst A. The relationship of pleural pressure to symptom development during therapeutic thoracentesis. Chest. 2006;129(6):1556–60.
52. Josephson T, Nordenskjold CA, Larsson J, Rosenberg LU, Kaijser M. Amount drained at ultrasound-guided thoracentesis and risk of pneumothorax. Acta Radiol. 2009;50(1):42–7.
53. Mayo PH, Goltz HR, Tafreshi M, Doelken P. Safety of ultrasound-guided thoracentesis in patients receiving mechanical ventilation. Chest. 2004; 125(3):1059–62.
54. Rahman NM, Singanayagam A, Davies HE, et al. Diagnostic accuracy, safety and utilisation of respiratory physician-delivered thoracic ultrasound. Thorax. 2010;65(5):449–53.
55. Moulton JS. Image-guided management of complicated pleural fluid collections. Radiol Clin North Am. 2000;38(2):345–74.
56. Keeling AN, Leong S, Logan PM, Lee MJ. Empyema and effusion: outcome of image-guided small-bore catheter drainage. Cardiovasc Intervent Radiol. 2008;31(1):135–41.
57. VanSonnenberg E, Nakamoto SK, Mueller PR, et al. CT- and ultrasound-guided catheter drainage of empyemas after chest-tube failure. Radiology. 1984;151(2):349–53.
58. Moulton JS, Moore PT, Mencini RA. Treatment of loculated pleural effusions with transcatheter intracavitary urokinase. Am J Roentgenol. 1989; 153(5):941–5.
59. Moulton JS, Benkert RE, Weisiger KH, Chambers JA. Treatment of complicated pleural fluid collections with image-guided drainage and intracavitary urokinase. Chest. 1995;108(5):1252–9.
60. Westcott JL. Percutaneous catheter drainage of pleural effusion and empyema. Am J Roentgenol. 1985;144(6):1189–93.
61. Maskell NA, Medford A, Gleeson FV. Seldinger chest drain insertion: simpler but not necessarily safer. Thorax. 2010;65(1):5–6.
62. Rahman NM, Maskell NA, Davies CW, et al. The relationship between chest tube size and clinical outcome in pleural infection. Chest. 2010; 137(3):536–43.
63. Maskell NA, Davies CW, Nunn AJ, et al. U.K. Controlled trial of intrapleural streptokinase for pleural infection. N Engl J Med. 2005;352(9):865–74.
64. Rahman NM, Maskell NA, West A, et al. Intrapleural use of tissue plasminogen activator and DNase in pleural infection. N Engl J Med. 2011;365:518–26.
65. Casola G, vanSonnenberg E, Keightley A, Ho M, Withers C, Lee AS. Pneumothorax: radiologic treatment with small catheters. Radiology. 1988;166(1 Pt 1):89–91.

Index

J. P. Kanne (ed.), *Clinically Oriented Pulmonary Imaging*,
Respiratory Medicine, DOI: 10.1007/978-1-61779-542-8,

MIX
Papier aus verantwortungsvollen Quellen
Paper from responsible sources
FSC® C105338

If you have any concerns about our products,
you can contact us on
ProductSafety@springernature.com

In case Publisher is established outside the EU,
the EU authorized representative is:
Springer Nature Customer Service Center GmbH
Europaplatz 3, 69115 Heidelberg, Germany

Printed by Libri Plureos GmbH
in Hamburg, Germany